T0302086

DRUGS IN THE MEDIEVAL MEDITERRANEAN

In this volume a distinguished international team of scholars examines the history of drugs within all the major medical traditions of the medieval Mediterranean, namely Byzantine, Islamicate, Jewish, and Latin, and in so doing analyses a considerable number of previously unedited or barely explored texts. A Mediterranean-wide perspective permits a deeper understanding of broader phenomena, such as the transfer of scientific knowledge and cultural exchange, by looking beyond single linguistic traditions or political boundaries. It also highlights the diversity and vitality of the medieval Mediterranean pharmacological tradition, which, through its close links with cookery, alchemy, magic, religion, and philosophy, had to adapt to multiple contexts, not least to changing social and political realities, as in the case of drugs as diplomatic gifts.

PETROS BOURAS-VALLIANATOS is Associate Professor of History of Science at the National and Kapodistrian University of Athens. He has published widely on Byzantine medicine and pharmacology. His most recent monograph, *Innovation in Byzantine Medicine: The Writings of John Zacharias Aktouarios (c.1275–c.1330)* (Oxford, 2020), has been awarded the Prize for Young Historians by the International Academy of the History of Science.

DIONYSIOS STATHAKOPOULOS is Assistant Professor in Byzantine History at the University of Cyprus. His main research focus is on Byzantine social history. His publications include *Famine and Pestilence in the Late Roman and Early Byzantine Empire* (Aldershot, 2004), *The Kindness of Strangers: Charity in the Pre-modern Mediterranean* (London, 2007), and *A Short History of the Byzantine Empire* (London, 2014, rev. ed. 2023).

DRUGS IN THE MEDIEVAL MEDITERRANEAN

Transmission and Circulation of Pharmacological Knowledge

EDITED BY

PETROS BOURAS-VALLIANATOS

National and Kapodistrian University of Athens

DIONYSIOS STATHAKOPOULOS

University of Cyprus

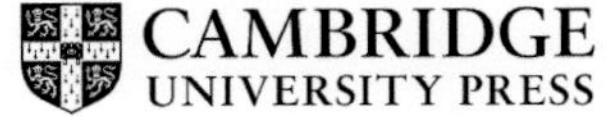

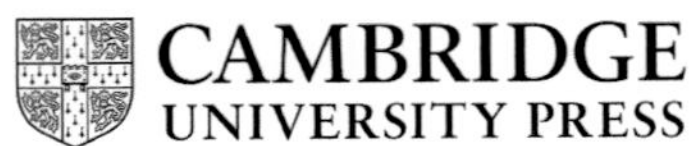

Shaftesbury Road, Cambridge CB2 8EA, United Kingdom

One Liberty Plaza, 20th Floor, New York, NY 10006, USA

477 Williamstown Road, Port Melbourne, VIC 3207, Australia

314–321, 3rd Floor, Plot 3, Splendor Forum, Jasola District Centre, New Delhi – 110025, India

103 Penang Road, #05–06/07, Visioncrest Commercial, Singapore 238467

Cambridge University Press is part of Cambridge University Press & Assessment, a department of the University of Cambridge.

We share the University's mission to contribute to society through the pursuit of education, learning and research at the highest international levels of excellence.

www.cambridge.org
Information on this title: www.cambridge.org/9781009389754

DOI: 10.1017/9781009389792

First published 2024

A catalogue record for this publication is available from the British Library.

A Cataloging-in-Publication data record for this book is available from the Library of Congress

ISBN 978-1-009-38975-4 Hardback

Contents

Figures

Tables

Contributors

ZOHAR AMAR is Full Professor in the Department of Land of Israel Studies and Archaeology at Bar-Ilan University. His research comprises natural history in ancient times and the history of medicine and ethnopharmacology, as well as the material culture and realia of daily life in the Middle Ages. Amar is the author of many books, including *Flora of the Bible* (Jerusalem, 2012), (with Efraim Lev) *Practical* Materia Medica *of the Medieval Eastern Mediterranean According to the Cairo Genizah* (Leiden, 2008), (with Efraim Lev) *Arabian Drugs in Early Medieval Mediterranean Medicine* (Edinburgh, 2016), and 120 articles.

PETROS BOURAS-VALLIANATOS is Associate Professor of History of Science at the National and Kapodistrian University of Athens and Honorary Fellow in History at the University of Edinburgh. He has published widely on Byzantine medicine and pharmacology, cross-cultural medical exchanges in the Eastern Mediterranean, the reception of the classical medical tradition in the Middle Ages, and Greek palaeography, including the first descriptive catalogue of the Greek manuscripts at the Wellcome Library in London. His most recent publications are: *Innovation in Byzantine Medicine: The Writings of John Zacharias Aktouarios (c.1275–c.1330)* (Oxford, 2020) and 'Cross-Cultural Transfer of Medical Knowledge in the Medieval Mediterranean: The Introduction and Dissemination of Sugar-Based Potions from the Islamic World to Byzantium', *Speculum* 96.4 (2021): 963–1008. He has also (co)-edited *Greek Medical Literature and Its Readers: From Hippocrates to Islam and Byzantium* (London, 2018), *Brill's Companion to the Reception of Galen* (Leiden, 2019), and *Exploring Greek Manuscripts in the Library at Wellcome Collection in London* (London, 2020).

LEIGH CHIPMAN (PhD, 2006, philosophy, Hebrew University of Jerusalem) is an independent scholar, editor, and translator based in

Jerusalem. She studies aspects of the social and intellectual history of medicine and the sciences in the medieval Islamicate world and has published numerous articles on these topics, as well as two books – *The World of Pharmacy and Pharmacists in Mamlūk Cairo* (Leiden, 2010) and *Medical Prescriptions in the Cambridge Genizah Collections: Practical Medicine and Pharmacology in Medieval Egypt* (co-authored with Efraim Lev, Leiden, 2012). She is currently working on a project on the afterlife of medieval pharmacy in the late Ottoman and colonial Middle East.

JEFFREY DOOLITTLE received his PhD in history at Fordham University in New York City. He is interested in the history of medicine in the early Middle Ages as well as the study of the Beneventan script. He has published articles on Gregory of Tours and the medieval commemoration of Charlemagne, and another article on the medical manuscripts of southern Italy is currently under review. His dissertation focused on the medical culture of the monastery of Montecassino in the ninth century, and he is now working on a transcription of the recipe collections of Montecassino, Archivio dell'Abbazia, cod. 69.

KORAY DURAK is an associate professor at the Department of History, Bogazici University, Istanbul, Turkey. His main areas of research interest include Byzantine and medieval Islamic trade, history of Byzantine pharmacology, and geographical imagination in the Middle Ages. Among his publications are 'From the Indian Ocean to the Markets of Constantinople: Ambergris in the Byzantine World', in *Life Is Short, Art Long: The Art of Healing in Byzantium – New Perspectives* (ed. Brigitte Pitarakis, Istanbul, 2018) and 'Commercial Constantinople', in *Cambridge Companion to Constantinople* (ed. Sarah Basset, Cambridge, 2022).

SIVAN GOTTLIEB is a Marie Sklodowska Curie fellow at the University of Granada under the guidance of Professor Carmen Caballero Navas. She was a Harry Starr fellow in Judaica at the Center for Jewish Studies at Harvard University (2022–3) and a postdoctoral researcher at Halpern Center for the Study of Jewish Self Perception at Bar Ilan University, Israel (2021–2). Her main research interests focus on illuminated Hebrew manuscripts from the Middle Ages and their connections to non-Jewish cultures, with a particular focus on the visual language used in the production of scientific and medical manuscripts. She received her PhD from the Hebrew University of Jerusalem, Israel, in

September 2021, under the supervision of Professor Sarit Shalev-Eyni on the subject of 'The Art of Medicine: Illuminated Hebrew Medical Manuscripts from the Late Middle Ages'. Her publications include an article in *Ars Judaica* on the Sereni Passover Haggadah and an article with Daniella Zaidman-Mauer on a magic spell in Yiddish for catching a thief.

RICHARD GREENFIELD is Professor of History at Queen's University, Kingston, Ontario. He is also co-editor of the Dumbarton Oaks Medieval Library, Greek Series. His work focuses on aspects of Byzantine popular religion. Book-length publications include *Traditions of Belief in Late Byzantine Demonology* (Amsterdam, 1988), *The Life of Lazaros of Mt. Galesion: An Eleventh-Century Pillar Saint* (Washington, DC, 2000), *The Life of Symeon the 'New' Theologian by Niketas Stethatos* (Cambridge, MA, 2013), *Holy Men of Mount Athos* (with Alice-Mary Talbot, Cambridge, MA, 2016), and *Animal Fables of the Courtly Mediterranean: The Eugenian Recension of Stephanites and Ichnelates* (with Alison Noble and Alexios Alexakis, Cambridge, MA, 2022). He is also the author of many articles and chapters on Byzantine sorcery, demonology, and monasticism.

FABIAN KÄS is a postdoctoral research fellow at the Martin Buber Institute for Jewish Studies of the University of Cologne. His publications in the fields of classical Arabic medicine and mineralogy include *Die Mineralien in der arabischen Pharmakognosie* (2 vols., Wiesbaden, 2010; PhD thesis University of Munich 2008), *Die Risāla fī l-Ḫawāṣṣ des Ibn al-Ǧazzār* (Wiesbaden, 2012), and *Al-Maqrīzīs Traktat über die Mineralien* (Leiden, 2015). He is co-author of *Marwān ibn Janāḥ: On the Nomenclature of Medicinal Drugs* (2 vols., Leiden, 2020).

EFRAIM LEV is Full Professor in the Department of Israel Studies at the University of Haifa. He was trained both as a historian and as a field biologist and therefore his academic work has always had a strong interdisciplinary focus. Currently his research focuses on ethno-pharmacology and the history of medicine in the medieval Middle East with particular emphasis on the medical documents in the Cairo Genizah. More specifically, he is reconstructing the inventory of the practical *materia medica*, studying original practical prescriptions and lists of *materia medica* and medical notebooks. Lev is the author of ten books, including (with Zohar Amar) *Practical* Materia Medica *of the Medieval Eastern Mediterranean According to the Cairo Genizah* (Leiden,

2008), (with Leigh Chipman) *Medical Prescriptions in the Cambridge Genizah Collections: Practical Medicine and Pharmacology in Medieval Egypt* (Leiden, 2012), (with Zohar Amar) *Arabian Drugs in Early Medieval Mediterranean Medicine* (Edinburgh, 2016), *Jewish Medical Practitioners in Medieval Muslim Territories: A Collective Biography* (Edinburgh, 2021), ten book chapters, and ninety articles.

PAULINA B. LEWICKA is Professor of Arabic and Islamic studies at the Faculty of Oriental Studies, University of Warsaw. For a number of years her research has been focused on various aspects of cultural and social history of the medieval Near East and, more particularly, of the Mamluk period. Her publications include *Šāfiʿ Ibn ʿAlī's Biography of the Mamluk Sultan Qalāwūn: Introduction, Edition, and Commentary* (Warsaw, 2000) and *Food and Foodways of Medieval Cairenes: Aspects of Life in an Islamic Metropolis of the Eastern Mediterranean* (Leiden, 2011). Currently she is involved in a project focusing on the social and cultural contexts of medicine in premodern Egypt.

PHILLIP I. LIEBERMAN is Associate Professor and Chair of Classical and Mediterranean Studies, Associate Professor of Jewish Studies and Law, Associate Professor of Religious Studies, and Affiliated Associate Professor of Islamic Studies and History at Vanderbilt University. His publications include *The Business of Identity: Jews, Muslims, and Economic Life in Medieval Egypt* (Stanford, CA, 2014) and *The Fate of the Jews in the Early Islamic Near East: Tracing the Demographic Shift from East to West* (Cambridge, 2022). He is editor of the Cambridge History of Judaism, volume 5 (*Jews in the Medieval Islamic World*, Cambridge, 2021), and served as a section editor of the *Encyclopedia of Jews in the Islamic World* (2010). In partnership with Lenn Goodman, also of Vanderbilt, he has completed a new translation of Maimonides' *Guide to the Perplexed*, to be published by Stanford University Press in 2024.

MATTEO MARTELLI (PhD, Greek philology, 2007; PhD history of science, 2012) is Professor of History of Science at the University of Bologna. His research focuses on Graeco-Roman and Byzantine science – in particular on alchemy and medicine – and its reception in the Syro-Arabic tradition. His publications include *L'alchimista antico* (Milan, 2019), *The Four Books of Pseudo-Democritus* (Leeds, 2014), and *Collecting Recipes: Byzantine and Jewish Pharmacology in Dialogue* (edited with Lennart Lehmhaus, Berlin, 2017). He is the principal investigator of the European Research Council project *AlchemEast* and he is currently working on a critical edition of the Syriac alchemical books ascribed to Zosimos of Panopolis.

MARIA MAVROUDI is Professor of Byzantine History and Classics at the University of California–Berkeley. In her first publication, *A Byzantine Book on Dream Interpretation* (Leiden, 2002), she focused on a tenth-century Byzantine book on dream interpretation that had been widely received in Latin and the European vernaculars and counted as the most important Christian dreambook of the Middle Ages. She showed that while it was generally viewed as a Byzantine invention partly based on the second-century manual of Artemidorus, it was a Christian adaptation of Arabic Islamic material and one among a larger group of texts originally written in Arabic or Persian and received into Greek between the ninth and the fifteenth centuries. During the next two decades, she worked on identifying the place of these translations within Byzantine literary culture and its reception in 'East' and 'West' during the medieval and early modern period. This begs reconsidering the position of the ancient Greek classics within the Byzantine, Arabic, and Latin intellectual traditions, as well as the supposed marginality of Byzantium within a broader medieval intellectual universe. Her most recent publications include 'The Byzantine Reception of Homer and His Export to Other Cultures' and 'Homer after Byzantium, from the Early Ottoman Period to the Age of Nationalisms', in *The Cambridge Guide to Homer* (ed. Corinne Pache, Cambridge, 2020); 'The Modern Historiography of Byzantine and Islamic Philosophy', in *al-Masaq* (2020); 'Astrological Texts among the Byzantine Translations from Arabic into Greek' (in Turkish), in *Toplumsal tarih* (2021); and 'The Modern Study of Selfhood in Byzantium compared with Medieval Europe and the Islamic World', in *Palaeoslavica* (2022).

ATHANASIOS RINOTAS is a PhD student and a Research Foundation – Flanders fellow at the Catholic University of Leuven in Belgium. He is interested in ancient Greek and medieval philosophy and their relation to magic, alchemy, and astrology. He has published various articles on Albertus Magnus and on ancient Greek and medieval alchemy. His PhD dissertation focuses on Albertus Magnus (1200–80) and explores the epistemological status of magic and alchemy in Albertus' work and how both magic and alchemy relate to his natural philosophy.

YARON SERRI is Lecturer in the Department of History, Philosophy and Jewish Studies at the Open University of Israel. He specialises in the history of medieval Arabic medicine including medical literature, and especially lexicography. Serri is the author of two books – (with Zohar Amar) *The Land of Israel and Syria according to al-Tamīmī's Description* (Ramat Gan, 2004) and (with Zohar Amar) *Maimonides' Treatise on Poisons and the Protection against Lethal Drugs (al-Maqālah al-Fāḍiliyyah)* (Kiryat, Ono, 2019) – and twenty-three articles.

DIONYSIOS STATHAKOPOULOS is Assistant Professor in Byzantine History at the University of Cyprus. His main research focus is on Byzantine social history. His publications include *Famine and Pestilence in the Late Roman and Early Byzantine Empire* (Aldershot, 2004), *The Kindness of Strangers: Charity in the Pre-modern Mediterranean* (London, 2007), and *A Short History of the Byzantine Empire* (London, 2014, rev. ed. 2023). His current project is a monograph on wealth, consumption, and inequality in the late Byzantine world.

KATHLEEN WALKER-MEIKLE specialises in premodern medical history and animal-human relationships. Her monograph *Medieval Pets* (Suffolk, 2012) is the first study of companion animals in the late medieval period. She has written articles and chapters on the use and meaning of animals in medieval medicine and medieval animal toxicology and is currently working on a project examining zoonotic encounters in the premodern period, along with further research on animal *materia medica*. She is currently the grants research manager at the Science Museum Group.

Acknowledgements

This book arose from an international conference, 'Drugs in the Medieval World', which took place at King's College London's (KCL) Strand Campus on 7–8 December 2018. The event was funded by the Wellcome Trust in the framework of the research project 'Experiment and Exchange: Byzantine Pharmacology between East and West (ca. 1150–ca. 1450)', led by Petros Bouras-Vallianatos (200372/Z/15/Z). The editors would like to warmly thank the Wellcome Trust for its substantial financial support and the Arts and Humanities Research Institute team at KCL for organisational support. We are thankful to all the speakers, chairs (†William Maclehose, Barbara Zipser), and participants who contributed to the lively discussions; special thanks are owed to Peregrine Horden for his ingenious concluding remarks. We are grateful to Ayman Atat, Heinrich Evanzin, Arsenio Ferraces Rodríguez, Grigory Kessel, Michael Stanley-Baker, and Ronit Yoeli-Tlalim for their stimulating papers, although these do not appear in the present volume. We are also thankful to the anonymous Cambridge University Press readers for their insightful suggestions and comments on an earlier version of this manuscript, and especially to our editor, Michael Sharp, for his expertise and care in the production of this book. Special thanks go to Pam Scholefield for compiling the index of this volume, and to the National and Kapodistrian University of Athens and the University of Cyprus for covering the relevant costs. Petros Bouras-Vallianatos would also like to express his gratitude to the rector of the University of Athens, Prof. Meletios-Athanasios Dimopoulos.

Petros Bouras-Vallianatos, Athens   Dionysios Stathakopoulos, Nicosia

Note to the Reader

Proper names of ancient Greek authors follow the *Liddell and Scott Greek–English Lexicon* (9th ed., 1940; revised supplement, 1996). The spelling of Late Antique and Byzantine names follows, in most cases, *The Oxford Dictionary of Byzantium* (1991) – for example, 'Aetios of Amida' instead of 'Aetius of Amida'. Transliteration of Greek terms follows the Library of Congress system (www.loc.gov/catdir/cpso/romanization/greek.pdf, accessed 19 January 2021) – for example, 'physis' not 'phusis', but 'euros' not 'eyros'. Transliteration of Arabic and Hebrew terms generally follows the Library of Congress system (www.loc.gov/catdir/cpso/romanization/arabic.pdf and www.loc.gov/catdir/cpso/romanization/hebrew.pdf, accessed 19 January 2021), but with a few variations in individual chapters. Where the original word or an implied word needs to be made explicit for reasons of clarity, it is supplied within parentheses and square brackets respectively – for example, 'From the Byzantine Empire (*al-Rūm*) [are imported] gold and silver utensils, dinars of pure gold, drugs (*ʿaqāqīr*), *buzyūn* [i.e. a fine silk]'. Page(s) is abbreviated to p(p.), folio(a) to f(f.), note(s) to n(n.), chapter(s) to ch. and chs, and number(s) to no. and nos.

Medieval Mediterranean Pharmacology

Petros Bouras-Vallianatos

> [R]ecipe for the small *tryphera*; beneficial for internal haemorrhoids, pain, and weakness of the stomach due to the accumulation of moistness; it also preserves health and is used for a great number of diseases. Take one part each of the bark of Chebulic myrobalan, or, if you want, use the Indian [myrobalan] instead, beleric and emblic [myrobalans]. Chop up, strain, and add rose oil; mix with scummed honey and place [the mixture] in a vessel made of fine pottery; the dosage is two to three *hexagia*[1] of this [mixture] along with tepid water.[2]

Called *tryphera* in Greek, and mostly known as *triphalā* in Sanskrit or *iṭrīfal* in Arabic, it was an extremely popular drug in the Middle Ages, from India to Baghdad and Cairo, and from Constantinople to Salerno and Paris, while various versions of it are still used nowadays in Ayurvedic medicine.[3] The recipe given above provides the short version of this composite drug, including five distinct categories of data: a) title or name of drug – that is, small *tryphera*; b) indications for its use, including for the treatment of various kind of ailments such as haemorrhoids and pain; c) list of

I am grateful to Dionysios Stathakopoulos and the anonymous reviewers for their constructive comments on an earlier draft of this chapter. Special thanks are owed to the Wellcome Trust for supporting the research project [214961/Z/18/Z: 'Making and Consuming Drugs in the Italian and Byzantine Worlds (12th–15th c.)'] from which this chapter has arisen.

[1] One *hexagion* is equal to 4.444 grams. See Schilbach (1970: 183, 276).

[2] *Ephodia tou apodēmountos*, 4.19, Vaticanus gr. 300, f. 145v, ll. 4–13: ' . . . στήλη τῆς μικρᾶς τρυφερᾶς, ὠφελοῦσα εἰς τὰς ἐσωχάδας καὶ εἰς πόνον στομάχου και ἀδυναμίαν αὐτοῦ, ἀπὸ τοῦ πλήθους τῆς ὑγρότητος, καὶ φυλάττει τὴν ὑγείαν, ἀποπέμπεται δὲ εἰς χρῆσιν πλῆθος ἀρρωστιῶν· λαβὼν τὸν φλοιὸν τοῦ μυροβαλάνου τοῦ κέπουλι· καὶ ἀντὶ τούτου εἰ θέλεις θὲς τὸ ἰνδικόν· καὶ πελίλιζ καὶ ἔμλεζ, ἀνὰ ἑνὸς μέρους· κόψας σήσας (correxi: σείσας cod.) ἀνάμιγε (an ἀνάμισγε?) μετὰ ῥοδελαίου καὶ φύρασον σὺν μέλιτι ἀπαφρισμένῳ· καὶ ἀπόθου εἰς κορούπιν λεῖον· ἡ δὲ πόσις ἐξ αὐτοῦ δύο ἑξάγ., μέχρι τριῶν μετὰ ὕδατος χλιαροῦ'. For the original Arabic version, see Suwaysī et al. (1999) I.376–8. All translations from Greek are mine, unless otherwise stated. All transcriptions from Greek retain the same spelling and punctuation as in the relevant codex, apart from the fact that I have supplied the iota subscript.

[3] On the importance of myrobalans in premodern medical practice across Eurasia, see Yoeli-Tlalim (2021: 63–84).

ingredients – that is, three kinds of myrobalan fruits, rose oil, and honey, along with posological details; d) method of preparation; and e) information about the administration – that is, it should be consumed with tepid water – and dosage.[4] This example has been taken from a twelfth-century Southern Italian or Sicilian manuscript of the unedited Greek translation of an Arabic medical work by Ibn al-Jazzār (fl. tenth century), *Zād al-musāfir wa-qūt al-ḥāḍir* (*Provisions for the Traveller and Nourishment for the Sedentary*/Gr. *Ephodia tou apodēmountos*), better known by its Latin title, *Viaticum*.[5]

The recipe for this panacea medicine can be discussed in a variety of overlapping contexts. First, the geographical and the transcultural. An originally Indian medicine, it was introduced to the Mediterranean through the Islamicate medical tradition and naturalised in various environments, becoming a common therapeutic agent for people all around the Mediterranean and transcending linguistic, regional, and political boundaries. In this case, it was part of a large manuscript, Vaticanus gr. 300, containing texts connected with the medical practice of Greek-speaking physicians in the multicultural milieu of southern Italy and Sicily. In other words, Mediterranean cultures – whether Byzantine, Islamicate, Jewish, or Latin – shared common elements of *materia medica* that defined pharmacological knowledge and practice. The substances themselves, in this case the myrobalans, originated in Asia (e.g. India and the Indochinese Peninsula) and, apart from being ingredients in compound drugs, they were commodities that travelled long distances before they were mixed with local Mediterranean ingredients, such as honey.[6] The long distances these substances travelled illustrate the global connections between the peoples of the Mediterranean and Eurasia as a whole and shows the interrelation of medicine and pharmacology with other fields, such as trade.[7]

Second, there is the textual and therapeutic context. A recipe is a textual entity which may have undergone several stages of editing, transmission (including translation), and elaboration as a result of scribal activity, often

[4] A long version, the so-called large great *tryphera* ('μεγάλη τρυφερά'), including a large number of additional ingredients, is found just after the recipe for the small one in the Greek translation in Vaticanus gr. 300, f. 146r, l. 10–f. 146v, l. 15.

[5] On Vaticanus gr. 300, see Lucà (1993: 36–63), who argues that the manuscript was copied, most probably in the area of Messina in Sicily, around 1130/40. On the Greek translation, which remains unedited, see Miguet (2017). On Ibn al-Jazzār and his work, see Bos (1993: 296–7) and Bos, Käs. and McVaugh (2022: 1–29).

[6] On the various kinds of myrobalan, see Amar and Lev (2017: 83–8).

[7] On the medieval spice trade, see Freedman (2012).

informed by the practical knowledge of experimentation by practitioners. A large number of pharmacological texts remain unedited or are available only in outdated and inadequate editions. Thus, we still know very little about the transmission of these treatises and their audiences. At the same time, a drug could be made up and used as a therapeutic agent in daily practice, thus defining pharmaceutical techniques in a hospital, at an apothecary's shop, in a domestic setting (e.g. a patient's home), or in other contexts.

The third context is non-medical. Studying pharmacological substances in non-medical texts can provide an excellent way to explore how pharmacological knowledge had to be adapted to such contexts. A recipe, for example, might contain methods of preparation that originated in cooking or alchemy or indeed the derivation might be the other way around. Furthermore, drugs, whether simple or composite, were often associated with magic, religion, philosophy, and even diplomacy, thus adding an interdisciplinary aspect to the study of medieval pharmacology.

I.1 Towards a Holistic Study of Pharmacological Knowledge in the Mediterranean

This volume explores medieval Mediterranean pharmacological knowledge or 'drug lore' by focusing on simple and compound drugs (i.e. those consisting of more than one ingredient) and their applications in contemporary societies. It aims to construct a Mediterranean-wide view for understanding more general medieval phenomena, such as the cross-cultural exchange of knowledge in the field of pharmacology from the ninth/tenth century to the fifteenth.[8]

For the purpose of this volume, the term 'Mediterranean' includes evidence from places across the Mediterranean, whether in Europe, the Middle East, or Africa, but it is not a merely geographical designation.[9] It is something broader because, culturally speaking, even places that did not

[8] Cross-cultural exchange often works on many levels and was invariably influenced by the relevant social and cultural milieus. In this I follow the approach of Brentjes, Fidora, and Tischler (2014: 30–3), who considered the 'cross-cultural exchange of knowledge as a way of life, not merely a linear act of translating'. Determining the multifaceted interactions involved and 'their loci of contact, transfer, transport and transformation and their participants either as identifiable individuals or as a representative of a social, professional, cultural, linguistic or other group' is an important element in the process.

[9] The use of 'Mediterranean' as a geographical expression is a modern construction and goes back to the nineteenth century. On this and the study of the 'Mediterranean' as a region, see Horden and Purcell (2000: 530–4).

have access to the Mediterranean were predominantly informed by its cultures. Thus, the volume also includes evidence from people not geographically situated in the Mediterranean, but who had very close links with it. One chapter, for example, concentrates on Abbasid Baghdad (Chapter 1), which is an inland region, but through its political status as the capital of the Abbasid caliphate was nevertheless an important centre for charting and understanding cultural exchange in the Mediterranean.

This book seeks to move away from past prejudices in the study of Mediterranean medical traditions, which often valued one tradition over another. It thus aims to promote the practice of studying the entire region simultaneously by initiating a dialogue between scholars of diverse traditions and disciplines without focusing on or privileging one tradition at the expense of another or highlighting the influence of one tradition on others. The volume is divided into two parts: the first includes studies on the transmission of pharmacological knowledge across cultures and regions and deals with a wide variety of medical texts and contexts; the second concentrates on pharmacology's interaction with other areas, such as alchemy, cooking, magic, and philosophy. The thirteen chapters in this volume include contributions focusing on the Byzantine, the Islamicate, the Jewish, and the Latin traditions. These labels often tend to be reductive. Nevertheless, this book does not set out to solve the complicated issues related to the definition of the various medieval traditions. The use of 'Byzantine' and 'Latin' in this volume mainly relates to the language in which the available sources are written – that is, Greek and Latin – rather than to defined geographical spaces. The term 'Islamicate' medical tradition is employed with reference to authors and practice in regions where Muslims were culturally dominant.[10] Lastly, the term 'Jewish' is used for evidence related to people identified as Jews, but who might often write in languages other than Hebrew, such as Arabic, and who could be situated in any region of the Mediterranean.[11]

It is hard to define a starting point for any study of the transmission, circulation, and adaptation of pharmacological knowledge in the wider medieval Mediterranean. Two significant parameters must be considered: first, the

[10] The term was coined by Hodgson (1974: 59), who states that '"Islamicate" would refer not directly to the religion, Islam, itself, but to the social and cultural complex historically associated with Islam and the Muslims, both among Muslims themselves and even when found among non-Muslims'.

[11] On Jewish medical authors and practice, see Caballero-Navas (2011). On Jewish authors who specifically wrote in Arabic, see Chipman (2013). For a recent critical survey of views about 'Jewish medicine' in general and about 'Jewish medicine' in the medieval era, see Lehmhaus (2021a: 9–20) and (2021b: 39–49), respectively.

reception of the classical medical knowledge, and, second, the introduction of new knowledge from the Islamicate world, especially from the eleventh century onwards. By the ninth century, as part of the large corpus of Greek medical texts that were translated into Arabic, Greek pharmacological knowledge had been combined in a unique way with Indian pharmacological lore in Abbasid Baghdad. Classical pharmacological knowledge, based on work by authors such as Dioscorides (fl. first century CE)[12] and Galen (129–216/17 CE),[13] was elaborated with the addition of new vegetal and animal substances from Asia, such as myrobalans, sandalwood, musk, and ambergris.[14] Also, some medical authors in the Islamicate world introduced their own pharmacological theories often based on experimentation – for example, al-Kindī (d. 873), who instigated a new theory of calculating the degrees of primary qualities of composite drugs (hot, cold, dry, moist) and modified earlier corresponding Galenic concepts.[15] Pharmacological knowledge from the Islamicate world reached other Mediterranean traditions by the eleventh century, initiating a period of assimilation and adaptation that lasted for many decades, even centuries in some cases.

The introduction of Islamicate pharmacological lore in the Byzantine, Jewish, and Latin medical traditions and their interaction with one another was neither a unified nor a simultaneous phenomenon, but rather showed a variety of patterns of adaptation and reception. First, it is evident that there was piecemeal introduction of oriental *materia medica* even before the tenth century.[16] For example, in the Byzantine and Latin traditions, one can see the steady introduction of ingredients such as musk, ambergris, galangal, camphor, and sugar, including new forms of sugar-based recipes/ingredients from the ninth century onwards in medical and non-medical

[12] On Dioscorides, see Riddle (1985).

[13] For an overview of Galenic pharmacology, see Vogt (2008). On Galenic pharmacological theories, see the comprehensive study by Harig (1974).

[14] Kahl (2019). See, for example, the cases of Al-Ṭabarī's (fl. *c.*830–50), *Firdaws al-ḥikma* (*Paradise of Wisdom*), and the *Kitāb al-ḥāwī* (*Comprehensive Book*) by Al-Rāzī (d. *c.*925), who wrote medical works attesting to the merging of Greek and Indian medicine. Greek texts were translated either directly into Arabic or via Syriac, while Sanskrit texts were translated either directly into Arabic or via Persian. On al-Ṭabarī, see Meyerhof (1931) and Kahl (2020); on al-Rāzī, see Kahl (2015). See also Amar, Lev, and Serri (2014), who discuss the case of Ibn Juljul (d. after 994).

[15] Pormann (2011); Chipman (2019).

[16] The term 'oriental' is used to refer to ingredients originating from India and the Far East. The term has been used with reference to the importation of spices from Asia to the Mediterranean by Jacoby (2016: 196).

works.[17] The most significant medium for the introduction of Arabic medical knowledge into the wider Mediterranean world was translation. The huge and systematic job of translating Arabic medical works into Latin by Constantine the African (d. before 1098/9) in the late eleventh century led to the creation of new medical compendia in Latin, such as the *Articella*, which remained the main textbook for Latin medical teaching in Europe until the sixteenth century.[18] The period was marked by the rediscovery of classical and late antique works,[19] which were combined with new knowledge from the Islamicate tradition. To give a few characteristic examples from the area of pharmacology, two important Latin *antidotaria* had appeared by the end of the eleventh century. The so-called *Antidotarium magnum*, which is a large collection of composite drugs that can number up to 1,300 recipes in some manuscripts, shows a unique elaboration of earlier pharmacological lore with newly introduced oriental substances. A certain Nicolaus created a much smaller and more user-friendly work, the *Antidotarium Nicolai*, by excerpting the most commonly used recipes from the *Antidotarium magnum*.[20] By the twelfth century an influential and very well-circulated Latin work on simple drugs, the *Circa instans*, had been put together in Salerno, which became the centre of medical activity in the western Mediterranean from then

[17] On the Byzantine and Latin traditions, see Bouras-Vallianatos (2021) and Burridge (2020: 235–7), respectively. The issue of theoretical versus actual *materia medica* is relevant here, or, in other words, whether the ingredients mentioned in medical works were actually in circulation before the tenth/eleventh centuries. In fact, there are non-medical sources that confirm the presence of oriental ingredients in the wider Mediterranean world in this period. For example, that galangal was supplied every year as far afield as the Abbey of St. Bertin in north-west France is confirmed in a charter of 867 (see Gysseling and Koch (1950) I.68.11–12). In the Byzantine world, the appendix to the *Book of Ceremonies*, ascribed to Emperor Constantine VII Porphyrogennetos (sole r. 945–59), includes, for example, musk, ambergris, and sugar, among the spices that the emperor would have with him when he went on campaign. See Constantine VII Porphyrogennetos, *What Should Be Observed When the Great and High Emperor of the Romans Goes on Campaign*, ed. Haldon (1990) 108.219–22. Another important work which makes early references to oriental *materia medica* is *Hippiatrica*, a Byzantine horse medicine manual, emphasising the importance of a more holistic assessment of medieval medical literature, including veterinary works. Its tenth-century recension (in Berolinensis Phillippicus 1538) includes notable mentions of ingredients such as ambergris and galangal. On this, see McCabe (2009: 288–90).

[18] We know very little about the life of Constantine the African. There is no doubt that he made his translations in Montecassino, where he lived as a monk. On Constantine the African and the transformation of Latin medicine in the late eleventh century, see Green (forthcoming) with further recent bibliography.

[19] For example, late antique Latin translations of Dioscorides' and Alexander of Tralles' (*c.*525–*c.*605) works or Theodore Priscianus' (fl. later fourth/early fifth century) Latin handbook, as well as new translations from Greek, such as Paul of Aegina's (fl. first half of the seventh century) *Epitome*. See Green (2008).

[20] On the *Antidotarium magnum*, which remains unedited, see Green (2019). Francesco Roberg is preparing a new edition of the *Antidotarium Nicolai*. See Roberg (2007).

onwards; this treatise shows significant influence from the Islamicate pharmacological tradition.[21] An abundance of evidence from Hebrew commercial documents (dated to the eleventh and twelfth centuries) in the so-called Genizah collection in Cairo shows the intense links between India and Egypt, including references to the importation of thirty-six spices, aromatics, varnishing plants, and medicinal plants to the Mediterranean.[22] This is particularly important since it confirms that the transfer of knowledge through translation was not just theoretical, but that oriental ingredients were simultaneously spreading across the Mediterranean.[23]

By the third quarter of the eleventh century, Symeon Seth, a Greek scholar active in Constantinople, who knew Arabic and most probably came from Antioch, had composed his *Treatise on the Capacities of Foodstuffs*, addressed to the Byzantine emperor Michael VII Doukas (r. 1071–8), which provides details on a large number of aliments and their properties. In this work, Symeon made a systematic attempt to introduce new data and codify Islamicate medical knowledge, which had been slowly infiltrating Byzantine medical circles in Greek since the tenth century.[24] It is worth noting that Symeon was an exact contemporary of Constantine the African, although his work is not comparable with the latter's grand-scale translation project. Southern Italy and Sicily played a significant role in introducing Islamicate pharmacological lore to the wider Byzantine world as well, which inevitably leads us to reconsider the role of Greek-speaking communities outside Byzantium proper. The *Ephodia tou apodēmountos* had been translated in the same area by the early twelfth century, along with other Arabic medical works, such as *On Purgative Drugs*, most probably from an Arabic treatise by Pseudo-Yūḥannā ibn Māsawayh (d. 857).[25] These treatises were abundantly copied and used by Byzantine medical authors in later centuries, thus enhancing

[21] The work survives in 138 manuscripts. See Ventura's (2016) comprehensive study of the text.

[22] Goitein and Friedman (2008: 16). See also Yoeli-Tlalim (2021: 71–3). Commodities from India reached Egypt (Alexandria) via the Gulf of Aden. Of course, there were other trade routes between India and the Mediterranean – for example, the overland routes from Baghdad (via Siraf on the Persian Gulf) to Trebizond and Constantinople. See Durak (2021).

[23] Cf. Ventura (2016: 379–81). On the debate about theoretical versus actual/practical *materia medica*, see note 17, and Lev and Amar (2007).

[24] Harig (1967); Bouras-Vallianatos (2021: 979–82).

[25] The earliest surviving manuscript of this translation is Vaticanus gr. 300, ff. 273v–284v, where it is attributed to St John of Damascus. See Bouras-Vallianatos (2021: 987, n. 125). This was most probably due to these two historical figures having the same name in Arabic – that is, Yūḥannā = John. The same confusion is also attested in the Latin tradition; see De Vos (2013: 683). On the Latin version of this treatise, see Ventura (2021: 185–99).

the dissemination of Islamicate pharmacological knowledge.[26] Further pharmacological works from the Islamicate world were translated into Byzantine Greek, including some Persian *antidotaria*, which led to a significant diffusion of oriental *materia medica* and new forms of composite drugs in the Greek-speaking eastern Mediterranean world.[27]

A number of important contemporaneous developments can be seen in the field of Jewish medical tradition. It is worth noting that no medical works were written in Hebrew until the end of the twelfth century.[28] Jews often wrote in Arabic in medieval Islamicate milieus. For example, Ibn Biklārish, a Jewish physician and pharmacist who lived in the Spanish city of Almeria, wrote a pharmacological work in Arabic, *Kitāb al-Mustaʿīnī* for al-Mustaʿīn (r. 1085–1109), the Hūdid ruler of Saragossa, in around 1106. The work includes a long list of 704 simple drugs and their properties in tabular form, along with their names in various languages. The author refers to earlier Greek and Arabic works by authors such as Dioscorides, Galen, Ibn Māsawayh, al-Kindī, and al-Bīrūnī (d. after 1050), and follows the Galenic principles of the degrees of intensity of primary qualities.[29] Meanwhile, by the end of the twelfth century, the first translations of Arabic works from Latin into Hebrew were being made in the Western European Christian world, in particular Provence. Further translations directly from Arabic into Hebrew in subsequent centuries promoted the writing of Hebrew texts, including the dissemination of Islamicate pharmacological knowledge in Hebrew, thus coinciding with contemporaneous translation work in other parts of the Mediterranean.[30] Lastly, an interesting collection of pharmacological recipes in Greek had been produced by a certain – most probably Greek-speaking – Jew called Benjamin

[26] See, for example, Bouras-Vallianatos (2020: 152–7). On Arabo/Persian-Byzantine medical translations, see Touwaide (2016).

[27] See, for example, the two Persian *antidotaria* translated into Greek by Gregory Chioniades and Constantine Melitiniotes in the fourteenth century. On these, see Bouras-Vallianatos (2021: 998–1002) and Kousis (1939), respectively.

[28] Caballero-Navas (2011: 1–2). There are two notable exceptions. The first is the so-called *Sefer ʾAsaph* (*Book of Asaph*), composed in the Middle East by the eighth to ninth centuries, which includes a section on *materia medica*. See Yoeli-Tlalim (2021: 26–34). The second was written by Shabbetai Donnolo (913–*c*.982), who was active in Byzantine southern Italy. He wrote a medical book in Hebrew, *Sefer Mirqaḥoth* (*Book of Remedies*), consisting of recipes for composite drugs. See Sharf (1995: 160–77) and Ferre (2004). It is worth noting that this treatise contains only limited references to oriental *materia medica*, such as cinnamon, ginger, myrobalan, and zedoary (*Sefer Mirqaḥoth* (*Book of Remedies*), 9, ed. Ferre (2004): 7).

[29] Burnett (2008). See also Bos and Käs (2016), who discuss the case of Marwān ibn Janāḥ's (d. second quarter of the eleventh century) *Kitāb al-Talkhīṣ* (*Book of the Commentary*).

[30] Caballero-Navas (2011: 324–35).

by the fourteenth century.[31] Unfortunately, we cannot identify where this author lived and worked. The work shows considerable influence from the Islamicate pharmacological tradition and must be seen as a piece of the multifarious puzzle that is the study of Jewish medical authors in the medieval Mediterranean.

This volume discusses examples of the transmission and circulation of medieval pharmacological knowledge in the Mediterranean, and aims to help us reconsider often neglected or little known stages in this process and ultimately to understand the entire area in a more holistic way. The chapters in both parts of this volume have not been arranged in chronological order; nevertheless, an attempt has been made to group together chapters dealing with the same tradition or a similar topic. My discussion of the chapters of this volume does not necessarily follow the order of the chapters in the table of contents.

Jeffrey Doolittle (Chapter 2) examines a group of oral and dental recipes transmitted as part of several Latin medieval medical compilations based on the *Natural History* by Pliny the Elder, including the *Medicina Plinii* as well as five witnesses of a later extended version, the *Physica Plinii*, dated to between the ninth and the fifteenth centuries. He shows how recipe collections relied on common sources, and how subtle but meaningful differences are observed in each version. Doolittle then argues that by the ninth/tenth centuries, ingredients coming from outside the Mediterranean, such as myrrh, pepper, and clove are increasingly recommended. The number of ingredients from Asia is even higher in the PP Flor-Prag manuscript of the *Physica Plinii*, which dates to the fourteenth/fifteenth century, thus confirming the significant spread of Islamicate pharmacological knowledge. This coincides with the facilitation of overland trade from Asia under the unified Mongol Empire, especially after 1304.[32]

The various translations of pharmacological works from one language to another resulted in introducing new terms that were previously unknown to its native speakers. Authors and translators of medical works often made considerable effort to provide synonyms for the *materia medica* for the convenience of readers throughout the Mediterranean.[33] I have already referred to the work of Ibn Biklārish, who in his work on simple drugs included equivalents for the names of ingredients in Syriac, Persian,

[31] The work is unedited and survives in three manuscripts, the earliest dated to the fourteenth century. See Bouras-Vallianatos (2020: 145, n. 23). I am currently preparing its *editio princeps* along with an English translation.

[32] Biran (2015: 551–2).

[33] Burnett (2016).

ancient and medieval Greek, Arabic, and *ʿajamiyyah* (Latin and Romance languages). Fabian Käs (Chapter 1) focuses on the unedited *Kitāb quwā l-adwiyah* (*Book on Simple Drugs*) by Ibn al-Tilmīdh (b. *c.*1073), a Christian physician active in the famous ʿAḍudī hospital in Baghdad, who provides synonyms for simples in Arabic, Syriac, Greek, and Persian. Käs argues that including these terms in multiple languages had a practical aim in the multicultural environment of Baghdad, namely to help physicians cross-check entries on *materia medica* in Syriac works or Arabic translations of Greek works. The Persian terms, on the other hand, might have been helpful to merchants involved in trading ingredients across greater Iran.

Kathleen Walker-Meikle (Chapter 3) deals with the unexplored Latin translation of an Arabic text on animal *materia medica*, the so-called *De sexaginta animalibus* (*On Sixty Animals*). In the Latin text, one finds extensive use of Arabic terminology for the names of the animals themselves and for units of measurements. The Latin term is often found alongside the Arabic term in transliteration (e.g. the Arabic *al-dhiʾb*, here *ozib*, is followed by the Latin term *lupo*, thus *De ozib lupo*). Terms for exotic animals were sometimes left untranslated; for example, the cheetah, *al-fahd* in Arabic, is rendered as *alphet* or *alfat* in Latin. These examples are a vivid testimony to the ongoing process of assimilation and naturalisation of foreign terms in the field of pharmacology – in this case, within the Latin tradition – as the result of the intensified transfer of knowledge, especially from the Islamicate world.

Maria Mavroudi (Chapter 4) discusses the presence of annotations with Greek plant names in Dioscoridean herbals in Arabic and of Arabic terms, written either in Arabic script or transliterated into Greek characters, in Greek medical manuscripts containing multilingual lexica of pharmacological substances. For example, the Greek terms 'μῆλα' and 'κυδώνια', written in a fluent eleventh-century hand, are provided in the margins for the Arabic *mālā* ('apples') and *qūdhūniā* ('quince') that appear in the main text in Leidensis or. 289, a codex originating in Samarkand in the late eleventh century. On the other hand, one can find Greek transliterations of Arabic terms, such as 'φαίχισεν' for *al-fāhisha*, which is given as an equivalent for the Greek 'καστόριον' ('castoreum') in late Byzantine dictionaries of synonyms. These cases attest to the intense interaction between the Byzantine and Islamicate pharmacological traditions and the progressive familiarisation of contemporary practitioners with foreign terms for *materia medica*.

The use of Greek – for example, 'τουτίαν' (cadmia) for the Arabic *tūtiyā* – or even Latin loanwords in Greek transliteration is highlighted by Matteo Martelli (Chapter 11), who discusses the interrelationship between pharmacology, alchemy, and cooking by focusing on an unedited recipe book of the fourteenth/fifteenth century in Parisinus gr. 2314. Martelli shows that the inclusion of such terms provides vital evidence on the process of tracing the interconnections between the diverse medieval medical traditions and the complicated patterns of transmission of medieval pharmacological knowledge.

Another interesting case is presented by Sivan Gottlieb (Chapter 6), who explores a unique group of medical texts – the so-called alchemical herbals – which are characterised by illustrations of plants and their roots (geometric, zoomorphic, or anthropomorphised). She particularly focuses on the Hebrew codex Parisinus 1199 (fifteenth century) from northern Italy, where the text accompanying each plant is a translation from a Latin source. Here, the translator adapted the Latin sources to suit the sensibilities of its Jewish audience; for example, references to Christ were rendered with Hebrew terms for God, while sometimes terms were completely omitted, such as the Latin *Sanctus*/*Sancta* (Saint). Moreover, each illustration is captioned with the name of the plant in Hebrew and Latin or Italian in Hebrew transliteration, whereas in some cases the Latin version may appear in Latin letters as well, thus adding another example of the complexities of transmitting pharmacological knowledge among Mediterranean linguistic communities.

Zohar Amar, Yaron Serri, and Efraim Lev (Chapter 5) discuss the production of a particular composite drug, theriac, in the eastern Mediterranean between the tenth and fifteenth centuries. Theriac was first composed by Andromachus, physician to the Roman emperor Nero (r. 54–68 CE) and was considered a sort of panacea antidote, especially in cases of poisoning by venomous animals. It attained great popularity in the wider Mediterranean in subsequent centuries and also became a famous antidote in the Islamicate world. The authors of this chapter examine testimonies connected with the Syro-Palestinian region, including certain treatises on the subject written by local authors, such as al-Tamīmī (d. *c.*960), who practised in Ramle before he moved to Egypt and wrote works on how to produce different kinds of theriac. The recipes for theriac were often modified by the use of local ingredients, such as asphalt from the Dead Sea, the venom of a particular snake from the same area, and wild plants from the mountains of Jerusalem (e.g. yellow bugle and moon carrot), attesting to notable cases of cross-fertilisation.

I.2 Pharmacological Texts and Contexts

I have already given some examples of texts related to the study of pharmacology in the medieval Mediterranean. A brief example from Vaticanus gr. 300, the manuscript from where the *triphalā* recipe cited in the opening epigraph originates, will further illustrate the urgent need for editions of unpublished and unexplored texts as well as the importance of studying previously neglected versions/redactions of certain treatises. Vaticanus gr. 300 is the earliest surviving copy of the *Ephodia tou apodēmountos* and was copied by four hands; four additional hands annotated the codex in the margin or in the main body of the text. Santo Lucà has convincingly argued for the identification of hand *d* with that of the most likely commissioner of the codex, a physician from Reggio, one Philip Xeros.[34] In fact, this copy of the *Ephodia tou apodēmountos* is unique since it is elaborated with supplemental material, showing Philip's personal involvement.

First, the scribes copied several additional recipes by Philip in various chapters of the translation in the main body of the text, thus constituting an integral part of the *Ephodia tou apodēmountos* in this witness. In some of these Philip addresses his son ('τέκνον'), also a physician, in a didactic tone, as, for example, in the case of a potion made with bugloss for the treatment of melancholy and heart affections.[35] These recipes would not have been printed/included in a conventional critical edition or at best some of them could have been provided in the *apparatus criticus* or in an appendix to the edition, thus not adequately representing the various additional layers/redactions of the text. In this case, these recipes are a rare testimony to Xeros' personal engagement with this copy of the *Ephodia tou apodēmountos* and also give us a glimpse of the medicines Philip most probably used in daily practice.

Second, the study of a particular text is not complete without an understanding of the paratextual elements – for example, marginal or interlinear notes and any diagrams that may accompany the text in the

[34] Lucà (1993: 50–6). See also Ieraci Bio (2006); Bouras-Vallianatos (2021: 982–8). Philip Xeros is also the co-author of a recipe book surviving in Parisinus gr. 2194 (fifteenth century), ff. 454r–464v. The title reads as follows: Βιβλίον περιέχον συνθέσεις συναχθὲν καὶ πειραθὲν παρὰ Εὐφημίου Σικελοῦ τοῦ θαυμασιωτάτου· καὶ Φιλίππου Ξηροῦ τοῦ Ῥηγινοῦ (correxi: Ῥιγινοῦ cod.), τῶν θαυμασίων ἰατρῶν (*Book Containing Recipes Compiled and Tested by the Most Marvellous Euphemios of Sicily and Philip Xeros of Reggio, [Who Are] among the Marvellous Physicians*).

[35] Vaticanus gr. 300, f. 91r, ll.15–17: '. . . ὠφέλιμον (correxi: ὠφέλημον cod.) ἐστὶ πρὸς μελαγχολίας καὶ τὰς καρδιακὰς διαθέσεις, καθὼς λέγει τέκνον Φίλιππος ὁ ἰητρὸς καὶ σὸς πατὴρ ὁ Ξηρός'. See Mercati (1917: 10–17), who offers transcriptions of these interventions throughout the codex.

various manuscripts.[36] In the previous case, there are marginal annotations or notabilia, some added by Philip Xeros himself. There are various categories of data given. For example, quite often Philip recommends his readers look at other recipes found in Paul of Aegina's *Epitome*, a seventh-century medical handbook which remained extremely popular throughout the entire Byzantine period – that is, on f. 244v, he refers to the chapter on erysipelas in Paul's work, which attests to the use of other medical texts by contemporary physicians in southern Italy and Sicily.[37] At the same time, Philip creates a complementarity between the *Ephodia tou apodēmountos* and Paul's text, which did not exist in the original Arabic treatise. Another interesting set of recommendations provides further information on certain recipes or details about a particular therapeutic procedure connected with the administration of a drug, thus enhancing the codex's usefulness to practitioners/readers. For example, on f. 173r, we read: 'first of all seek to purge',[38] and on f. 27r, Philip recommends his son not administer medicines that can be smelt, perhaps referring to medicines in the form of incense, since ingredients such as roses, camphor, and musk could strengthen the stomach.[39] The advice is related to the contents of the main text, in which a certain recipe is given in order, inter alia, to purge the stomach.[40] Lastly, a third group of annotations is related to the provision of synonyms in Greek intended to familiarise the reader with the Arabic terms given in Greek transliteration in the main body of the text. For example, in the margin of f. 198r, Philip adds two synonyms in Greek for the Arabic term given in Greek transliteration in the main text.[41] The Greek synonyms are 'βάλσαμον' and 'σισύμβριον', which are both terms used for various species of mint.[42] The Arabic term, 'νεμμέμ', a transliteration of one of the Arabic words for mint (i.e. *nammām*), is highlighted in the text with an asterisk, and the adverb 'ἀραβιστί' is used

[36] 'Paratext' is a term Gérard Genette (1997: 2) coined to refer to the material surrounding a printed text, including titles, prefaces, introductions, and footnotes. Genette's literary interpretation has more recently been applied to the study of manuscripts; see, for example, Cooper (2015).

[37] Vaticanus gr. 300, f. 244v (left margin): 'ζήτει καὶ ἑτέραν πύλην ἐρυσιπέλατος εἰς τὸν Παῦλον'. 'Πύλη' is found throughout the Greek translation of the *Ephodia tou apodēmountos* and corresponds to the Arabic *bāb*, the term for chapter.

[38] Vaticanus gr. 300, f. 173r (right margin): 'ζήτει ἐν πρώτοις τὴν κάθαρσιν'.

[39] Vaticanus gr. 300, f. 27r (right margin): 'μὴ ἐπιδώσῃς ὀσφραντὰ τέκνον ἐν καιρῷ βοηθήματι, τὰ γὰρ ὀσφραντὰ εἰσπνεόμενα, τονοῦσι τὸν στόμαχον, ὡς ῥόδα, νύμφας, μυρσίνας, καὶ τὰ ὅμο[ια] καὶ λευκοῖα, ἡ (correxi: ἢ cod.) καφορά, καὶ ὁ μόσχος'.

[40] Vaticanus gr. 300, f. 27r, ll. 1–4: 'ἐν τούτοις στήλη ἱερᾶς . . . καὶ καθαίρει δὲ καὶ τὸν στόμαχον'.

[41] Vaticanus gr. 300, f. 198r (right margin): 'βάλσαμον τὸ λεγόμενον σισύμβριον (correxi: σεισήμβριον cod.), ἀραβιστὶ δέ'.

[42] LSJ, s.v. βάλσαμον, II: costmary; σισύμβριον: bergamot-mint. Cf. Delatte (1939: II.392.10–11): 'σισύμβριον ἤτοι τὸ βάλσαμον'.

here to denote the Arabic version. This example is an emphatic reminder of the gradual dissemination and reception of the translations of Arabic medical texts throughout the Mediterranean from the eleventh century onwards.

Having outlined potential outcomes from the study of unedited and very little explored medieval pharmacological texts, I would like to add comments on the nature of the available primary sources. It is quite difficult to categorise medieval pharmacological texts. For example, Henry Sigerist, writing in 1958, attempted to create a categorisation of pharmacological literature by dividing the relevant early medieval Latin texts into four large groups: a) 'materia medica', which mainly includes texts on simple drugs,[43] often accompanied by illustrations, thus adding an art historical perspective to the study of medieval pharmacological texts;[44] b) 'collections of recipes', further subdivided into '*antidotaria*' (lists of composite drugs with many ingredients) and '*receptaria*' (lists of simple recipes); c) 'hermeneumata', brief glosses about pharmacological ingredients or lists of synonyms; and d) 'treatises on weights and measures', which he considered an essential appendix to each collection of recipes.[45] Sigerist's categorisation can also be applied to the output of the various Mediterranean traditions between the ninth/tenth and fifteenth centuries. But rather than attempting to find a way of categorising pharmacological texts, I would like to point out trends that marked the period under examination.

First, vast reference works were created that attempted to systematise previous knowledge, often elaborated with knowledge derived from practical experience. I have already referred to the late eleventh-century Latin collection of recipes, the so-called *Antidotarium magnum*. By the early fourteenth century, the vast *Dynameron* by the so-called Nicholas Myrepsos had been composed in Greek, providing a long list of 2,650 recipes of composite drugs, making it the most extensive medieval work on the topic.[46] The *Dynameron* is not a list of official recipes aimed at regulating pharmaceutical activity, as was the case for the Latin *Ricettario Fiorentino*, the first European pharmacopoeia, which was published in Florence in 1499,[47] although it could be seen as the first Byzantine

[43] On medieval collections of *materia medica*, see the thought-provoking study by Ventura (2017).

[44] The Greek treatise of Dioscorides, *De materia medica*, and its versions and translations constituted the main source of influence on Mediterranean pharmacological traditions. For a comprehensive introduction to the topic, see Collins (2000).

[45] Sigerist (1958: 144). See also the more detailed categorisation by Touwaide (2005).

[46] The text has recently been edited by Valiakos (2020).

[47] See Colapinto (1993).

pharmacopoeia that attempted to systematise the composition of drugs and offer a reference manual of standardised recipes. Another notable example is *al-Jāmiʿ li-mufradāt al-adwiyah wa-l-aghdhiyah* (*Collector of Simple Drugs and Foodstuffs*) by the Andalusian Arab Ibn al-Bayṭār (d. 1248), who provides a description of 1,400 simples in alphabetical order based on more than 150 ancient and medieval authors as well as his own observations.[48]

Second, this period also saw the production of practical manuals for daily practice – for example, collections of the most useful and 'tested' recipes, often connected with the activity of one or more practising physicians and apothecaries or a particular place of healing, such as a hospital. One can point to several examples of the so-called *iatrosophia*[49] in Byzantine Greek or the collections of recipes connected with Byzantine hospitals, the so-called *xenōnika*;[50] the Arabic equivalents are the *aqrābādhīnat*.[51] There are also recipe books from the medieval Latin tradition, including those connected with hospitals,[52] or those associated with apothecaries.[53]

Third, the large number of Arabic works translated into Greek, Hebrew, and Latin and the existence of diverse multicultural milieus in the Mediterranean created a real need for glossaries of pharmacological ingredients. These can vary from just one folio to massive tomes. Perhaps the most prominent Latin witness of this process is the thirteenth-century *Clavis sanationis* (*Key to Healing*) by Simon of Genoa, which is written in narrative form. It is a huge work (there are 770 entries starting with 'A' alone), and about 75 per cent of its content is pharmacological, providing details about simples (etymological date, descriptive date, healing uses), including synonyms in Greek and Arabic.[54] A large number of bilingual and multilingual glossaries also survive, which provide synonyms for terms in one or more languages, usually arranged alphabetically in parallel columns.[55] These are usually given in transliteration using the alphabet

48 Cabo Gonzalez (1997).

49 The term may be applied to the treatise itself, even to a manuscript that contains a collection of practical medical treatises, including both diagnostic and therapeutic information. On Byzantine examples, see Touwaide (2007) and Zipser (2019).

50 Bennett (2017).

51 On examples of hospital formularies from Byzantium and the Islamicate worlds, see Horden (2013). On recipe books in the medieval Islamicate world, see Álvarez Millán (2020–1: 248–68).

52 See, for example, the *Ricettario* of the hospital of Santa Maria Novella in Florence as preserved in Florentinus Magliabechianus XV.92. Although the codex dates to 1515, it contains many recipes dating back to the fifteenth century. Henderson (2006: 297–300) suggests that it may have been copied from existing collections.

53 Silini (2001).

54 Bouras-Vallianatos (2013).

55 On medieval medico-botanical synonym lists, see the traditional introduction to the topic by Steinschneider (1892).

of the source language (e.g. Arabic, Latin, and Ottoman Turkish synonyms for Greek terms in Greek transliteration or even more complicated examples, including synonyms in Latin, Romance, and Arabic in Hebrew characters, but without any lexical material, in Hebrew, and so on).[56] Similarly one can also find lists of substitute drugs, which were often appended to pharmacological works in manuscripts and which may have had a highly practical value in medieval societies where some of the substances were not always readily available.[57]

Some of the contributions to this book discuss a significant number of previously little studied and/or unedited pharmacological texts. Fabian Käs (Chapter 1) provides the first critical presentation of the contents of the unpublished work *Book on Simple Drugs* by Ibn al-Tilmīdh by looking at the two surviving manuscripts – that is, Londiniensis BL or. 8294 and Wellcomensis or. 9. The work contains 287 entries, which provide a wealth of information arranged in five sections.

The first section provides synonyms for the Arabic terms in various languages. The next two deal with the primary qualities and degrees of intensity of the drugs concerned, and the fourth deals with therapeutic information. Käs notes the influence of Ibn Sīnā's *Qānūn fī al-ṭibb* (*Canon of Medicine*) on Ibn al-Tilmīdh's work, in particular on sections two and three, thus confirming the authority Ibn Sīnā's work had in the Islamicate medical tradition.

Perhaps the most interesting section is the last one – that is, the fifth part – where the author provides information about the use of each ingredient in the composite drugs administered in the ʿAḍudī hospital in Baghdad. This is a unique reference where the author makes a connection between the theoretical details he provides about pharmacological ingredients and their place in the daily routine of a medieval medical institution.

Leigh Chipman (Chapter 10) writes about the thirteenth-century *Minhāj al-dukkān* [*How to Run a Pharmacy*], a manual for pharmacists in Arabic by an otherwise unknown Jewish druggist from Cairo, al-Kūhīn al-ʿAṭṭār. By comparing preparations from *Minhāj al-dukkān* and an anonymous fourteenth-century cookbook from Cairo *Kanz al-fawāʾid fī tanwīʿ al-mawāʾid* (*Treasure Trove of Benefits and Variety at the Table*), she found a large number of almost identical recipes. Interestingly, the pharmacological manual often provides additional details, including an earlier written source and a brief attestation of efficacy, such as the term

[56] For examples from the Greek and Hebrew traditions, see Touwaide (1999) and Bos and Mensching (2005), respectively.

[57] On these kinds of texts, see Touwaide (2012).

mujarrab ('tried and tested'). Efficacy statements had often been added to pharmacological recipes since antiquity, aimed to attest the validity of the therapeutic effect of the recipe to later readers.[58] They may have been added by an author or a later scribe in the form of an annotation, and sometimes became an integral part of the text. Although it is unclear whether those who added such statements had actually tested a recipe, such additions nevertheless were clearly an indicator of the most effective drugs. Similar statements are also found in Arabic medical self-treatment compendia discussed by Paulina Lewicka (Chapter 9), as well as in Latin medieval recipes or the accounts of simple drugs in Hebrew discussed by Jeffrey Doolittle (Chapter 2) and Sivan Gottlieb (Chapter 6), where statements such as *ualde prodest* ('very beneficial') and *baḥun* ('tested') respectively are found.

There is evidence of a growing specialisation on the part of apothecaries in the twelfth and thirteenth centuries across the Mediterranean, and not only in Mamluk Egypt, as suggested in the discussion earlier in this introduction.[59] Apothecaries formed guilds in various Italian cities, as the large number of surviving statutes suggests. It was mainly for the doctor to diagnose and prescribe and for the apothecary to prepare and deliver the drugs.[60] An example from guild statutes in fourteenth-century Venice attests that apothecaries were neither allowed to make drugs without the consent of doctors nor even to treat the injured although there was considerable variation in this respect among Italian cities.[61] Furthermore, specific state mechanisms were developed to control the production of important composite drugs, including theriac.[62] On the Byzantine side, evidence suggests the operation of guilds by the so-called *myrepsoi* by the thirteenth century – for example, in the city of Thessaloniki.[63] Strict regulations were also imposed on the preparation of drugs and the administration of poisons in Byzantium. We are informed of great concern about deaths caused by poisonous drugs made by apothecaries, something considered more serious than a death caused by the sword.[64]

[58] On efficacy statements, see Jones (1998) and Totelin (2011). See also Álvarez Millán (2020–1: 216–24), who discussed drug testing in the Islamicate medical tradition.

[59] For example, the separation of the profession of physicians from apothecaries by an edict of Frederick II (r. 1220–50), promulgated in 1231 in Melfi. On apothecaries' practice in the western Mediterranean, see Bénézet (1999).

[60] On the interaction between apothecaries and physicians, see Moulinier (2006).

[61] Ciasca (1927: 316, n. 6). [62] Moulinier (2006: 121–3).

[63] Kislinger (1988: 117). On pharmacy-related professions in Byzantium, see Varella (2007).

[64] See the fourteenth-century legal synopsis of the statements of canon and civil law by Matthew Blastares, *Treatise in Alphabetical Arrangement*, ed. Potlis and Rallis (1859) 361.

As regards the practice of apothecaries and the preparation and selling of drugs, interdisciplinary study of the surviving apothecaries' jars (*albarelli*) and bottles (*unguentaria*) remains a *desideratum*.[65] An excellent example of the wealth of information that one can derive from combining historical and archaeological data comes from the study of an *albarello*, a bottle, and a ceremonial cup found in the thirteenth-century burial of a Turkic prince in southern Ukraine. Renata Holod and Yuriy Rassamakin have argued for a Mediterranean origin for the *albarello* and the bottle, while the palynological (i.e. concerning the study of pollen dust and particles) and botanical analyses of the cup revealed a large amount of vegetal ingredients from the steppe.[66]

Jeffrey Doolittle (Chapter 2) points out the urgent need for palaeopathological studies when discussing medieval Latin dental recipes. Dental evidence could provide useful information on diet and social stratification, which in turn could help us understand the access of the lower classes to medicines. Doolittle provides a transcription of *Physica Plinii*, chapters 28–41, on oral and dental health from Montecassino Cod. 69, Archivio dell'Abbazia, and emphasises the importance of consulting different manuscripts of the *Physica Plinii* when studying a particular text, which was continuously modified and elaborated in the Middle Ages. The principal trajectory of these changes reflects gradual increases, not only in the number of recipes themselves, but also in the attention given to signs of precision – including the use of formal pharmaceutical nomenclature and metrological units and symbols – and the inclusion of a diverse range of new ingredients. These recipes also reveal shifting and patterned uses for particular medical ingredients and substances described by classical authorities and provide insight into the ways that medieval medical writers were reading, interpreting, and adapting their sources. The recipes can be very short, containing just one or two ingredients, as in the case of a preparation for teething in infants, where the use of goat's milk and/or rabbit brain is recommended, while at other times, as in the case of the recipe for a dentifrice, it has up to seven ingredients, i.e. cloves, African mastic, oyster shells, pumice, burned bread, galingale, and vinegar.

Kathleen Walker-Meikle (Chapter 3) focuses on the manuscript transmission of the *De sexaginta animalibus* and shows that it is a translation of an Arabic work on the properties of the body parts of animals by an

65 On examples from Florence, Thessaloniki, and Ayyubid Syria, see respectively Cora (1973), Antonaras (2010: 408–13), and Jenkins-Madina (2006: 132 and passim).

66 Holod and Rassamakin (2012).

eleventh-century physician, ʿUbaydallāh ibn Bukhtīshūʿ, by comparing the text with the *manāfiʿ* (usefulness) section from an Arabic bestiary by the same author. She also argues for the existence of two recensions by studying the manuscript tradition of the work for the first time and comparing each entry in both recensions with Ibn Bukhtīshūʿ's text and ʿĪsā ibn ʿAlī's *Book on the Useful Properties of Animal Parts: De sexaginta animalibus* details the medical uses of animal ingredients, sometimes juxtaposed with information with magical connotations with no separation between the two. The text contains about fifty-six chapters and starts with man and the quadrupeds, followed by birds, vermin, and aquatic creatures. Each animal entry then includes different sections on various pharmacological ingredients, such as blood, bile, fat, liver, and urine. A significant number of ingredients were particularly popular in medieval pharmacological recipes. Fat from pigs, goats, and sheep was an essential ingredient for the preparation of various kinds of unguents, a prominent dosage form for local application to the skin. Some animal ingredients, such as musk and ambergris, could originate from as far away as India and the Far East, having to be transported across large areas, which was reflected in their remarkably high price. The famous Venetian merchant traveller Marco Polo (*c.*1254–*c.*1324) refers to musk as an extremely expensive substance.[67]

Maria Mavroudi (Chapter 4) is concerned with the very little known and poorly edited Byzantine *Lexikon tōn Sarakēnōn* (*Lexicon of Saracens*), which consists of around 400 entries. It is a bilingual lexicon of mainly animal and plant substances. Arabic names for *materia medica* transliterated in Greek characters are accompanied by the equivalent Greek terms. Mavroudi shows that this lexicon was actually composed as an essential companion to the Greek translation of Ibn al-Jazzār's aforementioned Arabic *Ephodia tou apodēmountos.* Intriguingly, one can also find words of Latin origin, thus confirming that the translation was made in a place where Latin was also in use. Mavroudi argues that the transliteration of the Arabic terms was not only provided for reasons of accuracy – that is, so that the Greek-speaking reader would be aware of the exact Arabic terms – but it also had practical significance: contemporary Greek practitioners had to be familiar with the names of pharmacological substances in Greek, Arabic, and Latin in order to acquire them in multicultural southern Italy and Sicily. Another example given by the author of this chapter enlightens us

[67] Jacoby (2006: 201–3). See also King (2017: 219–69). On ambergris, see the comprehensive case study by Durak (2018).

further on the role not just of the written but also of the oral transmission of medieval pharmacological knowledge. An eleventh-century Greek copy of Paul of Aegina's medical handbook, Parisinus gr. 2205, transmits Greek notes referring to oral consultations with a Muslim inhabitant of the city of Veroia in the southern Balkans in order to identify plants such as 'σάμψυχον' ('marjoram'). This note provides us with an insight into the other business associated with the practice of medicine in a medieval context, including obtaining, processing, and transporting *materia medica*.

Sivan Gottlieb (Chapter 6) discusses the texts of the herbal Parisinus hébr. 1199. Each entry gives details in Hebrew and Latin about the use of one plant; various parts of the plant may be used as simple drugs or can form a compound with the addition of other ingredients such as eggs, milk, honey, wine, or even bear fat. Pharmacological information is often associated with details about the geographical distribution of the plant and its habitat. The most common references to therapeutic uses are for wounds and eye affections, both quite common in the Middle Ages. The texts sometimes include the names of physicians who had confirmed the usefulness of a certain recommendation, including very famous medical authorities such as the thirteenth-century pioneer physician and founder of academic medical training in Bologna, Taddeo degli Alderotti.[68] Intriguingly, these references have been removed from the Hebrew versions. We are particularly fortunate in being able to identify a distinct group of marginal annotations by someone who was most probably a past owner of the manuscript. This person provided brief, additional material for certain entries, including efficacy statements (e.g. *kvar badukḳ*/'already verified') or additional uses – for example, *le-ke'evey ḥaze ṿe-'isṭumakha*, *le-ke'evey shinayim* (i.e. for pains in the chest and stomach, for toothache), thus confirming that the manuscript was used by later readers and actively connecting the material of the codex with medical practice. Most interestingly, this manuscript includes illustrations for seventy-two of the ninety-eight plants mentioned. Although the illustrations do not represent the plants accurately, they give an essential visual overview of their parts. In many cases, the depiction of the plants is associated with their uses – for example, the anthropomorphised illustration of mandrake as a female figure is connected with the plant's use as a fertility agent, thus highlighting its gynaecological significance.

Paulina Lewicka (Chapter 9) examines two previously fairly unexplored self-treatment manuals written in Arabic, Ibn al-Akfānī's (d. 1349) *Ghunyat*

68 On Taddeo degli Alderotti, see Siraisi (1981).

al-labīb fī mā yusta'mal 'inda ghaybat al-ṭabīb (*Wealth of Information for the Intelligent Man When the Doctor Is Not Around*), originating in Mamluk Egypt; and al-Qurashī's *Ghunyat al-labīb ḥaythu lā yūjad al-ṭabīb* (*The Richness of Information for the Intelligent Man When the Doctor Is Not Around*), which remains unedited and for which we have no details about the dates and provenance of its author.

Self-treatment compendia go back to the Graeco-Roman world, where, for example, in the first century AD Rufus of Ephesus, among others, wrote a medical work addressed to the layman, which no longer survives. The Islamicate medical tradition comprises a considerable number of self-treatment manuals, and the earliest surviving example is by al-Rāzī (*Man lā yaḥḍuruhu al-ṭabīb*/*For the One Who Is Not Attended to by a Doctor*), who emphasised the need for a book to provide instructions on how to prepare affordable and easily procurable drugs. Ibn al-Akfānī prioritises ensuring a regulated diet over the use of drugs, which, according to him, should be as simple as possible and not include too many ingredients. Among the compound drugs he nevertheless discusses are references to popular medicaments such as rose syrup, barley water, and oxymel. Lewicka argues that most of the recipes for composite drugs derive from either al-Rāzī's *Kitāb al-ḥāwī* or Ibn Sīnā's *Qanūn fī al-ṭibb*, both very influential works in the medieval Islamicate world. Al-Qurashī was concerned in his treatise to provide advice on 'well-known and easily available ingredients', thus recalling al-Rāzī and echoing the well-known notion of the so-called *euporista*, simple and compound drugs that could be obtained easily.[69]

A last point of interest is the unusual types of ingredients often suggested by both authors. For example, al-Qurashī recommends blood of hoopoe to remove a leucoma from the eye or burnt lung of a wild donkey or horse mixed with honey or pomegranate syrup to treat a heavy cough. In both cases, these ingredients clearly derived from folk or occult medical practices. In fact, in both manuals one finds magical and religious content interwoven with medical advice.

I.3 Boundaries of Pharmacology

This volume aims to play a decisive role in promoting the study of non-medical texts as sources of information about medieval pharmacology and its entanglement with magic, religion, philosophy, cooking, alchemy, and

[69] On *euporista*, see now Brodersen (2020).

diplomacy. A useful critical examination of the medieval concept of drugs as therapeutic agents in light of Byzantine sources on sorcery is presented by Richard Greenfield (Chapter 7). He first sets out a case study of the use of a vegetal substance, the asphodel, which was widely used by ancient and medieval medical authors as an expectorant, an emmenagogue, and for a variety of affections, including kidney and urinary. Asphodel also appears in the popular magico-therapeutic treatise *The Magical Treatise of Solomon*, where it is recommended for various ailments, including headache and dysentery. It could also be used for expelling demons or protecting against the evil eye. Nevertheless, the drug is not connected with the theories of humoral pathology but is presented as having attained its properties due to its planetary connection with Saturn. There are further superstitious details about the gathering of the plant, which may include a Christian prayer and the invocation of magical names.

The connection of astral bodies with the properties of simple or composite drugs is also emphasised by Paulina Lewicka (Chapter 9); by examining Ibn al-Akfānī's medico-pharmacological self-treatment compendium, she shows that it often includes chapters that discuss the occult or magical properties (*khawāṣṣ*) of certain ingredients.[70] For example, the effectiveness of a mixture of the gall of a mountain goat with wild lettuce in protecting against poisons is said to be enhanced if consumed when the sun enters Aries.

The 'sacred' or 'magical' character of therapeutic material is even more obvious in the case of amulets. Greenfield gives an example from *Kyranides*, a widely circulated Greek magico-medical textbook dated to the fourth century, which records that, if someone wears an amulet made of rocket, nightingale, sea urchin, and a gemstone, along with an image of Venus, they will be well-liked/loved and will be avoided by wild animals. This operates on the principles of sympathetic magic, for example, by evoking the alluring song of the bird or the involvement of Venus, a symbol of love, sex, and fertility.

Similarly, in a Christian context in Byzantium, pious believers trusted that someone who wore an amulet containing a holy image or the relic of a certain saint or even oil from a lamp or wax from a candle from a shrine would receive effective therapy. Such was the popularity of 'sacred' substances that the use of holy water or holy oils is not only mentioned in Christian miracles, but they could often be found as ingredients in

70 On occult science in the Byzantine and Islamicate traditions, see Mavroudi (2006) and Saif and Leoni (2021), respectively.

composite drugs in Byzantine medical recipe books where superstitious elements were usually present.[71] Overall, Greenfield argues that amulets with magical or religious connotations and used as therapeutic agents could be seen as a substitute for drugs.

In fact, the use of amulets containing animal, mineral, and vegetal ingredients for therapeutic purposes had been quite widespread since antiquity and corresponding advice is even found in the works of physicians such as Galen and Alexander of Tralles. In his *On the Capacities of Simple Drugs* Galen recommended an amulet made of peony root be hung around the neck of an epileptic child. He attempted to explain it in a rational way by suggesting the patient may inhale particles from the root.[72] Similarly, Alexander of Tralles, writing in the sixth century, recommends the use of a large number of amulets for the treatment of epilepsy and gout but, although he accepted from his own experience (*peira*) that they might sometimes work, he never attempted to give a rational explanation. He grouped this kind of advice in separate sections of his works under the so-called *physika* (natural remedies, i.e. alternative or occult therapeutic practices, including the use of amulets, incantations, etc.).[73] Details about the use of certain simples as amulets were often intertwined with pharmacological or magical properties. For example, in the alchemical herbal examined by Sivan Gottlieb (Chapter 6) are eighteen references to the use of amulets, and the same applies in Kathleen Walker-Meikle's discussion of animal *materia medica* (Chapter 3), where each entry contains medicinal and magical properties side by side.

In another context, Phillip Lieberman (Chapter 8) examines the views of the well-known Jewish rabbi, philosopher, and physician Moses Maimonides (1138–1204), who worked in Morocco and Egypt, on the use of amulets. In his *Dalālat al-ḥāʾirīn* (*The Guide to the Perplexed*) Maimonides accepts the use of magical remedies, which may be also found in rabbinic literature or Arabic medical literature such as al-Tamīmī's *Kitāb al-murshid* (*The Guide*), including the use of amulets made of vegetal, mineral, animal, or even human parts (e.g. fox's tooth,

[71] On the use of holy water in Byzantine healing miracles, see Narro (2019). For examples in Byzantine medical recipe books, see John Archiatros, *Iatrosophion*, 208.א, ed. Zipser (2009) 164.29–30: 'ἁγιάσματος τῶν ἁγίων θεοφανίων' ('Epiphany water', i.e. holy water sanctified with special blessings on the Feast of Epiphany) and *Therapeutikai*, 38, ed. Bennett (2003) 423.4: 'ἁγίου ἐλαίου τῆς ἁγίας Ζηναΐδός' ('holy oil of St Zenais').

[72] Galen, *On the Capacities of Simple Drugs*, 6.3, ed. Kühn (1826) XI.859–60. Cf. Jouanna (2011). On the reception of this recommendation in Byzantine and post-Byzantine prayer books (*euchologia*), see Stathakopoulos (2020: 77–9).

[73] Bouras-Vallianatos (2014); Grimm-Stadelmann (2020: 103–18).

the nail of one who has been hanged, peony, dog dung, marcasite). Interestingly, Maimonides allows these remedies to be recommended – 'even if not prescribed by reason' – once there is adequate experience confirming their effectiveness, which reminds us of Alexander of Tralles' empirical approach to the use of *physika*. Similarly, Lewicka provides examples of the use of amulets (e.g. coconut for malarial fevers, ruby for plague) where Ibn al-Akfānī often confirms that their suitability as curatives has been tested by experience.

Athanasios Rinotas (Chapter 12) addresses a closely related topic by focusing on the medico-philosophical approaches of the thirteenth-century philosopher and theologian Albertus Magnus. Although not a practising physician, Albertus wrote about medicine. In his work *On Minerals* Albertus refers to certain stones in the form of amulets worn around the neck as capable of treating diseases such as epilepsy and melancholy. Yet Albertus does not touch upon or refer explicitly to how these stones could act. The Dominican master adopted the notion of the medical properties of stones from authorities of the past, such as Pliny the Elder and Dioscorides, mainly through the works of Arnold of Saxony (fl. 1225) and Thomas of Cantimpré (*c.*1200–*c.*1270), and he often put great weight on experience, especially as regards the powers of stones, most probably influenced by Ibn Sīnā's Latin translation of the *Canon of Medicine*.

Rinotas argues that in dealing with epilepsy and melancholy, Albertus attempted to philosophise the knowledge of stones. He accepts a humoral understanding of disease (e.g. connecting phlegm with epilepsy and black bile with melancholy) and uses his theory of colours to give a philosophical explanation. For example, the hot and dry nature of red stones could control the moistness and coldness epilepsy causes in the human body. Similarly, the blackness of onyx could be a factor in increasing the symptoms of melancholy.

This volume also shows that the fields of cooking and alchemy can often be very close to that of pharmacology and their comparative study can be beneficial in contextualising various pharmacological recommendations. Leigh Chipman (Chapter 10) explores common recipes for compounds in al-ʿAṭṭār's pharmacological work *Minhāj al-dukkān* and the anonymous cookbook *Kanz al-fawāʾid fī tanwīʿ al-mawāʾid*. For example, a recipe for a snack to go with alcoholic drinks in the cookbook is labelled as a recipe for strengthening the digestion in the pharmacopoeia. In the case of a recipe for an oxymel of chewy candy, the cookbook even refers to humours and qualities, thus giving more medical information than the

Minhāj al-dukkān. Chipman argues that a certain recipe can take on a particular meaning in a particular context. Thus, a recipe in the cookbook that is surrounded by recipes for drinks and food dishes has a purely nutritional character, while the same recipe in a pharmacological context stresses its healing rather than its nutritional effect. In another case Chipman shows how the dietary advice on consuming sour grape juice and pickled almonds at the end of a recipe from the Genizah collection, T-S Ar. 30.305, can be better contextualised by studying *Kanz al-fawāʾid*, which contains a large number of recipes of dishes 'for the nourishment of the sick'.

Matteo Martelli (Chapter 11) critically examines unedited manuscripts with examples of pharmacological recipes intermixed with alchemical formulae. For example, in Bononiensis 1808, a medical miscellany, recipes for composite drugs appear side by side with procedures for making metallic, black, and coloured inks; two of them on silver ink in particular very closely resemble techniques of preparation used in pharmacological recipes (e.g. grinding ingredients up in a mortar). In another example from Vaticanus gr. 1174, which includes a large compilation of mainly alchemical texts, four alchemical recipes (e.g. on making gold, or on how to polish adulterated silver) are followed by a pharmacological recipe for a salt ascribed to St Gregory the Theologian.

Byzantine medical manuscripts contain unedited recipes for salts which have been attributed to a variety of sacred figures, including St Luke, St Gregory the Theologian, and others. In this case, the recipe consists of eleven ingredients, including vegetal ones (e.g. Cretan hyssop, pennyroyal) and minerals (e.g. common salt), without, however, providing any indications for the recipe's use. Martelli has managed to find a similar recipe for a salt in Nicholas Myrepsos' *Dynameron*, which is recommended for improving vision and sharp-sightedness, thus giving us a new appreciation of pharmacological recipes found in alchemical collections. In fact, goldsmiths were often affected by eye conditions and early Byzantine medical sources (e.g. Oribasios, Aetios of Amida) report the use of eye salves to treat them, as Martelli aptly shows.

Koray Durak's study (Chapter 13) views medieval evidence on medicines from a highly interesting angle. He deals with diplomatic exchanges in the form of gifts, and, in particular, of simple and composite drugs carried out between Byzantium and its neighbour states. By exploring a large number of medical and non-medical sources from the Byzantine and the Islamicate worlds – letters, hagiographical and historiographical works, and works on trade and commerce – Durak shows how medicines could effectively support diplomacy and extracts useful details about the high price and availability of certain spices, such as pepper, and composite drugs – for example, theriac.

Interestingly, Durak also points out the usefulness and practical value of drugs as healing substances for members of royal families or even for the animals of royal hunting establishments, such as hawks and falcons, compared to merely decorative gifts or 'objects of display', such as wall hangings or gold vessels and coins. For example, theriac was considered an invincible antidote against poisons; *moumie* (bitumen or asphalt/ Ar. *mūmiyā'*), a rare panacea simple drug, is recommended for any kind of fractured limbs, whether human or animal; and a certain unnamed stone of triangular shape was used to treat dropsy. The latter is actually the only documented simple drug/ingredient sent from Byzantium to an Islamicate court: the vast majority of the evidence shows diplomatic gifts going in the other direction. Durak demonstrates that the study of diplomatic gifts can give us a better understanding of the multidimensional patterns in the introduction and dissemination of various rare substances from the Islamicate world to Byzantium and the wider Mediterranean, including vegetal (e.g. aloeswood, camphor, saffron), animal (e.g. ambergris, musk), and mineral ingredients (e.g. *mūmiyā'*).

In the case of compound drugs, the prestigious nature of theriac, along with the rarity of some of its ingredients, allowed it to enter the diplomatic arena. Apart from its role as a powerful antidote, theriac was also used prophylactically as a drug for the preservation of health. It was included with luxurious liturgical objects Ignatios, Patriarch of Constantinople, gave to Pope Adrian II in 871 and to the king of the Anglo-Saxons, Alfred the Great (r. 871–*c.*886). It was among the gifts sent by Byzantine emperors with embassies to both the West and the Islamicate world. It was also among the gifts Abbasid and Mamluk rulers sent to the Byzantines and other states, thus confirming its prominent status in various Mediterranean regions and showing that the same drugs or elements of *materia medica* often characterised the pharmaceutical practices of the entire Mediterranean.

This book is the best proof that advances in the study of medieval pharmacology cannot happen in isolation but only through careful interdisciplinary research, a true dialogue of equals among specialists in the Byzantine, Islamicate, Jewish, and Latin traditions. The fascinating insights afforded by the contributions included in this volume corroborate the links between these traditions and the complex ways in which knowledge was transferred though translations, annotations, and adaptations.

While the importance of the Islamicate medical and pharmacological tradition and how it became familiar to the rest of the medieval Mediterranean world is undeniable, the transfer of knowledge was not a one-way street. Nor did the development of the pharmacological tradition within each cultural sphere happen in isolation from medical practice or from other fields such as cooking, alchemy, and magic. All these factors contributed to the process that this collection of essays dynamically outlines and explores. Finally, this volume makes clear that to move forward, it is necessary to produce new and improved editions of texts – to study and comment on their origins, date, formation, sources, and use. Only then can we hope to do justice to this complex and fascinating aspect of medieval science, scholarship, and practice.

REFERENCES

Álvarez Millán, C. 2020–1. 'Drugs Testing, Tested Remedies and Medical-Literary Genres in Medieval Islam', *Suhayl* 18: 205–73.

Amar, Z., Lev, E., and Serri, Y. 2014. 'On Ibn Juljul and the Meaning and Importance of the List of Medicinal Substances Not Mentioned by Dioscorides', *Journal of the Royal Asiatic Society* 24: 529–55.

Amar, Z., and Lev, E. 2017. *Arabian Drugs in Early Medieval Mediterranean Medicine*. Edinburgh: Edinburgh University Press.

Antonaras, A. C. 2010. 'Early Christian and Byzantine Glass Vessels: Forms and Uses', in F. Daim and J. Drauschke (eds.), *Byzanz: Das Römerreich im Mittelalter, vol. 1: Welt der Ideen, Welt der Dinge*. Mainz: Römisch-Germanisches Zentralmuseum, 383–430.

Bénézet, J.-P. 1999. *Pharmacie et médicament en Méditerranée occidentale (XIIIe–XVIe siècles*. Paris: H. Champion.

Bennett, D. 2003. '*Xenonika*: Medical Texts Associated with Xenones in the Late Byzantine Period'. PhD thesis, Royal Holloway, University of London.

Bennett, D. 2017. *Medicine and Pharmacy in Byzantine Hospitals: A Study of the Extant Formularies*. Abingdon: Routledge.

Biran, M. 2015. 'The Mongol Empire and Inter-civilizational Exchange', in B. Z. Kedar and M. E. Wiesner-Hanks (eds.), *Expanding Webs of Exchange and Conflict, 500 CE–1500 CE*. Cambridge: Cambridge University Press, 534–58.

Bos, G. 1993. 'Ibn al-Jazzār on Women's Diseases and Their Treatment', *Medical History* 37: 296–312.

Bos, G., and Käs, F. 2016. 'Arabic Pharmacognostic Literature and Its Jewish Antecedents: Marwān ibn Ǧanāḥ (Rabbi Jonah), Kitāb al-Talḫīṣ', *Aleph* 16: 145–229.

Bos, G., Käs, F. , and McVaugh, M. R. eds. and trans. 2022. *Ibn al-Jazzār's Zād al-musāfir wa-qūt al-ḥāḍir: Provisions for the Traveller and Nourishment for the Sedentary. Books I and II: Diseases of the Head and the Face*. Leiden: Brill.

Bos, G., and Mensching, G. 2005. 'The Literature of Hebrew Medical Synonyms: Romance and Latin Terms and Their Identification', *Aleph* 5: 169–211.

Bouras-Vallianatos, P. 2013. 'Simon of Genoa's *Clavis Sanationis*: A Study of Thirteenth-Century Latin Pharmacological Lexicography', in B. Zipser (ed.), *Simon of Genoa's Medical Lexicon*. Berlin: De Gruyter, 31–48.

Bouras-Vallianatos, P. 2014. 'Clinical Experience in Late Antiquity: Alexander of Tralles and the Therapy of Epilepsy', *Medical History* 58: 337–53.

Bouras-Vallianatos, P. 2020. *Innovation in Byzantine Medicine: The Writings of John Zacharias Aktouarios (c.1275–c.1330)*. Oxford: Oxford University Press.

Bouras-Vallianatos, P. 2021. 'Cross-Cultural Transfer of Medical Knowledge in the Medieval Mediterranean: The Introduction and Dissemination of Sugar-Based Potions from the Islamic World to Byzantium', *Speculum* 96.4: 963–1008.

Brentjes, S., Fidora, A., and Tischler, M. M. 2014. 'Towards a New Approach to Medieval Cross-Cultural Exchanges', *Journal of Transcultural Medieval Studies* 1: 9–50.

Brodersen, K. 2020. *Gut beschaffbare Heilmittel (Euporista)*. Stuttgart: Anton Hiersemann.

Burnett, C. ed. 2008. *Ibn Baklarish's Book of Simples: Medical Remedies between Three Faiths in 12th-Century Spain*. Oxford: Oxford University Press.

Burnett, C. 2016. 'The *Synonyma* Literature in the Twelfth and Thirteenth Centuries', in S. Brentjes and J. Renn (eds.), *Globalization of Knowledge in the Post-Antique Mediterranean, 700–1500*. London: Routledge, 131–9.

Burridge, C. 2020. 'Incense in Medicine: An Early Medieval Perspective', *Early Medieval Europe* 28: 219–55.

Caballero-Navas, C. 2011. 'Medicine among Medieval Jews: The Science, the Art, and the Practice', in G. Freudenthal (ed.), *Science in Medieval Jewish Cultures*. Cambridge: Cambridge University Press, 320–42.

Cabo Gonzalez, A. M. 1997. 'Ibn a̱l-Bayṭār et ses apports à la botanique et à la pharmacologie dans le Kitāb al-Ǧāmiʿ', *Médiévales: Langue, Textes, Histoire* 33: 23–39.

Chipman, L. 2013. 'The Jewish Presence in Arabic Writings on Medicine and Pharmacology during the Medieval Period', *Religion Compass* 7/9: 394–401.

Chipman, L. 2019. 'The Reception of Galenic Pharmacology in the Arabic Tradition', in P. Bouras-Vallianatos and B. Zipser (eds.), *Brill's Companion to the Reception of Galen*. Leiden: Brill, 304–16.

Ciasca, R. 1927. *L'arte dei medici e speziali nella storia e nel commercio fiorentino dal sec. XII al XV*. Florence: Olschki.

Colapinto, L. 1993. 'The "Nuovo Receptario" of Florence', *Medicina nei Secoli* 5: 39–50.

Collins, M. 2000. *Medieval Herbals: The Illustrative Traditions*. London: British Library.

Cooper, C. E. 2015. 'What Is a Medieval Paratext?', *Marginalia: Journal of the Medieval Reading Group at the University of Cambridge* 19: 37–50.

Cora, G. 1973. *Storia della maiolica di Firenze e del contado: secoli XIV e XV*, 2 vols. Florence: Sansoni.

Delatte, A. ed. 1939. *Anecdota Atheniensia et alia*, vol. II. Paris: Droz.

De Vos, P. 2013. 'The "Prince of Medicine": Yūḥannā ibn Māsawayh and the Foundations of the Western Pharmaceutical Tradition', *Isis* 104.4: 667–712.

Durak, K. 2018. 'From the Indian Ocean to the Markets of Constantinople: Ambergris in the Byzantine World', in B. Pitarakis and G. Tanman (eds.), *Life Is Short, Art Long: The Art of Healing in Byzantium. New Perspectives.* Istanbul: Istanbul Research Institute, 201–25.

Durak, K. 2021. 'The Commercial History of Trebizond and the Region of Pontos from the Seventh to the Eleventh Centuries: An International Emporium', *Mediterranean Historical Review* 36.1: 3–41.

Ferre, L. 2004. 'Donnolo's *Sefer ha-Yaqar*: New Edition with English Translation', in G. Lacerenza (ed.), *Šabbeṯay Donnolo: scienza e cultura ebraica nell'Italia del secolo X.* Naples: Università degli studi di Napoli L'Orientale, 1–20.

Freedman, P. 2012. 'The Medieval Spice Trade', in J. M. Pilcher (ed.), *The Oxford Handbook of Food History*. Oxford: Oxford University Press, 324–40.

Genette, G. 1997. *Paratexts: Thresholds of Interpretation*, trans. J. E. Lewin. Cambridge: Cambridge University Press. [Originally published in French as *Seuils*. Paris: Editions du Seuil, 1987.]

Goitein, S. D., and Friedman, M. A. 2008. *India Traders of the Middle Ages: Documents from the Cairo Geniza ('India Book')*. Leiden: Brill.

Green, M. H. 2008. 'Rethinking the Manuscript Basis of Salvatore De Renzi's *Collectio Salernitana*: The Corpus of Medical Writings in the "Long" Twelfth Century', in D. Jacquart and A. Paravicini Bagliani (eds.), *La 'Collectio Salernitana' di Salvatore De Renzi*. Florence: SISMEL/Edizioni del Galluzzo, 15–60.

Green, M. H. 2019. 'The *Antidotarium magnum*: A Short Description'. www.academia.edu/4611623/Antidotarium_magnum_-_An_Online_Edition (accessed 15 September 2021).

Green, M. H. forthcoming. 'In and beyond the Beneventan Zone: The Transformation of Latin Medicine in the Late Eleventh Century', in A. J. Irving and R. Gyug (eds.), *Brill's Companion to the Beneventan Zone*. Leiden: Brill.

Grimm-Stadelmann, I. 2020. *Untersuchungen zur Iatromagie in der byzantinischen Zeit: Zur Tradierung gräkoägyptischer und spätantiker iatromagischer Motive*. Berlin: De Gruyter.

Gysseling, M., and Koch, A. C. F. eds. 1950. *Diplomata Belgica ante annum millesimum centesimum scripta*. 2 vols. Brussels: Belgisch Inter-Universitir Centrum voor Neerlandistiek.

Haldon, J. F. ed. 1990. *Constantine Porphyrogenitus: Three Treatises on Imperial Military Expeditions*. Vienna: Verlag der Österreichischen Akademie der Wissenschaften.

Harig, G. 1967. 'Von den arabischen Quellen des Simeon Seth', *Medizinhistorisches Journal* 2: 248–68.

Harig, G. 1974. *Bestimmung der Intensität im medizinischen System Galens: Ein Beitrag zur theoretischen Pharmakologie, Nosologie und Therapie in der Galenischen Medizin.* Berlin: Akademie-Verlag.

Henderson, J. 2006. *The Renaissance Hospital: Healing the Body and Healing the Soul.* New Haven, CT: Yale University Press.

Hodgson, M. G. S. 1974. *The Venture of Islam: Conscience and History in a World Civilization, vol. I: The Classical Age of Islam.* Chicago, IL: University of Chicago Press.

Holod, R., and Rassamakin, Y. 2012. 'Imported and Native Remedies for a Wounded "Prince": Grave Goods from the Chungul Kurgamn in the Black Sea Steppe of the Thirteenth Century', *Medieval Encounters* 18: 339–81.

Horden, P. 2013. 'Medieval Hospital Formularies: Byzantium and Islam Compared', in B. Zipser (ed.), *Medical Books in the Byzantine World.* Bologna: Eikasmos, 145–64.

Horden, P., and Purcell, N. 2000. *The Corrupting Sea: A Study of Mediterranean History.* Oxford: Blackwell.

Ieraci Bio, A. M. 2006. 'La medicina greca dello Stretto (Filippo Xeros ed Eufemio Siculo)', in F. Burgarella and A. M. Ieraci Bio (eds.), *La cultura scientifica e tecnica nell'Italia meridionale Bizantina.* Soveria Mannelli: Rubbettino, 109–24.

Jacoby, D. 2006. 'Marco Polo, His Close Relatives, and His Travel Account: Some New Insights', *Mediterranean Historical Review* 21: 193–218.

Jacoby, D. 2016. 'Constantinople As Commercial Transit Center, Tenth to Mid-Fifteenth Century', in P. Magdalino, N. Necipoğlu, and I. Jevtić (eds.), *Trade in Byzantium.* Istanbul: Koç Üniversitesi, Anadolu Medeniyetleri Araștirma Merkezi, 193–210.

Jenkins-Madina, M. 2006. *Raqqa Revisited: Ceramics of Ayyubid Syria.* New York: Metropolitan Museum of Art.

Jones, C. 1998. 'Efficacy Phrases in Medieval English Medical Manuscripts', *Neuphilologisches Mitteilungen* 99: 199–209.

Jouanna, J. 2011. 'Médecine rationnelle et magie: Le statut des amulettes et des incantations chez Galien', *Revue des Études Grecques* 124: 47–77.

Kahl, O. 2015. *The Sanskrit, Syriac and Persian Sources in the* Comprehensive Book *of Rhazes.* Leiden: Brill.

Kahl, O. 2019. 'On the Transmission of Indian Medical Texts to the Arabs in the Early Middle Ages', *Arabica* 66: 82–97.

Kahl, O. 2020. '"From the Writings of an Indian Woman": Pharmaceutical Fragments of a Lots Ayurvedic Text on Gynecology, Preserved in a Ninth-Century Arabic Medical Compendium', *Pharmacy in History* 62: 150–8.

King, A. 2017. *Scent from the Garden of Paradise: Musk and the Medieval Islamic World.* Leiden: Brill.

Kislinger, E. 1988. 'Gewerbe im späten Byzanz', in *Handwerk und Sachkultur im Spätmittelalter*. Vienna: Österreichischen Akademie der Wissenschaften, 103–26.

Kousis, A. 1939. 'Quelques considérations sur les traductions en grec des oeuvres médicales orientales et principalement sur les deux manuscrits de la traduction d'un traité persan par Constantin Melitiniotis', *Πρακτικὰ Ἀκαδημίας Ἀθηνῶν* 14: 205–20.

Lehmhaus, L. 2021a. 'Defining or Defying Jewish Medicine? Old Problems and New Questions', in L. Lehmhaus (ed.), *Defining Jewish Medicine: Transfer of Medical Knowledge in Premodern Jewish Cultures and Traditions*. Wiesbaden: Harrasowitz, 3–26.

Lehmhaus, L. 2021b. 'The Academic Quest for "Jewish Medicine": A Survey of the Field', in L. Lehmhaus (ed.), *Defining Jewish Medicine: Transfer of Medical Knowledge in Premodern Jewish Cultures and Traditions*. Wiesbaden: Harrasowitz, 27–55.

Lev, E., and Amar, Z. 2007. 'Practice versus Theory: Medieval Materia Medica according to the Cairo Genizah', *Medical History* 51: 507–26.

Lucà, S. 1993. 'I Normanni e la 'Rinascita' del sec. XII', *Archivio Storico per la Calabria e la Lucanica* 60: 1–91.

Mavroudi, M. 2006. 'Occult Science and Society in Byzantium: Considerations for Future Research', in P. Magdalino and M. Mavroudi (eds.), *The Occult Sciences in Byzantium*. Geneva: La Pomme d'or, 39–95.

McCabe, A. E. 2009. 'Imported *Materia Medica*, 4th–12th Centuries, and Byzantine Pharmacology', in M. Mundell Mango (ed.), *Byzantine Trade, 4th–12th Centuries*. Farnham: Ashgate, 273–92.

Mercati, G. 1917. 'Filippo Xeros Reggino, Giovanni Alessandrino iatrosophista e altri nel codice Vaticano degli "Ephodia"', in G. Mercati, *Notizie varie di antica letteratura medica e di bibliografia*. Rome: Tipografia poliglotta vaticana, 9–41.

Meyerhof, M. 1931. 'Ali aṭ-Ṭabarī's "Paradise of Wisdom": One of the Oldest Arabic Compendiums of Medicine', *Isis* 16: 6–54.

Miguet, T. 2017. 'Premiers jalons pour une étude complète de l'histoire du texte grec du *Viatique du Voyageur* (Ἐφόδια τοῦ ἀποδημοῦντος) d'Ibn al-Ǧazzār', *Revue d'Histoire des Textes* 12: 59–105.

Moulinier, L. 2006. 'Médecins et apothicaires dans l'Italie médiévale: Quelques aspects de leurs relations', in F. Collard and E. Samama (eds.), *Pharmacopoles et apothicaires: Les "pharmaciens" de l'Antiquité au Grand Siècle*. Paris: L'Harmattan, 119–34.

Narro, Á. 2019. 'Holy Water and Other Healing Liquids in the Byzantine Collections of Miracles', in J. J. Pomer Monferrer and H. Rovira (eds.), *Aigua i vi a les literatures clàssiques i la seua tradició*. Reus (Tarragona): Editorial Rhemata, 121–43.

Pormann, P. E. 2011. 'The Formation of the Arabic Pharmacology between Tradition and Innovation', *Annals of Science* 68: 493–515.

Potlis, M., and Rallis, G. A. eds. 1859. *Σύνταγμα τῶν θείων καὶ ἱερῶν κανόνων . . . ἐκκλησιαστικὴν κατάστασιν διεπούσαις διατάξεσι*, vol. VI. Athens: Ek tou Typographeiou tēs Augēs.

Riddle, J. 1985. *Dioscorides on Pharmacy and Medicine*. Austin: University of Texas Press.

Roberg, F. 2007. 'Text- und redaktionskritische Probleme bei der Edition von Texten des Gebrauchsschrifttums am Beispiel des Antidotarium Nicolai (12. Jahrhundert): Einige Beobachtungen. Mit einem Editionsanhang', *Mittellateinisches Jahrbuch* 42: 1–19.

Saif, L., and Leoni, F. 2021. 'Introduction', in L. Saif, F. Leoni, M. Melvin-Koushki, and F. Yahya (eds.), *Islamicate Occult Sciences in Theory and Practice*. Leiden: Brill, 1–40.

Schilbach, E. 1970. *Byzantinische Metrologie*. Dusseldorf: Brukken.

Sharf, A. 1995. *Jews and Other Minorities in Byzantium*. Jerusalem: Bar-Ilan University Press.

Sigerist, H. E. 1958. 'The Latin Medical Literature of the Early Middle Ages', *Journal of the History of Medicine and Allied Sciences* 13.2: 127–46.

Silini, G. 2001. *Umori e Farmaci: Terapia medica tardo-medievale*. Gandino: Iniziative Culturali.

Siraisi, N. 1981. *Taddeo Alderotti and His Pupils: Two Generations of Italian Medical Learning*. Princeton, NJ: Princeton University Press.

Stathakopoulos, D. 2020. 'The Boundaries between Possession and Disease: Medical Concepts in Byzantine and Post-Byzantine Exorcisms', in C. Dietl, N. Metzger, and C. Schanze (eds.), *Wahnsinn und Ekstase Literarische Konfigurationen zwischen christlicher Antike und Mittelalter*. Wiesbaden: Reichert, 69–81.

Steinschneider, M. 1892. 'Zur Literatur der "Synonyma"', in I. L. Pagel (ed.), *Die Chirurgie des Heinrich von Mondeville*. Berlin: A. Hirschwald, 582–95.

Suwaysī, M. et al. eds. 1999. *Zād al-musāfir wa-qūt al-ḥāḍir*. 2 vols. Tunis: al-Majmaʿ al-Tūnisī lil-ʿUlūm wa-l-Ādāb wa-l-Funūn, Bayt al-Ḥikmah.

Totelin, L. 2011. 'Old Recipes, New Practice? The Latin Adaptations of the Hippocratic Gynaecological Treatises', *Social History of Medicine* 24: 74–91.

Touwaide, A. 1999. '*Lexica medico-botanica byzantina*: Prolégomènes à une étude', in L. Pérez Castro, F. Adrados, and L. de Cuenca (eds.), *Τῆς φιλίης τάδε δῶρα: Miscelánea léxica en memoria de Conchita Serrano*. Madrid: Consejo Superior de Investigaciones Científicas, 211–28.

Touwaide, A. 2005. 'Pharmaceutical Handbooks', in T. Glick, S. J. Livesey, and F. Wallis (eds.), *Medieval Science, Technology and Medicine: An Encyclopedia*. Abingdon: Routledge, 393–4.

Touwaide, A. 2007. 'Byzantine Hospital Manuals (*Iatrosophia*) As a Source for the Study of Therapeutics', in B. S. Bowers (ed.), *The Medieval Hospital and Medical Practice*. Aldershot: Ashgate, 147–75.

Touwaide, A. 2012. '*Quid pro Quo:* Revisiting the Practice of Substitution in Ancient Pharmacy', in A. van Arsdall and T. Graham (eds.), *Herbs and Healers from the Ancient Mediterranean through the Medieval West: Essays in Honor of John M. Riddle*. London: Routledge, 19–62.

Touwaide, A. 2016. 'Agents and Agencies? The Many Facets of Translation in Byzantine Medicine', in F. Wallis and R. Wisnovsky (eds.), *Medieval Textual Cultures*. Berlin: De Gruyter, 13–38.

Valiakos, I. ed. 2020. *Nikolaos Myrepsos' Dynameron. Critical Edition*. Heidelberg: Propylaeum.

Varella, E. 2007. 'Pharmacy Related Professions in Byzance', *Medicina nei Secoli* 19: 653–66.

Ventura, I. 2016. 'Medieval Pharmacy and Arabic Heritage: The Salernitan Collection *Circa Instans*', *Impact of Arabic Sciences in Europe and Asia* [Micrologus 16], 339–401.

Ventura, I. 2017. 'Classification Systems and Pharmacological Theory in Medieval Collections of *Materia Medica*: A Short History from Antiquity to the End of the 12th Century', in T. Pommerening and W. Bisang (eds.), *Classification from Antiquity to Modern Times: Sources, Methods, and Theories from an Interdisciplinary Perspective*. Berlin: De Gruyter, 101–66.

Ventura, I. 2021. 'Sulla trasmissione vernacolare dello "Schriftencorpus" attribuito allo Ps.-Mesue: Per una ricognizione delle traduzioni tra XIII e XVI secolo', *Carte Romanze* 9.2: 183–265.

Vogt, S. 2008. 'Drugs and Pharmacology', in R. J. Hankinson (ed.), *The Cambridge Companion to Galen*. Cambridge: Cambridge University Press, 304–22.

Yoeli-Tlalim, R. 2021. *ReOrienting Histories of Medicine: Encounters along the Silk Roads*. London: Bloomsbury Academic.

Zipser, B. ed. 2009. *John the Physician's* Therapeutics*: A Medical Handbook in Vernacular Greek*. Leiden: Brill.

Zipser, B. 2019. 'Galen in Byzantine *Iatrosophia*', in P. Bouras-Vallianatos and B. Zipser (eds.), *Brill's Companion to the Reception of Galen*. Leiden: Brill, 111–23.

PART I

Transmission of Pharmacological Knowledge

Texts and Contexts

CHAPTER 1

Ibn al-Tilmīdh's Book on Simple Drugs

A Christian Physician from Baghdad on the Arabic, Greek, Syriac, and Persian Nomenclature of Plants and Minerals

Fabian Käs

Amīn al-Dawla Hibatallāh ibn Ṣāʿid Ibn al-Tilmīdh was born in Baghdad around the year 1073 CE into a family of Christian physicians. After years of travel in Persia, he returned to his home town, where he served several Abbasid caliphs as their personal physician. These entrusted him with high-ranking positions, namely that of 'head of physicians' and of director of the renowned ʿAḍudī hospital. Ibn al-Tilmīdh was also a prominent member – according to his Muslim biographers a 'priest and head' – of the Nestorian community of Baghdad, where he died in AH 560/1165 CE aged over ninety.[1]

Ibn al-Tilmīdh wrote about twenty books[2] and treatises, including collections of his own Arabic poems and letters. Most of his medical works were commentaries and abridgements of Greek and Arabic classics – for example, Galen's commentaries on Hippocrates' *Aphorisms* and his *Prognostic*. One of his abridgments hitherto deemed to be lost – that of Miskawayh's book on beverages – could recently be identified in a manuscript kept in Ankara.[3] His most renowned writings are his

[1] For a concise account of Ibn al-Tilmīdh's life and work, see Kahl (2007: 7–19). The most important original sources are Ibn Abī Uṣaybiʿah, *ʿUyūn al-anbāʾ fī ṭabaqāt al-aṭibbāʾ* (*Sources of Information on the Classes of Physicians*), ed. Savage-Smith, Swain, and van Gelder (2020, online version), chapter 10, biography 64 = ed. Müller (1882) I.259–76; Yāqūt, *Muʿjam al-udabāʾ* (*Dictionary of Learned Men*), ed. Rifāʿī (1936) XIX.276–82; and Ibn Khallikān, *Wafayāt al-aʿyān* (*Obituaries of Famous Persons*), ed. ʿAbbās (1968) VI.69–77; cf. Kahl (2007: 7, n. 17).

[2] See the two lists of works given in Ibn Abī Uṣaybiʿah, *ʿUyūn al-anbāʾ fī ṭabaqāt al-aṭibbāʾ* (*Sources of information on the classes of physicians*), 10.64.20, ed. Savage-Smith et al. (2020, online version) = ed. Müller (1882) I.276 and Yāqūt, *Muʿjam al-udabāʾ* (*Dictionary of learned men*), ed. Rifāʿī (1936) XIX.278–9; cf. Kahl (2007: 13); Iskandar (1977); Iskandar (1981); Kahl (2010); Ibn al-Tilmīdh, *Maqālah fī al-faṣd* (*Treatise on phlebotomy*), ed. Ḥammāmī (1997).

[3] Ankara, Library of the Arts Faculty, MS Saib 2057, ff. 1–9 (cf. Örs, Tuzcu, and Hekimoğlu (2006–8)). Fuat Sezgin (1970: 336), who examined this fragmentary, horribly misbound, and often damaged manuscript in the 1970s, was not able to identify the author of these *Ikhtiyārāt min kitāb Miskawayh fī al-ashribah* (*Excerpts from Miskawayh's Book on Beverages*). In fact, on f. 9r there is a colophon,

Aqrābādhīn (*Dispensatory*), which consists of twenty chapters, and a concise treatise on phlebotomy.

Ibn al-Tilmīdh's main work on simple drugs is little known and has not yet been edited. The *Kitāb quwā l-adwiyah* (*Book on the Faculties of Simple Drugs*) or *al-Maqālah al-Amīniyyah fī al-adwiyah al-bīmāristāniyyah* (*Amīn [al-Dawlah's] Treatise on the Drugs of the Hospital*) is preserved in two manuscripts, both kept in London (British Library Or. 8294 and Wellcome Library, WMS Or. 9). Because of their divergent titles, most modern authors erroneously assumed that the manuscripts represent two different books. The text consists of 287 alphabetically arranged entries on medicinal plants, minerals, and a few animal products. The drugs mentioned are all well known, many from antiquity on. While some Arabic authors dealing with this topic tried to collect information on as many drugs as possible,[4] Ibn al-Tilmīdh confined himself to those practically used in Baghdad in his time. This fact allows some conclusions, especially on drugs imported from abroad – for example, from India. Each entry of the book is divided into five sections, dedicated to synonyms, descriptions, 'faculties', benefits of the simple drug, and its use in compound remedies at the ʿAḍudī hospital.[5]

The most interesting of these sections is the first, since Ibn al-Tilmīdh mentioned there not only the usual Arabic names of plants and minerals and their synonyms. Instead, he regularly listed the drugs' Syriac (written

according to which the sign *lī* for comments found throughout the text refers to the 'author of the *Ikhtiyārāt* (*Excerpts*), namely Amīn al-Dawlah known as Ibn al-Tilmīdh al-Baghdādī'. Since the preceding lines are dedicated to varieties of *nabīdh*, the colophon certainly belongs to the excerpts from the book on beverages. A few pages earlier, there is a misbound colophon indicating the end of Ibn al-Tilmīdh's excerpts from al-Rāzī's *Ḥāwī* (*Comprehensive Book*). This abridgment was also listed by Ibn Abī Uṣaybiʿah, *ʿUyūn al-anbāʾ fī ṭabaqāt al-aṭibbāʾ* (*Sources of Information on the Classes of Physicians*), 10.64.20 (ed. Savage-Smith et al. (2020, online version), no. 5 = ed. Müller (1882) I.276: *Ikhtiyār kitāb Miskawayh fī al-ashribah* (*Selections from Miskawayh's Book of Beverages*)); and Yāqūt (ed. Rifāʿī (1936) XIX.278: *Mukhtaṣar kitāb al-ashribah li-Miskawayh* (*Abridgment of Miskawayh's Book of Beverages*)).

[4] Ibn al-Bayṭār, *al-Jāmiʿ li-mufradāt al-adwiyah wa-l-aghdhiyah* (*Collector of Simple Drugs and Foodstuffs*), written one century later, has more than 2,300 entries. He incorporated, for example, all drugs mentioned by Dioscorides into his own work. Needless to say, all too many of these were unknown to the Arabs of his time. Copying these pieces of information certainly had no value for the practitioners. By contrast, Ibn Jazlah's *Minhāj al-bayān* (*The Clear Method*) and Ibn Sīnā's *Qānūn fī al-ṭibb* (*Canon of Medicine*), which were important sources of Ibn al-Tilmīdh's simple drugs, also focus on the drugs' practical use and availability.

[5] The most renowned hospital (*bīmāristān*) of Baghdad was founded in 372/982 by the Buwayhid ruler ʿAḍud al-Dawla (Dunlop (1960: I.1224–5)). It flourished until the Mongol conquest in 1258. Ibn al-Tilmīdh's works are closely related to this hospital. His dispensatory replaced that by Sābūr ibn Sahl formerly used there and his book on simple drugs is, in some respects, a supplement to the former. This relation to the ʿAḍudī also explains the relatively small number of manuscripts circulating outside of it.

in Syriac characters in one manuscript), Persian, and Greek names. Because of his Christian education and his long sojourn in Iran, he certainly mastered Syriac and Persian. One of his biographers even mentions his knowledge of Greek, which seems unlikely for Baghdad in the twelfth century. He rather may have found these synonyms in Syriac lexica or the Arabic versions of Greek medical books, especially the translations of Dioscorides' *De materia medica.*[6] These synonyms have indeed practical value, since Ibn al-Tilmīdh's fellow Christian physicians were still able to check Syriac books on pharmacognosy. The original Greek names also appear in the oriental translations and the Persian terms were, apparently, important for merchants active in Iran and India trade.

This chapter aims to contribute to the study of the exchange of pharmacological knowledge between various medieval traditions with a focus on the names of plants and minerals. On another level, it makes several observations on how earlier knowledge on drugs was received and adopted in the multilingual milieu of twelfth-century Baghdad.

1.1 Manuscripts of the *Kitāb quwā l-adwiyah*

Ibn al-Tilmīdh's book on simple drugs is, to our knowledge, preserved in two copies only. Since the manuscripts bear different titles, several authors assumed that they represent different works by Ibn al-Tilmīdh, which is not the case.[7] Manuscript A is entitled *Kitāb quwā l-adwiyah al-mufradah allatī yakthuru istiʿmāluhā fī tarkībāt al-bīmāristān* (*Book on the Faculties of Simple Drugs That Are Often Used in Compound Remedies of the Hospital*, f. 1r). The problematic colophon of MS B reads *al-Maqālah al-Amīniyyah fī al-adwiyah al-māristāniyyah*, which is also confirmed by Ibn al-Tilmīdh's biographers.[8] It is, despite this, not certain that the latter was indeed the original title, since Arabic authors do not normally mention themselves in

6 On annotations related to *materia medica* in Greek and Arabic manuscripts of Dioscorides, see Mavroudi (Chapter 4) in this volume.

7 Ullmann (1970: 306); Kahl (2007: 13); but Käs (2010: I.119–23). The author of this chapter was able to prove that both manuscripts represent the same text in his unpublished master's thesis 'Untersuchungen zum *Kitāb Quwā l-adwiya* des Ibn at-Tilmīḏ', written in 2001 under the auspices of the late Munich professor Rainer Degen (1941–2010).

8 Ibn Abī Uṣaybiʿah, *ʿUyūn al-anbāʾ fī ṭabaqāt al-aṭibbāʾ* (*Sources of Information on the Classes of Physicians*), 10.64.20, ed. Savage-Smith et al. (2020, online version), no. 3 = ed. Müller (1882) I.276; Yāqūt, *Muʿjam al-udabāʾ* (*Dictionary of Learned Men*), ed. Rifāʿī (1936) XIX.278–9. Both list the title *al-Maqālah al-Amīniyyah fī al-adwiyah al-bīmāristāniyyah.* The translation by Savage-Smith et al. – 'A treatise for Amīn on drugs for hospitals' – is incorrect since it is a 'treatise *by* Amīn on drugs *used in (sc. the ʿAḍudī) hospital*'.

their headings. For practical reasons, I shall use in what follows the shortened title *Quwā*.

Manuscript (MS) A: London, British Library, Or. 8294[9] (226 folia, 13 lines, text: 16.5 × 14.5 cm, elegant, almost fully vocalised *naskhī*).[10] The manuscript contains the full text of the *Quwā* only. According to the colophon on f. 224r it was completed in Baghdad in *Shawwāl* 654/1256 by a certain Christian doctor, named Yaʿīsh ibn Jadāʾ al-Naṣrānī *al-mutaṭabbib* al-Irbīlī. On the margin of the colophon there is a note, according to which the text was compared with the autograph of the author (*nuskhat muʾallifihī* [the second word is barely legible]) in *Rajab* 655/1257. It is likely that this Yaʿīsh was also the scribe of a famous illuminated manuscript of al-Ghāfiqī's *Kitāb al-adwiyah al-mufradah* (*Book on Simple Drugs*) copied a few months earlier.[11]

Manuscript (MS) B: London, The Library at Wellcome Collection, Or. 9, ff. 149v–234r. (234 folia, 17 lines, size: 23 × 17 cm, text: 19 × 11 cm, *naskhī*). This collective volume also contains Abū Bakr al-Rāzī's *al-Aqrābādhīn al-ṣaghīr* (*Small Dispensatory*; ff. 4r–26r), the treatise *Man lam yaḥḍurhū al-ṭabīb* (*Who Has No Physician to Attend Him*) by the same (ff. 27v–68v), Ibn al-Tilmīdh's *Maqālah fī al-faṣd* (*Treatise on Phlebotomy*; ff. 70r–78r), and his *Aqrābādhīn* (*Dispensatory*, ff. 79r–148r).[12] Because of their bad state, several folia were replaced in 1228/1871 by modern copies by a certain physician of Damascus, named Tūmā Buṭrūs Jibāra. On f. 234r he copied the old colophon, according to which the volume was written in 597/1200 by Ibrāhīm ibn Naṣr ibn Ibrāhīm ibn Muḥammad ibn al-Ḥasan ibn Ibrāhīm ibn Munīr al-Kindī.[13] In our case, the folia 169, 170, 211, 220, and 229–34 are modern substitutes. Tūmā was in fact not able to reconstruct the whole of the text of the *Quwā*. After f. 170 the end of the letter

[9] www.qdl.qa/en/archive/81055/vdc_100048368830.0x000001 (accessed 1 January 2019).

[10] Hamarneh (1975: 139, no. 158); Edwards (1922: 139, no. 19).

[11] Cf. Käs (2016: 261, n. 8).

[12] Iskandar (1967: 79, 224–5, 130, 78); cf. Kahl (2007: 20). The untitled last folia of this section do not obviously belong to the *Aqrābādhīn*. On f. 148r the main copyist wrote *tammat Ikhtiyārātu . . . Amīni l-Dawlati . . . bni l-Tilmīdhi* and on f. 146r the copyist of the modern pages stated *tamma mā khtārahū . . . Amīnu l-Dawlati . . . l-maʿrūfu bi-bni l-Tilmīdhi min Kitābi J.[ālīnūsa]*. Ibn al-Tilmīdh wrote several treatises entitled *Ikhtiyār* or *Mukhtār* (Ibn Abī Uṣaybiʿah, *ʿUyūn al-anbāʾ fī ṭabaqāt al-aṭibbāʾ* (*Sources of Information on the Classes of Physicians*), 10.64.20, ed. Savage-Smith et al. (2020, online version) = ed. Müller (1882) I.276). Since most of these pages are concerned with substitute drugs, they might represent fragments of the *Mukhtār min Kitāb abdāl al-adwiyah li-Jālīnūs* (*Selections from the Book on Substitute Drugs by Galen*), also listed by Ibn Abī Uṣaybiʿah. In a similar manner, another manuscript of the *Aqrābādhīn* (MS London, British Library, Or. 8293, ff. 164r–165v) contains a fragment entitled *Mukhtār min abdāl Jālīnūs* (*Selections from Galen's Substitute Drugs*). Other fragmentary statements on the use of drugs in MS B (cf. f. 143r *qāla Shaykhunā . . . l-maʿrūfu bi-bni l-Tilmīdhi*) cannot, however, originate from that treatise.

[13] Iskandar (1967: 78).

bā' and the beginning of the letter *tā'* and after f. 288 most of the letters *lām*, *mīm*, and *nūn* are missing. The text bears no title and the original table of contents is lost. The replaced colophon of f. 234r reads *tammat al-Maqālah al-Amīniyyah fī al-adwiyah al-māristāniyyah.*

1.2 Contents

Each of the 287 entries of the *Quwā* is divided into five sections. The first three are arranged in parallel columns in both manuscripts. The first section, which includes the lemma written in larger characters, is dedicated to the Arabic and foreign-language names of the drug. The middle column deals with the description of the drug and its varieties. Occasionally, the choice quality is indicated. The left column is dedicated to the 'quality' (hot, cold, moist, dry) and the 'degree' (I–IV) of the drug according to the humoral theory. The second and third sections were apparently influenced by Ibn Sīnā's (d. 1037) *Qānūn fī al-ṭibb* (*Canon of Medicine*),[14] where similar and also schematised accounts of the description (*al-māhiyyah*), the humorist quality and degree (*al-ṭab'*), and the choice quality (*al-ikhtiyār*) were given at the beginning of each entry. The fourth section is dedicated to the therapeutic uses of the simple drug. The length of these accounts varies from a few lines up to one or two pages. Unlike Ibn Sīnā, who followed a strict scheme of possible uses,[15] Ibn al-Tilmīdh arranged this material rather arbitrarily.

The fifth section has a unique character, since no other Arabic book on pharmacognosy contains similar detailed lists of the pharmaceutical use of simple drugs. At the end of each entry, Ibn al-Tilmīdh lists the 'compound remedies of the hospital' (*al-murakkabāt al-bīmāristāniyyah*), in which the respective drug is used as an ingredient. This *bīmāristān* is, of course, the famous 'Aḍudī hospital of Baghdad, where Ibn al-Tilmīdh served for many years as head physician (*sā'ūr*).[16] One can certainly interpret these mentions of *al-murakkabāt al-bīmāristāniyyah* as cross-references to a written formulary. It is, however, not clear which book he meant here. Until it was

[14] Ibn Sīnā, *Qānūn fī al-ṭibb* (*Canon of Medicine*), ed. (1877) I.243–470.

[15] Ibn Sīnā, *Qānūn fī al-ṭibb* (*Canon of Medicine*), ed. (1877) I.239–42.

[16] See Kahl (2007: 8–9). Our author meant here certainly not hospitals in general. Of the few mentions of the word *bīmāristān* in his *Aqrābādhin* (*Dispensatory*, ed. Kahl (2007) 30, no. 66) only two (ed. Kahl (2007) 54, 59, nos. 21, 34) are concerned with hospitals in general. In most cases, the adjective *bīmāristānī* is part of the name of the remedy (ed. Kahl (2007) 58, 62, 67, 73, 89, 118, 132, 143, nos. 33, 230, 49, 67, 84, 137, 277, 310). Like in his *Quwā*, he apparently meant that this compound drug is used – or was invented – in the hospital of Baghdad. Two mentions are of particular interest in our context, since Ibn al-Tilmīdh alludes there to a 'copy of the hospital' (*nuskhat al-bīmāristān*).

replaced by Ibn al-Tilmīdh's own *Aqrābādhīn*, a special recension of Sābūr ibn Sahl's (d. 255/869) dispensatory was used in the ʿAḍudī hospital.[17] As the two specimens below will show, not all of the remedies listed in the *Quwā* are actually found there, whereas they all appear in Ibn al-Tilmīdh's own book. Since we do not know which of his two treatises was written first, there are two possible solutions for this problem. If the *Aqrābādhīn* predate the *Quwā*, *al-murakkabāt al-bīmāristāniyyah* may simply be an alternative title of his own dispensatory. In the other – more probable – case, Amīn al-Dawlah may have referred to the contemporary 'official formulary' of the hospital – certainly an enlarged version of Sābūr's book – which could be regarded as *travaux préparatoires* of the *Aqrābādhīn*. One can only speculate as to why Ibn al-Tilmīdh included these unusual fifth sections in his *Quwā*. One practical use may have been that the physicians of the ʿAḍudī hospital knew which compound drugs cannot be mixed when the ingredient is not at hand.

As a first specimen, I will edit here the fourth entry of the letter *alif* dedicated to the 'sky-blue iris' (A f. 16r–v/B f. 158r–v). It should be noted that the passage on the therapeutic use of its root and the oil obtained from it is rather short in comparison with many other entries. Ibn al-Tilmīdh did not explicitly mention his sources here. It is, however, likely that he copied most of the text verbatim from Ibn Sīnā's *Qānūn fī al-ṭibb* (ed. 1877, I.255–6, s.v. *īrisā*), since almost all statements are found there too. Only a few identical pieces of information were given by Ibn Jazlah (493/1100) in his *Minhāj al-bayān* (*The Clear Method*, f. 35r–v, s.v. *īrisā*; cf. f. 28r, s.v. *aṣl al-sawsan al-asmānjūnī*). Some of Ibn Sīnā's statements and descriptions can be traced back to Iṣṭifān's translation of Dioscorides' *De materia medica*, 1.1.

أصل السوسن الأسمانجوني، ويسمّى[18] باليونانية إيرس وبالسريانية[19] ܐܝܪܣܐ[20] وبالفارسية[21] بن سوسن[22] أسمانجوني.[23]
هو أصل عقد له ورق دقاق[24] وزهر مختلف الألوان من بياض وصفرة وأسمانجونية وفرفرية.
حارّ يابس في آخر الثانية.
ينضج ويفتّح ويجلو[25] وينقّي ويسكّن وجع الكبد والطحال الباردين، ولذلك ينفع من الاستسقاء ومن[26] السموم، ودهنه يزيل الأبردة والنافض.
ويستعمل من المركّبات المارستانية في[27] ٢: في أقراص الكبر، وأقراص السوسن، وهما[28] أقراص لصلابة الطحال.

[17] Kahl (2009: 1–7). On Sābūr ibn Sahl, see also Chipman (Chapter 10) in this volume.
[18] om. A ويسمّى باليونانية [19] om. A وبالسريانية [20] B إيرسا A ܐܝܪܣܐ [21] A هز B وبالفارسية
[22] A شوس B سوسن [23] B أسمانجون A سمانجوني corr. أسمانجوني [24] om. B دقاق
[25] A ويجلوا B ويجلو [26] B وينفع من A ومن [27] om B. في ٢
[28] B وأقراص لصلابة A وفي قرص ينفع من صلابة corr. وهما أقراص لصلابة

Root of the sky-coloured iris (*aṣl al-sawsan al-asmānjūnī*). It is called in Greek *īris*,[29] which means 'rainbow', in Syriac *īrisā*,[30] and in Persian *bun-i sūsan-i asmānjūnī*.[31]

It is a knotty root with fine leaves and flowers with diverse colours, namely white, yellow, sky-coloured, and purple.

It is hot and dry at the end of the second [degree].

It brings to ripeness, opens, cleans, purifies, and alleviates the pain of the liver and the spleen, if they are affected by coldness. For this reason, it is beneficial for dropsy and poisoning. Its oil helps patients suffering from coldness and shivering.[32] In the dispensatory of the hospital it is used in 2 [recipes]: The caper pastilles[33] and the iris pastilles[34] – both pastilles for sclerosis of the spleen.

The second specimen is of particular interest since Ibn al-Tilmīdh gives here his own Syriac etymology of an Arabic name for purslane (A f. 34r–v/B f. 167v). His statements on the description (*ma'rūf*), the degrees, and the therapeutic use have, again, striking parallels in Ibn Sīnā's *Qānūn fī al-ṭibb* (ed. 1877, I.275, s.v. *baqlat al-ḥamqā'*). The unusual lemma *bizr* (!) *al-baqlah al-ḥamqā'* was perhaps inspired by Ibn Jazlah who had chosen the same catchword in his *Minhāj al-bayān* (f. 31v).

بزر[35] **البقلة الحمقاء**، ويسمّى الفرفح وهو معرّب من[36] السرياني ويسمّى الرجلة، ܦܪܦܚܝܢܐ[37]، وبالفارسية[38] دندان ساي[39] وتخم فرفهن. **معروف**.

[29] *Īris* is the usual Arabic transcription of Greek 'ἶρις'. It is already to be found in Iṣṭifān's translation of Dioscorides' *De materia medica* (1.1, ed. Wellmann (1907) I.5, ed. Dubler and Terés (1952) II.11), where it was also explained as 'rainbow' (*qaws Quzaḥ*; cf. Dietrich (1988) I.1). The same gloss was also given by Ibn Sīnā (*Qānūn fī al-ṭibb* (*Canon of Medicine*), ed. (1877) I.255.22) and Ibn Jazlah (*Minhāj al-bayān* (*The Clear Method*), MS London, British Library, Add. 5934, f. 35r.ult.).

[30] Syriac ܐܝܪܝܣܐ is a common transcription of the Greek name. See Löw (1881: no. 21); Bar Bahlūl, ed. Duval (1890) I.147.8. *Īrisā* was also the lemma of the relevant entries of Ibn Sīnā's *Qānūn fī al-ṭibb* (*Canon of Medicine*, ed. (1877) I.256) and Ibn Jazlah's *Minhāj al-bayān* (*The Clear Method*, f. 35r).

[31] Persian *bun-i sūsan-i asmāngūnī* means 'root of the sky-coloured lily'. See Steingass (1930: 200b): *bun* – 'root'; Steingass (1930: 709a): *sūsan-i asmāngūnī* – 'A variegated kind of lily, yellow, white, and blue'. The word *asmāngūnī*, composed of *asmān* 'sky' and *gūn* 'colour', was written in both manuscripts with *jīm* instead of *gāf*, perhaps since *asmānjūnī* is a common Arabicised loanword. The Persian form *sūsan* is in turn a Semitic loanword attested as early as in Pahlavi (Middle Persian); see MacKenzie (1971: 75): *sōsan* – 'lily'; Löw (1881: no. 323).

[32] Ibn Sīnā, *Qānūn fī al-ṭibb* (*Canon of Medicine*), ed. (1877), I.256.12; cf. Dioscorides, *De materia medica*, 1.1.2, ed. Wellmann (1907) I.7.4; transl. Beck (2011) 6: '(sc. it helps) hypothermics or shiverers'; ed. Dubler and Terés (1952) II.12.14: *wa-yanfa'u mina l-baradi wa-l-nāfiḍi*.

[33] Ibn al-Tilmīdh, *Aqrābādhīn* (*Dispensatory*), ed. Kahl (2007) 51, 181, no. 9: *qurṣ al-kabar li-ṣalābat al-ṭiḥāl*; Sābūr ibn Sahl, *Aqrābādhīn* (*Dispensatory*), ed. Kahl (2009) 26, 122, no. 7.

[34] Ibn al-Tilmīdh, *Aqrābādhīn* (*Dispensatory*), ed. Kahl (2007) 53, 184, no. 19: *qurṣ al-sawsan li-ṣalābat al-ṭiḥāl*; Sābūr ibn Sahl, *Aqrābādhīn* (*Dispensatory*), ed. Kahl (2009) 31, 128, no. 24.

[35] B بقلة A بزر البقلة الحمقاء [36] B الفرفح A من السرياني [37] om. B ܦܪܦܚܝܢܐ

[38] B ويسمّى A وبالفارسية [39] A دنداب ساى وىحم فرفهن B دندان ساي وتخم فرفهن

بارد في الثالثة، رطب في الثانية.

عصارتها نافعة من الحمّيات الحادّةوالتهاب الكبد والأحشاء بأسرها، وتمنع[40] القيء المرّي، وفيها قبض تمنع به النزف والسيلانات، وتنفع[41] من السحج والإسهال المراري شربًا وحقنًا، وتنفع من قروح المثانة والكلى وأوجاعهما، وتنفع من نفث الدم، وتقطع شهوة الجماع إلّا فيمن يغلب على مزاج حشاه الحرّ، وتنفع[42] من نزف الرحم، وعصارتها تخرج حبّ القرع وذلك بتطفئتها الحرارة العفنية التي عنها يتكوّن[43]، وتشفي الضرس بلزوجتها، وتذهب[44] الثآليل إذا حكّت بها بخاصّية فيها.

ويستعمل[45] من المركّبات المارستانية[46] في ١١: قرص الأميرباريس الصغير، وقرص[47] الكافور، وقرص الغافت، وقرص الخشخاش، وقرص الكهرباء، ومسهل[48] ماء الجبن، ومطبوخ الزوفا، وبنادق البزور[49] لقروح المثانة، والمطبوخ المارستاني[50]، وسفوف لأصحاب السعال، وبرود[51] الورد، وفي سفوف الطين.

Purslane seed (*bizr al-baqlah al-ḥamqāʾ*). It is also called *al-farfaḥ*,[52] which is a loanword from Syriac and it is also called *al-rijla*.[53] [In Syriac] *parpaḥinē*[54] and in Persian *dandān-sāy* and *tukhm-i farfahan*.[55]

It is well-known.

Cold in the third degree; moist in the second degree.

Its juice is beneficial for acute fevers and inflammations of the liver and the entire intestines. It prevents bilious vomiting. Its astringency prevents haemorrhages and flows. Drunk or applied as a clyster, it is beneficial for abrasion of the intestines and bilious diarrhoea. It is beneficial for ulcers and pain of the bladder and the kidneys as well as for spitting of blood. It stops the desire for sexual intercourse, unless the temperament of the [patient's] intestines is dominated by heat. It is beneficial for discharges from the uterus. Its juice expels tapeworms by extinguishing the putrid heat that generates them. With its viscosity, it heals molar teeth. With a sympathetic virtue, it removes warts, when rubbed on them.

40 A ويمنع B وتمنع   41 A وينفع B وتنفع   42 A وينفع B وتنفع
43 A تتكوّن ويشفي B يتكوّن وتشفي   44 A ويذهب B وتذهب   45 B وتستعمل A ويستعمل
46 om. A المارستانية   47 A قرص B وقرص   48 AB مدل corr. مسهل
49 A البزور المثانية B لقروح المثانة corr. البزور لقروح المثانة   50 A البيمارستاني B المارستاني
51 om. B وبرود الورد وفي سفوف الطين

52 There are several spelling varieties of this loanword, the most common of which is *farfakh*; see Dietrich (1988: 271, n. 3). In both manuscripts, it is consequently written *farfaḥ* with *ḥāʾ* – MS A even adds a *muhmal*. This form may indeed go back to the author, since the alleged Syriac etymon is also written with ܚ. It is not clear if *farfaḥ* is indeed a Syriac loanword, since both forms may have been borrowed from Persian *parpahan* independently (cf. Bos et al. (2020: no. 751)).

53 *Al-baqlah al-ḥamqāʾ* (lit. 'the stupid vegetable') and *rijlah* are common Arabic names of purslane; cf. Dietrich (1988: 106); Bos et al. (2020: nos. 125, 751).

54 For Syriac ܦܪܦܚܝܢܐ, see Brockelmann (1928: 604a). MS A indicates here the plural form also often attested (Löw (1881: 320, no. 264)). MS B does not give a correct transcription of the Syriac word; instead it repeats the Arabic form, *al-farfaḥ*.

55 Steingass (1930: 538a): *dandān-sā* – 'purslain'; 289a: *tukhm* – 'seed'; 921a: *farfahan* – 'purslain'; 240a: *parpahan* – 'purslain'.

In the dispensatory of the hospital, it is used in eleven[56] [recipes]: The small barberry pastille,[57] the pastille with camphor,[58] the agrimony pastille,[59] the poppy pastille,[60] the amber pastille,[61] the purgative with cheese-water,[62] the hyssop decoction,[63] the seed 'hazelnuts' for vesical ulcers,[64] the hospital decoction,[65] the powder for those who suffer from cough,[66] the rose coolant,[67] the bole powder.[68]

1.3 Languages Employed by Ibn al-Tilmīdh

Table 1.1 lists all entries of the letter *alif* and the Arabic, Greek, Persian, and Syriac terms mentioned there. The list is mainly based on MS A, since MS B omitted many of the foreign-language terms.[69]

It is a characteristic phenomenon that most of the lemmas are not genuine Arabic terms (except for nos 16, 18, 21). Ibn al-Tilmīdh certainly did not invent this system. The choice of his lemmas was clearly influenced by his main sources, especially Ibn Sīnā's *Qānūn fī al-ṭibb* and Ibn Jazlah's *Minhāj al-bayān* – the rare spelling variety *abrank* of no. 28 may have been copied from al-Rāzī's (d. *c.*925) *al-Ḥāwī* (*Comprehensive Book*).[70] One reason for the preponderance of foreign names was the fact that many of

[56] Both manuscripts give the numeral 11, while MS A lists 12 and MS B 10 remedies. All of them are also to be found in Ibn al-Tilmīdh's dispensatory.

[57] Ibn al-Tilmīdh, *Aqrābādhīn* (*Dispensatory*), ed. Kahl (2007) 49, 179, no. 3; Sābūr ibn Sahl, *Aqrābādhīn* (*Dispensatory*), ed. Kahl (2009) 24, 120, no. 3.

[58] Ibn al-Tilmīdh, *Aqrābādhīn* (*Dispensatory*), ed. Kahl (2007) 50, 180, no. 7; Sābūr ibn Sahl, *Aqrābādhīn* (*Dispensatory*), ed. Kahl (2009) 25, 121, no. 5.

[59] Ibn al-Tilmīdh, *Aqrābādhīn* (*Dispensatory*), ed. Kahl (2007) 50, 181, no. 8; Sābūr ibn Sahl, *Aqrābādhīn* (*Dispensatory*), ed. Kahl (2009) 25, 122, no. 6.

[60] Ibn al-Tilmīdh, *Aqrābādhīn* (*Dispensatory*), ed. Kahl (2007) 51, 181, no. 10; Sābūr ibn Sahl, *Aqrābādhīn* (*Dispensatory*), ed. Kahl (2009) 26, 122, no. 8.

[61] Ibn al-Tilmīdh, *Aqrābādhīn* (*Dispensatory*), ed. Kahl (2007) 52, 183, no. 15; Sābūr ibn Sahl, *Aqrābādhīn* (*Dispensatory*), ed. Kahl (2009) 30, 127, no. 21.

[62] Ibn al-Tilmīdh, *Aqrābādhīn* (*Dispensatory*), ed. Kahl (2007) 73, 204, no. 86.

[63] Ibn al-Tilmīdh, *Aqrābādhīn* (*Dispensatory*), ed. Kahl (2007) 108, 249, no. 224; Sābūr ibn Sahl, *Aqrābādhīn* (*Dispensatory*), ed. Kahl (2009) 33, 131, no. 35.

[64] Ibn al-Tilmīdh, *Aqrābādhīn* (*Dispensatory*), ed. Kahl (2007) 64, 194, no. 53: *banādiq li-ḥarqat al-bawl wa-qurūḥ al-mathāna*; Sābūr ibn Sahl, *Aqrābādhīn* (*Dispensatory*), ed. Kahl (2009) 62, 163, no. 129: *safūf li-ḥarqat al-bawl wa-yusammā banādiq al-buzūr*.

[65] Ibn al-Tilmīdh, *Aqrābādhīn* (*Dispensatory*), ed. Kahl (2007) 118, 252, no. 230; Sābūr ibn Sahl, *Aqrābādhīn* (*Dispensatory*), ed. Kahl (2009) 76, 181, no. 165.

[66] Ibn al-Tilmīdh, *Aqrābādhīn* (*Dispensatory*), ed. Kahl (2007) 71, 203, no. 79.

[67] Ibn al-Tilmīdh, *Aqrābādhīn* (*Dispensatory*), ed. Kahl (2007) 163, 296, no. 385; Sābūr ibn Sahl, *Aqrābādhīn* (*Dispensatory*), ed. Kahl (2009) 91, 198, no. 199.

[68] Ibn al-Tilmīdh, *Aqrābādhīn* (*Dispensatory*), ed. Kahl (2007) 71, 202, no. 76.

[69] On the use of medical terms in various languages in the same text, see also Walker-Meikle (Chapter 3), Mavroudi (Chapter 4), and Martelli (Chapter 11) in the present volume.

[70] Al-Rāzī, *al-Ḥāwī* (*Comprehensive Book*), ed. (1962) XX.93.

Table 1.1 *Specimens of foreign-language terms*

No.	Lemma	Arabic synonyms	Greek	Persian	Syriac	English
1	*asārūn*		*asārūn* (ἄσαρον)		ܐܣܪܘܢ	asarabacca
2	*afyūn*		*afyūn* (ὄπιον)		ܐܦܝܘܢ/ܫܠܝܚܐ ܕܚܫܚܫܐ	opium
3	*aqāqiyā*	*ʿuṣārat al-qaraẓ*	*aqāqiyā* (ἀκακία)		ܐܩܐܩܝܐ/ܐܪܚܝ ܕܘܪܛܐ	gum Senegal
4	*aṣl al-sawsan al-asmānjūnī*		*īris ay qaws quzaḥ* (ἶρις, i.e. ‘rainbow’)	*bun-i sūsan-i asmān-jūnī*	ܐܝܪܣܐ	sky-coloured iris
5	*anīsūn*	*bizr al-raziyānaj al-rūmī*	*anīsūn* (ἄνησσον)	*raziyānaj rūmī*	ܐܢܝܣܘܢ	anise
6	*afsintīn*	*shīḥ*	*afsintīn* (ἀψίνθιον)		ܐܦܣܢܬܝܢ	absinth wormwood
7	*ushshaq*	*lizāq al-dhahab*		*ushshaq*	ܐܘܫܩ	gum ammoniac
8	*isfīdhāj al-raṣāṣ*	*ānuk mujaffaf*		*isfīdhāj*	ܐܣܦܝܕܓ	ceruse
9	*aghārīqūn*		*aghārīqūn* (ἀγαρικόν)		ܐܓܪܝܩܘܢ	agaric
10	*ihlīlaj*			*ihlīlaj*	ܗܠܝܠܓܐ	myrobalan
11	*amlaj wa-shīr-amlaj*			*amlaj, shīr-amlaj*	ܐܡܠܓ	emblic jam
12	*ās*	*rand*		*mūrd*	ܐܣܐ	myrtle
13	*usṭūkhūdhūs*		*usṭūkhūdhūs* (στοιχάδος), *stukhās* (στοιχάς)		ܣܛܘܟܘܕܘܣ	French lavender

14	*afithīmūn*		*afithīmūn* (ἐπίθυμον)		ܐܦܬܝܡܘܢ	epithyme
15	*usqūlūfandriyūn*		*usqūlūfandriyūn* (σκολοπένδριον)		ܐܣܩܘܠܘܦܢܕܪܝܘܢ	rusty-back fern
16	*abhul*	*thamarat al-ʿarʿar*			ܒܪܘܬܐ	savin juniper
17	*amīrbārīs*			*zirishk*		barberry
18	*idhkhir*	*fuqqāḥ al-idhkhir*	*skhīnūn* (σχοῖνος)		ܓܠܐ ܕܓܡܠܐ	camel grass
19	*utrujj*			*turunj*	ܐܬܪܘܓܐ/ܫܘܪܐ ܡܥܐ	lemon
20	*ijjāṣ*			*ālū, shāhalūj*	ܚܫܐ	plum
21	*iklīl al-malik*				ܟܠܝܠ ܡܠܟܐ	melilot
22	*aruzz*					rice
23	*iqlīmiyā fiḍḍī wa-iqlīmiyā dhahabī*		*qadmiyā* (καδμεία)	*shakht* (fort. *shūkhtah*)		silver calamine and gold calamine
24	*ithmid*	*kuḥl Sulaymān*			ܟܘܚܠܐ ܕܫܝܢܐ	antimony
25	*ushnah*			*duwālak*	ܥܒܬܐ	tree moss
26	*anzarūt*			*anzarūt*	ܐܢܙܪܘܬ	sarcocolla
27	*anjurah*	*qurrayṣ*		*anjurah*	ܦܪܝ ܚܒܬܐ	Roman nettle
28	*abrank Kābulī*			*abrank*		white-flowered embelia

the officinal plants employed by the ancient Greek physicians and featuring in the dispensatory of the ʿAḍudī hospital were unknown on the Arabian Peninsula in pre-Islamic times. The translators of books on *materia medica* therefore often only transcribed the Greek phytonyms (nos 1–3, 5, 6, 9, 13–15, 23).[71] Most of the Greek terms mentioned here were well known to the Arab pharmacologists[72] and the occasional explanations of their literal meanings (no. 4) are also often attested.[73] There are two interesting exceptions in the letter *alif*. French lavender (no. 13) was usually referred to as *usṭūkhūdhūs*, allegedly a transcription of the Greek genitive case 'στοιχάδος'.[74] Ibn al-Tilmīdh lists the synonym *stukhās* (MS A; *stkhʾws* MS B) – obviously a transcription of the nominative case 'στοιχάς' – which is not otherwise attested in the usual Arabic literature.[75] Instead, the almost identical (ܛ vs. ܬ) Syriac transcription ܣܛܘܟܐܣ can be found in Bar Bahlūl's lexicon.[76] A similar case is the spelling variety *skhīnūn* (no. 18) for Greek 'σχοῖνος', which corresponds to the form ܣܟܝܢܘܢ listed by the glossographer Bar ʿAlī.[77] These and several other examples show that Ibn al-Tilmīdh must not necessarily have spoken Greek himself. It is rather likely that he took his information on Greek words from the Syriac lexica.

Another important source for Arabicised names of plants (nos 5, 7, 10, 11, 17, 19, 26–8) and minerals (no. 8) was Persian. The reason for this was again that most cultivated plants and exotic spices were unknown to the Bedouins and the pre-Islamic resident population of the Arabian Peninsula. The frequent use of Persian loanwords as lemmas in the pharmacognostic literature was certainly also influenced by the fact that important authors, such as Ibn Sīnā and al-Rāzī, were of Iranian descent.

[71] It should also be stressed that the predominance of Greek loanwords in the letter *alif* is more extreme than in other letters, since all words beginning with a vowel were transcribed with an *alif*.

[72] For example, Ibn Sīnā, *Qānūn fī al-ṭibb* (*Canon of Medicine*), ed. (1877), I.248 (*asārūn*); I.256 (*afyūn*); I.246 (*aqāqiyā*); I.243 (*anīsūn*); I.244 (*afsintīn*); I.464 (*ghārīqūn*); I.252 (*usṭūkhudhūs*); I.251 (*afitīmūn*); I.386 (*sqūlūfandriyūn*).

[73] An interesting example is the entry dedicated to the marshmallow (*khiṭmī*, A f. 76r/B f. 180r). Ibn al-Tilmīdh states that its Greek name (sc. 'ἀλθαία') – which he actually did not mention – means 'full of benefits' (*al-kathīr al-manāfiʿ*). That synonym was already listed by Ibn Sīnā (*Qānūn fī al-ṭibb* (*Canon of Medicine*), ed. (1877) I.453), who gave no explanation of it. Ibn al-Tilmīdh adds in this entry a quotation from Galen's *Tafsīr li-aymān Buqrāṭ wa-ʿahdihī* (*Commentary on the Hippocratic 'Oath'*), according to which the rod of Asclepius is a marshmallow stem because of its many benefits (*li-kathrat manāfiʿihī*; cf. 'ἀλθαίνω' ('to heal')). That text is only known from its Oriental tradition; cf. Fichtner (2017: no. 390).

[74] Dietrich (1988) 374.

[75] Only al-Bīrūnī mentions the similar form *stūkhas* in his book on simple drugs entitled *al-Ṣaydanah* (*The Pharmacy*), ed. Zaryāb (1991) 44, no. 40.

[76] Bar Bahlūl, ed. Duval (1890) II.1330.1.

[77] Gottheil (1908: II.169.3).

We know from his biographers that Ibn al-Tilmīdh spent several years in Persia and there is no doubt he acquired a certain knowledge of Persia's language. Besides the terms copied from his usual sources, Ibn al-Tilmīdh often mentions Persian synonyms, especially of well-known things (nos 12, 20).[78] Sometimes he adds to Arabicised loanwords the original Persian forms.[79] The most interesting features in this context are certainly Ibn al-Tilmīdh's etymologies of loanwords, many unattested in other sources.[80] Two of them were cited by Ibn al-Bayṭār (d. 646/1248), who explicitly mentioned 'Amīn al-Dawlah Ibn al-Tilmīdh' as his source.[81]

The Persian terms of the *Quwā* represent, with a few exceptions, standard modern Persian forms. Ibn al-Tilmīdh only 'Arabicised' the orthography by writing *kāf* instead of *gāf*, *bā'* instead of *peh*, and *jīm* instead of *chīm*. Terms loaned at an early date preserve the Pahlavi ending *-ag* Arabicised as *-aj* (nos 5, 8, 10, 11), *-ak* (nos 25, 28), or *-aq* (no. 7). Ibn al-Tilmīdh uses these traditional along with modern forms – for example, in the case of the terms *ālū* ('plum', no. 20) and *shāhalūj* ('king's plum'). Although the overwhelming number of synonyms represents literary Persian, some terms that could not be identified might also be dialectal words Ibn al-Tilmīdh heard during his stay

78 Other such examples are the Persian names of iron (*ḥadīd/āhan*; A f. 64v/B f. 174v), raisins (*zabīb/mawīz* A f. 96v/B f. 189r), wax (*sham'/mūm* A f. 134r/B f. 204v), honey (*'asal/angubīn*; A f. 151r/B f. 212v), milk (*laban/shīr* A f. 195r/om. B), apricots (*mishmish/zard-ālū* A f. 202r/om. B), and quicklime (*nūrah/āhak* A f. 217r/om. B).

79 Good examples are the names of polypody (*basfāyij/bas-bāy*, i.e. *bas-pāy*; A f. 41r/om. B), manna (*taranjubīn/ṭall-ankubīn*, i.e. *ṭall-angubīn*; A f. 50r/om. B), sebesten fruits (*safistān/sak-bistān*, i.e. *sag-pistān*; A f. 120v/B f. 199r), and musk (*misk/mushk*; A f. 198v/om. B).

80 Examples are the names of lemon balm (*bādharanjbūyah/al-utrujjī al-rā'iḥah* 'citron-scented'; A f. 38r/B f. 169v), tamarisk fruits (*kazmāzaj/'afṣat al-ṭarfā'* 'tamarisk gallnuts'; A f. 57v/B f. 171r), cucumbers (*khiyār-bādharanj/khiyār utrujjī* 'citron-shaped cucumber'; A f. 75v/B f. 180r), bishop's weed (*nānakhwāh/ṭālib al-khubz* 'beggar for bread'; A f. 213r/om. B), or water lilies (*nīlūfar/al-nīlī al-ajniḥah, al-nīlī al-aryāsh* 'having blue wings/feathers'; A f. 213v/om. B).

81 Ibn al-Bayṭār, *al-Jāmi' li-mufradāt al-adwiyah wa-l-aghdhiyah* (*Collector of Simple Drugs and Foodstuffs*), ed. (1874) IV.173, s.v. *nānakhwāh* (= A f. 213r/om. B); IV.185, s.v. *nīlūfar* (= A f. 213v/om. B). The *Jāmi'* contains two more explicit quotations: II.135, s.v. *rāziqī* (= A f. 152v/B f. 213v); IV.185, s.v. *nūshādir* (= A f. 215r/om. B). Depending on Ibn al-Bayṭār, the explanation of the term *nīlūfar* was incorporated by al-Nuwayrī (d. 733/1333) into his encyclopaedia *Nihāyat al-arab fī funūn al-adab* ((*The Ultimate Ambition in the Arts of Erudition*), ed. Sha'īrah et al. (1929–92) XI.219). Another early user of the *Quwā* was Ibn al-Tilmīdh's contemporary al-Sharīf al-Idrīsī (d. 559/1165), who explicitly mentioned him several times in his *al-Jāmi' li-ṣifāt ashtāt al-nabāt wa-ḍurūb anwā' al-mufradāt* (*Compendium of the Properties of Diverse Plants and Various Kinds of Simple Drugs*) facs.-ed. Sezgin et al. (1995) II.523, index, s.v. Ibn al-Tilmīdh). The unusual multilanguage lists of synonyms found in the *Ṣifāt* (Ullmann (1970: 278); Käs (2010: I.123–9)) may, at least to a certain extent, have been inspired by the *Quwā*. Another model was obviously the section of the 'tables' of al-Rāzī's *al-Ḥāwī* (*Comprehensive Book*), ed. (1962) XXII.

in Iran. On one occasion (A f. 62v/om. B, s.v. *tūdharī*), he stated that the inhabitants of Isfahan called the hedge mustard *ḥ'kḥy*, which could not be retrieved from the lexica.

The systematic notation of Syriac terms in Ibn al-Tilmīdh's *Quwā* is unique in the history of the Arabic pharmacology. Although a considerable number of Arabic phytonyms are ultimately Aramaic loanwords (e.g. nos 12, 20),[82] they were rather neglected by authors on the nomenclature of drugs. Writers from the East – such as al-Rāzī in the tables of volume XXII of his *al-Ḥāwī* or al-Bīrūnī in his *al-Ṣaydanah* (*The Pharmacy*) – often noted Syriac terms, but the classics of this genre – such as the lists of synonyms by Ibn Juljul, Ibn Janāḥ, al-Ishbīlī, Maimonides, or the anonymous *Dioscurides triumphans* – were written in the West, where Aramaic was absolutely unimportant. Ibn al-Tilmīdh regularly adds at the end of the first column one or more Syriac terms, written in Estrangelo characters in MS A. As in the case of the Arabic names of drugs, only a minority of these are genuine Syriac terms (see nos 2, 3, 12, 18–21, 24, 27).[83] The others are Persian loanwords (nos 7, 8, 10, 11, 26) or transcriptions of Greek terms (nos 1–6, 9, 13–15). Ibn al-Tilmīdh's terms certainly do not represent the spoken dialect of his Christian community in Baghdad. Instead, he drew on written sources in classical Syriac, either books on medicine or glossographical sources, such as the lexica by Bar ʿAlī or Bar Bahlūl, where parallels can regularly be found. For the possible use of such a text by Ḥunayn, see later in this chapter. Furthermore, some Greek words show clear signs of systematised transcriptions typical for the lexica.[84]

MS B almost completely omitted the Syriac terms. They appear only when the term was allegedly written in Arabic characters in Ibn al-Tilmīdh's autograph. This happened when he quoted from Arabic sources already containing the Syriac foreign word (see no. 4).[85] This of course raises the question of whether these terms are authentic. In principle, the Syriac words may also have been added by a later copyist. However, their use parallels that of the Persian terms, which were regularly copied by the

[82] Fraenkel (1886: 139). Besides loans of genuine words, Greek and Persian terms also came to the Arabs via Aramaic intermediary forms – for example, *utrujj* (no. 19).

[83] In the letter *alif* only nos 22, 23, and 28 list no Syriac synonym. Mistakes of the scribe of MS A cannot be excluded, since in no. 23 he also omitted the Greek and Persian synonym preserved in MS B.

[84] In the case of ܗܘܦܪܒܝܘܢ (A f. 161v), for 'εὐφόρβιον', ܗ serves only as usual transcription of 'ε'.

[85] In the entry *ḥarmal* (A f. 71r/B f. 178r), he quotes from the Arabic translation of Dioscorides, *De materia medica* (ed. Dubler and Terés (1952) II.261.14), according to which the Syrians call this kind of rue *bashāshā*. This word appears in both MSS in Arabic characters. MS A adds the Syriac form ܒܫܫܐ..

scribe of MS B. There is one more argument for the authenticity of these synonyms: On four occasions, MS A contains in the main text short passages in Syriac. These are concerned with the lethal dosage of colocynth pulp (A f. 130r/B f. 203r), resin spurge (A f. 162/B f. 217r), coriander (A f. 178v/B f. 224r), and February daphne (A f. 208v/MS B is lacunose here). It is not clear if Ibn al-Tilmīdh quoted from a Syriac book on poisons, or if he used Syriac here as a secret code. In two out of the three cases that can be compared, MS B omitted these statements completely. In the entry on resin spurge, MS B has an Arabic translation of this sentence, which allows the following conclusions. The four passages are not later additions and were apparently 'encrypted' by Ibn al-Tilmīdh himself. The scribe of the prototype of MS B then translated one passage only into Arabic. As a consequence, the copyist of MS B – who perhaps simply did not master Syriac[86] – had to omit the other two passages. This assumption would also explain why all synonyms in Syriac characters are missing from this manuscript.

One of only four explicit quotations from the *Quwā* in Ibn al-Bayṭār's (d. 1248) *al-Jāmiʿ li-mufradāt al-adwiyah wa-l-aghdhiyah* (*Collector of Simple Drugs and Foodstuffs*, IV.185.30) is concerned with the Syriac name of the water lily. Ibn al-Tilmīdh stated that the meaning of this term is 'water cabbage' (*wa-rubbamā summiya bi-l-Suryāniyyati mā maʿnāhu kurunbu l-māʾi wa-huwa* ܟܪܘܒܐ ܕܡܝ̈ܐ A f. 214r/ om. B). Ibn al-Bayṭār – who certainly had no knowledge of this language – copied the Arabic translation but omitted the Syriac term, perhaps since it was also written in Estrangelo characters in the copy he used.

Other languages were not treated in the *Quwā*, with one remarkable exception: in the entry *wajj* (sweet flag, A f. 220r/B f. 232r), he stated that the plant is called in Turkish *akīr* – that is, modern Turkish *eğir*.[87] Since this term does not appear in Ibn al-Tilmīdh's usual sources, it is not clear why he mentioned it here.

[86] This assumption is supported by the fact that he occasionally left blank spaces for Syriac terms in the first column (B f. 203r/A f. 130r), sometimes even preceded by *bi-l-Suryāniyyah* (A f. 151r/B f. 212v; B f. 221r/A f. 170v). In the entry dedicated to the pomegranate (B f. 185v/A f. 88v), no space is left, but the sentence *wa-yusammā l-muzzu † ayi l-ladhīdhu* ('it is called *al-muzz* ... which is to say "delightful"') makes no sense without the term ܗܢܝܐܐ ('delightful') as preserved in MS A.

[87] Cf. Redhouse (1890: 178a): اكير *éyír* – The sweet flag, *acorus calamus*.

1.4 Sources

Ibn al-Tilmīdh only occasionally named his sources. These quotations are furthermore misleading, since his most important sources were almost never explicitly indicated. As shown in the case of the aforementioned two edited specimens, almost all pieces of information included in the *Quwā* are also found in Ibn Sīnā's *Qānūn fī al-ṭibb*. Although Ibn Sīnā was mentioned four times,[88] there is no doubt the *Qānūn* was Ibn al-Tilmīdh's main source. Furthermore, we know that he highly appreciated this work and that he wrote marginal commentaries (*ḥawāshī*) on it, which are partially preserved as an autograph.[89] Ibn al-Tilmīdh was also acquainted with al-Rāzī's monumental *al-Ḥāwī*, which he abridged in a treatise entitled *Mukhtaṣar al-Ḥāwī* (*Abridgment of the Comprehensive Book*) or *Ikhtiyār kitāb al-Ḥāwī* (*Selections from the Comprehensive Book*), mentioned by his biographers and fragmentarily preserved in a few manuscripts.[90] The *Quwā* contain only two explicit quotations from al-Rāzī.[91] Despite this, he likely made more use of the *Comprehensive Book* without mentioning it. The extent of this dependence can hardly be determined, since already the *Qānūn* depended widely on al-Rāzī.[92] An important manual on simple drugs often used by medical practitioners and preserved in many copies is the *Minhāj al-bayān* by Ibn Jazlah. Ibn al-Tilmīdh also wrote apparently lost marginal commentaries on this book. Although he never mentioned the *Minhāj* in his *Quwā*, he likely used it as well. It is a unique feature of Ibn Jazlah's book that the drugs are often alphabetically arranged according to the part used (e.g. seed, root, leaves etc.) and not according to the actual name of the plant. In the cases of the entries *aṣl al-sawsan al-asmānjūnī* and

88 MS A f. 24v/B f. 162v (= Ibn Sīnā, *Qānūn fī al-ṭibb* (*Canon of Medicine*), ed. (1877) I.386); A f. 149v/B f. 212r (= I.396); A f. 194r/om. B (= I.352); A f. 210v/om. B. (= I.362).

89 Edwards (1922: no. 23); Iskandar (1977); Iskandar (1981).

90 Ibn Abī Uṣaybiʿah, *ʿUyūn al-anbāʾ fī ṭabaqāt al-aṭibbāʾ* (*Sources of Information on the Classes of Physicians*), 10.64.20, ed. Savage-Smith et al. (2020, online version), no. 4 = ed. Müller (1882) I.276; Yāqūt, *Muʿjam al-udabāʾ* (*Dictionary of Learned Men*), ed. Rifāʿī (1936) XIX.278. About a quarter of the text is preserved in MS Berlin, Staatsbibliothek Preußischer Kulturbesitz, Ahlwardt 6260 (Wetzstein 1188). In the misbound and fragmentary manuscript Ankara, Üniversitesi Dil ve Tarih-Coğrafya Fakültesi Kütüphanesi, Saib 2057, there is on f. 6v.7 a colophon indicating the end of *Ikhtiyārāt al-Ḥāwī* (*Selections from the Comprehensive Book*) by *Amīn al-dawlah . . . al-maʿrūf bi-Ibn al-Tilmīdh al-Baghdādī*.

91 The statement on the provenance of balsam of A f. 47v/om. B is ascribed to a *Kitāb al-ṣaydanah fī al-ṭibb* (*Book of the Pharmacy on Medicine*). Since it is missing from the entry *balasān* of the identically named chapter of al-Rāzī's *al-Ḥāwī* (*Comprehensive Book*), ed. (1962) XXII.12–13, it may have been taken from a lost monograph entitled *K. al-Ṣaydanah* mentioned by al-Rāzī's biographers (Sezgin (1970: 291)). The description of the therapeutic benefits of burned scorpions of A f. 146r/B f. 210r could not be traced in the pharmacological sections of the *Ḥāwī*.

92 Cf. Fellmann (1984).

bizr al-baqlah al-ḥamqāʾ, we have seen that reminiscences of this unusual system can be observed in the *Quwā*.

Another possible source is the chapter on simple drugs[93] of the *Kitāb al-miʾah* (*Book of the Hundred [Chapters]*) by Abū Sahl al-Masīḥī (d. 401/1010). Ibn al-Tilmīdh knew this book and wrote a marginal commentary (*ḥawāshī*)[94] on it, as well as an abridgement (*mukhtār*), both listed by his biographers. There is only one explicit mention of 'the author of the *Kitāb al-miʾah*'[95] in the *Quwā* and anonymous quotations can hardly be traced since this book was presumably one of the sources of Ibn Sīnā, who was a disciple of al-Masīḥī. Ḥunayn ibn Isḥāq (d. 260/873) was cited a few times.[96] In only two cases, Ibn al-Tilmīdh mentioned the title of the work used; one was his book on substitute drugs (*Kitāb al-abdāl*).[97] On A f. 221r/om. B, Ibn al-Tilmīdh stated that Ḥunayn had explained a Syriac term in his *Jamhara*. Such a title is not attested for Ḥunayn; it can nevertheless not be excluded that Ibn al-Tilmīdh indeed had access to such a glossographical work ascribed to Ḥunayn.[98] The other quotations[99] were presumably taken from his diverse translations, where he sometimes gave explanations of foreign-language words. Another Syriac term ascribed to Jibrīl (sc. Ibn Bukhtīshūʿ, fl. 212/817), may also originate from the glossographical literature (A f. 203v/om. B). The *Quwā* contain two more mentions of Jibrīl: one is concerned with the therapeutic use of scammony (A f. 116r/197v) and the other with a synonym of the term *faranjamushk*.[100] Other early Arabic authors on

93 Masīḥī, *Kitāb al-miʾah* (*Book of the Hundred*), ed. Sanagustin (2000) I.267–306 (chapter 31).

94 According to a note found on the Internet, which could not be checked, these *Ḥawāshī* seem to be preserved in a manuscript kept in Tehran: *Majlis-i shūrā-ʾi Islāmī*, no. 6335, *Catalogue* XIX.351, previously no. 61228 (cf. www.aghabozorg.ir/showbookdetail.aspx?bookid=100419, accessed 31 July 2021).

95 In the entry for *ʿinab* (grape; A f. 152v/B f. 213v), Ibn al-Tilmīdh mentioned explanations of the word *rāziqī* by 'Abū Sahl al-Masīḥī *ṣāḥib Kitāb al-miʾah*', by ʿUbaydallāh [*sic*] ibn Yaḥyā *ṣāḥib al-Ikhtiṣārāt al-arbaʿīn* (Sezgin (1970: 256–7)), the author of the *Kitāb al-bulghah* (*The Sufficient Book*; several texts bearing this title are attested), and al-Sukkarī (a grammarian). This passage is absolutely unusual for the *Quwā* and may have been copied from an intermediary source. It is actually not found in the *Kitāb al-miʾah* (*Book of the Hundred*) as edited by Sanagustin (2000).

96 According to his biographers, Ibn al-Tilmīdh also wrote a commentary on Ḥunayn's *Masāʾil fī al-ṭibb* (*Questions on Medicine*), but there is no evidence that he used it for the *Quwā*.

97 A f. 204r/om. B; cf. Sezgin (1970: 255, no. 12).

98 Fragments of such a glossary referred to as '*Thabat*' were preserved by al-Rāzī (Kahl (2011: 387)) and especially Bar Bahlūl (ed. Duval (1890): III.xviii, III.vii, III.xi).

99 A f. 24r/B f. 162r; A f. 136v/B f. 206r; A f. 170v/B f. 221r.

100 A f. 163r/B f. 217v. This passage is also interesting since Ibn al-Tilmīdh mentions there that Qudāmah ibn Jaʿfar (d. *c*.337/948) used the same synonym in his *Kitāb al-kharāj wa-ṣināʿat al-kitābah* (*Book of the Land Tax and the Art of the Secretary*). Unfortunately, I was unable to locate this quotation in al-Zubaydī's (1981) edition of this fragmentarily preserved book.

medicine mentioned in the *Quwā* are Ibn Māsawayh (d. 243/857),[101] Ibn Māssa (d. *c*.275/888), and Masīḥ (al-Dimashqī, d. 225/839).[102] Ibn al-Tilmīdh did certainly not always consult the originals of their works, instead most quotations could have been borrowed secondarily from his usual sources.[103]

As we have seen, the number of explicit quotations from Arabic sources is rather small, which is typical for the Eastern school of pharmacognosy. Authors from the West and especially from al-Andalus, such as Ibn Samajūn, Ibn Janāḥ, or Ibn al-Bayṭār, consequently named all their sources. While al-Rāzī often mentioned his authorities in *al-Ḥāwī*, Ibn Sīnā did this only occasionally. Authors depending on the *Qānūn* – for example, Ibn Jazlah and Ibn al-Tilmīdh – followed his model. The only names regularly occurring in Ibn Sīnā's book are those of the unrivalled Greek physicians. As a consequence, Ibn al-Tilmīdh also often cites Dioscorides for descriptions of plants and the like.[104] The person named most frequently in the *Quwā* is Galen.[105] The overwhelming part of these quotations originates from *On the Capacities of Simple Drugs*, which is explicitly mentioned twice.[106] On one occasion, he also quoted from *On the Composition of Drugs according to Kind*.[107] Other Greek authorities were only mentioned occasionally: Hippocrates

101 A f. 61r/B f. 172v; A f. 69r/B f. 177r; A f. 69v/B f. 177v.

102 A f. 126r/B f. 201v. Ibn al-Tilmīdh states that the quotation is from Masīḥ's *Aqrābādhīn* (*Dispensatory*). Since a monograph bearing that title is not known, he may have meant the section on compound remedies of his *Kunnāsh* (*Handbook*); cf. Sezgin (1970: 228).

103 The only statement ascribed to ʿĪsā ibn Māssa (A f. 172v/B f. 221v) is, for example, already present in al-Rāzī's *al-Ḥāwī* (*Comprehensive Book*), ed. (1962) XXI.305, and Ibn Sīnā's *Qānūn fī al-ṭibb* (*Canon of Medicine*), ed. (1877) I.421.

104 A f. 19v/B f. 160r; A f. 24r/B f. 162r; A f. 26r/B f. 163r; A f. 27v/B f. 164r; A f. 28v/B f. 164v; A f. 47v/om. B; A f. 52v/om. B; A f. 61r/B f. 173r; A f. 62r/B f. 173v; A f. 73r/B f. 179r; A f. 102r/om. B; A f. 118r/B f. 198r; A f. 158v/B f. 215r; A f. 170v/B f. 221r; A f. 190r/om. B.

105 A f. 14v/B f. 157v; A f. 15r/B f. 157v; A f. 24r/B f. 162r; A f. 28v/B f. 164v; A f. 46v/om. B; A f. 70v/B f. 178r; A f. 75r/B f. 179v; A f. 76r/B f. 180r; A f. 77v/B f. 180v; A f. 92r/B f. 187r; A f. 96v/B f. 189r; A f. 97r/B f. 189v; A f. 107r/B f. 193v; A f. 122v/B f. 200r; A f. 129r/B f. 202v; A f. 134v/B f. 205r; A f. 141r/B f. 208r; A f. 142r/B f. 208r; A f. 146r/B f. 210r; A f. 149v/B f. 212r; A f. 156v/B f. 212v; A f. 174v/B f. 222v; A f. 177v/B f. 223v; A f. 191r/om. B; A f. 214v/om. B. Ibn al-Tilmīdh certainly did not always consult the originals of Galen's books. His quotation of A f. 149v/B f. 212r is, for example, also found in Ibn Sīnā's *Qānūn fī al-ṭibb* (*Canon of Medicine*), ed. (1877) I.399, and al-Rāzī's *al-Ḥāwī* (*Comprehensive Book*), ed. (1962) XXI.198.

106 A f. 46v/om. B; A f. 134v/B f. 205r: *fī Kitābihī fī al-adwiyah al-mufradah* (*In His Book on Simple Drugs*).

107 A f. 134v/B f. 205r *fī Kitābihī fī tarkīb al-adwiyah bi-ḥasab ajnāsihā* (*In His Book on the Composition of Drugs according to Kind*). Another explicit quotation is problematic since the manuscripts give divergent titles (A f. 174v/B f. 222v). MS A reads *fī Kitābihī l-maʿrūf bi-ārāʾ Buqrāṭ wa-Falāṭun* (*On the Doctrines of Hippocrates and Plato*), while MS B has the variety *fī Kitābihī l-maʿrūf bi-l-adwiyah al-muqābilah li-l-adwāʾ* (*On Antidotes*). For the only quotation from the commentary on the Hippocratic *Oath*, see note 73.

featured only once in the *Quwā*,[108] Paul of Aegina twice,[109] and Rufus of Ephesus three times.[110]

REFERENCES

ʿAbbās, I. ed. 1968–77. *Aḥmad ibn Muḥammad ibn Khallikān, Wafayāt al-aʿyān wa-anbāʾ abnāʾ al-zamān*. 8 vols. Beirut: Dār Ṣādir.

Beck, L. Y. tr. 2011. *Pedanius Dioscorides of Anazarbus:* De materia medica. Second, revised, and enlarged edition. Hildesheim: Olms.

Bos, G., Käs, F., Lübke, M., and Mensching, G. eds. 2020. *Marwān ibn Janāḥ: On the Nomenclature of Medicinal Drugs (Kitāb al-talkhīṣ)*. 2 vols. Leiden: Brill.

Brockelmann, C. 1928. *Lexicon syriacum*. Halle: Niemeyer.

Dietrich, A. 1988. *Dioscurides Triumphans. Ein anonymer arabischer Kommentar (Ende 12. Jahrh. n. Chr.) zur Materia medica, 2. Teil: Übersetzung und Kommentar*. Gottingen: Vandenhoeck & Rupprecht.

Dubler, C. E., and Terés, E. eds. 1952–9. *La 'Materia medica' de Dioscórides: Transmisión medieval y renacentista*. 5 vols. (vol. II: Dubler, C. E., *Kitāb Diyāsqūrīdūs wa-huwa Hayūlā al-ṭibb fī al-ḥashāʾish wa-l-sumūm. Tarjamat Iṣṭifān ibn Bāsīl*). Barcelona/Tetuan: Tipogr. Emporium.

Dunlop, D. M. 1960. 'Bīmāristān. I. Early Period and Muslim East', in H. A. R. Gibb et al. (eds.), *Encyclopaedia of Islam: New Edition*, vol. I. Leiden: Brill, 1222–4.

Duval, R. ed. 1890–1901. *Lexicon syriacum auctore Hassano bar Bahlule*. 3 vols. Paris: National Printing Office.

Edwards, E. 1922. 'Some Rare and Important Manuscripts from the Collections of Ḥājjī ʿAbdu'l-Majīd Belshāh; Now Either in the British Museum or in the Private Collection of Professor Edward G. Browne', in T. W. Arnold (ed.), *A Volume of Oriental Studies Presented to Edward G. Browne, M.A., M.B., F.B. A., F.R.C.P., Sir Thomas Adams's Professor of Arabic in the University of Cambridge . . . on His 60th Birthday (7 February 1922)*. Cambridge: Cambridge University Press, 137–49.

Fellmann, I. 1984. 'Ist der *Qānūn* des Ibn Sīnā ein Plagiat des *Kitāb al-ḥāwī* von ar-Rāzī?' *Zeitschrift für Geschichte der arabisch-islamischen Wissenschaften* 1: 148–54.

Fichtner, G. 2017. *Corpus galenicum: Bibliographie der galenischen und pseudogalenischen Werke. Erweiterte und verbesserte Ausgabe 2017/05* (http://cmg.bbaw.de/online-publikationen/Galen-Bibliographie_2017-05.pdf, accessed 31 December 2019).

Fraenkel, S. 1886. *Die aramäischen Fremdwörter im Arabischen*. Leiden: Brill.

108 A f. 44r/om. B; cf. [Hippocrates], *On Regimen*, 2.45, ed. Littré (1849) VI. = 542–4 = ed. Joly and Byl (2003) 166–8.

109 Ibn al-Tilmīdh had apparently no access to his book. The quotation of A f. 192v/om. B was copied from al-Rāzī's *al-Ḥāwī* (*Comprehensive Book*), ed. (1962) XXI.473, and also the second passage is explicitly marked as a secondary quotation (f. A f. 107r/B f. 193v: *dhakara baʿḍuhum ʿan Fūlus*).

110 A f. 102r/om. B; A f. 179v/B f. 224r (cf. al-Rāzī, *al-Ḥāwī* (*Comprehensive Book*), ed. (1962) XXI.334); A f. 182r/B f. 225r (= al-Rāzī, *al-Ḥāwī*, ed. (1962) XXI.386).

Gottheil, R. J. H. ed. 1908. *The Syriac-Arabic Glosses of Īshōʿ bar ʿAlī, Part II.* Rome: Lincean Academy.

Hamarneh, S. M. 1975. *Catalogue of Arabic Manuscripts on Medicine and Pharmacy at the British Library.* Cairo: Les éditions universitaires d'Egypte.

Ḥammāmī, Ṣ. M. ed. 1997. *Ibn al-Tilmīdh, Maqālah fī al-Faṣd.* Aleppo: Jāmiʿat Ḥalab.

Ibn al-Bayṭār, Ḍiyāʾ al-Dīn ʿAbdallāh ibn Aḥmad. 1874. *al-Jāmiʿ li-mufradāt al-adwiyah wa-l-aghdhiyah.* 4 vols. Bulaq.

Ibn Sīnā, Abū ʿAlī al-Ḥusain ibn ʿAbdallāh. 1877. *Kitāb al-qānūn fī al-ṭibb.* 3 vols. Bulaq.

Iskandar, A. Z. 1967. *A Catalogue of Arabic Manuscripts on Medicine and Science in the Wellcome Historical Medical Library.* London: Wellcome Historical Medical Library.

Iskandar, A. Z. 1977. 'An Autograph of Ibn al-Tilmīdh's Marginal Commentary on Ibn Sīnā's "Canon of Medicine"', *Le Muséon* 90: 177–236.

Iskandar, A. Z. 1981. 'Another Fragment from the Autograph of Ibn al-Tilmīdh's "Marginal Commentary on Ibn Sīnā's Canon of Medicine"', *Bulletin of the School of Oriental and African Studies* 44: 253–61.

Joly, R. (in collaboration with S. Byl). ed. 2003. *Hippocratis de diaeta.* Berlin: Akademie Verlag.

Kahl, O. ed. 2007. *The Dispensatory of Ibn at-Tilmīḏ: Arabic Text, English Translation, Study and Glossaries.* Leiden: Brill.

Kahl, O. ed. 2009. *Sābūr ibn Sahl's Dispensatory in the Recension of the ʿAḍudī Hospital.* Leiden: Brill.

Kahl, O. 2010. 'Two Antidotes from the "Empiricals" of Ibn al-Tilmīdh', *Journal of Semitic Studies* 55: 479–96.

Kahl, O. 2011. 'The Pharmacological Tables of Rhazes', *Journal of Semitic Studies* 56: 367–99.

Käs, F. 2010. *Die Mineralien in der arabischen Pharmakognosie.* 2 vols. Wiesbaden: Harrassowitz.

Käs, F. 2016. 'Review of F. J. Rageb and F. Wallis, eds. The Herbal of al-Ghāfiqī. A Facsimile Edition of MS 7508 in the Osler Library of the History of Medicine, McGill University, with Critical Essays. Montreal: McGill-Queen's University Press 2014', *Orientalistische Literaturzeitung* 111: 259–62.

Littré, É. ed. 1839–61. *Oeuvres complètes d'Hippocrate: Traduction nouvelle avec le texte grec en regard, collationné sur les manuscrits et toutes les éditions; accompagnée d'une introduction, de commentaires médicaux, de variantes et de notes philologiques; suivie d'une table générale des matières.* 10 vols. Paris: J.-B. Baillière.

Löw, I. 1881. *Aramäische Pflanzennamen.* Leipzig: Engelmann.

MacKenzie, D. N. 1971. *A Concise Pahlavi Dictionary.* London: Oxford University Press.

Müller, A. ed. 1882–4. Muwaffaq al-Dīn Aḥmad ibn al-Qāsim ibn Abī Uṣaybiʿah: *ʿUyūn al-anbāʾ fī ṭabaqāt al-aṭibbāʾ.* 2 vols. Cairo: al-Maṭbaʿah al-Wahbiyyah.

Örs, D., Tuzcu, K., and Hekimoğlu, M. 2006–8. *Ankara Üniversitesi Dil ve Tarih-Coğrafya Fakültesi Kütüphanesi yazmalar kataloğu.* 2 vols. Ankara: Ankara Üniversitesi Dil ve Tarih Coğrafya Fakültesi.

al-Rāzī, Abū Bakr. 1962–79. *Kitāb al-ḥāwī fī al-ṭibb.* 23 vols. Hyderabad: Dāʾirat al-maʿārif al-ʿuthmāniyyah (vol. I–X, ²1974–9; vols. XI–XXXIII, ¹1962–70).

Redhouse, J. W. 1890. *A Turkish and English Lexicon.* Constantinople: Boyajian.

Rifāʿī, A. ed. 1936–8. Yāqūt al-Rūmī: *Muʿjam al-udabāʾ/Irshād al-arīb ilā maʿrifat al-adīb.* 20 vols. Cairo: Maktabat ʿĪsā al-Bābī al-Ḥalabī.

Sanagustin, F. ed. 2000. *Abū Sahl ʿĪsā ibn Yaḥyā al-Masīḥī, Kitāb al-miʾah fī al-ṭibb.* 2 vols. Damascus: Institut français d'études arabes.

Savage-Smith, E., Swain, S., and van Gelder, G. J. eds. 2020. *A Literary History of Medicine: The ʿUyūn al-anbāʾ fī ṭabaqāt al-aṭibbāʾ of Ibn Abī Uṣaybiʿah.* 5 vols. Leiden: Brill (https://scholarlyeditions.brill.com/reader/urn:cts:arabicLit:0668IbnAbiUsaibia.Tabaqatalatibba.lhom-ed-ara1:10.64 and https://scholarlyeditions.brill.com/reader/urn:cts:arabicLit:0668IbnAbiUsaibia.Tabaqatalatibba.lhom-tr-eng1:10.64, accessed 21 January 2022).

Sezgin, F. 1970. *Geschichte des arabischen Schrifttums*, vol. III. Leiden: Brill.

Sezgin, F., Amawi, M., and Neubauer, E. eds. 1995. *Muḥammad ibn Muḥammad al-Idrīsī: Kitāb al-jāmiʿ li-ṣifāt ashtāt al-nabāt wa-ḍurūb anwāʿ al-mufradāt.* 2 vols. Frankfurt: Institute for the History of Arabic-Islamic Science at the Johann Wolfgang Goethe University.

Shaʿīrah, M. ʿA., Ziyāda, M. M., and Ibrāhīm, M. A. eds. 1929–92. *Aḥmad ibn ʿAbd al-Wahhāb al-Nuwayrī: Nihāyat al-arab fī funūn al-adab.* 31 vols. Cairo: Markaz taḥqīq al-turāth.

Steingass, F. 1930. *A Comprehensive Persian-English Dictionary.* 2nd ed. London: Routledge.

Ullmann, M. 1970. *Die Medizin im Islam.* Leiden: Brill.

Wellmann, M. ed. 1907. *Pedanii Dioscuridis Anazarbei De materia medica libri quinque.* 3 vols. Berlin: Weidmann.

Zaryāb, ʿA. ed. 1991. Abū l-Rayḥān Muḥammad ibn Aḥmad al-Bīrūnī: *Kitāb al-ṣaydanah fī al-ṭibb.* Tehran: Markaz-i Nashr-i Dānishgāhī.

al-Zubaydī, M. Ḥ. ed. 1981. *Qudāmah ibn Jaʿfar: Kitāb al-kharāj wa-ṣ-ṣināʿat al-kitābah.* Baghdad: Wizārat al-thaqāfa.

CHAPTER 2

Drugs, Provenance, and Efficacy in Early Medieval Latin Medical Recipes

Jeffrey Doolittle

Medical recipes in Latin are valuable witnesses to a nexus of intellectual interests of the people who recorded them – individual recipes provide evidence of grammatical education, familiarity with classical geography and metrological units, and, of course, the depth of engagement with other medical texts such as herbals and theoretical treatises. However, since early medieval pharmacological texts in the Latin tradition have long been viewed as problematic or debased, many are yet unedited and the relationships between extant texts remain relatively unexplored. As a result, scholars have had a very difficult time approaching these recipes as cultural artifacts and using them as historical sources. The variations observed between different copies of medieval Latin medical recipe collections, for example, remain notoriously difficult to interpret. A few examples of a kind of *dentifricium*, or toothpaste, found across several copies of an early medieval medical compilation called the *Physica Plinii*, itself based on a passage from the *Natural History* by Pliny the Elder, highlight basic interpretive issues (see Table 2.1).

In these three recipes, the key ingredient of the dentifrice changes. Pliny's *Natural History* describes the medicinal qualities of the burnt ankle bones of a cow and specifies that the ashes (*cinis*) of the bones, when mixed with myrrh, can be used as a *dentifricium*.[1] An adaptation of this recipe, found in a late eighth-century collection copied at the monastery of Lorsch, has simpler wording with no mention of myrrh, and instead specifies that the *dentifricium* can be made also of ashes, but here of

Heartfelt thanks go especially to Richard Gyug and Monica Green, who read earlier drafts of this chapter, and also to Eliza Glaze, Arsenio Ferraces Rodríguez, and many others with whom I discussed important aspects of this research.

[1] Pliny, *Natural History*, 28.49.179, ed. Mayhoff (1897): 336. Pliny actually gives two dental remedies here, only one of which survives in the early medieval collections. The first part of the remedy, intended for strengthening painful loose teeth, does not appear in the *Physica Plinii* derivations, but the dentifrice, minus the myrrh, does.

Table 2.1 *Comparison of* dentifricium *recipes based on Pliny the Elder's* Natural History *(key ingredient in bold)*

Recipe	Source
Talus bubulus *accensus eos, qui labent cum dolore, admotus confirmat; eiusdem cinis cum murra dentifricium est.* (The ankle bones of a cow, ignited and applied to loose and painful teeth, will strengthen them; the ashes of the bones with myrrh are a dentifrice.)	Pliny, *Natural History* 28.49.179 (s. i)[1]
Plumbi albi *cinis dentifricium est.* (The ashes of white lead (tin) are a dentifrice.)	*Physica Plinii,* c. 39, Bamberg, Staatsbibliothek, Msc. Med. 1 (s. viii ex/ix in)[2]
Item. ***uulbi. albi.*** *cinis. dentifricium est.* (Likewise, the ashes of a white bulb are a dentifrice.)	*Physica Plinii,* c. 39, Montecassino, Arch. dell'Abbazia, cod. 69 (s. ix ex)[3]

1 Pliny, *Natural History*, 28.49.179, ed. Mayhoff and Jan (1897): 336.
2 Stoll (1992: 146).
3 Montecassino, Arch. dell'Abbazia, cod. 69, p. 49b (c. 39).

a substance called *plumbi albi* ('white lead' or tin).[2] In another version of the recipe from a late ninth-century manuscript produced at the abbey of Montecassino, an almost identically worded preparation calls yet again for ashes, but this time of another substance identified as *uulbi albi* (a 'white bulb', perhaps a kind of onion), a rough anagram of the *plumbi albi* in Bamberg 1.[3]

If we focus on the many changes in this one recipe, apart from the inclination to see the *Natural History* recipe and its recommendation of *talus bubulus* as the correct version, it is difficult to see any one of these ingredients as more or less plausible than the others. These changing ingredients might simply be mistakes, perhaps made by scribes who were unfamiliar with the material or working from poor exemplars.[4] Or as Linda Voigts has argued, these changes could instead be evidence of deliberate

2 See Stoll (1992: 146).

3 Pliny's *Natural History*, the original source for many of the recipes in these particular collections, contains descriptions for substances labelled as *plumbi albi* and *uulbi* (although none specifically labelled 'white'). See the indispensable index to the Latin text by Schneider (1967). This and other oral and dental remedies from MC 69 have been transcribed for the first time in the appendix to this chapter.

4 See, for example, Stannard (1999c, 1999d, 1999e), who also argues that mistakes in medical texts became codified as authorities repeated them.

ingredient substitutions made by scribes who were much more knowledgeable and creative than we give them credit for.[5] In the collection of medical texts deriving from Pliny's encyclopaedia (especially the texts known to scholars as the *Medicina Plinii* and *Physica Plinii*, from which our examples were drawn), assessing the differences between these possibilities is difficult, largely due to the work required: the tradition encompasses thousands of individual recipes, the philological relationships between the extant texts require much more study, and several key witnesses remain unedited.[6] However, a quantitative assessment of the contents of a grouping of recipes from this tradition, especially focusing on ingredients and efforts at specification, helps us avoid getting lost in the weeds of the changes in individual recipes such as those just mentioned. Recent research has shown that medieval medical collections, including the *Physica Plinii*, were not static creations, but adapted and rearranged as needs and contexts changed; consequently, a quantitative approach to recipes and their contents can shed much-needed light on changes from recipe to recipe and collection to collection.[7]

This chapter cannot encompass all the medical remedies from the *Natural History* found in medieval collections, but will instead explore a smaller yet still representative subset of preparations dealing with issues of oral and dental health (stomatology) drawn from six different versions of these recipe collections: the edited text of the *Medicina Plinii* and five further witnesses of the *Physica Plinii* surviving in manuscripts from the late eighth through fifteenth centuries.[8] Collectively, these six versions of the text can provide at least an impressionistic view of pharmacological change in a complicated Latin tradition that has to this point received very little scholarly attention.

Although these Plinian collections remained somewhat insulated from the more dramatic changes in Mediterranean and European *materia medica* of the eleventh centuries and later, significant transformations still occur between the older and newer witnesses.[9] After surveying the

[5] Voigts (1979). See also more recent reconsiderations of the value and meaning of medieval medicine in Vázquez Buján (1984), Van Arsdall (2007), and Horden (2009).

[6] Scarborough (1986: 59–60) voiced many of these same concerns.

[7] Fischer (2000: 242) has distinguished the receptary, or recipe collection, from other kinds of medical writing, as a collection of pharmaceutical remedies without information regarding diagnosis, one of the most popular types of medical text. The scholarship on this point is considerable. See foundational works on the topic of Latin recipes by Riddle (1974), Voigts (1979), and Cameron (1993). For a broad overview of botanical texts (including recipes) with bibliography, see Touwaide (2010).

[8] The textual tradition of these Plinian medical materials is, of course, far older (and wider), stretching from shortly after the completion of the *Natural History* itself. For an overview, see the entries in Sabbah, Corsetti, and Fischer (1987: 113–14, 127–9, and 131–5).

[9] Still, it is worth mentioning that some *Medicina Plinii*/*Physica Plinii* copies do contain ingredients associated with the changing medical sensibilities of the third quarter of the eleventh century

manuscript tradition of these related collections and the place of stomatological recipes within it, this chapter will review several broad changes observed in the structure and contents of remedies. The first, and perhaps most apparent, is that the number of simple remedies tends to decrease as a proportion of the whole while the number of compound remedies increases; the second is that new remedies added to the collection show an emphasis on markers of precision, as medical nomenclature and metrological units become more prevalent in recipes; and the third is that the kinds of ingredients employed in oral and dental applications diversify considerably over time. The principal trajectory observed in these six Latin medical recipe collections is one of gradual accretion, which not only suggests changes in thinking about recipes as a medical genre, but also gives us a glimpse of the changing attitudes about *materia medica* and efficacy.

Based on the comparison and analysis of some of the recipes in these collections, a striking change over time occurred in the Plinian tradition as added remedies are increasingly seen to require complicated instructions, precise quantities and names, and more 'exotic' ingredients. These subtle shifts, witnessed over the course of centuries, reflect changing scholarly expectations for what pharmaceutical recipes in written collections should look like, perhaps as a result of a growing engagement with *materia medica* in general, including those sourced from farther and farther from the Mediterranean zone.

2.1 The Place of Dental Remedies in the Works of 'Dr Pliny'

As the flurry of excitement about the discovery of fragments of lapis lazuli in the dental calculus of a middle-aged woman from the eleventh or twelfth century has shown, interest in questions pertaining to the oral and dental health of medieval people has exploded in recent years.[10] Modern

(sometimes in copies produced well before, in fact), such as *myrobalanus* (in Bamberg cod. Med. 2, ed. Önnerfors (1975) 107, 110–11, 113, and 117), and *camphora* (as *caphora*, in the Plinian collection of eye remedies in Ivrea, Biblioteca Capitolare 87, ed. Giacosa (1886) 15). Opsomer (1989) remains an essential starting point for tracing ingredients in early medieval medical texts, although there are some discrepancies between her catalogue, which is based on editions, and texts as they appear in manuscripts. For discussion of broader eleventh-century changes, see Riddle (1965), Stannard (1974), Freedman (2008), and Amar and Lev (2017), as well as the other chapters in this volume.

[10] According to Radini et al. (2019), this individual, identified as a monastic woman, may have processed lapis lazuli in her mouth in preparation for decorating a medieval manuscript. According to the authors' interpretations ('Scenario 3'), there is also a possibility that the individual may have been using lapis lazuli medicinally, a practice attested in European medical texts from the eleventh century and later. See Lev (2007) and Glaze (2018) for more on the medical use of lapis lazuli.

researchers have come to recognise the centrality of oral and dental health in humans as an indicator of general health, and, as a result, some of the compelling stories locked inside of historical dental remains are just beginning to be told.[11] As Robin Fleming has shown in her work and Clare Pilsworth has summarised for a specifically northern Italian context, the osteoarchaeological investigation of human dentition reveals a great deal of information about the lived experiences of premodern individuals, including profound facts about age, diet, migration, morbidity, and other general health conditions.[12] Claire Burridge has also recently suggested that archaeologically attested problems in dental health and hygiene, including tooth decay, caries, and other assorted issues constituted a very real practical concern for medieval people that may have played a much more direct role in shaping the compilation and copying of collections of dental remedies than we have understood up to this point.[13]

Despite these recent developments regarding the immense scientific and historic value of teeth, the therapeutic recipes that medieval people recorded to care for their stomatological problems remain understudied.[14] When medical historians discuss oral or dental recipes at all, it is often only in derision.[15] Part of this is no doubt related to the fact that no classical Greco-Roman treatise specifically focusing on issues of dental health survives, and dental recipes themselves do not

[11] See also Witwer-Backofen and Engel (2019: 84), who explain that 'oral health is a window to overall health because it interacts with almost all body functions'. Other significant works on premodern dentistry and oral health include Holst and Coughlan (2000) on the dental health of victims of the Battle of Towton (1461); Kondor (2007), who interpreted dental evidence as evidence for diet as well as social stratification; and Becker (2014), who studied a set of Roman tooth extractions discovered in a collection. And while not specifically related to dental health or hygiene, it is also significant that many of the astounding discoveries relating to the identification of historic and prehistoric outbreaks of the bubonic plague are founded upon the interpretation of ancient genetic evidence found within teeth. This is not the place for a full bibliography of that rapidly developing field, but see Little (2011) and Green (2014), which is open access (https://scholarworks.wmich.edu/medieval_globe/1, accessed 15 March 2020), for an introduction to some of the literature.

[12] Fleming (2006); Pilsworth (2014: 62–8). [13] Burridge (2019).

[14] For the purposes of this chapter, a 'dental and oral remedy' refers to a preparation included under a specific chapter in one of the six recipe collections of this study that appears to be applied to problems of the mouth and teeth. These chapters occur as a group in close proximity to one another in all collections, with more or less clear labels. These preparations include those intended to treat oral and dental diseases and conditions such as bad breath, ulcerations of the mouth, gum diseases, toothache, infant teething, loose teeth, and caries, as well as instructions for the formulation of various freshening, whitening, and strengthening powders, rinses, and toothpastes. See Wynbrandt (1998) for a more general and rather negative history of dentistry (and Pliny the Elder). See also the brief discussion of dental health and oral medicine in the Roman Empire in Jackson (1988).

[15] Indeed, if the medicine of the early Middle Ages has a negative reputation (see Baader (1984)), it seems that the dental knowledge of the early Middle Ages is often regarded as several steps worse. See Jackson (1988: 120) and Wynbrandt (1998: 3).

seem to have been transmitted independently.[16] Perhaps tellingly, Isidore of Seville, the author of *The Etymologies*, the most prominent encyclopaedia of the early Middle Ages, did not include oral or dental problems as part of his widely copied schema of human diseases and health problems.[17] The difficulty of situating dental treatments in a medical framework reflects the strongly 'do-it-yourself' nature of dental care in the ancient and medieval worlds.[18] This may also suggest, as Lynda Coon has argued, a deep anxiety over the nature of the mouth (along with other orifices of the body) as a transitional point between the interior and exterior of the body, as well as the place of the mouth, teeth, and tongue as the intermediary between thought and practice.[19] Although these concerns and difficulties persisted, dental preparations became an important, even sizable, component of many late antique and early medieval receptaries, especially those arranged *a capite ad calcem* ('from head to heel'), including those deriving from the *Natural History* of Pliny the Elder.[20]

Although Pliny was not writing a medical book, he devotes a considerable amount of space in his *Natural History* to practical medical matters, and perhaps as a consequence of that practical bent, dental concerns play a significant part.[21] Pliny's dental remedies (of which there are at least 240 in the text) are included as part of his larger holistic goals to provide a means to

16 Beccaria (1956), contains no references to an independent work of dental preparations; similarly, nothing is listed specifically for teeth in other catalogues on medical manuscripts by Wickersheimer (1966) or the catalogue of medical texts in Sabbah, Corsetti, and Fischer (1987).

17 Isidore, whose book on medicine was often excerpted and circulated in early medieval medical manuscripts, divided health issues into three general categories: acute and chronic conditions and problems that affected the surface of the body. He did not discuss dental issues at all but did discuss the nature of teeth more generally in Book XI in the context of the human body. See Sharpe (1964).

18 Jackson (1988).

19 Coon (2011: 88–96) alludes to the anxiety in Benedictine writing about the mouth and teeth as needing special regulation as a 'treacherous orifice' that both utters slander and prayer and also complicates the boundary between physical and spiritual.

20 Other Greco-Roman medical authors also treat matters of dental health within larger works. Celsus, *On Medicine*, 7.12, tr. Spencer (1938) III.366–71 gives perhaps the most detailed instructions for a tooth extraction and discusses other dental issues. See the Latin edition by Marx (1915). See also the passage on dental health in Cassius Felix, *On Medicine* 32.1–14, ed. Fraisse (2002) 73–8.

21 See Bostock and Riley (1855), Healy (1999), Beagon (2005), and Doody (2010). Most prominently in Pliny, *Natural History*, 7.15.68, ed. Mayhoff (1875) 17–18: 'Some facts concerning teeth'. After identifying exceptional or shocking cases of dental abnormalities from Greek and Roman myth and history, Pliny discusses the unique properties of teeth and gives the often-cited 'fact' that women have fewer teeth than men. He is also most intrigued by the contradiction in teeth as being exceptionally strong, yet especially weak at the same time: although he says teeth are the part of the body most resistant to fire, they are also often the first part of the human body to fail. He highlights the singularly important roles teeth play in mastication as well as speech, and also introduces prognostications based on teeth.

care for the human body using natural substances, as well as to express a comprehensive understanding of the important qualities of the given plants, animals, or minerals that he discusses.[22] The majority of the medical recipes in the *Natural History* concentrates between Books 20 and 32, but additional remedies can be found scattered throughout the entire work.[23] Rather significantly for later compilers, Pliny concentrated most of his oral and dental remedies in a few discrete points in his book; the remedies found in the *Medicina Plinii*, philologically the oldest compilation of Plinian remedies, are almost entirely drawn from these ready-made collections.[24] In addition to his recommendations on the therapeutic properties of natural and crafted substances as well as instructions for concocting thousands of remedies, Pliny commented on a variety of other medical issues, including basic matters of anatomy and physiology, the role of medicine in society, pathology and epidemiology, the origins and sources of pharmaceutical compounds, Greek and Latin systems of weights and measures, and many other things which found their way into early medieval medical manuscripts.[25]

Pliny's medical remedies made their way into several different collections that in time developed their own transmission histories and also influenced each other in a fascinating series of late antique cross-pollinations.[26] Alf Önnerfors, the editor of several of these Plinian

[22] Pliny is careful to quantify this effort at every opportunity: in his preface, he states that he has assembled 20,000 facts drawn from 200 books by 100 authors. Each chapter and subsection are further quantified in terms of the number of remedies that Pliny has assembled, although sometimes his numbering is a little difficult to follow. As Gudger (1924) states, the number of authorities Pliny uses is actually 473 (146 Roman and 327 Greek authors).

[23] For a good overview, see Stannard (1965, 1999a).

[24] These compilations are almost ready to excerpt as is, and are scattered in the second half of the encyclopaedia. Pliny, *Natural History*, Books 20–37, ed. Mayhoff (1892–7). They focus on tooth diseases and toothache remedies, and several concentrate on the diseases of infants, which focus primarily on teething and are amassed in Books 25 (remedies from wild plants), 28 (medicinal uses of living creatures, including humans), 30 (remedies from animal products), and 32 (remedies from aquatic creatures). Beyond these concentrations, Pliny provides dental preparations more widely scattered in Books 20 (on garden plants), 23 (on cultivated trees), and 24 (on wild trees). Pliny's 240 remedies are split almost perfectly evenly between remedies deriving from plants and those deriving from animals (including humans).

[25] Pliny, *Natural History*, ed. Mayhoff (1875–1906). See especially several essays in French and Greenaway (1986) for several aspects of the late antique medical adaptations, including those by Morton (1986), Nutton (1986), and Scarborough (1986).

[26] In the fifth/sixth century CE, a number of other compilations of the *materia medica* drawn from Pliny, Dioscorides, and other sources also appeared. One of these, the *Herbarium*, was credited to a certain 'Apuleius Platonicus', but other texts included the *Curae quae ex hominibus* edited by Ferraces Rodríguez (2015), and others. This particular grouping often travelled together and developed a separate textual tradition and seems to have drawn on slightly different versions of the Plinian recipes that appeared in the *Medicina*/*Physica* trajectory. See study and commentary by

compilations, proposed that at some point no later than the fourth century, the name 'Plinius Secundus Iunior' was attached to an otherwise anonymous medical compilation of 1,100 prescriptions drawn primarily from the *Natural History*, reorganised into three books of chapters arranged mostly *a capite ad calcem*, thus creating a collection modern scholars have named the *Medicina Plinii*.[27] This text, as D. R. Langslow pointed out, was the first *euporista* ('easy to procure remedy collection') composed in Latin since that of Scribonius Largus, and was extraordinarily influential.[28] It has survived in a number of manuscripts of its own, but portions of it also made their way into a number of other early medieval medical texts; the late fourth- or early fifth-century Marcellus of Gaul in his *De medicamentis liber* cites as sources Pliny the Elder and 'the other Pliny' (*uterque Plinius*), likely a reference to his indebtedness to both the *Natural History* and the medical compilation based on it.[29] Then, at some point between the fifth and sixth centuries, independently of Marcellus' work, another enlargement based on the *Medicina Plinii* was made, likely in Italy; modern scholars have labelled this collection the *Physica Plinii*, and it too was copied in a number of manuscripts. It survives in three major recensions.[30]

Pradel-Baquerre (2013). To this constellation of Plinian medical works should also be added the *Additamenta* which were appended to a copy of Theodore Priscianus' *Euporiston*. The remedies are at least partially Plinian in origin and have been edited by Rose (1894).

[27] The text of the *Medicina Plinii* has been edited several times. Rose (1875) provided the first modern edition based primarily on two manuscript witnesses while Önnerfors (1964) more fully consulted the wider tradition and developed a stemma. Önnerfors' dating of the text of the *Medicina Plinii* collection to the third or fourth century is based on both its strong resonances in terms of language and vocabulary with the *Natural History* as well as the *Medicina Plinii*'s relative textual conservatism. See also Rose (1874), Önnerfors (1963), Sabbah, Corsetti, and Fischer (1987: 113–14), Opsomer (1989: xiii), Stoll (1992: 16–24), and Langslow (2000: 64). See also the English translation by Hunt (2020) based on Önnerfors' Latin text.

[28] Langslow (2000: 64–5).

[29] Marcellus is sometimes also surnamed 'Empiricus' (after his in-text explanation of how he compiled his work) or 'of Bordeaux', but was probably not from there. Marcellus primarily drew upon Scribonius Largus' *Compositiones* as well as Vindicianus, but he utilised a similar *a capite ad calcem* structure as the *Medicina Plinii*, and he also incorporated a number of Plinian remedies. An early edition of *De medicamentis liber* by Helmreich (1889) has been superseded by that of Niedermann and Liechtenhan (1968). For further bibliography, see Stannard (1973), Sabbah, Corsetti, and Fischer (1987: 111–13), and Langslow (2000: 66).

[30] These three branches are each named for their principal manuscript witnesses (*Bambergensis*, *Sangallensis*, and *Florentino-Pragensis*). See especially Önnerfors (1963), Sconocchia (1989, 1992), and Fischer (1986, 1993) for an overview of the tradition. Altogether, there are at least two other branches of the *Physica* tradition. The first, which survives in excerpts only, is the *Physica Plinii Eporediensis* (Ivrea, Biblioteca Capitolare, cod. 87, s. x/xi), ed. Giacosa (1886), although Fischer (1986) established its relationship to the *Physica* tradition. See also Beccaria (1956: 284–5). Ivrea 87 contains primarily remedies for the eyes and no dental preparations. The second additional branch, as detailed in Cameron (1983a, 1983b) and Adams and Deegan (1992), is the *Physica* version used by the compiler/translator of Bald's *Leechbook*, a ninth-century Old English recipe collection.

The dental remedies found in the early medieval *Medicina Plinii* compilation and five of the fullest *Physica Plinii* enlargements (all detailed in Table 2.2) provide an excellent opportunity to analyse pharmacological changes in Latin medicine. These five witnesses of the *Physica Plinii* share much common material with the *Medicina Plinii*, but there are some key differences between the texts. To summarise, the *Medicina Plinii* chapters and recipes are more philologically consistent from copy to copy compared to the much wider degree of variability seen in the several witnesses of the *Physica Plinii*.[31] Part of this may be related to the names and authors given for the collections, and the divergent auras of authority they each developed. The most comprehensive witnesses of the *Medicina Plinii*, of which the ninth-century manuscript St Gallen, Stiftsbibliothek, Cod. 752 is the earliest, are almost all entitled *De medicina*, ascribed to 'Plinius Secundus Iunior', and contain a prologue by Pliny, or at least *a* Pliny, an arrangement which may have invited a more conservative treatment of the text.[32]

The five witnesses of the *Physica Plinii*, on the other hand, as described in Table 2.2, reveal significant mutability, reflected in a series of modifications in organisation, attributions, and *tituli*. The earliest extant version of the *Physica* tradition, and the second recipe collection of this study, is from one of the most famous medical manuscripts of the earlier Middle Ages, the *Lorscher Arzneibuch* (Bamberg Staatsbibliothek, Msc. Med. 1, or 'Bamberg 1'), produced around 800 at the Carolingian monastery of Lorsch.[33] Unlike the *Medicina Plinii*, this manuscript copy bears no explicit connection to Pliny whatsoever. It is instead identified as the work of Caelius Aurelius *medicus* and the Plinian collection in three books is presented as one, which constitutes just one part of a larger five-book receptary.[34] The third collection, found in St Gallen,

[31] This is simply seen in the publication history of the two respective collections. The *Medicina Plinii* has been published as a single edition of the various manuscript witnesses, whereas the dramatic differences between the textual branches of the *Physica* have forced publication of that collection witness by witness.

[32] Önnerfors (1963). The *De Medicina* might be a better name for the collection than the somewhat artificial *Medicina Plinii*. For the edition of the *Medicina Plinii*, see Önnerfors (1964). See also Doody (2010: 139).

[33] The 'Lorsch Pharmacopeia', Bamberg, Staatsbibliothek Msc. Med. 1 was named as part of UNESCO's 'Memory of the World Register' in 2013 (www.unesco.org/new/en/communication-and-information/memory-of-the-world/register/full-list-of-registered-heritage/registered-heritage-page-5/lorsch-pharmacopoeia-the-bamberg-state-library-mscmed1, accessed 15 January 2022). See Beccaria (1956: 193–7), Platte and Platte (1989) for selected studies and texts, and Keil and Schnitzer (1991). Stoll (1992) provided a transcription of the manuscript. See also Fischer (2010) for an overview of the debates surrounding this manuscript.

[34] The *Physica* in Bamberg 1 generally reflects the same *a capite ad calcem* structure seen in the *Medicina Plinii* but has numbered the chapters as a single book.

Table 2.2 *Comparison of date, origin, attribution, and title of the* Medicina Plinii *and* Physica Plinii *witnesses used for this study*

Witness	Date and Origin	Attribution and Title
Medicina Plinii (ed. *Önnerfors*)	s. iv; (MS copies from s. ix, St. Gall)	**Plinius Secundus Iunior,** *De Medicina* (as in Sang. 752)
***Physica* Copies**		
Bamb. 1: Bamberg, Staatsbibliothek, Msc. Med 1 (*Physica Plinii*)	s. viii ex/ix in.; Lorsch	**Caelius Aurelius**; 'Explicit liber excerptus de libro Caelii Aurelii medici, cuius libros laudasse probatur Cassiodorus' (f. 35v)
Sang. 751: St. Gallen, Stiftsbibliothek, cod. 751 (*Physica Plinii*)	s. ix; N. Italy	**Plenus/Plinius/Filinus**; 'pleni secundum ep*istu*la medicinalis explicit' (p. 183); 'FILINI SECDI EPS[L] MEDICINE' (p. 184); 'plini secondi de fisicis LIBER EXPLICIT' (p. 201)
MC 69: Montecassino, Archivio dell'Abbazia, cod. 69 (*Physica Plinii*)	s. ix ex; S. Italy (Montecassino)	**No name**; acephalous
Bamb. 2: Bamberg, Staatsbibliothek, Msc. Med. 2 (*Physica Plinii*)	s. ix/x, N. Italy	**Paulus**; 'INCIP*IT* LIB*ER* PAUU' (f. 93v); 'INCIP*IT* LIB*ER* PAULI' (f. 95v)
PP Flor-Prag: *Physica Plinii Florentino-Pragensis* (ed. Winkler, Wachtmeister, and Schmitz)	s. xiv/xv; Italy	**Plinius**; 'Prologus Plinii in Physicam'; **Plinius Secundus**; 'Proemium in medicinam C. Plinii Secundi'

Stiftsbibliothek 751 ('Sang. 751'), originally from a scriptorium of northern Italy in the ninth century, is in a similar three-book arrangement as the *Medicina Plinii*.[35] This copy, also edited by Önnerfors and believed to

[35] For St Gall 751, see Beccaria (1956: 372–81) and Sabbah et al. (1987: 129).

have been based on a reworking of the *Medicina/Physica* text done during the sixth or seventh century with many magical interpolations, is called *Liber fisicum medicinalis* but is anonymous.[36] It is also the most divergent among the six collections.[37] The fourth witness, the unedited late ninth-century copy in Montecassino, Archivio dell'Abbazia, cod. 69 ('MC 69'), likely produced at the abbey of Montecassino, is the most comprehensive version of the text, but is acephalous and arranged as a single book (see the appendix to this chapter for a transcription of the dental remedies).[38] A text very similar to the MC 69 redaction found in late ninth- or early tenth-century northern Italian manuscript, now known as Bamberg, Staatsbibliothek Msc. Med. 2 ('Bamberg 2'), is called the *LIBER PAULI* in one location and even more confusingly, *LIBER PAUU* (perhaps, as Fischer has suggested, a corruption of 'Plini') in another.[39] The sixth Plinian collection for this study, deriving from another reworking of the *Medicina* and *Physica Plinii* made in the thirteenth or fourteenth centuries, has been edited by Joachim Winkler, Walter Wachtmeister, and Günter Schmitz.[40] The edition is based on the three closely related fourteenth- and fifteenth-century manuscripts of Önnerfors' *Florentino-Pragensis* branch ('PP Flor-Prag), which consistently reference both the *Physica* name and a connection to Pliny.[41]

The oral and dental remedies are all found as a group of related chapters in each of these collections, even if those chapters are organised slightly differently

36 See the full edition of the *Physica Plinii Sangallensis* in two volumes by Önnerfors (2006–7). Önnerfors (2004) also published the chapter on dental recipes separately. Another fragmentary copy in St Gallen 217/1396 is entitled *De fisicis liber* (and variously ascribed to Pleni, Plini, or Filini. See also the entry in Beccaria (1956: 381–3).

37 Önnerfors (2006–7).

38 See catalogue entries and bibliography for Montecassino 69 in Beccaria (1956: 293–7); Lowe and Brown (1980: II.63); see also Adacher (1984) for a study of Montecassino's medical manuscripts. Sconocchia (1989: 515–19) identified Montecassino as a particularly full exemplar of the *Bambergensis* branch and proposed a new edition, although that has not been completed.

39 Bamberg 2 has also been edited by Önnerfors (1975). Fischer (2008) has convincingly shown this spelling of PAUU to be most likely a corruption of the name *Plini*, and not a mistaken attribution to Paul of Aegina as some commentators have surmised. This title of *Liber Pauli* is also attached to a brief excerpt of several *Physica Plinii* chapters on cures for the breast found in Vendome 175, as identified by Green (2000: Appendix, p. 26).

40 Each editor, closely following Önnerfors as a model, took responsibility for one of the three books of the *Physica*. Winkler (1984) completed Book I, Wachtmeister (1985) managed Book II, and Schmitz (1988) completed Book III. See also Langslow (2000: 69).

41 These five witnesses are drawn from three of the main branches of the tradition. The *Physica Plinii* texts in Bamberg 1, Bamberg 2, and MC 69 are from the Bambergensis branch; Sang. 751 is from the Sangallensis branch; the PP Flor-Prag edition is from the three manuscripts of the Florentino-Pragensis branch. See Önnerfors (1963), Fischer (1986), Deegan and Adams (1992), and Sconocchia (1992) for more on the manuscript tradition.

between the *Medicina Plinii* and each of the five redactions of the *Physica Plinii*. With the exception of the Sang. 751 copy, which combines all the oral and dental remedies into two chapters, the fuller *Physica* witnesses echo the *Medicina Plinii* structure, but divide each of the *Medicina*'s three large chapters into subordinate ones each on a more specific oral or dental affliction.[42] As Table 2.3 illustrates, the compiler of the *Physica Plinii*, at least according to the oldest witness in Bamberg 1, divided the recipes of the *Medicina Plinii*'s chapter *De oris vitiis* (ch. 12) between seven new chapters dealing with mouth ailments (chs. 28–34), and the *Medicina* chapter *Dentibus* (ch. 13) between six on dental preparations (chs. 35–40). The collection in Bamberg 1 replicated the third short chapter from the *Medicina Plinii* devoted to children's teething (ch. 41: *Dentioni*). The organisational sensibilities are based largely on key words in the recipes which are then usually excised from the recipe in the *Physica* copies.[43] The later *Physica Plinii* texts found in MC 69, Bamberg 2, and the PP Flor-Prag all followed the same general chapter arrangement as the *Physica Plinii* copy in Bamberg 1.[44]

Unlike the *Medicina*, the five *Physica* collections are diverse in more ways than simply *tituli*, authorship, and chapter arrangements; such diversity makes them particularly useful to make a comparative study of pharmacological changes through the Middle Ages.

2.2 Oral and Dental Recipes: Continuity and Change

Although briefly surveyed, these six medieval receptaries remain unique witnesses with their own production contexts and subsequent histories. With such considerations in mind, direct comparison of the dental recipes taken from the *Medicina Plinii* and five witnesses of the *Physica Plinii* tradition poses significant methodological problems. While there does not seem to be any direct evidence of one of these copies being used to make another, there are close relationships between the texts nonetheless, and focusing on a discrete grouping of recipes through different versions of

42 Sang. 751 instead features all mouth remedies in one chapter and all the dental remedies in another; the recipes for teething are located in the general dental chapter.

43 Thus, a recipe's inclusion in either the chapter on 'defects' (*uitia*), 'sores' (*ulcera*), 'wounds' (*uulnera*), or 'putrefaction' (*putredinem*) of the mouth, for example, owes a great deal to the language employed in the earlier versions of the recipe than any specific typological distinctions. Langslow (2000: 148), however, at least in Celsus and Cassius Felix, sees evidence of some 'semantic oppositions at work' in the use of these terms, rather than simply a case of *variatio sermonis*.

44 This should also be compared to Fischer (1986) as well as Sconocchia (1989, 1992) regarding the main changes between versions of the *Physica Plinii*.

Table 2.3 *Structure and contents of the sections on oral health between the copy of the* Medicina Plinii *and the oldest extant recension of the* Physica Plinii *(Bamberg 1). The* Physica *copies in MC 69 and PP Flor-Prag have replicated the chapter arrangement in Bamberg 1.*

Medicina Plinii	Bamberg 1 (*c.*800)
12. Oris uitiis (For defects of the mouth)	28. Ad vitium oris (For a defect of the mouth) 29. Ad ulcera oris (For sores of the mouth) 30. Ad tumorem gingiuarum uel uitium oris (For swelling of the gums or a defect of the mouth) 31. Ad putredinem oris (For putrefaction of the mouth) 32. Ad foetorem oris (For bad breath) 33. Ad os saliuosum et libidum (For a salivating and livid mouth) 34. Ad os et labra (For the mouth and lips)
13. Dentibus (For the teeth)	35. Ad dentium dolore (For tooth pain) 36. Ad dentes si nimio capitis reumate capitis laxauerint (For teeth that become loose from excessive rheuma of the head) 37. Ad dentium molariorum dolorem (For pain of the molars) 38. Ad dentes uitiosos aut cauos (For rotten teeth and cavities) 39. Ad dentes candidandos (For whitening teeth)[1] 40. Ad dentes molares uel ad omnes ut sint incorrupti et inpassibiles inmobilesque (For stabilising and protecting molars and all teeth)[2]
14. Dentioni infantium (For teething of infants)	41. Ad dentionem (For teething)

1 This is presented as Chapter 40 in the capitula table.

2 This is presented as Chapter 39 in the capitula table and is reported there as *Ad omnes dentes ut fiant firmi*. However, this is the title in the text of the chapter, which accords with the titles of the chapter found elsewhere.

a text gives an impressionistic view of broader changes in medical thinking. The oral and dental recipe chapters show evidence of reorganisation and simplification, although the general inclination is towards growth. The specifics of that growth, however – whether defined as the kinds of recipes that are being incorporated into the tradition, changes in approaches to precision, or the diversity and numbers of ingredients required – all suggest changing attitudes and expectations about remedies, their presentation, and perhaps also their efficacy.

Scholars have had a difficult time even agreeing on the form and definition of a medical recipe in these texts.[45] Where possible, in identifying what the scribes intended as recipes, physical manuscript evidence should guide modern scholars – the scribes may not have always understood the words they were copying, but they undoubtedly intended the written forms and arrangements we can now observe in manuscripts. Consequently, several design details help in identifying and distinguishing recipes from one another. Jerry Stannard, Debby Banham, and others have pointed to the all-important *Item* opening ('likewise' or 'also') as an aid in differentiating successive pharmaceutical preparations in a list.[46] Additional details in the manuscript include patterns in uses of colour or rubrication; initials or *litterae notabiliores* placed at the start of new remedies; numerals, spaces, punctuation, and other special marks similarly used as dividers; as well as considerations of the scribe's planned *mise en page*, but unfortunately, many of these details are not recorded in editions. As might be expected, these patterns are easier to see in some witnesses than others, but it is worth mentioning that the strategies employed in arranging the information on a manuscript page can be quite diverse even for similar kinds of texts, which may provide yet further insights into the intellectual cultures of the centres that produced the manuscripts. One of the main features of the transmission of these chapters through the centuries is the slow accretion of supplementary recipes from other sources, as evidenced

[45] The evolution in organisation and numbering systems in the *Physica Plinii* editions put forth by Önnerfors demonstrate these changing sensibilities, but ultimately highlight the basic difficulty in navigating these recipe collections. In his early editions, such as the *Medicina Plinii* (1964), Önnerfors would indicate numbering of the recipes in the margins but seems to have relied more on connections to Pliny's *Natural History* to draw his boundaries. His later editions of Bamberg 2 (1975) included numeration that followed the codicological evidence a bit more closely. Finally, his most recent edition of Sang. 751 (2006–7) abandoned numbering of the recipes altogether, favouring a system that recorded manuscript page and line numbers only.

[46] Voigts (1979), Stannard (1999b, 1999f), Banham (2011), and others have introduced aspects of the typology of early medieval medical recipes. Langslow (2000: 31) also includes a brief discussion of the language of the recipe genre through an analysis of a medical parody found in Plautus' *Mercator*.

Table 2.4 *Main comparison of numbers of recipes for oral problems, dental problems, and children's teething*

Recipe Type	Med. Plin.	Bamb. 1	Sang. 751	MC 69	Bamb. 2	Flor-Prag
Oral recipes	22	17	7	36	38	50
Dental recipes	30	19	45	46	49	80
Teething recipes	5	2	0	5	5	7
Total	57	38	52	87	92	137

through the expansion of the dental health sections as witnesses across the centuries (see Table 2.4):

Aude Doody has surmised that much of this accretion may have been in the form of appendices or marginal additions to a text which were then copied en masse from a manuscript when a new copy was prepared, thus becoming part of the 'official' text.[47] The *Medicina Plinii* contains fifty-seven oral and dental remedies, but the five witnesses in the *Physica* tradition show considerable fluctuations in size.[48] From thirty-eight total recipes found in Bamberg 1, Sang. 751 contains fifty-two, MC 69 and Bamberg 2 each contain around ninety, and the PP Flor-Prag is the largest collection with 137 total recipes in all the oral and dental chapters. Altogether, nearly 500 oral and dental remedies are found across these six different collections.

[47] Doody (2010). This tendency may also account for some of the more significant variations between the different branches of the Plinian recipe collections as regional additions were slowly creating very different texts. Perhaps a stage of Doody's process is shown in the margins of MC 69. In the thirteenth century a reader added a number of marginal recipes directly related to the medical topics treated in the main text, many of them drawn from *De Herba Bettonica* by Pseudo-Antonius Musa and *Herbarius* by Pseudo-Apuleius. A copyist who used this manuscript to make a new copy of the recipe collection might have taken down all the recipes on the page, merging the *Physica* with the Antonius Musa/Herbarius elements to create a new recipe collection. This may also help explain the characteristic arrangement of old and new remedies observed in different witnesses. Older remedies tend to be found in small contiguous groups, with new remedies interspersed here and there between them. This arrangement may indicate a copyist including an original text of older remedies with new remedies added in margins at the bottom of the page.

[48] In his edition of the text, Önnerfors (1964) was more interested in facilitating comparison with the *Natural History* than in presenting recipes as they appear in his manuscript witnesses. Investigation of *Medicina Plinii* copies in Sang. 752 (s. ix), Leiden, Universiteitsbibliothek Voss. Lat. O. 92 (s. x) and London, British Library, Royal MS 12 E XX (s. xii) reveals the regular employment of majuscules in tandem with small *puncti*, sometimes a bit elevated, which rather consistently divide the recipes into much smaller, recognisable units.

2.3 Simple and Compound Remedies

In the *Natural History*, Pliny himself contrasted between simple remedies of a few ingredients and the more complicated preparations composed of multiple ingredients, which he often lampooned; in the dental remedies of the six subsequent adaptations, the simple preparations Pliny would likely have favoured tend to dwindle, as more complicated preparations increase.[49] As Table 2.5 shows, the *Medicina Plinii*, which contains a prologue extolling the virtues of simple, cheap remedies, features a dental section in which nearly 90 per cent of the remedies are either one- or two-ingredient preparations. In the subsequent *Physica* collections, there is a proportional decrease in the number of simplest recipes and a corresponding increase in more complicated preparations of three or more ingredients. The *Physica* copies in Bamberg 1 and Sang. 751 show slight decreases in the number of their simplest recipes to only 80 per cent of the total, with more complicated preparations up to around 20 per cent of their totals.[50] In the late ninth-century and early tenth-century witnesses in MC 69 and Bamberg 2, simples constitute no more than 66 per cent of the total, and more complicated remedies comprise 34 per cent of the more complicated recipes.[51] The numbers level off for the PP Flor-Prag, but still the complicated remedies number around one-third of the total.

Despite the declining numbers, one- to two-ingredient recipes constitute the majority in all collections.[52] A good representative example is a rather unassuming preparation for teething in infants involving the application of either goat milk or rabbit brain on the gums with a clear antecedent in the *Natural History*:

> ***Natural History*** **(28.78.259)**: *Lacte caprino aut cerebro leporum perunctae gingivae faciles dentitiones faciunt.*[53]

[49] See Healy (1999). Pliny's antagonism towards complicated medicines is especially pronounced in the opening chapters of Book 29, especially 29.8 in Pliny, *Natural History*, ed. Mayhoff (1897) 367–77. Pliny in particular lampoons the crafting of *theriace* with its 600 ingredients and the *Mithridatium antidotum*, which has 54, equating the loss of Roman public morals with the increase in medical chicanery, and instead supports the simple remedies of someone like Cato, as *vatem et oraculum* ('prophet and oracle'). On theriac, see also Amar, Serri, and Lev (Chapter 5) in the present volume.

[50] Most of this growth is actually in three-ingredient recipes, as 13 per cent of the total recipes in Bamberg 1 and 19 per cent of the total recipes in Sang. 751 are of the three-ingredient variety.

[51] In contrast to the growth in Bamberg 1 and Sang. 751, most of these new multi-ingredient recipes are actually those containing four or more, with the largest recipes in both MC 69 and Bamberg 2 containing eleven unique ingredients.

[52] There may also be something especially useful or valued in the two-ingredient recipes characterised by a 'X *uel* Y' formula, as they feature a built-in substitution. In fact, while one-ingredient recipes show such a dramatic decrease through the various redactions of the text, it is noteworthy that two-ingredient recipes, many following this formulaic structure, always constitute just slightly more than a third of the total in any given witness.

[53] Pliny, *Natural History* 28.78.259, ed. Mayhoff (1897) 364.

Table 2.5 *Distributions of one-, two-, and 3+ ingredient recipes in the dental and oral health chapters of the six recipe collections, with percentages*

Collection	Recipes	1 ing.	%	2 ing.	%	1+2 ing.	%	3+ ing.	%
Med. Plinii[1]	57	29	0.51	21	0.37	50	0.88	5	0.09
Bamberg 1	38	15	0.39	16	0.42	31	0.82	7	0.18
Sang. 751[2]	52	20	0.38	20	0.38	40	0.77	10	0.19
MC 69	87	24	0.28	32	0.37	56	0.65	31	0.35
Bamberg 2	92	28	0.30	33	0.36	61	0.66	31	0.34
PP Flor-Prag.	137	44	0.32	52	0.38	96	0.70	41	0.30

1 The *Medicina Plinii*, ed. Önnerfors (1964) also contains two remedies with no ingredients.
2 The *Physica Plinii Sangallensis*, ed. Önnerfors (2006–7) also contains two remedies with no ingredients.

(Goat's milk or rabbit brain smeared on the gums renders dentation easier.)

Medicina Plinii **(1.14.2)**: *Lacte caprino aut leporino cerbello gingiuae perfricantur.*[54]

(Goat's milk and/or rabbit brain are rubbed all over the gums.)

Bamberg 1 (c. 41, f. 25r): *Lacte caprino et leporis cerebro gingiuae perfricantur.*[55]

(Goat's milk and rabbit brain are rubbed all over the gums.)

Sang. 751 (c. 8, p. 200): *Caprino lactae uel leporis cerebello gingiuas refrica.*[56]

(Rub goat's milk or rabbit brain on the gums.)

MC 69 (c. 41, p. 49b): *Lacte caprino et leporis. cerebro. gingiue. perfricantur.*[57]

(Goat's milk and rabbit brain are rubbed all over the gums.)

Bamberg 2 (c. 41.1, f. 150r): *Lacte caprinum et leporis cerebrum gingiue perfricantur.*[58]

(Goat's milk and rabbit brain are rubbed all over the gums.)

PP Flor-Prag (1.42.1): *Lacte caprino et leporis cerebro gingiue perfricantur.*[59]

(Goat's milk and rabbit brain are rubbed all over the gums.)

This recipe shows a basic formula ('*X uel Y* + *verb*') that is also seen in many other examples: it is a spare listing of two basic ingredients given in an either/or pattern, with a single verb of instruction and a brief clause detailing how the ingredients are to be used.[60] This recipe is one of the few found in all six collections as well as the *Natural History*.[61] As the similarities in the various redactions show, even in the more erratic witness in Sang. 751, this recipe was rather resistant to change, a feature aided no doubt by the readily

[54] *Medicina Plinii*, ed. Önnerfors (1964) 22. See Langslow (2000: 324) for a discussion of the use of *cerebellum* (as 'animal brain') as opposed to *cerebrum* ('human brain').

[55] Stoll (1992: 146). [56] Önnerfors (2006–7: 16).

[57] Montecassino, Arch. dell'Abbazia, cod. 69, p. 49b. [58] Önnerfors (1964: 60).

[59] Winkler (1984: 192).

[60] The only thing out of character in this particular example is the missing *Item* which usually begins preparations.

[61] Indeed, this is itself a statement on the very mutability of these collections, and what appears to be a rather high level of choice in copying portions of text as space, time, interest, and so on allow. It also alludes to the undoubtedly large number of copies of recipes that likely existed in the early Middle Ages that unfortunately have not survived.

understood and perhaps even easily procured ingredients and simple instructions. Considering the short *Natural History* passage from which this recipe was adapted, the subsequent redactions have trimmed the language even further.[62]

However, despite the fact that simple one- and two-ingredient recipes remain the majority in all copies of the *Physica Plinii*, there is a considerable shift from such simple recipes in favour of three- and four-plus ingredient recipes. The recipe detailed next is not found in the either the *Medicina Plinii* or the *Physica Plinii* copies in Bamberg 1 or Sang. 751, but it does appear in the *Physica* tradition in MC 69 and Bamberg 2 copies of the late ninth and early tenth centuries as well as the PP Flor-Prag redactions:

> **MC 69 (c. 36.7, p. 47b)**: *Item. denti. fricium. ad idem. folii. ÷ I. ungelle. marine. ÷ I. masticis. afre. ÷ I. ostrearum. testa. numero. IIII. pumicis. ÷ I. panis. conbusti. ÷ I. cyperu. ÷ I omnia. in puluerem. redacta commiscis. ex eo. dentes. fricas.*[63]
>
> (Another dentifrice for the same: cloves, 1 ounce; 'sea hoof', 1 ounce; African mastic, 1 ounce; 4 oyster shells; pumice, 1 ounce; burned bread, 1 ounce; galingale, 1 ounce; with everything reduced to a powder, mix together and rub the teeth with it.)
>
> **Bamberg 2 (c. 36.8, f. 147r–v)**: *Item dentifricium addidem: folii ÷ I, ungelle marine ÷ I, masticis afre ÷ I, ostreorum testa numero IIII, pumicis ÷ I, panis conbusti ÷ I, ciperu ÷ I: omnia in puluere redacta commiscis, ex eo dentes fricas.*[64]
>
> (Another dentifrice for the same: cloves, 1 ounce; 'sea hoof', 1 ounce; African mastic, 1 ounce; 4 oyster shells; pumice, 1 ounce; burned bread, 1 ounce; galingale, 1 ounce; with everything reduced to a powder, mix together and rub the teeth with it.)
>
> **PP Flor-Prag (1.37.8)**: *Item dentifricium ad hec: folii unciam I, yo unciam I, masticis afre I, ostree testas numero IIII, pumicis unciam I, panis combusti I, cyperi I: omnia in puluerem redacta commisces, et ex aceto dentes fricabis.*[65]

[62] In a process which was outlined earlier in this chapter, this trimming is compensated by the chapter heading *Dentitioni* or something similar, so the meaning is not lost. However, in Sang. 751, the dental recipes are all in a single chapter, so in that collection, it is not clear that this remedy is for teething in infants; therefore, unless the reader was familiar with other exemplars, this recipe has simply become another general recipe for gums/teeth.

[63] Montecassino, Arch. dell'Abbazia, cod. 69, p. 47b.

[64] Önnerfors (1975: 58).

[65] Winkler (1984: 182–3).

(Another dentifrice for this purpose: cloves, 1 ounce; violet, 1 ounce; African mastic, 1 ounce; 4 oyster shells; pumice, 1 ounce; burned bread, 1; galingale, 1; with everything reduced to a powder, mix it together and with a bit of vinegar, rub the teeth.)

This particular recipe is substantively different from the example above in both format and content. It is a specific medicament, provided with a more formal pharmaceutical name, here identified as a *dentifricium*, and contains a more complex arrangement of seven ingredients, each with specified amounts and symbols for units of measurement (*unciae*), as well as decidedly more complicated instructions for preparation and administration involving several steps. There are some more exotic-sounding *materia medica* present, from the difficult-to-identify *folium*, evidently some kind of aromatic leaf, perhaps clove, to the specification of 'African' mastic (*masticis afre*).[66] There are also several marine *materia medica*, including oyster shells and the enigmatic *ungelle marine* (literally, 'sea hoof') in both the MC 69 and Bamberg 2 versions.[67]

The PP Flor-Prag edition of the later medieval witnesses contains several even more complicated recipes of multiple ingredients not found in any of the earlier witnesses. The recipe that follows includes a formal nomenclature identifying the preparation as an *acopum calefactorium* (warming pain reliever/anodyne), two attestations of its value and efficacy (*ualde summum* and elsewhere *ualde prodest*), a listing of multiple medical applications for the remedy, and a long list of required ingredients:[68]

PP Flor-Prag (1.38.3): *Item acopum calefactorium et ualde summum, facit enim ad eas ualitudines que diuturne sunt: ad paraliticos, scyaticos*[69] *et*

[66] See Everett (2012: 231, n. 1) for discussion of *folium*. Everett gives 'leaf of Malabar' as a translation but is uncertain. He also summarises the disagreement among scholars as to what this ingredient is, as the term seems to alternately indicate a number of different aromatic plants, including patchouli, and spikenard, in addition to malabar. Green (2001: 279) translates *folium* as clove in the *Trotula*. On *folium* in Latin/'φύλλον' in Greek, see Kokoszko and Rzeźnicka (2018), who argue that this should be identified with Malabar leaf.

[67] See the compelling discussion on the meaning of *ungella marina* by Burridge (2020: 234–5). There, in a discussion of different animal-based aromatics, she suggests that *ungella marina* is a kind of mollusc and might be linked to *onycha*, one of the ingredients of the consecrated incense used in the Temple of Solomon. Perhaps the *ungella marina* refers to the operculum, or 'trap door' of some sea snails. The early modern Italian scientist and medical thinker Antonio Vallisneri commented on a pharmaceutical material called *unghia marina*, which he connected to the Latin forms *ungula marina* and Greek *sōlēn* and described as a bivalve mollusc that resembles a fingernail or hoof in colour and material. See Vallisneri (1733: 477). Pliny mentions the *sōlēn*, also called the *onychas* at several points; see *Natural History*, 32.32.103 and 32.53.151, ed. Mayhoff (1897) 84 and 102.

[68] Langslow (2000: 494). On efficacy statements, see also Gottlieb (Chapter 6), Lewicka (Chapter 9), and Chipman (Chapter 10) in this volume.

[69] See Langslow (1991: 567 and 2000: 486): *Ischiadicus* meaning sciatica or a disease of the hip.

opistotonicos[70] *sed et neruorum contractiones et arteticos*[71] *et ad omnem dolorem totius corporis et turpitudinem; ualde prodest. Recipit herbe bratee*[72] *dragmas XLVIII, samsuci dragmas CCLXXXVIII, rute seminis XXIIII, cardamomi XXIII, squinantii XII, cacrii*[73] *XXIIII, baccarum lauri dragmas XXIIII, piretri XXIIII, cyperi XXIIII, meliloti uncias III; hec omnia tundes et cribrabis grosso cribello et infundes in uino summo per dies tres, quarta die uero mittes oleum sauinum uel spanum*[74] *et omnia suprascripta coques cum oleo diligenter molli igne; postea exprimes omnia et in oleum mittes ceram et omnia reliqua in oleum mitti debent; postea tolles myrre et stactis dragmas XVI, cere rubee libras III, terebentine uncias VI, calami aromatici III, costi III, styracis III, yu III, piperis albi III, piperis communis III, nitri III, sinapis dragmas XLVIII, spicanardi uncias III, folii unam, afronitri III, opobalsami*[75] *sex, adipis urtuli marini VI, medulle ceruine VI, gutte ammoniace III, olei nardini libram I, olei sauini ueteris libras II, olei cyprini pondo III, olei herini pondo III, olei laurini II, olei styracini libram I; ista sequentia aromatica tundes et cribrabis et commiscebis cum omnibus suprascriptis, et cum opus fuerit uteris et super maxillam impositum sanat dentes molares.*[76]

(A warming pain reliever and certainly the best, made for those illnesses that last for a long time: for paralytics, sciatics and opisthotonics, but also contractions of the nerves, and arthritics and for all pain of the whole body and turpitude; it truly works. Take: the herb savin, 48 drachmas; marjoram, 288 drachmas; rue seed, 23; cardamom, 23; camel grass, 12; *cachrys*, 24; laurel berries, 24 drachmas; pyrethrum, 24; galingale, 24; clover, 3 ounces. Grind and sift everything through a wide sieve and pour into the best wine for three days. On the fourth day, add Sabine or Spanish oil; cook all of the above with the oil carefully with a gentle flame. Afterward, squeeze everything; place wax in the oil and all the rest should be cast in oil. After that, take myrrh and stacte, 16 drachmas; red wax, 3 pounds; terebinth, 6

[70] See Langslow (2000: 488): *Opisthotonus*: 'one of three kinds of tetanus in which the body is drawn rigidly backward'.

[71] See Langslow (1991: 491 and 2000: 479). *Arthriticus*: 'Arthritis; a sufferer from arthritis'.

[72] *Bratheos*: likely a reference to *sabinum/sauinum* – a kind of juniper. See MacKinney (1944). See also Pliny, *Natural History*, 24.61.102 ed. Mayhoff (1897) 87–8, who says *sabina* is the same as the Greek *brathy*, and useful as a substitute for frankincense. He does not mention a dental application. Note that *oleum sabinum* also appears twice in this recipe, which seems to be a geographical reference to oil from Sabinia (south-central Italy) in one instance and a reference to the aromatic oil of savin in the second based on its immediate contexts.

[73] See Pliny, *Natural History*, 24.60.101 ed. Mayhoff (1897) 87. According to Pliny, there are many different kinds of *cachrys*, which are a kind of growth found in certain plants. Again, he does not mention a dental use.

[74] MacKinney (1944: 276–88).

[75] Secretion from a balsam tree. See Green (2001: 285).

[76] Winkler (1984: 186–8). Although the recipe is unique in the *Physica Plinii* tradition, earlier collections include other examples of preparations called *acopum/acopa*, as in MC 69 with five other examples, mostly for sciatics. This particular recipe also shows some similarity to an *Acopum* recipe in the MC 69 antidotary (not part of the *Physica Plinii* text in that manuscript), pp. 350b–351a. However, the introduction of an *acopum* in the dental section in PP Flor-Prag is noteworthy.

ounces; sweet flag, 3; costus, 3; storax, 3; violet, 3; white pepper, 3; common pepper, 3; nitrum, 3; mustard, 48 drachmas; spikenard, 3 ounces; folium, 1; afronitrum, 3; opobalsamum, 6; seal fat, 6; deer marrow, 6; drops of ammoniac, 3; nard oil, 1 pound; aged savin oil, 2 pounds; cypress oil, 3 in weight; *olei herini*, 3 in weight; bay laurel oil, 2; storax oil, 1 pound. Grind and sift that arrangement of aromatics and mix together with everything written above. Use it when necessary; placed upon the cheek, it heals painful molars.)

In fact, although this *acopum* is listed as part of the chapter on molar pain, the preparation is not strictly, nor indeed even primarily for teeth. It is also recommended for a whole range of other afflictions, including paralysis, sciatica, a kind of tetanus, contractions of the nerves, arthritis, pains of the whole body, and even turpitude; the acknowledgement that it is for a dental issue at all comes only at the very end of the recipe.[77] Continuing some of the trends in pharmaceutical substances seen in the previous set of recipes, this single remedy calls for a demanding series of upwards of thirty-seven ingredients in significant quantities. Many of these ingredients also seem to strongly hint at an exotic provenance: included here are *materia medica* like cardamom, myrrh/stacte, styrax, two different kinds of pepper, afronitrum, opobalsamum, and nard oil among others. Similarly, preparation of this recipe requires several successive steps over the course of several days.

2.4 Signs of Precision

As in the recipe examples just discussed, the longer recipes of three or more ingredients often contain a range of different markers of precision than the simple one- or two-ingredient preparations. A wider consideration of patterns in the use of these markers of precision, including the employment of specific medical nomenclature for certain types of preparations and use of metrological units and their symbols, bolsters arguments about changing sensibilities in recording medical remedies.[78] The use of these two markers of precision shows an upward trajectory through the various witnesses. This trend highlights the rather unique mutability of the *Physica Plinii* tradition.[79] The *Physica Plinii*

[77] See Langslow (2000) for identification and references for these specialised terms.

[78] There are other markers too, such as the use of quantification, classical place names, non-pharmaceutical materials referenced in recipes, provision of synonyms for ingredients, and so on, but space restricts the discussion to these two listed here.

[79] In other words, this pattern does not seem to be replicated in other Pliny-derived medical texts. Copies of the *Medicina Plinii* survive from the ninth century through the later Middle Ages, and do

Table 2.6 *Relative frequencies of named preparations/medicaments, metrology, and the numbers of recipes containing such features*

Marker	*Med. Plin.*	Bamb. 1	Sang. 751	MC 69	Bamb. 2	Flor-Prag.
Nomenclature	1	3	2	10	11	15
Metrology	3	8	1	42	41	63
# of Recipes with these specifications	4 recipes	6 recipes	3 recipes	18 recipes	17 recipes	30 recipes
Percentage of total recipes	7%	16%	6%	21%	18%	22%

witnesses, however, as a malleable collection of remedies, show not only a decided transition from simple remedies to the more complex, but also corresponding changes in the use of these two markers of precision, as Table 2.6 demonstrates.[80]

As shown in Table 2.6, the dental chapters in the *Medicina Plinii* contain very few markers of precision, and the two oldest *Physica* copies in Bamberg 1 and Sang. 751 are similar in that regard. In each of these collections only 6–16 per cent of the total recipes show *any* use of medical nomenclature or metrological measurements. The fifty-seven dental recipes from the *Medicina Plinii* text feature only a single instance in which a specific pharmaceutical name was employed (a reference to a *dentifricium*) and three units of measure. Sang. 751 is more or less the same as the *Medicina Plinii* though with more metrological units, and

not seem to have such considerable shifts in terms of recipe complexity – most recipes in all witnesses seem to have a consistent simplicity. At the other end of the spectrum, *De medicamentis liber* by Marcellus contains formal pharmaceutical names, quantities and metrology, but again, little change over the course of the textual tradition; early medieval and later medieval copies of these other Plinian texts do not evince as much change over time as the *Physica Plinii*.

80 A brief comment on methodology: this is as simple as counting instances of these situations. In terms of nomenclature, I counted any references to specific names for therapeutic preparations. These were usually as recipe headings (as in *Item dentifricium*), although I also counted instances where a recipe indicated that something should be used 'like' a specific preparation or otherwise referenced a more formal medicament name. I measured metrological precision again simply by counting. I included metrological symbols as well as words for units in the Greco-Roman system of weights and measures. I did not count vague statements of measure, such as handfuls, bunches, or other similar cases. For more on medical nomenclature, see Langslow (1991, 2000). For metrology and the use of Greco-Roman system of weights and measures in medieval medical manuscripts, see Platte and Platte (1989: 76–8), and bibliographic essays by Jones (1996: 418–19) and Zupko (1996: 443–6) in Mantello and Rigg (1996). For more general notes and bibliography, see Zupko (1981).

Bamberg 1 contains a few more of these signs of precision in each category. The only formal nomenclature used in the oral and dental remedies in these three collections is the term *dentifricium*, a Latin (and not Latinised Greek) medical term.[81] The few measures, encountered as both words and symbols, tend to be Latin ones.[82]

The later receptaries in MC 69, Bamberg 2, and the Florence-Prague edition demonstrate that as the more complicated remedies proliferate, there are corresponding increases in the use of all three markers of specification, found in 23–27 per cent of the total recipes in each. The employment of a formal nomenclature of Latin and Latinised Greek therapeutic labels, especially in rubricated headings, provides a very different scholarly tone, and perhaps even something of a hierarchy of recipes in the contexts where it is used.[83] In the three later receptaries, MC 69 contains references to ten, Bamberg 2 eleven, and the Florence-Prague edition fourteen different named preparations.[84] *Dentifricia* remain the most common named medicament in the oral and dental sections in all three collections, but several other therapeutics are also introduced. The collections in MC 69 and Bamberg 2 each include the same instructions for two different kinds of tablets for toothache (*trocisci*; all are specified *ad dolorem dentis*), a recipe for a powder for humours of the teeth (*puluis ad humore dentium*).[85] A further comparison is made in one of the *trociscus* recipes to using the medicine 'in the manner of a *collyrium*' (*in modum colliri*).[86] The Florentino-Pragensis version of the text contains upwards of fourteen uses of specific therapeutic nomenclature, including all of the instances seen in the earlier MC 69 and Bamberg 2 collections, with further remedies for another powder (*pulvis ad reuma dentium*), a preparation known as a *gera*, and two remedies for *acopa* (pain relievers/anodynes); one of the latter was noted earlier as the most extensive recipe in the oral/dental section in any of the six collections.[87]

[81] Langslow (2000: 276–7) identifies *dentifricium* as one of five similar compound medical terms in Latin ('tooth' + 'rub' + '-*ium*') and explains it as a Latin calque of the Greek *odontotrimma*, a particularly early example in the development of Latin as a medical language.

[82] These measures include the *sextarius*, attested in all three receptaries, the weight of the *denarius*, and the ounce (*uncia*); there is a reference to the Greek measure *obolus* as a dosage in Bamberg 1.

[83] Langslow (2000: 76–139) provides a typology and overview of the different meanings of Greek medical terms in Latin medical texts by Celsus, Scribonius, Theodorus Priscianus, and Cassius Felix, some of which are also found in Plinian medical collections.

[84] Many of these therapeutics concentrate in the chapter titled *Ad dentes laxos* (MC 69), *Si dentes nimio capitis reumate laxaverint et dolor fuerit infesus* (Bamberg 1), or *Ad dentes laxatos* (PP Flor-Prag). This is Chapter 36 in MC 69 and Bamberg 1, but 37 in PP Flor-Prag.

[85] Langslow (2000: 510) defines a *trochiscus* as a round pill and nods to its Greek origin.

[86] See Langslow (2000: 498); a collyrium is typically an eye salve and is also from a Greek word.

[87] The recipe for the *gera* is found in the chapter on gums but is also recommended for a number of other complaints: *Item gera que facit ad os cui reuma molestum est, et ad gingiuas reumatizantes, siue ad*

The increased use of Greco-Roman metrological units and their symbols in MC 69, Bamberg 2, and even more so in PP Flor-Prag, also changes the look of the collections.[88] Metrological precision in the dental remedies of MC 69 (which contains forty-two units), Bamberg 2 (forty-one) and PP Flor-Prag (sixty-three) tends to concentrate in the same recipes that also have formal therapeutic names.[89] In these three collections, metrological precision is expressed through a combination of symbols and words for a wide range of units. In all three, the *uncia* (ounce) is most frequently attested, followed by the *semuncia* (half-ounce) in MC 69 and Bamberg 2 and the *dragma* (drachma or dram) in the PP Flor-Prag edition. Other units for dry and liquid weight such as the *obolus* (obol), *libra* (pound), *cyatus*, *sextarius*, *scripulus* (scruple), and *cotila*/*cotyla* are also present, but less frequently encountered.

2.5 *Materia Medica*

The oral and dental remedies in these six receptaries exhibit considerable changes in the number, type, and quality of the ingredients they recommend. Using a series of tables, three principal observations regarding these changes are briefly summarised: (1) the number of ingredients and kinds of *materia medica* employed in dental remedies tends to increase in later collections; (2) the majority of ingredients are recommended only once, but that majority decreases over time; and (3) certain ingredients come to be favoured over others, appearing in a number of different dental preparations in later collections. All of these trends suggest that compilers seem to prize not only a diversity of the kinds of ingredients recommended, but also a subtly developing emphasis on certain ingredients that have distinctive similarities, both in terms of perceived geographic origin and therapeutic qualities, as particularly effective in oral and dental applications. In short, the ingredients that become the most prevalent in these remedies are those with exotic origins and a combination of astringent, styptic, and calefacient properties.

The first important observation, demonstrated in Table 2.7, is that the number of ingredients and types of *materia medica* employed in dental and

uuam, uel quibus pus exit de auribus. Langslow (2000: 503) says *hiera*, another Latinised Greek word meaning 'sacred', was 'a name given to various antidotes', as reported in Scribonius and elsewhere.

88 Weddell (2010: 897–919) gives a good bibliographic overview.

89 The need for interpreting these metrological units and making conversions between them is also seen in some of these manuscripts by the inclusion of treatises on weights and measures. Montecassino 69, for example, contains an elaborate set of metrological conversions between Greco-Roman units in a series of short treatises on pages 537a–544a.

Table 2.7 *Numbers of ingredients overall in the oral/dental chapters (total) in comparison with number of unique ingredients (individual* materia medica *substances counted separately) referenced in each collection*

Collection	*Med. Plin.*	Bamb. 1	Sang. 751	MC 69	Bamb. 2	Flor-Prag.
Total number of recipes	57	38	52	87	92	137
Total ingredients	92	73	90	228	231	368
Individual *materia medica*	60	58	62	111	115	204

oral recipes increases significantly and at a rate faster than the increase of remedies themselves from collection to collection, which seems to indicate that compilers are seeking out pharmaceutical diversity over time. As might be expected, the recipe collections that contain larger numbers of recipes not only recommend more ingredients overall, but also a more diverse array of substances.[90] Altogether, at least 1,084 ingredients are prescribed in the oral and dental chapters in these six collections, but many of these are obviously repeated from copy to copy and even recipe to recipe. Whereas dental chapters in the *Medicina Plinii* and the early *Physica Plinii* copies in Bamberg 1 and Sang. 751 each contain around 60 unique *materia medica*, these 60 items are recommended about ninety times in the recipes of both (92 ingredients in *Medicina Plinii* and 90 in Sang. 751), but only seventy-three times in Bamberg 1. The *Physica Plinii* copies in MC 69 and Bamberg 2 both have between 111 and 115 different *materia medica* in each collection that are prescribed a total of around 230 times in recipes. Finally, the dental remedies of PP Flor-Prag reference 204 unique types of *materia medica*, all recommended a total of 368 times.

The second important point about changes in the ingredients of all six collections, shown in Table 2.8, is that most of the *materia medica* in each

[90] There are several further methodological problems. As the example of the dentifrice at the beginning of the chapter demonstrates, a single ingredient can change in subsequent redactions to very different things. In such situations, I have erred on the side of diversity and counted these as separate ingredients rather than trying to second-guess the many, many scribes' possible intentions. Further, some things occupy a grey area between *materia medica* and tools, instruments, and vessels. For example, references to objects such as linen cloth as a bandage or to bowls and other dishes can be found both in the dental remedies and elsewhere, but unless there is an explicit reference to these objects' use as a material component in a remedy, I have tended not to count them.

Table 2.8 *Ingredients that appear only once in the collection of dental and oral remedies, expressed as figures and percentages*

Collection	*Med. Plin.*	Bamb. 1	Sang. 751	MC 69	Bamb. 2	Flor-Prag.
Individual *materia medica*	60	58	62	111	115	204
Ingredients appearing only once	44	41	47	71	78	115
Percentage of Total	73%	71%	76%	64%	68%	56%

collection are recommended only once, but the number of such one-off ingredients as a percentage of the whole declines over time, which suggests that the interest in ingredient diversity alluded to earlier has a limit. In the *Medicina Plinii*, and then also in the *Physica* copies in Bamberg 1 and Sang. 751, just under three-quarters of the total number of recommended ingredients for dental preparations appear only once in each collection. In the *Physica* copies of MC 69 and Bamberg 2, this frequency is slightly lower, at just 64 per cent in the former and 68 per cent in the latter. Finally, in the PP Flor-Prag version, although the number of one-off ingredients is 115 out of 378 total ingredients, the total percentage of such ingredients is only 56 per cent, a significant drop.

As the frequency of one-off ingredients tends to decline as a percentage in the dental sections of later receptaries, the third observation is that there is a corresponding increase in the frequency of recommendations for certain ingredients over others. In all collections, the most prevalent ingredients are liquids, including wine, vinegar, and honey, all used as bases for other materials. As Table 2.9 shows, the *Medicina Plinii*, Bamberg 1, and Sang. 751 are all similar in that they feature very few repeated recommendations for any of their *materia medica*. In the dental preparations in the *Medicina Plinii*, the most prevalent ingredient is mulberry (but with only four citations), followed by common plantain, worms, and goose fat.[91] The dental section of Bamberg 1 contains even fewer repeated

[91] Ingredient identification is obviously difficult and approximate, but an incredible array of resources are now available. Opsomer (1989) has provided a directory of *materia medica* in early medieval Latin medical texts; Everett (2012) has provided identification of the ingredients in the *Alphabetum Galieni*

recommendations; no ingredients are recommended more than twice, in fact, and in Sang. 751, the only ingredient cited more than twice is lentisk (*lentiscus*, with five references). The three collections of dental remedies in MC 69, Bamberg 2, and PP Flor-Prag all show divergent patterns. They each contain an array of ingredients that are prescribed multiple times in different recipes. The most frequently prescribed *materia medica* in the dental prescriptions in these latter copies of the text include myrrh (*murra*), saffron (*crocus*), salt (*sal*), pepper (*piper*), and nut-gall (*galla*), but also, a bit less frequently, pomegranate (*malum granatum*), mastic (*mastiche*), *folium*, and *costus*.[92] Alum (*alumen*, especially in the copies in Bamberg 2 and PP Flor-Prag) and pennyroyal (*pulegium*, especially in MC 69) are additional ingredients that are employed with increasing frequency in the collections.[93]

These particular *materia medica* that become the most prevalent in the latter three collections follow very deliberate patterns as well: in the first place, they are items that largely appear to be exotic in origin (at least from an Italian/northern Mediterranean perspective).[94] While it is undeniable that most of the ingredients in any of these collections appear to be local, a quick review of the items recommended the most in the dental preparations in MC 69, Bamberg 2, and PP Flor-Prag in Table 2.9 shows an unmistakeable emphasis on items that may have rather more distant provenance. Establishing what 'exotic' or 'local' actually means in a medieval recipe collection copied from late antique sources is fraught with a multitude of complications, but other popular herbal literature of the Middle Ages such as the *Alphabetum Galieni* can give an idea of the geographical associations of certain *materia medica*.[95] Nut galls are usually specified as Alexandrian, African, or Asian/Syrian in the

with additional bibliography and commentary. Another resource is the *materia medica* list for the remedies in the *Trotula* in Green (2001: 137–64).

92 This assumption is based on the geographic origin of the extant manuscripts of the *Physica Plinii*.

93 These changes in ingredients in the *Physica Plinii* can be compared to other findings on trade and movement of ingredients in the medieval Mediterranean, as, for example, in Lev (2007), who studied Genizah documents from the eleventh through fourteenth centuries and noted the most prevalent ingredients held and sold by Jewish merchants of Cairo included myrobalans, pepper, saffron, lentisk, almond, basil, rose, rosemary, cattle products, camphor, and spikenard.

94 While Scarborough (1986: 61) assumes an Italian milieu for the perspective on ingredients in the *Natural History*, it is best not to universalise this to all the recipe collections based on Pliny. Still, the context of production of manuscript copies of the *Physica Plinii*, where known, seems to indicate a primarily Italian environment.

95 See also McCormick (2001: 708–19) for more about changes in *materia medica* in medical manuscripts. Freedman (2008: 50–75) gives an overview of exotic spices as medicines. Everett (2012) is again helpful, as the *Alphabetum Galieni* often includes geographical information on its *materia medica*, which can demonstrate perceptions of exotic origins, and in some cases, even circulated in contexts very close to those of the *Physica Plinii*. See also the opening chapters of Miller (1969), which provides a census of spices and incense from around the Roman Empire and beyond but is based solely on classical-era sources. Other works on spices include Donkin (2003), Keay (2006), and Nabhan (2014).

Table 2.9 *The most common ingredients in the oral and dental remedies of each collection (with frequency of citations in each collection in parentheses)*

Collection	*Med. Plin.*	Bamb. 1	Sang. 751	MC 69	Bamb. 2	Flor-Prag.
Most common *materia medica*	Mulberry (4)	Plantain (2)	Lentisk (5)	Salt (7)	Salt (7)	Myrrh (11)
	Plantain (3)	Galls (2)	Myrtle (2)	Myrrh (6)	Myrrh (6)	Saffron (10)
	Worms (3)	Pepper (2)	Salt (2)	Saffron (5)	Saffron (5)	Salt (10)
	Goose fat (3)	Asparagus (2)	Arnoglossa (2)	Galls (5)	Galls (5)	Pepper (8)
	Goat milk (2)	Goat milk (2)	Plantain (2)	Ivy (5)	Ivy (5)	Galls (6)
	Amurca (2)		Goat milk (2)	Pepper (5)	Pepper (5)	Alumen (6)
	Lentisk (2)			Pomegranate (4)	Pomegranate (4)	Wild fig (3)
	Myrrh (2)			Pennyroyal (4)	Mastic (4)	Pumice (3)
				Mastic (4)	Folium (4)	
				Folium (4)	Costus (4)	
				Costus (4)	Alumen (4)	

recipes themselves.[96] But for many of the other more prevalent ingredients encountered in the dental remedies of the latter three collections, the *Alphabetum Galieni* suggests a long-distance provenance. As an example, myrrh (*murra*), which the *Alphabetum Galieni* says comes from Arabia (*quae maxime in Arabia inuenitur*), is employed twice in the *Medicina Plinii*, but is found six times in MC 69 and Bamberg 2, and then eleven times in PP Flor-Prag. Other ingredients show similar patterns, including pepper (*piper*) and *folium* which are understood to come from India (*quae in India nascitur*); mastic (*mastiche*), which comes from the island of Chios (*in Chio insula nascitur*); costus (*costum*), from a number of locations from around the Mediterranean and beyond; and alum, sourced from Melos (or Nylos, according to one manuscript copy), Egypt, and Macedonia.[97]

These more prevalent ingredients in the latter three *Physica Plinii* collections also show a second pattern: in addition to the emphasis on materials sourced from distant places, there is also a therapeutic consistency that seems to be developing in these particular ingredients as well. Again, using the *Alphabetum Galieni* to explain hidden theoretical assumptions of the recipe compilers, many of the prevalent ingredients in the six collections exhibit a narrow range of three therapeutic qualities as astringents, calefacients, and styptics.[98] Even in the *Medicina Plinii*, some of the repeated ingredients possess these same qualities; according to the *Alphabetum Galieni*, lentisk and myrrh are both styptic and warming, mulberry, and plantain are astringent, while *amurca* (amorge, or olive lees) is identified as styptic.[99] But this therapeutic emphasis is amplified considerably in the latter collections. Of the most prevalent ingredients in MC 69 and Bamberg 2, the *Alphabetum Galieni* identifies myrrh and folium as both calefacient and styptic, and pepper as both calefacient and astringent. Salt, pomegranate, costus, and alumen are all described as strongly astringent materials, along with the pennyroyal in MC 69. Mastic and costus are two further calefacients and saffron is identified as styptic.[100]

[96] The *Physica Plinii* copies sometimes give information on origins of certain *materia medica* in other recipes and chapters, as, for example, in c. 89 (*Ad uentrem temperandum*), where the ingredient *mirubalanus* is said to originate from Egypt.

[97] Myrrh (*AG*, 180, ed. Everett, 2012: 280–1); Pepper (*AG* 209: 306–7); Folium (*AG* 111: 230–1); Mastic (*AG* 186: 284–5); Costus is said to come from a number of places, and the *Alphabetum Galieni* ranks the quality based on geography: Crete, Egypt, Arabia, India, and Syria (*AG* 64: 194–5); Alum (*AG* 7: 148–9); Crocus (*AG* 44: 176–7).

[98] *Alphabetum Galieni*, ed. Everett (2012).

[99] Lentisk (*AG* 151, ed. Everett, 2012: 260–1); Myrrh (*AG* 180: 280–1); Mulberry (*AG* 194: 290–1); Plantain (*AG* 217: 312–3); Amurca (*AG* 18: 158–9).

[100] The chapter headings after all often address physical situations such as loose teeth or too much saliva in the mouth, which may have led to recipes full of ingredients known for their binding and

All of these patterns suggest that the ingredient changes we see are not random or mistakes, but that the compilers of the latter collections are including new recipes with ingredients that subtly express changing ideas regarding ingredient origins and their perceived effectiveness against assorted oral and dental maladies. Clearly, this pattern is most pronounced in the latest collection, PP Flor-Prag, written well after the eleventh-century introduction of the Arabic *materia medica*, as it contains the widest array of ingredients in the largest number of recipes. However, even the ninth- and tenth-century witnesses, especially MC 69 and Bamberg 2, contain a significant array of *materia medica* increasingly recommended for oral and dental remedies such as myrrh, pepper, saffron, and clove – items that could be procured only in Italy through long-distance Mediterranean trade networks.

2.6 Conclusion

Assumptions about remedies, precision, *materia medica*, and, ultimately, about efficacy, are changing in significant ways as reflected in these six redactions of Plinian-inspired recipe collections. While the *Medicina Plinii* remains a fairly conservative and consistent work in its own transmission history, the *Physica Plinii*, whether because of the more convoluted relationship with its source material in Pliny's *Natural History*, or further (mostly invisible) factors of its contexts of production, is a more changeable and dynamic collection. Still, reflecting on these investigations, two further observations on change and continuity in the tradition are worth mentioning.

The first observation is that much more work needs to be done to contextualise the different redactions of the *Medicina Plinii* and *Physica Plinii*. It is important to remember that while there are relationships between these collections, there is still much to explore and understand. Of course, we must not forget that the *Medicina Plinii* and its pithier remedies were themselves copied throughout the Middle Ages, and by no means died out with the proliferation of the expanded *Physica Plinii* productions. Beyond the story of the shifts in these ingredients is a deeper narrative of academic, practical, cultural choices being made at the centres that produced these various manuscript copies. What mechanisms governed the creation of a copy of the *Medicina Plinii* as opposed to the *Physica Plinii*, especially in the wake of the Carolingian Renaissance? Obviously, access to texts plays

astringent properties. Similarly, there is also the Hippocratic *Aphorism* (Section 5.18): 'Cold is bad for the bones, teeth, nerves, brain, and the spinal cord; heat is good for these structures.' See Lloyd (1978: 223).

a significant role, but so too does wealth, access to resources and power, intellectual/scholarly aspirations, and a host of other issues and concerns that demand further study.

The second observation is that despite all the fluctuations in the ingredients of dental remedies in the ninth-century collections and even later, very few of the materials, if anything (at least in these chapters), are actually completely 'new' to the Latin medical tradition even if they are gaining new applications in dental remedies. In fact, even with the new complicated recipes added to the PP Flor-Prag version, that collection retains a strongly Plinian character. Almost every ingredient charted in the dental remedies was already mentioned at some point somewhere in the *Natural History*, or at least in other *Physica Plinii* remedies for other conditions. But what is true in many of these new recipes added to the tradition is that older, known ingredients are being redeployed in new dental and oral applications whilst simultaneously being given new properties and purposes. As we have seen, some ingredients, such as myrrh, salt, pepper, and galls became strongly associated with dental remedies over the course of the six collections, even if they do not completely replace the remedies of local ingredients that came before them. This sort of creative rethinking and redeployment of ingredients that may have been relatively exotic in Pliny but still well known enough for other medicinal purposes was no doubt an important precursor to an even more substantial interaction with entirely new classes of ingredients in the eleventh century and after.

Appendix

Physica Plinii Chapters 28–41 on Oral and Dental Health from Montecassino, Archivio dell'Abbazia, Cod. 69. pp. 42b–49b

What follows is a transcription of the recipes of the fourteen chapters on oral and dental afflictions contained in the first receptary of Montecassino, Archivio Dell'Abbazia, Cod. 69 identified by Sergio Sconocchia as a witness of the *Physica Plinii.* There are obviously many variations between spellings of certain words, especially of names of diseases, herbs, or other medical ingredients, sometimes even in the same chapter or recipe.

In general, I have aimed at a diplomatic transcription, preserving the punctuation, spelling, and structure of the recipes as they are presented in the manuscript, and I have refrained from correction and interpolation except in particularly troublesome passages. Even then, my priority has been to capture what is present in the manuscript in my transcription, leaving my ruminations, reflections, and comparisons for the footnotes. I have only compared the lexicon with other editions when complications arose. I have opted to expand many abbreviations using orthographical conventions observed elsewhere, but I have left all units of measurement, numerals, and other symbols (with the exception of the ampersand, which is always expanded) exactly as they appear as in the text. The original recipe collection has numbered chapters, but the recipes within each chapter are unnumbered; I have taken the step of numbering these recipes (in brackets) to aid in future comparison and research and have relied strictly upon codicological cues in the manuscript as my guide for the delineation of each preparation.

Style guide

-*m*	Expansion of abbreviation
[1], [m]	Addition/correction/emendation not in manuscript
\ite/	Interlinear insertion
(10b)	Page and column
~~Capitis~~	Erasure

Common symbols and abbreviations

ɜ:	Denarius
Z, <, d. or dr:	Drachma
hb.:	Herba
lib.:	Libra
÷, scrip.:	Scripulus
Σ, £:	Semuncia
ff, or sext.:	Sextarius

XXVIII. Ad Uitium. Oris.[101]

[28.1] Sepiaru*m*. ossa. in cinere. (43a) redacta. et. ori sparsa. uitia. emendat.

[28.2] Item. coclearu*m*. uacuaru*m*. cinis. cu*m* murra. tritus. hac sparsus. uitia. oris. emendat.[102]

[101] Chapter numbers and titles are given in orange ink, written with uncial letters, with the main text of the recipes written in dark brown/black ink in Beneventan script. The first recipe of each chapter is given a hollow capital initial in brown outline infilled with solid compartments of green, orange, and cream of three to five lines in height (c. 32 *Ad fetorem oris* and c. 36 *Si dentes nimio capitis reumate laxaverint et dolor fuerit infestu* have the two largest initials at five lines each). Each successive recipe is accorded with a separate *littera notabilior*, usually an *I* for *Item* in the left margin in orange ink.

[102] Bamberg 2 (c. 31) has an additional preparation here: *Ad ranulam oris: eruginem campana, alumen cata modicum cum uino modicum: pone sub lingua, et gargarizet.*

[28.3] Item. sinapis. semen. siue. rafani. ex. uino. decoctu*m*. uno. obolo. datu*m*. emendat.

[28.4] Item. herba. ciclaminos. tritam. trociscos. facies. aequales. ex his. cu*m* opus. fuerit. ex aceto. ad crassitudinem. mellis. inlitu*m*. reprimet. sanat.

XXIX. Ad Ulcera. Oris.

[29.1] Caprinum. femu*m*. cu*m* melle. tritum. et litu*m*. sanat.

[29.2] Item. cucurbite. ortulane. exuste. puluere*m*. piper. sal. candidu*m*. rute. parum. satureiam. coriandri. mentam. exusta. similiter. caput. sarde. conbustu*m*. haec omnia. in puluerem. redacta. commisces. deinde. lauas. os. uino. ueteri. et sic. inponis.

[29.3] Item. plantaginis. sucus. emendat. uel. radix. com. mastucata. (43b)

[29.4] Item. hedere. uacas. cu*m* cassia. et murra. pari. pondere. ex uino. commanducata. ulcera. oris. emendant.

[29.5] Item. morenaru*m*. ex capite. earum. cinus. cum melle. inlinitur.

[29.6] Item. ulcera. et rimas. seuu*m*. bobis. et uituli. cu*m* adipe. anseris.

XXX. Ad Uulnera. Oris. Siue Tumore. Gingiuaru*m*.

[30.1] Aprotanum. uiridem. teris. diligenter. cu*m* melle. misces. tangis. loca. de intus. quae dolet. et de foris. ubi. tumor est. apponis. et mirabiliter. curat.

[30.2] Item. ad oris. uulnera. uel gingiuarum. in mustum. dulcem. recens. mittis. malum. granatu*m*. siccu*m*. plenu*m*. et alterum. uiride. cu*m* cortice. et coquis. in stagnato. ad carbones. ut spissitudinem. mellis. adsumat. Leuas. de foco. et addes. murre. et stiptiterice.[103] scistis. puluerem. tenuissimum. commiscis. ex eo. uulnera. linis. (44a)

XXXI. Ad Putredinem. Oris. Lingue. Siue Palati. Et Ad Gingibas. Que Ab Humore. Comeduntur.[104]

[31.1] Aluminis. scissi. ÷ I. galle. asiane. ÷ IS. murre. ÷ II. piperis. grana. XV. mellis dispumati. ÷ VIIII. colligis. et uteris.

[103] Bamberg 2 (c. 30) has *stiptirie* here.

[104] The table of capitula of this manuscript (p. 7b) gives a shortened chapter title: *XXXI. Ad putredinem oris lingue siue palati.*

[31.2] Item. ad usturam*m*. moris. ex humore. crocum. cu*m*. nucleo. et aqua. frigida. tritum. in ore. teneat. quod si uulnera. fecerit. paru*m* mellis. adiungis.

[31.3] Item. ad usturam. oris. aut angenarum. uel. gingiuarum. sucum. caulis. cum. mel. gargarizari. expedit. statim. ulcera. sanat.[105]

[31.4] Item. si. feruentia. os. exusserit. intus. continuo. sanatur. gargarizatione. lactis. canini.

[31.5] Item. cui. os. ab humore exusserit uel. papulatum cantabru*m*. coquito. eius. aqua. in ore. gargarizato. quod. si ardor. fuerit. cu*m*. ipsa. aqua crocu*m*. terito. (44b) si autem. et humor. habundauerit. rosa. sicca. cu*m* furfure. coquito. et ita gargarizato.

[31.6] Item. ad putredine*m*. oris. aloe. drag*ma*. I. uinu*m*. et mel. quantum. sufficit.

XXXII. Ad Fetorem. Oris.

[32.1] Folia. fagi. com. manducata. emendat.

[32.2] Item. poleium. et syrpillu*m*. siccum. co*m*manducatum. bene. facit.

[32.3] Item. uadens. dormitu*m*. aceto. bono. os. lauet.

[32.4] Item. mastice. commasticet. et uino. suaui. os colluat.

[32.5] Item. murinus. cinis. cu*m* melle. dentibus. infricatur.

[32.6] Item. folia. myrte. et lentisci. pari. pondere. et galle. syriace. dimidium. pondus. simul. tere. et asp*er* sauino. uetusto. matutinis. mandere.

[32.7] Item. si alitus. fetet. cu*m* dormitu*m*. uadit. aceti. boni. cyatu*m*. p*er* partes. sorbeat. prode est. quod si. et plenetico. hoc. dederis. in paucis. diebus. sanus erit. (45a)

[32.8] Item. hedere. bace. cum cassia. et murra. pari. pondere. ex uino.[106]

[32.9] Item. serpillu*m*. herba. quae gallice. lauriu. dicitur. ieiunus commanducet. et gluttiat.

[32.10] Item. ad eos. quibus. subitus humor. fetorem facit. siue. putridinem. gingiuarum. ita. ut dentes cadant. quod grece. elpe dicitur. hiu. ÷ I. cum mellis. ÷ VI. coquis. bene. tritum. et curabis.

105 Bamberg 2 (c. 32) has an additional preparation inserted here: *Item cepe manducantur, quia sanant.*

106 This recipe is the same as XXVIIII.4 above but note the words *commanducata. ulcera. oris. emendant* are missing.

XXXIII. Ad Ossa. Liuosu*m* Et Liuidum.[107]

[33.1] Lentisci. fasces. in umbra. siccatum. tunde. et cribla. de cortice. pini. trito. et criblato. tantundem. facis. miscis. et dentes. fricas.

[33.2] Item. origanu*m*. teris. cribras. et exinde. dentes. gingiuas. quae fricas. hoc et tumore*m*. gingiuaru*m*. et pallorem. easque. sanguinantes. emendant.

[33.3] Item. ad gingiuaru*m*. dolore*m*. (45b) et tumorem. camemelli. h*er*b*e*. tuse. puluere. uino. mixtum. coque. donec. ad dimidiu*m* ueniat. ex eo. os. conlauatur. statim. medetur.

XXXIV. Ad Os. Et Labra.

[34.1] Os. album. et teneru*m*. ne rugosu*m*. fiat. farina*m*. candidam. lacte. et oleo. aspargito. inde. cum dormitu*m*. ibis. labra. subungito.

[34.2] Item. labra. si fuerint. rupta. puleium. ex acito. misces. et cum. dormito. uadis. exinde. tangito.

[34.3] Item. adeps. ansarinus. aut. galline. rimas. labioru*m*. emendat.

[34.4] Item. membrana. ouoru*m*. uel. cruda. uel. cocta. detracta. labrorum. fissuris. medentur.

[34.5] Item. labroru*m*. ulcera. et lingue. hirundinis. sanat. in mulso. decocte.

XXXV. Ad Dentiu*m*. Dolorem.[108]

[35.1] Asparagi. siluatici. radix. in uino. dequoquitur. id. in ore continetur. et dolorem sedat. sucus eius. similiter facit.[109]

[35.2] Item. brassica. commasticatum dolorem. facillime. sedat.

[35.3] Item. hedere. radicem. coques. (46a) in mero. puro. quod in ore. tenes. et transit. dolor.

[107] The table of capitula gives *XXXIII Ad ossa liuosum et liuidum* without any puncti, but the orthography is the same as the heading here; this has been corrected in the Bamberg 2 edition to *Ad os saliuosum et liuidum*.

[108] The table of capitula is just slightly different: *XXXV. Ad dentiu*m *dolore*.

[109] Bamberg 2 (c. 35) and PP Flor-Prag. (c. 36) give *sucus eius similiter facit* as a separate remedy. Bamberg 1 (c. 35), however, is like MC 69 here in combining them into one.

[35.4] Item. sucu*m*. hedere. cu*m* aceto. et paruo. sale. in diuersa*m* narem. mittis.

[35.5] Item. tymu*m*. et pyretrum. pari. pondere. tusum. denti. adicies.

[35.6] Item. peretri. radix. et posca. et melle. gargarizatur. et tenetur. in ea. parte. qua dolet.

[35.7] Item. ad dentiu*m*. prioru*m*. dolorem. cupressi. pipulas.[110] in uino. decoctas. ex eodem uino. tepidum. in ore. tenetur. et sanatur.

[35.8] Item. cucurbite. satis bene. decocte. sucus. dolorem. inibet. et mobilitatem. stabili. tinore.[111] conpressus.

[35.9] Item. cyperi. puluerem. dentes. et gingiua. replet.

[35.10] Item. radix. pentafilli cu*m* aceto. aut. cu*m* uino. decocta. in ore. continetur.

[35.11] Item. quinquefoliu*m*. cu*m* sua. radice. in aceto. uel. uino. coctu*m*. dentibus. continetur.

[35.12] Item. adicies. in olla. acetum. satureiam. et \sale/ ~~in uno~~[112] in uno. ferueant. et maxilla. (46b) contenebis.

[35.13] Item. fenuculu*m*. uiridem. masticet. et sucum. conteneat.

[35.14] Item. tus. et bacelauri. in uino. deferbeant. et in ore. sustineat. quamdiu. potuerit.

[35.15] Item. stiptiria. < II. strutiu. < I. tere. et utere.

[35.16] Item. uiola*m*. siccam. ex uino. coques. et calidu*m*. ori. continebis.

[35.17] Item. uinu*m*. et piper. misces. et tepidu*m*. ore. continebis.

[35.18] Item. ortice. m\i/noris.[113] radice*m*. commasticet. et sucus. eius. ori. contineat. uel. acetu*m*. tepidum. gargarizet.

[35.19] Trociscus. ad dolorem. dentis. uel. ad laxatione. dentium. aluminis. scissi. ÷ II. aluminis rutundi. ÷ II. hius. ydia.[114] castorei. croci. murre. galle. aloes. uncias. binas. senopis. lib*ra*. I. uini. stiptici. quantu*m*. sufficit. ad colligendu*m*. hinc. facis. trociscos. quos. cum. opus. fuerit. resolutos. in uini. stiptico. in ore. tenebis. facit. et ad disintericos iniectus.

[110] Bamberg 2 (c. 35) gives *pilulas* here. PP Flor-Prag (c. 36) similarly gives *pillulas*.

[111] The punctus splits the words awkwardly here: *stabilit in ore* makes more sense.

[112] The second half of this line has been erased. A scribe has written in 'sale' over what was there earlier, which looks at least like a '-ri-' ligature, then perhaps *in uno* (which is then repeated on the next line). MC 69's corrected *et sale in uno ferueant* is identical to Bamberg 2 (c. 35): *et sale in uno ferueant* and similar to PP Flor-Prag (c. 36): *et salem ut in unum ferueat.*

[113] Small I inserted above M with punctus, perhaps by original scribe.

[114] Another wayward punctus seems to have split the ingredient *sydia* in half here: *Hiu. Sydia*, which has been corrected in Bamberg 2 (c. 35).

[35.20] Trociscos. ad dolorem. dentis. (47a) catmiae. ÷ I. calcitis. cocte. in carbonibus. ÷ IS. utru*m*q*ue* separatim. cu*m* aceto. acri. diligentissime. in modum collirii. teres. et co*m*misces. facisque. trociscus. quos in aceto. resolues. et tepefactum. in ore. tenes.

XXXVI. Si Dentes. Nimio. Capitis. Reumate. Laxauerint. Et Dolor Fuerit. Infestus.[115]

[36.1] Piretri. radicem. co*m*masticet. et ore. teneat. omne. reuma. decurrent. est. quidem. radix. uehemens. sed. postea. refrigerat.

[36.2] Item. anogallici. radicem. commasticabis. laxos. dentes. marrubii. fasciculos. tres. cum aqua. *ff.*[116] III. in olla. noua. coques. ad tertias. hinc. tepidu*m*. gargarizabis. mane. et meridie. p*er* dies. septem. post haec. semen. hber.[117] calicularis. quam. alii. dentalem. alii. simphoniaca*m* uocat. mittis. sup*er* carbones. et p*er* traiectorium. (47b) totum. fuma*m*. ore. trahis. omnes. gingiuas. ex siccat et humores. malos. p*er*ducit. et dentes. confirmat.

[36.3] Item. myrte. fasciculum. cimarum. rubis. fasciculum. et corticem. mali. granati. in aceto. dequoques. et inde. os. sepius. colis.

[36.4] Item. aristolocia. tusa. in puluerem. dentibus. laxis. iniecta. confirmat.

[36.5] Item. galle. syriae. ÷ I. istiptiriae.[118] ÷ I. corticis. granati. ÷ I. sicci. croci. ɜ. III. in puluerem subtilem. redigis. et gingiuis. inpones.

[36.6] Item. pulei. sine. fumo. lib*ra*. I. iris. ÷ VI. salis. amoniaci. ÷ III. haec tusa. et creta. pro denti. fricio. habebis.

[36.7] Item. denti. friciu*m*. ad idem. folii. ÷ I. ungelle. marine. ÷ I. masticis. afre. ÷ I. ostrearu*m*. testa. n*umero*. IIII. pumicis. ÷ I. panis. conbusti. ÷ I. cyperu. ÷ I omnia. in puluerem. redacta co*m*miscis. ex eo. dentes. fricas.

[36.8] Item. puluis. ad humore. dentiu*m*. farina. desicale. manus. duas. plenas. (48a) salis. tantundem. facies. pastam. et coques. ita ut in puluerem. possit. redigi. folii. £. costi. £. piperis. albi. grana. LX. satureie. £. pulei. £. caput. sarde. maioris. conbuste. £.

[115] The title in the table of capitula is much shorter: *XXXVI Ad dentes laxos.*

[116] The symbol for the sextarius.

[117] Abbreviated *hber*. Should likely be *hbe*, an abbreviation for *herbe*, as it is presented in Bamberg 1 (c. 36), Bamberg 2 (c. 36), and PP Flor-Prag (c. 37), as well as elsewhere in this manuscript.

[118] Bamberg 2 (c. 36) gives the spelling *stiptirie*; PP Flor-Prag (c. 37) does not include this ingredient.

auripimentum. £. cucurbite. sicce. conbuste. £. haec. omnia. in puluerem. redacta. et commixta. uteris. sic. tamen. ut prius. de uino. uetus. os lauet.[119]

[36.9] Item. dentifricium. ad reuma. quo omni. tempore. utaris. lucernas. sabinenses. III. imples. sale. quarum. foramina. cludes. de consparso. ordiacio. et mittis. sub carbones. in arulam. ita ut. triduo. iugiter. carbonibus. sint. operte. quas. tollens. in puluerem. mollissimum. redicis. addes. folii. £. costi. ÷ I. masticis. ÷ I. omnia. trita. cribrata. in unum. misces. et cotidie. uteris.

[36.10] Item. innula. A.[120] ieiunis. commanducata. dentes. confirmant.

[36.11] Item. acetum. in ore. continebis. gingiuas. constringis. et dentes. continet. (48b)

[36.12] Item. aqua. in qua. lentiscum. decoctum. est. dentes. mobiles. confirmat.

[36.13] Item. ruborum. in quibus. mora. nascuntur. pampini. decocuntur. in uino. austero. et commanducantur. id. qui uinum. ori. continetur.

XXXVII. Ad Dentium. Molariorum. Dolorem.[121]

[37.1] Proserpine. herbe. quam alii. camemellum. dicunt. sucus. in aurem. stillatus. sedat. dolorem.

[37.2] Item. ac peste.[122] lapatium est. quod. alii. romice. dicunt. radix. eius. commanducata. et sucus. in ore tentus. statim. dolorem. tollit. et cum. acetos. quinque decocta. in ore aceto tento. idem facit.

[119] Bamberg 2 (c. 36) presents this similarly, although PP Flor-Prag (c. 37) gives this as two separate remedies. The first is the powder for humours of the teeth: *Item puluis ad humorem dentium: farine de sigala duas manus plenas tolles ac salis tantundem; facies pastam et coques ita ut in puluerem possis redigere.* The long list of ingredients is then in a second remedy which follows it (with some rearrangement and abridgement): *Item costi semunciam, folii semunciam, capitis sardene maioris combusti semunciam, auripigmenti semunciam, cucurbite sicce semunciam; hec omnia in puluerem redacta et commixta uteris, sic tamen, ut prius de uino ueteri os laues.*

[120] Majuscule A with bar over. Bamberg 2 (c. 36) gives *Item enula am ieiunus conmanducata dentes confirmat*; PP. Flor-Prag (c. 36) gives *Item enula ab ieiunus commanducata dentes confirmat.*

[121] The table of capitula title is slightly different: *XXXVII. Ad dentium* molare *dolorem.*

[122] Bamberg 2 (c. 37): *hacreste*; PP Flor-Prag (c. 38): *agrestis.*

XXXVIII. Ad Dentes. Uitiosus. Aut Cabos.

[38.1] Gallas. alexandrinas. folium. quantum. sufficiat. costum. aeque. aduersus. gallas. masticis. ciae. grana. L. croci. parum. piper. grana. LX. balaustiu (49a) caliculos. V. flos rose quantum. sufficiat. haec omnia in puluerem redacta uteris.

[38.2] Item. ad dentes. cabos tytimalli. et caprici. lactis.[123] cu*m* galbano. resolutis. cabis. dentibus. inditi. tollunt. dolorem. ita. ut cera*m*. sup*er*ponat. nec lingua. aduratur.

[38.3] Item. cinis. murini. femi. indutus. prode est.

[38.4] Item. uermiu*m*. terrenorum. cinis. indutus. cera. opertus. ex. facili. eos. cadere. cogit. idem. cinis. inlitus. dolentiu*m* cauis. dentibus. iubat.

XXXIX. Ad Dentes. Candidos. Faciendos.

[39.1] Dentifriciu*m*. pumice. conbusto. et trito. dentifricium. utere.

[39.2] Item. conquilii. marini. testam. sale. plenam. conburis. tere. et dente. frica.

[39.3] Item. testa. sepie. tusa. et cribrata. cu*m* pumicis. farina. parte. dimidia. cum. costi. puluere. cottidie. dentes. fricato. et candidi. erunt. (49b)

[39.4] Item. uulbi. albi. cinis. dentifricium est.[124]

[39.5] Item. ossa. ex ungulis. suu*m*. conbusta. eundem. usu. prestant.

XL. Ad Dentes. Molares. Uel Ad Omnes. Ut Sint Incorrupti. Et Impassibiles. Inmobiles. Que. Magn*um* Remed*ium*.[125]

[40.1] Bitis. albe. butrionis. suco cotilis. duabus. mori radii. ces. cortices. coques. ad tertias. et in ore. teneat ac diluat. p*er*dies. VII. numquam dentes. doleuit.

[123] Bamberg 2 (c. 38) also gives *caprici lactis*, but PP Flor-Prag (c. 39) gives *caprifici lac*.

[124] See above at pp. 58–9 for more discussion. Bamberg 2 (c. 39) and PP Flor-Prag (c. 36) also give *bulbi albi*; Bamberg 1 (c. 39) gives *plumbi albi*. SG 751 (c. 8) gives *talum bubulum*, which is what appears in *Natural History*, 28.49.179, ed. Mayhoff (1897) 336.

[125] The table of capitula gives a shorter title: *XL. Ad dentes molares. ut ad omnes ut si\n/t incorrupti et inpossibiles*.

[40.2] Item. inuiolati. prestantur. dentes. si quis. cottidie. mane. ieiunos. habeat. sub lingua. salis. granum. donec. liquescat.

XLI. Dentioni

[41.1] Lacte caprino et leporis. cerebro. gingiue. p*er*fricantur.
[41.2] Item. delfini. dentium. cinis. cum. melle. gingiuis. inlinitur.
[41.3] Item. celebrum.[126] leporis. in cibo. datur.
[41.4] Item. foliis. hedere. prune. subponuntur.
[41.5] Item. butiru*m*. cu*m* melle. temperabis. ex inde gingiuas. ungis.

REFERENCES

Adacher, S. 1984. 'La trasmissione della cultura medica a Montecassino tra la fine del IX secolo e l'inizio del X secolo', *Miscellanea Cassinese* 55: 385–400.

Adams, J. N., and Deegan, M. 1992. 'Bald's *Leechbook* and the *Physica Plinii*', *Anglo-Saxon England* 21: 87–114.

Amar, Z., and Lev, E. 2017. *Arabian Drugs in Early Medieval Mediterranean Medicine*. Edinburgh: University of Edinburgh Press.

Arsdall, A. van 2007. 'Challenging the "Eye of Newt" Image of Medieval Medicine', in B. S. Bowers (ed.), *The Medieval Hospital and Medical Practice*. Aldershot: Ashgate, 195–205.

Baader, G. 1984. 'Early Medieval Latin Adaptations of Byzantine Medicine in Western Europe', *Dumbarton Oaks Papers* 38: 251–9.

Banham, D. 2011. 'Dun, Oxa and Pliny the Great Physician: Attribution and Authority in Old English Medical Texts', *Social History of Medicine* 24:1: 57–73.

Beagon, M. 2005. *The Elder Pliny on the Human Animal: Natural History Book 7*. Oxford: Oxford University Press.

Beccaria, A. 1956. *I codici di medicina del periodo presalernitano (secoli IX, X e XI)*. Rome: Edizioni di storia e letteratura.

Becker, M. J. 2014. 'Dentistry in Ancient Rome: Direct Evidence for Extractions Based on the Teeth from Excavations at the Temple of Castor and Pollux in the Roman Forum', *International Journal of Anthropology* 29(4): 209–26.

Bostock, J., and Riley, H. T. trans. 1855. *The Natural History of Pliny*. London: Henry G. Bohn.

Burridge, C. 2019. 'An Interdisciplinary Investigation into Carolingian Medical Knowledge and Practice'. Cambridge University: PhD Thesis.

Burridge, C. 2020. 'Incense in Medicine: An Early Medieval Perspective', *Early Medieval Europe* 28:2: 219–55.

[126] Bamberg 2 (c. 41) and PP Flor-Prag (c. 42) give *cerebrum*, although PP Flor-Prag specifies the animal as *pecudis*, rather than *leporis*.

Cameron, M. L. 1983a. 'Bald's *Leechbook*: Its Sources and Their Use in Its Compilation', *Anglo-Saxon England* 12: 153–82.

Cameron, M. L. 1983b. 'The Sources of Medical Knowledge in Anglo-Saxon England', *Anglo-Saxon England* 11: 135–55.

Cameron, M. L. 1993. *Anglo-Saxon Medicine*. Cambridge: Cambridge University Press.

Coon, L. L. 2011. *Dark Age Bodies: Gender and Monastic Practice in the Early Medieval West*. Philadelphia: University of Pennsylvania Press.

Donkin, R. A. 2003. *Between East and West: The Moluccas and the Traffic in Spices up to the Arrival of the Europeans*. Philadelphia, PA: American Philosophical Society.

Doody, A. 2010. *Pliny's Encyclopedia: The Reception of the Natural History*. Cambridge: Cambridge University Press.

Everett, N. ed. and tr. 2012. *The Alphabet of Galen: Pharmacy from Antiquity to the Middle Ages: A Critical Edition of the Latin Text with English Translation and Commentary*. Toronto: University of Toronto Press.

Ferraces Rodríguez, A. ed. 2015. *Curae quae ex Hominibus atque animalibus fiunt*. Santiago de Compostela: Andavira Editora.

Fischer, K.-D. 1986. 'Quelques réflexions sur la structure et deux nouveaux témoins de la Physica Plinii', *Helmantica* 37: 53–66.

Fischer, K.-D. 1993. 'Physica Plinii', in *Lexikon des Mittelalters*, vol. VI. Munich: Artemis, 2111a.

Fischer, K.-D. 2000. 'Dr. Monk's Medical Digest', *Social History of Medicine* 13:2: 239–51.

Fischer, K.-D. 2008. 'A Mirror for Deaf Ears? A Medieval Mystery', *Electronic British Library Journal*, Article 9. http://www.bl.uk/eblj/2008articles/article9.html, accessed 15 November 2018.

Fischer, K.-D. 2010. 'Das "Lorscher Arzneibuch" im Widerstreit der Meinungen', *Medizinhistorisches Journal* 45: 165–88.

Fleming, R. 2006. 'Bones for Historians: Putting the Body back into Biography', in D. Bates, J. Crick, and S. Hamilton (eds.), *Writing Medieval Biography, 750–1250: Essays in Honour of Frank Barlow*. Woodbridge: Boydell and Brewer, 29–48.

Fraisse, A. ed. 2002. *Cassius Felix. De la médecine*. Paris: Les Belles lettres.

Freedman, P. 2008. *Out of the East: Spices and the Medieval Imagination*. New Haven, CT: Yale University Press.

French, R., and Greenaway, F. eds. 1986. *Science in the Early Roman Empire: Pliny the Elder, His Sources and Influence*. Totowa, NJ: Barnes and Noble Books.

Giacosa, P. (ed.). 1886. 'Un ricettario del secolo XI esistente nell'Archivio capitolare d'Ivrea', *Memorie della Reale Accademia delle scienze di Torino* 2nd ser., 37: 643–63.

Glaze, F. E. 2018. 'Salerno's Lombard Prince: Johannes "Abbas de Curte" As Medical Practitioner', *Early Science and Medicine* 23: 177–216.

Green, M. H. 2000. 'Medieval Gynecological Texts: A Handlist', in *Women's Healthcare in the Medieval West: Texts and Contexts*, Appendix, pp. 1–36. Aldershot: Ashgate.

Green, M. H. ed. and tr. 2001. *The Trotula: A Medieval Compendium of Women's Medicine*. Philadelphia: University of Pennsylvania Press.

Green, M. H. ed. 2014. *Pandemic Disease in the Medieval World: Rethinking the Black* Death. *The Medieval Globe* 1. Open Access. https://scholarworks.wmich.edu/medieval_globe/1, accessed 15 March 2020.

Gudger, E. W. 1924. 'Pliny's *Historia naturalis*: The Most Popular Natural History Ever Published', *Isis* 6.3: 269–81.

Healy, J. F. 1999. *Pliny the Elder on Science and Technology*. Oxford: Oxford University Press.

Helmreich, G. ed. 1889. *Marcelli De Medicamentis Liber*. Leipzig: B.G. Teubner.

Holland, B. K. ed. 1996. *Prospecting for Drugs in Ancient and Medieval European Texts*. Amsterdam: Harwood Academic.

Holst, M., and Coughlan, J. 2000. 'Dental Health and Disease', in V. Fiorato, A. Boylston, C. Knusel, and R. Hardy (eds.), *Blood Red Roses: The Archaeology of a Mass Grave from the Battle of Towton AD 1461*. Oxford: Oxbow Books, 77–89.

Horden, P. 2009. 'What's Wrong with Early Medieval Medicine?', *Social History of Medicine* 24.1: 5–25.

Hunt, Y. trans. 2020. *The* Medicina Plinii*: Latin Text, Translation, and Commentary*. New York: Routledge.

Jackson, R. 1988. *Doctors and Diseases in the Roman Empire*. London: British Museum Press, 118–21.

Jones, P. M. 1996. 'Medicine', in F. A. C. Mantello and A. G. Rigg (eds.), *Medieval Latin: An Introduction and Bibliographical Guide*. Washington, DC: Catholic University of America Press, 416–21.

Keay, J. 2006. *The Spice Route: A History*. Berkeley: University of California Press.

Keil G., and Schnitzer, P. eds. 1991. *Das Lorscher Arzneibuch und die frühmittelalterliche Medizin*. Lorsch: Verlag Laurissa.

Kokoszko, M., and Rzeźnicka, Z. 2018. 'Malabathron (μαλάβαθρον) in Ancient and Early Byzantine Medicine and Cuisine', *Medicina nei secoli* 20: 579–616.

Kondor, K. 2007. 'Dental Pathology in Two Árpádian Age Cemeteries at Visegrád: Evidence for Diet and Social Stratification', *Annual of Medieval Studies at CEU* 13: 51–73.

Langslow, D. R. 1991. 'The Formation and Development of Latin Medical Vocabulary: A. Cornelius Celsus and Cassius Felix'. Wolfson College, Oxford University: PhD Thesis.

Langslow, D. R. 2000. *Medical Latin in the Roman Empire*. Oxford: Oxford University Press.

Lev. E. 2007. 'Drugs Held and Sold by Pharmacists of the Jewish Community of Medieval (11–14th centuries) Cairo According to Lists of *Materia Medica* Found at the Taylor–Schechter Genizah Collection, Cambridge', *Journal of Ethnopharmacology* 110: 275–93.

Little, L. 2011. 'Plague Historians in Lab Coats', *Past and Present* 213(1): 267–90.

Lloyd, G. E. R. ed. 1978. *Hippocratic Writings*. New York: Penguin.
Lowe, E. A., and Brown, V. 1980. *The Beneventan Script: A History of the South Italian Minuscule*, vol. II. Rome: Edizioni di Storia e Letteratura.
MacKinney, L. C. 1944. '"Oleum Savininum": An Early Medieval Synthesis of Medical Prescriptions', *Bulletin of the History of Medicine* 16, no. 3: 276–88.
Mantello, F. A. C., and Rigg, A. G. eds. 1996. *Medieval Latin: An Introduction and Bibliographical Guide*. Washington, DC: Catholic University of America Press.
Marx, F. ed. 1915. *A. Cornelii Celsi quae supersunt*. Leipzig: B. G. Teubner.
Mayhoff, K., and Jan, L. eds. 1875–1906. *C. Plinii Secundi Naturalis historiae libri XXXVII*. 5 vols. Leipzig: B. G. Teubner.
McCormick, M. 2001. *Origins of the European Economy: Communications and Commerce, A.D. 300–900*. Cambridge: Cambridge University Press.
Miller, J. I. 1969. *The Spice Trade of the Roman Empire: 29 B.C. to A.D. 641*. Oxford: Clarendon.
Morton, A. G. 1986. 'Pliny on Plants: His Place in the History of Botany', in R. French and F. Greenaway (eds.), *Science in the Early Roman Empire: Pliny the Elder, His Sources and Influence*. Totowa, NJ: Barnes and Noble Books, 86–97.
Nabhan, G. P. 2014. *Cumin, Camels, and Caravans: A Spice Odyssey*. Berkeley: University of California Press.
Niedermann, M., and Liechtenhan, E. eds. 1968. *Marcelli De medicamentis liber*. 2 vols. Second Edition. Berlin: B. G. Teubner.
Nutton, V. 1986. 'The Perils of Patriotism: Pliny and Roman Medicine', in R. French and F. Greenaway (eds.), *Science in the Early Roman Empire: Pliny the Elder, His Sources and Influence*. Totowa, NJ: Barnes and Noble Books, 30–58.
Önnerfors, A. 1963. *In Medicinam Plinii Studia Philologica: De memoria et uerborum contextu opusculi, de elocutione et aetate deque iis operibus, quibus medio aeuo conceptum est*. Lund: CWK Gleerup.
Önnerfors, A. ed. 1964. *Plinii Secundi Iunioris qui feruntur de Medicina libri tres*. Berlin: Akademie-Verlag.
Önnerfors, A. ed. 1975. *Physica Plinii Bambergensis (Cod. Bamb. Med. 2, fol. 93v–232r)*. Hildesheim: Georg Olms.
Önnerfors, A. ed. 2004. '*De Physica* q.u. Plinii Sangallensi annotationes aliquot cum capite prius inedito (Cap. VIII, Ad dentium dolorem remedia, pp. 197–200),' in S. Sconocchia and F. Cavalli (eds.), *Testi medici latini antichi: Le Parole de medicina: lessico e storia. Atti del VII Convegno Internazionale, Trieste, 11-13 ottobre 2001*. Bologna: Pàtron Editore, 197–210.
Önnerfors, A. ed. 2006–7. *Physica Plinii quae fertur Sangallensis (cod. Sang. 751 pp. 183–280)*. 2 vols. Lund: Lunds University.
Opsomer, C. 1989. *Index de la pharmacopée du Ier au Xe siècle*. 2 vols. Hildesheim: Olms-Weidmann.
Pilsworth, C. 2014. *Healthcare in Early Medieval Northern Italy: More to Life Than Leeches*. Turnhout: Brepols.
Platte, A., and Platte K. eds. 1989. *Das 'Lorscher Arzneibuch': Klostermedizin in der Karolingerzeit; Ausgewählte Texte und Beiträge*. Lorsch: Laurissa.
Pradel-Baquerre, M. 2013. 'Ps.-Apulée, "Herbier": introduction, traduction et commentaire. Archéologie et Préhistoire'. Université Paul Valéry, Montpellier III: PhD Thesis.

Radini, A., Tromp, M., Beach, A. et al. 2019. 'Medieval Women's Early Involvement in Manuscript Production Suggested by Lapis Lazuli Identification in Dental Calculus', *Science Advances* 5.1.

Riddle, J. M. 1965. 'The Introduction and Use of Eastern Drugs in the Early Middle Ages', *Sudhoffs Archiv für Geschichte der Medizin und der Naturwissenschaften* 49: 175–98.

Riddle, J. M. 1974. 'Theory and Practice in Medieval Medicine', *Viator* 5: 157–84.

Rose, V. 1874. 'Uber die Medicina Plinii', *Hermes* 8: 18–66.

Rose, V. ed. 1875. *Plinii Secundi quae fertur una cum Gargilii Martialis Medicina.* Leipzig: B. G. Teubner.

Rose, V. ed. 1894. *Theodori Prisciani: Euporiston, Libri III cum physicorum fragmento et additamentis pseudo-Theodoris.* Leipzig: B. G. Teubner.

Sabbah, G., Corsetti, P.-P., and Fischer, K.-D. eds. 1987. *Bibliographie des textes médicaux latins: antiquité et haut moyen âge.* Saint-Étienne: Publications de l'Université de Saint-Étienne.

Scarborough, J. 1986. 'Pharmacy in Pliny's Natural History: Some Observations on Substances and Sources', in R. French and F. Greenaway (eds.), *Science in the Early Roman Empire: Pliny the Elder, His Sources and Influence.* Totowa, NJ: Barnes and Noble Books, 59–85.

Schmitz, G. ed. 1988. *Physicae quae fertur Plinii Florentino-Pragenis liber tertius.* Frankfurt: Peter Lang.

Schneider, O. 1967. *In C. Plini Secundi Naturalis Historiae Libros Indices.* 2 vols. Hildesheim: Georg Olms.

Sconocchia, S. 1989. 'La medicina nella tarda antichità: Un nuovo testimone della cosiddetta *Physica Plinii Bambergensis*', in A. Garzya (ed.), *Metodologie della ricerca sulla tarda antichità: atti del Primo Convegno dell'Associazione di studi tardoantichi.* Naples: M. D'Auria Editore, 515–27.

Sconocchia, S. 1992. 'Per una nuova edizione della cosiddetta Physica Plinii Bambergensis', *Tradizione e ecdotica dei testi medici* 275–89.

Sharpe, W. D. 1964. 'Isidore of Seville: The Medical Writings. An English Translation with an Introduction and Commentary,' *Transactions of the American Philosophical Society* 54:2: 1–75.

Spencer, W. G. ed. 1938. *Celsus: De Medicina.* Loeb Classical Library, vol. III. Cambridge, MA: Harvard University Press.

Stannard, J. 1965. 'Pliny and Roman Botany', *Isis* 56.4: 420–5.

Stannard, J. 1973. 'Marcellus of Bordeaux and the Beginnings of Medieval Materia Medica', *Pharmacy in History* 15.2: 47–53.

Stannard, J. 1974. 'Eastern Plants and Plant Products in Medieval Germany', in *Actes du XIIIe Congrès International d'Histoire des Sciences, Moscou, 18–24 août 1971, Sections III & IV: Antiquité et Moyen Age*: 220–25.

Stannard, J. 1999a. 'Medicinal Plants and Folk Remedies in Pliny, *Historia Naturalis*', in J. Stannard, K. E. Stannard, and R. Kay (eds.), *Pristina Medicamenta: Ancient and Medieval Medical Botany.* London: Variorum, Essay 2, 3–23.

Stannard, J. 1999b. 'Aspects of Byzantine *Materia Medica*', In J. Stannard, K. E. Stannard, and R. Kay (eds.), *Pristina Medicamenta: Ancient and Medieval Medical Botany*. London: Variorum, Essay 9: 205–11.

Stannard, J. 1999c. 'Medieval Reception of Classical Plant Names', in J. Stannard, K. E. Stannard, and R. Kay (eds.), *Herbs and Herbalism in the Middle Ages and Renaissance*. Aldershot: Ashgate, Essay 1: 153–62.

Stannard, J. 1999d. 'Medieval Herbals and Their Development', in J. Stannard, K. E. Stannard, and R. Kay (eds.), *Herbs and Herbalism in the Middle Ages and Renaissance*. Aldershot: Ashgate, Essay 3: 23–33.

Stannard, J. 1999e. 'The Theoretical Bases of Medieval Herbalism', in J. Stannard, K. E. Stannard and R. Kay (eds.), *Herbs and Herbalism in the Middle Ages and Renaissance*. Aldershot: Ashgate, Essay 4: 1–9.

Stannard, J. 1999f. 'Rezeptliteratur as Fachliteratur,' in J. Stannard, K. E. Stannard, and R. Kay (eds.), *Herbs and Herbalism in the Middle Ages and Renaissance*. Aldershot: Ashgate, Essay 7: 59–73.

Stoll, U. 1992. *Das "Lorscher Arzneibuch": Ein Medizinisches Kompendium des 8. Jahrhunderts (Codex Bambergensis Medicinalis 1): Text, Übersetzung und Fachglossar*. Stuttgart: Franz Steiner.

Touwaide, A. 2010. 'Botany', in A. Classen (ed.), *Handbook of Medieval Studies: Terms – Methods – Trends*. Berlin: De Gruyter, 145–81.

Vallisneri, A. 1733. *Opere Fisico-Mediche Stampate e Manoscritte del Kavalier Antonio Vallisneri Raccolte da Antonio suo figliuolo*, vol. III. Venice: Sebastiano Coleti.

Vázquez Buján, M. E. 1984. 'Problemas generales de las antiguas traducciones médicas latinas', *Studi Medievali* 3.25: 641–80.

Voigts, L. 1979. 'Anglo-Saxon Plant Remedies and the Anglo-Saxons', *Isis* 70: 250–68.

Wachtmeister, W. ed. 1985. *Physicae quae fertur Plinii Florentino-Pragenis liber secundus*. Frankfurt: Peter Lang.

Weddell, M. 2010. 'Metrology', in A. Classen (ed.), *Handbook of Medieval Studies: Terms –Methods – Trends*. Berlin: De Gruyter, 897–919.

Wickersheimer, E. 1966. *Les manuscrits latins de médecine du haut moyen age dans les bibliothèques de France*. Paris: IRHT.

Winkler, J. ed. 1984. *Physicae quae fertur Plinii Florentino-Pragenis liber primus*. Frankfurt: Peter Lang.

Witwer-Backofen, U., and Engel, F. 2019. 'The History of European Oral Health: Evidence from Dental Caries and Antemortem Tooth Loss', in R. H. Steckel, C. S. Larsen, C. A. Roberts, and J. Baten (eds.), *The Backbone of Europe: Health, Diet, Work and Violence over Two Millennia*. Cambridge: Cambridge University Press, 84–137.

Wynbrandt, J. 1998. *The Excruciating History of Dentistry: Toothsome Tales and Oral Oddities from Babylon to Braces*. New York: St. Martin's Press.

Zupko, R. E. 1981. *Italian Weights and Measures from the Middle Ages to the Nineteenth Century*. Philadelphia, PA: American Philosophical Society.

Zupko, R. E. 1996. 'Weights and Measures', in F. A. C. Mantello and A. G. Rigg (eds.), *Medieval Latin: An Introduction and Bibliographical Guide*. Washington, DC: Catholic University of America Press, 443–6.

CHAPTER 3

De sexaginta animalibus

A Latin Translation of an Arabic Manāfiʿ al-ḥayawān *Text on the Pharmaceutical Properties of Animals*

Kathleen Walker-Meikle

This chapter discusses *De sexaginta animalibus* (*On Sixty Animals*), a little-studied Latin text that is a translation from the popular Arabic genre of properties of animals. This genre orders its contents by individual animals rather than the more usual pharmacological categorisation of individual ingredient component (simple), compound medicine, or ailment. The properties of each individual animal may be medical or magical and the text does not distinguish between the two.

It is notable for the extensive use of untranslated Arabic terminology and is a shining example of the cross-cultural transmission of pharmacological and linguistic knowledge across traditions. By raising its profile this can be an important contribution to the study of animal *materia medica* and the translation of medical texts across the medieval Mediterranean. The copious use of Arabic terminology, which is discussed in detail, raises the question whether multilinguism in texts is helpful for the reader or potential practitioner. *Sexaginta animalibus* appears to have been transmitted in the Latin tradition, from the thirteenth to the sixteenth centuries, with very little visible therapeutic application of its contents. But lack of practical application should not discount its importance to the wider phenomena of knowledge transfer and cultural exchanges. Medieval medical manuscripts could have other important uses other than purely practical ones, such as educational or pedagogical.[1]

In the second volume of *A History of Magic and Experimental Science*, Lynn Thorndike noted the existence of a work on the medicinal virtues of

Many thanks to Fabian Käs for reading an early draft of this chapter and his helpful suggestions and corrections to the Arabic.

[1] Horden (2013).

animals, asserting that it had been printed once (Venice, 1497) with the title *De proprietatibus iuvamentis et nocumentis sexaginta animalium* (*On the Healing and Harmful Properties of Sixty Animals*).[2] He gave some manuscript references, enlarged in Thorndike and Pearl Kibre's *A Catalogue of Incipits of Mediaeval Scientific Writings in Latin*, and remarked that it had been cited once in the thirteenth century by Albertus Magnus in regard to the complexion of the dog.[3] The text is composed of individual animal entries, in which the medicinal properties of just under sixty animals are detailed.

Although there is no resemblance in regard to content, transmission, or tradition, in structure the individual entries on each animal's medicinal and magical properties are similar to treatises such as the late antique Latin Ps. Sextus Placitus *Medicina ex animalibus* (*Medicine from Animals*) or the Greek *Kyranides* (books 2–4).[4] However, due to the proliferation of transliterations of Arabic animal names and units of measurement in the text, it was clear that it was a translation of an original Arabic treatise on animal *materia medica*. *Sexaginta animalibus* has been occasionally cited by scholars, without further study, as an unknown Latin treatise of Arabic origin, with the author identified as either unknown or ascribed to Abū Bakr al-Rāzī (Rhazes, d. *c*.925) due to the two sixteenth-century printed editions and several manuscripts ascribing the work to the latter.[5]

This chapter will attempt to place the Latin text in its original Arabic genre and make a claim of authorship, along with examples of the text itself, the animals covered, the use of transliterated Arabic terminology,

[2] Referred to as *Sexaginta animalibus* (*Sixty Animals*) in future.

[3] Thorndike (1923: 762) (Chapter LXIV Experiments and Secrets of Galen, Rasis, and others: 1. Medical and Biological) and Thorndike and Kibre (1963: 1688). The Albertus Magnus citation is *Dicitur autem in libro sexaginta animalium quod caro canis calida est et sicca* ('It is said, however, in the book of sixty animals that the flesh of the dog is hot and dry', *De animalibus* (*On Animals*) XXII ii 18). Albertus also cites the text in his entry on the *alzabo* and uses it extensively in Book XXII, which discusses quadrupeds. Albertus Magnus, *De animalibus* (*On Animals*), ed. Stadler (1916–20) II.1360 and 1367.

[4] Sextus Placitus, *Libri medicinae Sexti Placiti Papyriensis ex animalibus pecoribus et bestiis vel avibus Concordantiae* (*Books of Medicine of Sextus Placitus Papyriensis from Animals, Cattle and Beasts or Birds: Concordance*), ed. Segolini (1998); and *Kyranides*, ed. Kaimakis (1976).

[5] Ventura (2005: 221):

> Besides the mentioned texts, a *Liber de proprietatibus membrorum et de utilitatibus et nocumentis animalium* (known also as *Liber sexaginta animalium*) belonging to Abū Bakr al-Rāzī's writings, transmits some both medical and magical properties of 56 animals. Nothing is known about the transmission and the diffusion of this work, nor its possible role within the 'official' medicine of the thirteenth and fourteenth centuries. Its content, however, seems to mix scientific medicine and magic rituals and superstitions, and to show a certain 'popular' level.

The 1500 Venice edition is cited. Nagel (1999: 224 n. 37): 'è conosciuto solo attraverso la tradizione latina' ('it is known only through the Latin tradition'). Zonta (1996: 280 n. 62) is sceptical of Steinschneider's (1956: 728–9, §470/7) suggestion that various Hebrew treatises on animal properties are translations of this Latin work.

and its transmission and diffusion in the Latin West. Despite its eponymous title, I have not found any version of *Sexaginta animalibus* that covers more than fifty-six animals in either the surviving manuscripts or early printed editions of 1497, 1500, and 1544. The lion is usually the first entry, and most of the manuscripts have been identified by cataloguers via the *incipit*, which refers to a use of this animal's neck: *Verbum Aristotles et Diascoridis est* ('This is the word of Aristotle and Dioscorides').

The order of the animals is usually consistent, starting with the lion and other and wild domestic quadrupeds, followed by the large section on birds, ending with the uses for a man or a woman, with some smaller categories (aquatic animals) and other uncategorised animals (such as the spider) between these two large sections. This is consistent with the order of animal entries in Arabic treatises on properties, such as ʿĪsā ibn ʿAlī and ʿUbaydallāh ibn Bukhtīshūʿ, where the entries generally follow the pattern of man, quadrupeds, birds, vermin, and aquatic animals. The pattern in *Sexaginta animalibus* is very similar, apart from placing the entries for man and woman at the end: starting with quadrupeds, a few entries on aquatic animals and vermin, birds, man, and woman. Each animal entry in turn lists the pharmaceutical properties of its individual organs and fluids, such as blood, bile, heart, liver, flesh, urine, and eyes among others.

However, if the work starts in the middle of the text, rather than with the first entry on the lion and the usual incipit, it can be hard to identify. Wellcome Library MS.560 begins with the section on birds (f. 110r) with the incipit *Upupe caro frigida grossa austera est et in pullis* ('the flesh of the hoopoe is cold, thick and bitter and in the chicks'). It was likely identified thanks to the title *Sermo razi in uolatilibus irrationalibus* (*Al-Rāzī's Discussion on Irrational Flying Birds*) as it was printed in two major early modern editions of al-Rāzī's work. I have identified Winchester College MS.26 (ff. 67r–68v) and Balliol College MS.285 (ff. 41r–v, f. 66r) as partial copies of *Sexaginta animalibus*. The relevant section in Balliol College MS.285 starts with the entry on the wolf, which is normally the eighteenth animal of the text (incipit: *De ozib lupo. Caro eius frigida est et sic fetida grossa*, 'The *ozib* the wolf, its flesh is cold, thick and foul-smelling'). It is catalogued as *Anon de Carne quorundam animalium* (*Anonymous Work on the Flesh of Various Animals*).[6] Winchester College MS.26 (67r–68v) begins in the middle of the entry for the sheep, normally the fourth quadruped from the start of the text, and the catalogue merely gives the confusing incipit (which starts in the middle of a sentence) *Sanguinem*

[6] Mynors (1963: 302).

globatum et confert flagellatis iuuamento magno ('congealed blood and it is of great help for those who have been whipped') and states that the text consists of 'Medical properties of ram, goat, horse, ass, camel, elephant, hart, gazelle'.[7]

Regarding its translation, it must have been translated by the early thirteenth century at the latest as it is quoted extensively by Albertus Magnus in his *De animalibus* (*On Animals*) and copies of the manuscript survive from the mid-thirteenth century onwards. The 1544 Basel edition claims that Gerald of Cremona, the great twelfth-century translator in Toledo, translated the work; however, it is not among the list of works generally accepted to be his translations, and therefore the translator is unknown.[8] It is likely that the translation was carried out in Toledo around Gerald of Cremona's circle, as there are similarities in the use of Arabic transliterations of animal names as in other translated texts, such as Ibn Sīnā's *Liber canonis*, which will be discussed later under terminology.

The title *De sexaginta animalium* appears to have travelled with the text from the start, as Albertus Magnus cites it twice under that name in *De animalibus*.[9] The manuscript used as the basis for the 1497 printed edition uses the title *De sexaginta animalium*; nevertheless this title appears in only one of the surviving manuscripts.[10] Its origin likely lies in that the translated version by the thirteenth century either covered sixty individual animal entries or this was the title of the Arabic work, despite no manuscript or printed version covering more than fifty-six beasts. It is possible that the Arabic original that formed the basis for the translated versions included more entries as other Arabic texts on the properties of animals, such as ʿĪsā ibn ʿAlī or the Ibn Bukhtīshūʿ composite bestiaries have references to considerably more animals.[11] The original Arabic text that was translated as *Sexaginta animalibus* does have intriguing

[7] Ker and Piper (1992: 619–21).

[8] *Abubetri Rhazæ Opera exquisitiora per Gerardum Toletanum* (Basel, 1544) 567. The phrase *Gerado Toletano Cremonensis Interprete* (Gerald of Cremona, interpreter of Toledo) is used on the title page. For a list of works translated by Gerald of Cremona, see Burnett (2001: 249–88, esp. 273–4). Cf. Burnett (2002: 95–144), Salmòn Muñiz (2002: 631–46), and McVaugh (2009: 99–112).

[9] Albertus Magnus, *De animalibus* (*On Animals*), ed. Stadler (1916–20), uses the text extensively and refers to it by name on p. II.1360 and 1367 (under the entries for the *alzabo* and 'dog', respectively).

[10] Leiden, Universiteitsbibliotheek MS Vossianus Chym. Q. 27, which from its date (sixteenth century, before 1540), the scribe could have feasibly had access to the 1497 Bergamo edition which calls it by this title: *Liber Rasis ad almansorem et alia* (Bonetus Locatellus, for Octavianus Scotus).

[11] For example, 110 different animals in the three different versions of ʿĪsā ibn ʿAlī, *Kitāb al-manāfiʿ allatī tustafādu min aʿḍāʾ al-ḥayawān* (*Book of Useful Properties That Can Be Obtained from Parts of Animals*); see Raggetti (2018: VIII).

characteristics that sets it apart from similar texts on the properties of animals, which will be introduced when discussing possible authorship.

The entries in *Sexaginta animalibus* frequently cite ancient authorities by name, in particular Galen, Aristotle, and Dioscorides, who are common sources in Arabic texts on the properties of animals. Some Arabic authors of these texts (ʿĪsā ibn ʿAlī and Ibn Bukhtīshūʿ) do not mention their sources directly. Others, such as al-Rāzī or Ibn al-Jazzār in their *khawāṣṣ* (texts on occult properties) do at times cite sources, but always preferred to do so if they were from Greek or early Arabic texts.[12] However, many of these citations do not correspond to identified works of these authors but were likely merely used to confer authority. The first line of the text cites both Aristotle and Dioscorides with *Verbum Aristotles et Diascoridis est in collo leonis non est aliquid coniuncture sed unum est continuum* ('according to the word of Aristotle and Dioscorides the lion's neck has no vertebrae but is just one single bone'). While this is a correct attribution from Aristotle's *History of Animals*, this material does not appear at all in Dioscorides' *De materia medica*.[13] At the same time, most of the virtues for animals in *Sexaginta animalibus* are not attributed directly to authors. For example, for the single entry on the hedgehog and sea urchin, twenty-three virtues are listed for both of these animals.[14] The same word for both animals in ancient Greek ('ἐχῖνος'), Latin (*ericius*) and Arabic (*qunfudh*) caused great zoological confusion, and the Arabic natural history tradition involved discussions on whether hedgehogs laid eggs or were semi-aquatic.[15] Four of the virtues are from Dioscorides, ranging from drinking the flesh with oxymel for dropsy and kidney pains to rubbing the ashes of the hedgehog's skin on one's head to

[12] Named authorities appear in the entries for the horse, mule, camel, elephant, gazelle, wolf (two citations), leopard, a type of fish, duck, and cockerel. On *khawāṣṣ*, see also Lewicka (Chapter 9) in the present volume.

[13] Aristotle, *History of Animals*, 497b17–19.

[14] See Basel (1544) 578–9 for the Latin text. Nearly the entire text is very similar to the corresponding material in ʿĪsā ibn ʿAlī in Raggetti (2018: 280–7) and in the composite Ibn Bukhtīshūʿ bestiary, San Lorenzo del Escorial, Ar. 898, in Ruiz Bravo-Villasante (1980: 53–6).

[15] Kruk (1985: 205–34). Scribes of some of the manuscripts were aware of the confusion and have divided the material, with the first half for the hedgehog and the second half for the sea urchin. This is the case of Ms Palatina Latina 1211 (ff. 66r–72v) which has *De proprietatibus ericii* ('on the properties of the hedgehog') followed by *De ericio maritimo* ('on the sea urchin'). Prague MS V. B.22 adopts a similar strategy: while the entire chapter on hedgehogs/sea urchins is not divided in the text, a later marginal hand has added *De hericio hermacio* and *De hericio marino* to indicate division between the two animals (ff. 234r–235r).

stop hair loss, but there is no direct mention of this origin.[16] One virtue is ascribed to a Criton (*Alchriton*), likely a reference to Statilius Criton, Emperor Trajan's physician (and procurator) and the author of a book of simples, sections of which were quoted by Galen. It is a variation on one of Dioscorides' recipes (using a sea urchin rather than a hedgehog for a baldness recipe, with some extra ingredients). In addition, there is a translated Arabic book on cosmetics ascribed to Criton which may be the source for this baldness recipe.[17] The rest of the virtues are without attribution.

One of the most striking features of *Sexaginta animalibus* is the copious use of Arabic terminology. It is often used for terms of measurement – for example, *alkisat* (*qīrāṭ*), used twice for the arrow fish (chapter 28) and one for the elephant (chapter 10). Arabic is also used throughout for *materia medica*, such as *alkitran* (*al-qaṭrān*) for bitumen in the entry on ants (chapter 34) and *alkal* ('bone or tooth') in the entry for the elephant (chapter 10).[18] Regarding the names of the animals themselves, sometimes the transliterated Arabic term is used alone, sometimes the Latin translation, and on occasion both the transliterated Arabic and the translated Latin terms.[19] It is possible that the original translator did not always provide a Latin translation for each animal, which might explain that in most of the manuscripts a large proportion of the names for birds remained in transliterated Arabic.

However, I believe that, judging from the manuscript evidence, it is most likely that most of the titles for each entry originally included both the Arabic and the Latin. This would explain why the same entry in one manuscript might have the Arabic, the same in another only the Latin, and a third, both. For example, Balliol College MS.285, the entry on the wolf (chapter 18) is titled *De ozib lupo*, with *ozib* being the transliteration of the same term in Arabic (الذئب/*al-dhi'b*), along with the Latin term. In the same manuscript the entry for the crocodile (chapter 29) uses only the transliterated Arabic *De atincah* (from the Arabic التمساح/*al-timsāḥ*). However, most of the manuscripts and all the printed editions, use only the Latin for this animal. For example, in Vatican Pal. lat. MS.1211 the entry is titled *De*

16 Dioscorides, *De materia medica*, 2.1 and 2.2, ed. Wellmann (1907) 121.11–122.6, entries on sea urchin and hedgehog. On annotations related to *materia medica* in Greek and Arabic manuscripts of Dioscorides, see Mavroudi (Chapter 4) in this volume.

17 Sezgin (1970: 60ff.). Many thanks to Fabian Käs for this reference.

18 This is a reference to either *sinn al-fīl* ('elephant's tooth') or *'aẓm al-fīl* ('elephant's bone'). It is very unlikely to be a reference to ivory, which is *al-'āj*.

19 On the use of terms of ingredients in various languages in the same text, see also Käs (Chapter 1), Mavroudi (Chapter 4), and Martelli (Chapter 11) in the present volume.

proprietate cocodrilli. Similarly, for the entry on the gazelle (chapter 12), Balliol MS.285 uses only the Latin: *De damma*. In contrast for the same animal, Winchester College MS.26 uses only the Arabic *De algagel* (Arabic الغزال/*al-ghazāl*). The 1497 printed edition also keeps only the Arabic for this animal, with a slightly modification of spelling (*De agazelli*). The entire text in Prague Nat. Lib. MS.X.H.20 lacks chapter titles but calls the animal *agazel* in the entry (f. 233r), with a later marginal hand glossing it as *De capriolo silvestri* ('on the wild roe deer'). This same manuscript only uses the Latin for the wolf, with *caro lupi* in the entry and *De lupo* in the same later marginal hand (f. 234r). Erfurt Amplon F. 244 titled chapter 12, as *De gazele* (f. 136r), using the version with the definite article, *algazel*, accompanied by a later marginal note of *gazel et capriolo* ('roe deer'). As can be observed, the Arabic transliterations are not consistently spelled by scribes unfamiliar with the language. In the entry for the wolf, Erfurt Amplon F. 244 titles it *De ezip lupo* (f. 138r), using both the Arabic and Latin. Using both terms can help gloss the unfamiliar but using only the Arabic could be confusing. Kraków, Biblioteka Jagiellońska 817 might have for the gazelle the reassuring *De damna vel algazele* (f. 32r), with *algazel* used in the entry itself. However, the same manuscript can make the very familiar impossible to recognise: the entry for the hedgehog (chapter 23) is titled *De cambua* (f. 33r) using only the Arabic (قنفذ/*qunfudh*). But this does beg a question: what is the use of a text on the medical and magical properties of animals if the reader cannot identify the animals in the first place?

There is an argument to be made that the translator might have only translated into Latin animals that could be easily identified and left the 'exotic' or Middle Eastern animals in the original Arabic. For example, the cheetah, usually described as a hybrid between a lion and a leopard, is quite consistently termed with only the Arabic term *al-fahd*, called *alphet* in Vatican Pal. lat. MS.1211, *alfat* in Kraków BK 817, and *alpheib* in the 1497 Bergamo edition. But this does not explain why the crocodile or hedgehog, animals not unknown to Latin scholars, would appear with only its Latin name in one manuscript and only its Arabic name in another, or why the familiar wolf would need to be glossed as *ozib* or *ezip* along with its Latin name.

The confusion in animal terminology reaches its zenith in the entry on the hyena (chapter 17), which would be *al-ḍabʿ* (الضبع) in Arabic. The animal never appears in any of the manuscripts with the correct Latin translation (*iena*). Instead, the Arabic transliteration either appears alone (with a wide variety of spellings) or accompanied incorrectly by assorted different animals, such as the badger or wolf. Thus, it can be *De alboçao uel taxone* ('the badger') (Bergamo, 1497), *Albozoa vel taxone* (Basel, 1544), *de zabo* (Winchester Ms 26), titled *tebea* with *alzida* used in the entry (Vatican Palatina lat. MS.1211), *De lupo zabo* ('the wolf') (Balliol MS.285), *Sermo de alzaboa* (Prague MS.V.B.22 f. 98r), *alagabor vel lupe* in the text with a later marginal note of *De lupa* ('the female wolf') (Prague MS.X.H.20 f. 233v), *de alzabea* (Erfurt Amplon F. 244 f. 138r), and *De lupa* (Kraków BK 817 f. 33r). It does appear that the animal in the Latin translation was not accompanied by the correct translation, which accounts for the great confusion. When quoting *Sexaginta animalibus* in his work on animals, Albertus Magnus was clearly working from a manuscript that only had the transliterated Arabic term, as he creates a separate entry for the *alzabo* and does not give its properties to animals such as the badger, wolf, or hyena that all have separate entries in his text.[20]

Arabic terminology abounds in translated Latin medical texts, so it is possible that the translated text always had many untranslated transliterated animal names. By way of comparison, two other Arabic texts, translated in twelfth-century Toledo by Gerald of Cremona, have copious untranslated terms for animals and plants. Al-Rāzī's *Almansor*, when discussing the puncture wounds of spiders and scorpions, mentions the *akatereti* and *sibth*, both untranslated.[21] The *Liber canonis* (Ar. *Qānūn fī al-ṭibb*/*Canon of Medicine*) of Ibn Sīnā (Avicenna, d. 1037) abounds in untranslated terminology for animals, particularly when discussing toxicology. There are chapters on the *alharathati* ('when discussing wasps and scarabs'), the *cafezati et altararati* under snakes, or *de algerarat* (*al-jarrārah*, a kind of scorpion), under species of spiders.[22] The argument cannot be made that this translation strategy was only reserved for very unfamiliar species, as very familiar animals can appear untranslated in Ibn Sīnā. Such is the case of the wolf, for which like in some manuscript of *Sexaginta animalibus*, only the Arabic term is used. In two chapters, when discussing rabies, along with familiar animals such as the dog and the weasel, the wolf is merely called *adhib* (الذئب): *de morsu canis domestici*

[20] Ed. Stadler (1916–20) II.1360. [21] Abū Bakr al-Rāzī (Rhazes), *Almansor*, 8.4–5.

[22] Ibn Sīnā Book 4, Fen 6, Treatise 3, ch. 19, Treatise 3, ch. 40, and Treatise 5, ch. 4, respectively. Untranslated terms are not merely confined to animals. Assorted transliterated terms for plants appear such as *de alkebikengi* (possibly either *kabīkaj*, buttercup, or *kākanj*, winter cherry) and *de algilbehenech* (likely *jalbahnak*, mignonette). And not only confined to the natural world, such as the chapter on tattoos in Book 4, Fen 9, Treatise 2, ch. 7 which is titled de *alguassem* (الوشم/*al-washm*).

non rabiosi et morsu similiter adib et similium and de morsu canis rabiosi et adhib rabiosi et mustelle rabiose et aliorum ('on the bite of the non-rabid domestic dog and the similar bite of the *adib*; the bite of the rabid dog, the rabid *adhib* and the rabid weasel and others').[23]

However, this still does not explain why some manuscripts use Latin terms for an animal while others use only the Arabic term for the same entry. I believe that it is possible that a large proportion of the original Latin text had entries with both the Latin and Arabic terms. This would explain why the manuscripts share three different translation strategies: either only Latin, only Arabic, or both, all three used inconsistently in the text for all the manuscripts of Recension A (see list of manuscripts at end of this chapter).

The sole manuscript of Recension B consistently uses both Arabic and Latin for almost every entry.[24] This thirteenth-century manuscript, Oxford MS Rawlinson C-328, is the only illustrated copy of the text in the Latin tradition with each animal receiving a colourful depiction in the margin. The manuscript is illustrated throughout and includes a copy of the late antique Ps. Sextus Placitus' *Medicinae ex animalibus* with all of those individual animal entries illustrated as well, so there are two texts on animal *materia medica*, from very different traditions, in the same manuscript in the same hand. MS Rawlinson C-328 has forty-six animals, with a few repetitions, fewer than the fifty-six of the animals covered by Recension A, but it does have entries for animals that do not appear in the latter, such as the jerboa and the mole. In addition, this manuscript has different transliterations than the ones usually seen in Recension A, such as *ssaba* for wolf rather than *ozib*/*ezip*. Most of the animal entries are headed by both Latin and Arabic terms, such as *De bove et vaca de arthurz de albachar* ('the bull and the cow', *al-thawr*/*al-baqarah*), *de vulpe siue tabac* ('the fox' or *al-thaʿlab*), or *de leone leseet* ('the lion', *al-ʾasad*). Two entries use only Arabic terminology, and eight use only Latin. Recension B appears only once elsewhere, in a manuscript that contains most of Recension A: Wellcome Library MS.560. This manuscript begins with the section on the entries for the birds, before addressing quadrupeds and other animals, rather than the usual order of starting with quadrupeds, with the lion first. On one folio (f. 140r) near the end of the text, is an entry on the wolf. This animal had already been covered on f. 119r, under the title *Capitulum primum de*

[23] Ibn Sīnā Book 4, Fen 6, Treatise 4, chs. 4 and 5.

[24] Thorndike (1923: 761) introduces Oxford, Bodleian Library MS Rawlinson C-328, ff. 147–154v, as another text on medicinal animal virtues under its title of *Medicinal Secrets of Galen*, but it is a recension of *Sexaginta animalibus*.

propietatibus lupi ('The first chapter of the properties of the wolf') and was the first quadruped on a list, with the entry corresponding to the text for Recension A. However, another entry on the wolf appears on ff. 147v–148r, under the title *de lupo qui mihi veni in alium librum rex Regnati* ('on the wolf that came to me from the other book of the reigning king').[25] This entry corresponds to the entry on the wolf of Recension B of *Sexaginta animalibus.* Ironically, it uses only the Latin term without the corresponding Arabic transliteration, which is the characteristic of Recension B.[26]

Regarding authorship of the text, in the Latin tradition, there is a convention of ascribing it to al-Rāzī (Rhazes). The 1497 printing states, above the list on contents, that *Liber Rasis philosophi filii zacharie de proprietatibus membrorum et de utilitatibus et nocumentis animalium aggregatus ex dictis antiquorum secundum quod probaverunt antiqui, et continuit sermones* (*Book of Rhazes the Philosopher, Son of Zachariah, on the Properties and the Uses and Hazards of Animals Added from the Sayings of the Ancients Which Were Tested by the Ancients, and in Chapters*) and ends with *Et sic est finis Tractatus Rasis de animalibus* (*And This Is the End of the Treatise of Rhazes on Animals*). The 1544 edition affirms *Abubetri Rhazae Maomethi Scientia Peritia quae insignis medici, de facultatibus partium animalium* (*The Science and Knowledge of Abū Bakr Rhazes Muḥammad, with Medical Signs, on the Properties of Animal Parts*).[27] A fifteenth-century manuscript now in the Bibliotheca Apostolica Vaticana (Pal. lat. MS.1211) changes the usual incipit of *Verbum aristotelis et diascorides* (*The Word of Aristotle and Dioscorides*) to *Verbum rasis et dyascorides* (*The Word of Rhazes and Dioscorides*) with the title *Sermo razi*, even though a later hand ascribes it to Galen with the title *Incipit liber Galien de animalibus et plantis* (*Book of Galen on Animals and Plants*). *Sermo razi* also appears at the start of a late fifteenth-century manuscript now in the Wellcome Library (MS.560). An early fifteenth-century manuscript

[25] The title *Rex regnati* is very puzzling. It might be a misspelling of the name *Abubecri Rasis*, but this is very unclear. Ibn Sīnā is at times referred to as *princeps* ('prince') in the Latin tradition, based on his Arabic title *al-ra'īs* ('the master'). But that still does not make this citation any more comprehensible!

[26] Wellcome MS.560, ends with an entry on man (ff. 147r–148v) which does not correspond to any of the entries on man in both Recension A or B, and so must remain unattributed. The text ends with *Explicit liber de animalibus tam racionalibus quam in racionalibus. Deo gratio amen*. This is followed by an entry on the mole (f. 148v) titled *Capitulum de Talpa*. This comes from an early medieval compilation of animal properties extracted from Pliny the Elder's *Natural History*, the *Curae quae ex hominibus animalibus fiunt*. Edited as 48. *Curas quae de talpa fiunt*, pp. 214–15 in Arsenio Ferraces Rodríguez (2015), *Curae quae ex hominibus animalibus fiunt*: 214–15.

[27] (Venice, 1497) ff. 108r and 112v; and (Basel, 1544) 567.

now in Prague (MS.V.B.22) firmly ascribes it to *Rhasis filii Zacharie* as does a sixteenth-manuscript now in Leiden.[28] The fifteenth-century catalogue for St Augustine's Abbey, Canterbury, refers to a manuscript titled *Liber Rhasis et diascorides de naturis animalium* (*Book of Rhazes and Dioscorides on the Nature of Animals*), which is almost certainly a reference to *Sexaginta animalium.*[29] The Dominican Thomas in his early fourteenth-century *De essentiis essentiarum* (*On the Essences of Substances*) refers to a book titled *Rasis in libro de proprietatibus membrorum animalium* (*Rasis on the Properties of the Members of Animals*)[30] for an experiment involving creating a homunculus from semen (and then using its blood), which does not appear in either the Latin or Arabic versions (although there are entries for using human blood). It was ascribed to Galen twice, once under the confusing title *Liber medicinalis de secretis Galieni* (*The Medicinal Book of the Secrets of Galen*, Bodleian Library, MS Rawlinson C-328)[31] and once by a later hand with the title *Incipit liber Galien de animalibus et plantis* in Vatican Pal. lat. MS.1211 even though the original scribe of the text titles it at the start as *Sermo razi.* Ascribing the text to a 'great' authority is not novel, and as the manuscript usually travels with other medical texts, including those by Galen and al-Rāzī.

Regarding the authorship of the text itself, it is a translation of an Arabic text on the virtues of assorted animals. This is part of a genre of books on properties of animals, minerals, and plants, often titled on the 'useful' (*manāfiʿ*) or 'occult' (*khawāṣṣ*) virtues.[32] Specifically, I believe that the *Sexaginta animalibus* is on the whole a translation of a work on the properties of the body parts of animals by the eleventh-century physician ʿUbaydallāh ibn Bukhtīshūʿ. He came from a celebrated family of Nestorian physicians who had served the caliphs in Bagdad

[28] Wellcome Library, MS.560, f. 110r. Leiden, Universiteitsbibliotheek MS Vossianus Chym. Q. 27, f. 58v starts on the first folio with *Rases, de sexaginta animalium.*

[29] Thorndike (1923: 762, n. 3). However, it is not listed under Pseudo-al-Rāzī works in Ruska (1939: 31–94).

[30] *Rasis in libro de proprietatibus membrorum animalium ponit unum experimentum* (*Rasis on the Properties of the Members of Animals*). See Page (2013: 67 and 185), who cites van Lugt's (2009: 272–3) suggestion that Thomas is referring to the *Liber vaccae (Book of the Cow), a Translation of the Kitāb al-nawāmīs.* One manuscript of *Sexaginta animalibus* (Prague, Public and University Library MS.X.H.20, ff. 230v–238v) is erroneously titled *Liber vaccae.*

[31] Vatican, Pal. Lat. MS 1211, ff. 66r–72v, and Oxford, Bodleian Library MS Rawlinson C-328, ff. 147r–154v. The latter is titled *Liber medicinalis de secretis Galieni* (*Medical Book of the Secrets of Galen*). It should not be confused with the *Secretis Galieni ad Monteum* (*The Secrets of Galen Given to Monteus*), which is a completely different treatise and is printed with other Pseudo-Galenic works in *Spurii libri* (Venice, 1609), ff. 101–108v.

[32] For more on this genre, see the introduction in Raggetti (2018: XI–XXV). See also note 12 of the present chapter.

for many generations and who traced their medical pedigree back to the 'medical school' of Jundīshāpūr (now Shāhābād in Iran), although there is now considerable scepticism on the existence of such an institution, in which Greek texts were translated into Syriac.[33] He lived in Mayyāfāriqīn and died in AD 1058. His best-known work was the *Kitāb ṭabā'i' al-ḥayawān wa-khawāṣṣihā wa manāfi' a'ḍā'ihā* (*Book on the Characteristics of Animals and Their Properties and the Usefulness of Their Organs*), based on several sources, including Aristotle, Hippocrates, Galen, Dioscorides, and 'Īsā ibn 'Alī.

Comparing the entries in *Sexaginta animalibus* with the modern edition of 'Īsā ibn 'Alī's *Kitāb manāfi' a'ḍā' al-ḥayawān* (*Book on the Useful Properties of Animal Parts*), it is clear that the original Arabic had access to more than one recension of Ibn 'Alī, as entries unique to each one of the recensions abound throughout, which will be demonstrated in the analysis of one of the entries later in this chapter.[34] Ibn Bukhtīshū''s original treatise itself does not survive in the original Arabic, but it was used extensively in Arabic bestiaries of the Ibn Bukhtīshū' tradition.[35] Anna Contadini, in her work on British Library MS Or. 2784, a study of the earliest extant illustrated copy of an Arabic bestiary, which dates from the thirteenth century, concludes that it is a composite text, similar to all the other bestiaries of this tradition, although the text is not always the exact same. Most of the animal entries are composed of two distinct parts. The first details the characteristics of the animal in question and is likely derived from the sixth-century Pseudo-Aristotelian text *On Animals* by Timotheus of Gaza rather than from Aristotle's zoological texts directly.[36] The second part of most of the animal entries deals with the 'usefulness' (*manāfi'*) of the animal in question, and this material comes from Bukhtīshū''s treatise on the parts of animals.[37]

While the original Bukhtīshū' text does not survive in Arabic, as it was adapted and used in these bestiaries it is possible to compare the Arabic text on the medical and magical properties of each animal (derived from Ibn Bukhtīshū') with the Latin text *Sexaginta animalibus*, which had already

[33] There is now considerable scepticism on the existence of a Nestorian medical school per se at Jundīshāpūr, in which Greek texts were translated in Syriac. See Dols (1987).

[34] Raggetti (2018).

[35] Contadini (2012: 43–8), Contadini (1996: 142–7), Contadini (2003) and Contadini (1992).

[36] Contadini (2012: 48–50). The first three books of Aristotle's Zoology were translated into Arabic in the ninth century (*Kitāb al-ḥayawān*), which itself would be translated by Michael Scot in the early thirteenth century. The Arabic title for Timotheus' work is *Kitāb al-ḥayawān al-qadīm* although it is not quoted as such in the manuscripts. Also see van den Abeele (1999).

[37] Contadini (2012: 39–43).

been translated into Latin before the earliest surviving Arabic bestiary using the same material.[38]

In his edition of Ibn al-Jazzār's work on specific properties, Fabian Käs has commented how *Sexaginta animalibus* follows the tradition of this genre, in both ʿĪsā ibn ʿAlī and particularly ʿUbaydallāh ibn Bukhtīshūʿ.[39] Käs noted that al-Jazzār's treatise has ten statements on the properties of animals which he could not trace in any other Arabic source, including Ibn Bukhtīshūʿ, but which are found in *Sexaginta animalibus*.[40] The most likely solution for this conundrum is that the text which was translated as *Sexaginta animalibus* is an enlarged version of ibn Bukhtīshūʿ's treatise on properties, that contains sections taken from Ibn al-Jazzār's work.[41] This would not be unusual, for as Lucia Raggetti has noted in her edition of ʿĪsā ibn ʿAlī, one of the earliest authors of this genre, the tradition is very fluid and the very nature of a compilation of properties of individual animals means that some properties might be added or discarded.

A possible connection should also be noted between the original Arabic text of *Sexaginta animalibus* and the early twelfth-century Ibn Biklārish's *Kitāb al-adwiyah al-mufradah li-l-Isrāʾīlī* (*Book of Simple Medicines by al-Israʾili*). This text is usually referred to as the *Kitāb al-Mustaʿīnī* (in honour of the author's patron, the ruler of Saragossa). Unlike in *manāfiʿ* literature, where the contents are organised by individual animals, in the *Kitāb al-Mustaʿīnī*, material covering plants, minerals, and animals is organised alphabetically by components. Thus, the entry for blood will encompass the properties for blood for thirteen different animals. Anna Contadini has discussed the structural and specific differences (in regard to uses and preparation) between the *Kitāb al-Mustaʿīnī and manāfiʿ* literature (specifically ibn Bukhtīshūʿ), pointing out that it is difficult to gauge the relationship between this text and other *manāfiʿ* texts. The intriguing connection is that the number of animals mentioned in the *Kitāb al-Mustaʿīnī is fifty-eight,* which is very close to the fifty-six discussed

38 See Contadini (2012: 57) for a list of the extant sixteen manuscripts of bestiaries of the Ibn Bukhtīshūʿ tradition – thirteen in Arabic and three in Persian – with five illustrated copies in all. Also see Contadini (1989, 1994).

39 Käs (2012: 8–9). I am very grateful to Fabian Käs for our discussion and correspondence on this issue. In his edition of Ibn al-Jazzār, he also demonstrated how it was the main source for the Pseudo-Albertus Magnus *De mirabilibus mundi* (*The Miracles of the World*), along with a translation of the *Kitāb al-nawāmīs* (*Liber vaccae, Book of the Cow*). There does not, however, appear to be any direct connection between the Latin translation of Ibn al-Jazzār's work and *Sexaginta animalibus*; see Saif (2016: 1–48).

40 These are Käs (2012: nos. 16, 20a, 33, 62, 63, 64, 74, 75, 77, 101).

41 A definite solution will likely only be possible with an edition of *Sexaginta animalibus*, which I plan to undertake, and more work on the contents of Ibn Bukhtīshūʿ's corpus.

in the *Sexaginta animalibus*. Could Ibn Biklārish have used the lost Arabic text of *Sexaginta animalibus* when compiling his treatise on medical remedies? Unfortunately, while there are some overlaps, there are notable differences and omissions, and the list of animals does not appear to concord. But, as Contadini remarks when discussing the text with other *manāfiʿ* works, 'we remain faced with tantalizing hints of contact emerging out of a body of material that points to a general cultural agreement about methods of treatment, but all too frequently fails to agree on specifics'.[42] Remke Kruk has made the point that often a large proportion of uses of animals in *manāfiʿ* texts are unique to it, making clear-cut connections between texts and authors difficult.[43]

The following section will compare one animal entry in both recensions of *Sexaginta animalibus* with the *manāfiʿ* section from an Arabic Ibn Bukhtīshūʿ bestiary (British Library Ms Or. 2784, titled *Kitāb naʿt al-ḥayawān*) which follows a long section on the characteristics of the elephant.[44] It will also note the recension used from Ibn ʿAlī for each individual property if pertinent.[45] As a final point, the order of the different properties for each entry in all three texts is different.

Recension A (The Elephant)

1) *Sexaginta animalibus*: Its flesh is cold, heavy, fatty, and abominable (not in Ibn Bukhtīshūʿ nor Ibn ʿAlī).

[42] Contadini (2008: 133–59, quote from 150). Some of these questions regarding potential links between the *Sexaginta animalibus* and the *Kitāb al-Mustaʿīnī* will be aided with the critical edition of the latter, under preparation by Joëlle Ricordel.

[43] Kruk (2010: 49–64).

[44] Available digitised: www.qdl.qa/en/archive/81055/vdc_100023556967.0x000001, accessed 24 November 2019.

[45] The Latin is the following: *De elephante. Caro eius ponderosa frigida pinguis abhominabilis. Qui gustat ex ea cum aqua et sale cocta cum seminibus asquesimi: sanat tussim antiquam: quando coquitur et liquefit cum aceto et semine feni. Si autem pregnans potet ex iure illo proiicit quod habet in utero. Fel eius quando immittitur per nares ad pondus unius alkisat cum tantundem moschi valet contra caducum morbum. Additamentum epatis sumptum et comestum cum aqua sumach et foliis citranguli valet plurimum contra dolorem epatis. Stercus elephantis si inungatur cum eo corium in quo sint pediculi apparentes et dimittantur donec desiccentur supra ipsum non remanebunt pediculi sed statim egredientur. Sepum elephanti si cum eo inungatur patiens dolorem capitis curatur. Aristoteles. Cum potatur alkal id os elephantis ad pondus unius uncia tritum vel rasura bibitum ab eo quem primo tangit lepra cum decem uncia aqua mentastri montani confert ei. Stercus elephanti si fumigetur cum eo domus aut locus in quo sunt culices necat eas.* The text is based on Venice (1497) and Basel (1544), but it is quite consistent throughout Recension A. The Arabic translation of Ibn Bukhtīshūʿ (British Library MS Or. 2784) is from Contadini (2012: 86), with corrections by Fabian Käs. The Arabic translation of Ibn ʿAlī is from Raggetti (2018: 244–7).

2) *Sexaginta animalibus*: For one who eats it with water and salt, cooked with asafoetida/lovage seeds, it cures a chronic cough.[46]

Ibn Bukhtīshūʿ: Elephant meat, when cooked in water, salt, and lovage,[47] and the broth given to sip to someone with a chronic cough and asthma, cures him (Ibn ʿAlī Recension B).

3) *Sexaginta animalibus*: When it is cooked with vinegar and fennel seeds until it is liquefied, if a pregnant woman should drink it, she will cast out whatever is in her womb.

Ibn Bukhtīshūʿ: If it is cooked in vinegar and asafoetida until boiled down to shreds and drunk by a pregnant woman, it causes an abortion (Ibn ʿAlī Recension B, although the same property appears with little variation in Recension A and C as well).

4) *Sexaginta animalibus*: When its bile is put in the nose, a weight of one *alkisat* with some musk, it is good against epilepsy.

Ibn Bukhtīshūʿ: Its gall-bladder – When someone with epilepsy takes a *qīrāṭ* of it is as a nasal injection together with a like amount of musk, it cures him. (Ibn ʿAlī Recension B only. Although the property appears in Recension A and C, the former does not give a unit measurement while C uses *mithqāl*.)

5) *Sexaginta animalibus*: The liver appendage, if eaten with sumac water and citron leaves is good for liver pains.

Ibn Bukhtīshūʿ: Elephant liver – When someone with liver pain eats it with sumac juice and aubergine leaves it is beneficial for him (resembles Ibn ʿAlī Recension A, which refers to the liver only. However, Ibn ʿAlī Recension C refers specifically to the liver appendage, like *Sexaginta animalibus*, and the additional ingredients are basil leaves and sumac.

6) *Sexaginta animalibus*: If elephant dung is smeared on skin where lice can be seen, and left to dry, the lice will not remain but leave immediately.

Ibn Bukhtīshūʿ: Elephant – dung. It kills lice if smeared onto the body and left until dry (Ibn ʿAlī Recension B only).

7) *Sexaginta animalibus*: If elephant fat is smeared on a patient suffering a headache, he will be cured, Aristotle.

Ibn Bukhtīshūʿ: Elephant fat – When used to fumigate someone with a headache it cures him. (Here it is fumigation, not rubbing).

[46] These are *seminibus asquisimi* in Basel 1497 (called *seminibus alkasini* in Leiden Vossianus Chym. Q. 27, f. 63r), the Arabic for lovage is *kashim* (كاشم). Both Balliol MS 285, f. 66v, and Erfurt Amplon MS F. 244, ff. 135v, call them *seminibus ferule* ('asafoetida seeds') here, which is what these seeds are consistently called in the next property.

[47] Translated as Mediterranean moon carrot in Raggetti (2018: 244–7).

However, the property of rubbing elephant fat for a headache is in Ibn ʿAlī Recension A and C. There is no mention of Aristotle in both authors. The adscription of this property in *Sexaginta animalibus* to Aristotle, which does not appear of his accepted works, could come from the *Kitāb naʿt al-ḥayawān*, ascribed to Aristotle, which claims that elephant's gall cures headache, and could have been one of Ibn Bukhtīshūʿ sources, as several of the properties mentioned can be found in it.[48]

8) *Sexaginta animalibus*: If *alkal*, that is elephant bone in one ounce measure (after being ground up) is mixed with ten ounces of mountain mint water, and drunk by one whom the first signs of leprosy have touched, he will be cured.

Ibn Bukhtīshūʿ: Elephant bone, that is, ivory (*al-ʿāj*) – When a piece is taken and ground of filed and drunk with water it is beneficial against the onset of elephantiasis. It must be drunk with the juice of mountain mint, for it then arrests the onset of elephantiasis and prevents it from increasing (this property appears in all three recensions of Ibn ʿAlī. Recension C mentions the measurement of ten dirham with river sedge water, rather than mountain mint water/ juice).

9) *Sexaginta animalibus*: If a house or someplace where there are bugs is fumigated with elephant dung, they will die.

Ibn Bukhtīshūʿ: It removes leprosy and if used as a fumigant it drives bugs away (there is no mention of leprosy in either *Sexaginta animalibus* or Ibn ʿAlī. This property in *Sexaginta animalibus* most resembles Ibn ʿAlī Recension B).

Sexaginta animalibus Recension A does not cover all of the material in ibn Bukhtīshūʿ, which has three additional properties, one of which is from Ibn ʿAlī Recension C ('If a woman drinks it, she will never get pregnant').[49] This last property however does appear in *Sexaginta animalibus* Recension B, which covers only three properties.

[48] *Kitāb naʿt al-ḥayawān* (*Book on the Description of Animals*, Tunis, MS Bibliothèque nationale 16385, f. 35v). Many thanks to Fabian Käs for alerting me to this text. This property does not appear in Aristotle's *History of Animals*, *Generation of Animals*, *Parts of Animals*, or *Progression of Animals*.

[49] These other two Ibn Bukhtīshūʿ properties are: 'When a woman drinks a *mithqāl* of ivory filings, she conceives. Parings of it reduce pain in the fingernails when left on them. If the same weight of iron filings is added to them and they are dusted onto haemorrhoids, it cures them. If fragments of tusk are hung on a black thread around the necks of cattle, they will be safe from plague' (Contadini (2012: 86)).

Recension B (MS Rawlinson C-328)[50] (The Elephant)

1) Elephant fat, when used to fumigate someone, is good against headache (this resembles Ibn Bukhtīshūʿ more than Recension A, with the mention of fumigation rather than rubbing the patient. Only Ibn ʿAlī Recension B mentions rubbing, A and C refer to fumigation). See property 7 of Recension A of *Sexaginta animalibus*. Recension B does not mention Aristotle.
2) This crushed, pulverised (to the weight of bezants) and drunk frequently with rose water will help keep one developing elephantiasis (the disease is specified as in Ibn Bukhtīshūʿ and Ibn ʿAlī, while Recension A terms it *lepra*. The measurements and plant ingredients are different).
3) A measurement of one bezant of dung given to a woman to drink will not permit her to conceive (this property is not in Recension A but is in in Ibn Bukhtīshūʿ and Ibn ʿAlī. For the later, it resembles most Recension C of Ibn ʿAlī, which mentions the measurement of one *dāniq*).

Analysing entries of *Sexaginta animalibus* with a copy of an Ibn Bukhtīshūʿ bestiary shows that it is likely an enlarged version of Ibn Bukhtīshūʿ.[51] It does have particular characteristics, such as the frequent mention by name of ancient authorities, as discussed previously. As Ibn Bukhtīshūʿ's original Arabic text does not survive, a direct comparison will not be possible, as the comparison can only be made with later reworked versions. *Sexaginta animalibus* has fewer animal entries in total and in general there are less properties per animal than in Ibn Bukhtīshūʿ. Adding to the mix is the fact that *Sexaginta animalibus* exists in two recensions, with Recension B containing shorter entries and often preserving material from the Arabic text which does not appear in Recension A. There are also some adaptions and omissions between the Arabic and Latin. Ingredients and measurements often change. Thus, the entry for the horse in the Arabic mentions how horse sweat mixed with mare's milk will cause an abortion if

[50] MS Rawlinson C-328, f. 151v: *Pinguido elefantis ualet fumigata contra sonitum capitis. Hos tritum et pulueriçatum et potatum sepe ab elefantiatico ad pondus biçanciorum et cum suco rosarum lentisane conseruat in eodem stata. Stercus eius potatum a muliere cum uino ad pondus biçancii non ultra permixit eam concipe.*

[51] I did most of the comparison with the *Kitāb manāfiʿ al-ḥayawān* (*Book on the Usefulness of Animals*, Real Biblioteca of San Lorenzo del Escorial, MS Ar. 898), using the Ruiz Bravo-Villasante (1980) translation.

given to a pregnant woman, while *Sexaginta animalibus* states that the mixture is horse sweat and wine.[52]

In addition, the Latin translator might have decided not to include all properties from the Arabic text he had access to. For example, the entry on the hyena in Ibn Bukhtīshūʿ mentions that the animal's hairs have two virtues: firstly, the hairs of a male hyena, mixed with pitch, and anointed on the bottom of an effeminate man, will cure him of this condition. In contrast, the hairs of a female hyena, mixed with pitch and anointed on the bottom of a man, he will become effeminate.[53] All copies of *Sexaginta animalibus*, in the entry for the *alzabo* (as the hyena is termed) have the first property but never the second.[54]

In addition, the text overwhelmingly travels with other medical material in the manuscript tradition. For example, the other texts in Winchester College MS 26 include Bruno Longobardensis' *Cyrurgia*, Archimatheus' *Practica*, Trotula's *De passionibus mulierum* (*On the Diseases of Women*), *Secreta ypocratis* (*Secrets of Hippocrates*), Pseudo-Hippocrates' *Capsula eburnea* (*The Ivory Casket*), a short work on clysters, Richardus Anglicus' *Signi Ricardi* (*Signs of Richard*), a treatise on falconry in Old French, *Circa instans*, a commentary on the *Antidotarium Nicholai*, *Attonomia palemonis* (*Palemon's Anatomy*), Roger de Barone's *Rogerina minor* and *Rogerina maior*, *Practica Platearii*, and Iohannes de Sancto Paulo's *Liber de medicinarum virtutibus* (*Book on Simple Medicines*). Like most thirteenth- and fourteenth-century manuscripts of the *Sexaginta animalibus*, the contents are overwhelmingly medical. In contrast, fifteenth- and sixteenth-century manuscripts of the text tend to travel with both medical and magical material. The late fifteenth-century Wellcome Library MS 560 includes Peter of Spain *Liber de oculis* (*Book on the Eye*) and *De xii aquis* (*On 12 Waters*), Roland of Parma *Rolandina*, Maimonides *Aphorismi de cibis et potibus* (*Aphorisms on Food and Drink*), al-Zahrāwī (Albucasis) *Liber servitoris de preparacionibus medicinarum simplicium* (*Book on the Preparation of Simple Medicines*), *Kiranides*, Ps. Albertus Magnus *Liber aggregationis* (*Book of Additions*), Ps. Albertus Magnus *Secreta*

[52] MS Escorial Ar. 898, in Contadini (1996: 144). Basel (1497): *De equo Sermo VI. Sudor equi mistus cum uino potatus a muliere pregnante proiicit fetum.*

[53] MS Escorial Ar. 898 in Ruiz Bravo-Villasante (1980: 43). This property is only in ʿĪsā ibn ʿAlī Recension C but talks about the flesh of the hyena, not the hairs; Raggetti (2018: 53).

[54] Basel (1497): *De alboçao uel taxone Sermo XVII: Si sumatur pilus zabo de pilis qui sunt circa collum masculi, et comburatur, teratur cum pice, deinde iungatur cum eo anus sodomittae patientis, removetur ab eo vitium illud.*

Secretorum Alberti Magni, Ps. Arnold of Villanova, *De XII sigillis* (*On Twelve Seals*), Anonymous *Experimenta* (*Experiments*), Ps. Apuleius *De Herbarius* (*On Herbs*), ending with Sextus Placitus *Medicinae ex animalibus*. To conclude, *Sexaginta animalibus*, addressing every possible animal part (fat, urine, blood, bile, horn, claws, skin, flesh, brain, liver, testicles, excrement, marrow, etc.) for more than fifty animals, deserves consideration alongside more familiar sources of animal *materia medica* lore, and as a rare translated text from the Arabic genre of works on the properties of animals.

Appendix

Printed editions of *Sexaginta animalibus*

- Bergamo, 1497 *Liber Rasis ad almansorem et alia* (Bonetus Locatellus, for Octavianus Scotus). In a large collection of mostly works by al-Rāzī and those ascribed to him, such as *Liber Rasis ad almansorem*, *Divisiones*, *Liber de juncturarum egritudibus*, *Liber de egritudinibus puerorum*, *Capsula eburnea*, *Libellus zoar de cura lapidis*, etc., ff. 108r–112v.
- Venice, 1500 (Johannes Hamman) [same version as Bergamo edition, although slight variation in the al-Rāzī and Pseudo-al-Rāzī treatises printed in the text].
- Basel, 1544. *Opera omnia of al-Rāzī works*. Titled *Abubetri Rhazæ Opera exquisitiora per Gerardum Toletanum*. Edited by Alban Thorer. Minor differences between this version and the two other printings. Titled *De facultatibus animalibus*, pp. 566–90.

Manuscripts of *Sexaginta animalibus*

Usual incipit: *verbum aristoteles et dioscorides est in collo leonis* (first line for the entry on the lion)

· Identified in Thorndike and Kibre (1963, 1688)
+ Identified by author
* Identified in other manuscript catalogues

Recension A

* Cesena (Forlì-Cesena), Biblioteca Comunale Malatestiana, D. XXVI.1, ff. 178r-181v.[55]

* Erfurt, Wissenschaftliche Bibliothek, Amplonian Collection, Handschriften F. 244 ff. 133–43 (early fourteenth century).

· Erfurt, Wissenschafliche Bibliothek, Amplonian Collection, Handschriften F. 273 ff. 98v–100v (early fourteenth century) [incorrectly ascribed as *De signis celestibus*].

* Innsbruck, Universitäts- und Landesbibliothek Tirol (olim Universitätsbibliothek), 489, ff. 54r–56v. Incomplete.[56]

* Kraków, Biblioteka Jagiellońska 817 pp. 28–42 (Catalogued as 'Rasis, *De sexaginta animalibus*'). Dated 1483.[57]

* Leiden, Universiteitsbibliotheek MS Vossianus Chym. Q. 27, ff. 58v-79r. Titled *Rases de proprietatibus sexaginta animalium* (sixteenth century, before 1540). Incipit: Ex verbis Aristoteles et dioscorides.

* London, Wellcome Library MS.560 (Miscellanea Medica XXXVI) ff. 110r–148r (*c.*1475). First folio titled: *Sermo razi in volatilibus irrationalibus.* Incipit: *Upupe caro frigida grossa austera est et in pullis.*[58]

\+ Oxford, Balliol College Library, MS.285 f. 41r–v, f. 66r (thirteenth century). Incipit: *De ozib lupo.*

· Prague, Národni knihovna České republiky MS.V.B.22 (Y.II.5. n. 48) ff. 95r–103r.

· Prague, Národni knihovna České republiky MS.X.H.20, ff. 230v–238v (thirteenth century) [incorrectly ascribed as *Liber vaccae*].

\+ Winchester, Winchester College Library MS.26 ff. 67r–68v (late thirteenth/early fourteenth century) Incipit: *sanguinem conglobatum et confert* (halfway through the entry for the sheep).

· Vatican, Bibliotheca Apostolica Latina, Palatina lat. MS.1211 ff. 66r–72v (fifteenth century). Despite having as an incipit '*verbum rasis et dyascorides*' and the title '*sermo razi*' in the scribe's hand, at the top of the first folio, it is incorrectly ascribed to Galen by another hand (*Incipit liber Galien de animalibus et plantis*).

[55] Garfagnini et al. (1982: 96–100), via http://www.mirabileweb.it, accessed 30 September 2019.
[56] Mairhofer et al. (2008: 578–83), via http://www.mirabileweb.it, accessed 30 September 2019.
[57] Láng (2008: 323). [58] Moorat (1962–73: I.432–4).

Recension B

+ Oxford, Bodleian Library, MS.Rawlinson C-328, ff. 147r–154v (thirteenth century). Titled *Liber medicinalis de secretis Galieni*. Only illustrated copy.

List of animal entries in *Sexaginta animalibus*

(from the 1497 Basel printed edition, most manuscripts follow this order)

1. De leone (lion)
2. De alpheib (lion/leopard hybrid. Transliterated Arabic: cheetah)
3. De tauro (the bull)
4. De ove (the sheep)
5. De capra (the goat)
6. De equo (horse)
7. De mulo vel mula (mule)
8. De asino (the ass)
9. De camello (the camel)
10. De elephante (the elephant)
11. De cervo (the deer)
12. De agazelli (the gazelle)
13. De urso (the bear)
14. De cane (the dog)
15. De vulpe (the fox)
16. De lepore (the hare)
17. De alboçao vel taxone (the alzabo/hyena)
18. De lupo (the wolf)
19. De leopard (the leopard)
20. De furone (polecat)
21. De mustela (weasel)
22. De simia (the ape)
23. De ericio (the hedgehog/sea urchin)
24. De cancro (the crab)
25. De testudine (the tortoise)
26. De tortuca (the turtle)
27. De pisce sagittali (the arrow fish)
28. De lacerta (the lizard)
29. De cocodrillo (the crocodile)
30. De rana (the frog)

31. De gato silvestri (the wild cat)
32. De mure (the mouse)
33. De *yaraboath*
34. De formici (on ants)
35. De aldea locustis (the locust swarm)
36. De uppupa (the hoopoe)
37. De *alkalkan*
38. De columbis (the dove)
39. De aucha (the goose)
40. De grue (the crane)
41. De noticula (night-owl?)
42. De *açtore* vel *alkarvem*
43. De carnibus avium vel aliorum vel de gallo (on the flesh of birds and others and on the cockerel)
44. De pullis (on hens)
45. De laudis cristatis (tufted lark)
46. De finoris (the finch?)
47. De *assikakak* (passeris, i.e. sparrows in Vatican Palatina lat. MS 1211)
48. De *alkemo*
49. De anseribus (on geese)
50. De corvo (the raven)
51. De pica (the magpie)
52. De passeribus domorum (on house sparrows)
53. De vulture (the vulture)
54. De aranea (the spider)
55. De homine (the man)
56. De muliere (the woman)

List of animal entries in Oxford, Bodleian MS Rawlinson C- 328 ff. 147r–154v

Incipit: *Incipit liber medicinalis de secretis Galeni*

De hominis	Man
De leone leseet	Lion (*al-ʾasad*)
De lupo ssaba	Wolf (*al-dhiʾb*)
De vulpe siue tabac	Fox (*al-thaʿlab*)
De mustela	Weasel
De urso dub	Bear (*al-dubb*)
De clire de aliador	Gazelle

(*cont.*)

De porco de hanzir	Pig (*al-khinzīr*)
De bove vel de arthaur	Bull (*al-thawr*)
De equo et equa de alfaras de atramaca	Horse and mare (*al-faras*)
De mulo et mula de albachal de albachala	Mule (*al-baghl*)
De asinus de aimac	Ass (*al-ḥimār*)
De asinibus de chimara	Ass (*al-ḥimār al-ahlī*)
De onagro de aimaraluoso	Onager/Wild Ass (*al-ḥimār al-waḥshī*)
De camelis de elgemel	Camel (*al-jamal*)
De pecude de cuebse	Sheep/Ram (*al-kabsh*)
De capreis et ircis de alaarizi de maciza	Goat (*al-māʿiz*)
De bove et vaca de arthurz de albachar	Bull and Cow (*al-thawr/al-baqarah*)
Thaa	
De leopardo ingemer	Leopard (*al-namir*)
De elephante de alfil	Elephant (*al-fīl*)
De furetta eliiceps	Ferret (*ibn ʿirs*)
De mure silvestri vel stelione de adalib	Wild mouse [gerboa] and a lizard (*al-ḍabb*)
De bubalis de elegemus	Buffalo (*al-jāmūs*)
De murilego de elthit	Cat (*hirr*?)
De simiis de h'erd	Monkey (*al-qird*)
De lince de elfeet siue leocupuscula	Lynx/Cheetah (*al-fahd*)
De genere muris de baasis	A type of mouse
De ansera de eluece	Goose (*al-iwazz*)
Huuabar	Bustard (*ḥubārā*)
De ericio de canfut	Hedgehog (*al-qunfudh*)
De cane de Kelbe	Dog (*al-kalb*)
De talpa de *gelte*	Mole (*al-khuld*)
De starnis	Crane
De gallina duragi	Hen (*al-dajājah*)
De vulture heemesir	Vulture (*al-nasr*)
De muscis viridibus	Green flies
De ave cum cresta foathit	Crested bird
De Turture alguarasa de eliamin	Turtledove (*al-warashān/al-ḥamām*)
Laudula uel uupu de eleut ehut	Lark and hoopoe (*al-hudhud*)
Yrandine de athaer de ave habente capud nigrorum	Swallow (*al-ṭāʾir*?)/black-headed bird
De pasere de aliartan	Sparrow (*ʿaṣāfīr*?)
De apro aut uero	Boar
De bubone	Owl
De vulture	Vulture
De transmarina aquila	Sea-eagle

(followed by a short section on humoral complexions)

REFERENCES

Abeele, B. van den. 1999. 'Le "De animalibus" d'Aristote dans le monde latin: Modalités de sa réception médiévale', *Frühmittelalterliche Studien* 33: 287–318.

Burnett, C. 2001. 'The Coherence of the Arabic-Latin Translation Programme in Toledo in the Twelfth Century', *Science in Context* 14: 249–88.

Burnett, C. 2002. 'Filosofiá natural, secretos and magia', in L. Garcia Ballester (ed.), *Historia de ciencia y de la téchnica en la Corona de Castilla*, vol. I. Valladolid: Junta de Castilla y León, Consejería de Educación y Cultura, 95–144.

Contadini, A. 1989. 'The Kitāb Manāfiʿ al-ḥayawān in the Escorial Library', *Islamic Art* 3: 33–57.

Contadini, A. 1992. 'The Kitāb Naʿt al-ḥayawān and the Ibn Bakhtīshūʿ Illustrated Bestiaries'. SOAS, University of London: PhD thesis.

Contadini, A. 1994. 'The Ibn Buḫtīšūʿ Bestiary Tradition: The Text and Its Sources', *Medicina nei Secoli Arte e Scienza* 6(2): 349–64.

Contadini, A. 1996. 'The Horse in Two Manuscripts of Ibn Bakhtīshūʿ's Kitāb Manāfiʿ al-Ḥayawān', in D. Alexander (ed.), *Furusiyya*. Vol. I: *The Horse in the Art of the Near East*. Riyadh: King Abdulaziz Public Library, 142–7.

Contadini, A. 2003. 'A Bestiary Tale: Text and Image of the Unicorn in the Kitāb naʿt al-ḥayawān (British Library, or. 2784)', *Muqarnas* 2: 17–33.

Contadini, A. 2008. 'The Zoological-Medicinal Material in the Arcadian Library Manuscript', in C. Burnett (ed.), *Ibn Baklārish's Book of Simples: Medical Remedies between Three Faiths in Twelfth Century Spain*. Oxford: Oxford University Press, 133–59.

Contadini, A. 2012. *A World of Beasts: A Thirteenth-Century Illustrated Arabic Book on Animals (the Kitāb Naʿt al-Ḥayawān) in the Ibn Bakhtīshūʿ Tradition*. Leiden: Brill.

Dols, M. W. 1987. 'The Origins of the Islamic Hospital: Myth and Reality', *Bulletin of the History of Medicine* 61: 367–90.

Ferraces Rodríguez, A. ed. 2015. *Curae quae ex hominibus animalibus fiunt: Estudio y edicion critica*. Santiago de Compostela: Andavira.

Garfagnini, G. C., Pomaro, G., Rossi, P., and Velli, A. 1982. *Catalogo di manoscritti filosofici nelle biblioteche italiane*, vol. IV. Florence: Olschki.

Horden, P. 2013. 'The Uses of Medical Manuscripts', in B. Zipser (ed.), *Medical Books in the Byzantine World*. Bologna: Eikasmós: 1–6.

Kaimakis, D. ed. 1976. *Die Kyraniden*. Hain: Meisenheim am Glan.

Käs, F. ed. 2012. *Die Risāla fī l-Ḫawāṣṣ des Ibn al-Ǧazzār: Die arabische Vorlage des Albertus Magnus zugeschriebenen Traktats De mirabilibus mundi*. Wiesbaden: Harrassowitz.

Ker, N. R., and Piper, A. J. 1992. *Medieval Manuscripts in British Libraries*, vol. IV. Oxford: Oxford University Press.

Kruk, R. 1985. 'Hedgehogs and Their "Chicks": A Case History of the Aristotelian Reception in Arabic Zoology', *Zeitschrift für Geschichte der arabisch-islamischen Wissenschaften* 2: 205–34.

Kruk, R. 2010. 'Elusive Giraffes: Ibn Abi l-Ḥawāfir's Badāʾiʿ al-Akwān and Other Animal Books', in A. Contadini (ed.), *Arab Painting: Text and Image in Illustrated Arabic Manuscripts*. Leiden: Brill: 49–64.

Láng, B. 2008. *Unlocked Books: Manuscripts of Learned Magic in the Medieval Libraries of Central Europe*. University Park: Pennsylvania State University Press.

Lugt, M. van der. 2009. '"Abominable Mixtures": The *Liber Vaccae* in the Medieval West, or the Dangers and Attractions of Natural Magic', *Traditio* 64: 229–77.

Mairhofer D., Neuhauser W., Rossini M. et al. 2008. *Katalog der Handschriften der Universitätsbibliothek Innsbruck*, vol. V. Vienna: Verlag der Österreichischen Akademie der Wissenschaften.

McVaugh, M., 2009. 'Towards a Stylistic Grouping of the Translations of Gerard of Cremona', *Mediaeval Studies* 71: 99–112.

Moorat, S. A. J. 1962–73. *Catalogue of Western Manuscripts on Medicine and Science in the Wellcome Historical Medical Library*. 3 vols. London: Wellcome Institute for the History of Medicine.

Mynors, R. 1963. *Catalogue of the Manuscripts of Balliol College Oxford*. Oxford: Clarendon.

Nagel, S. 1999. 'Testi con due redazioni attribuite ad un medesimo autore: il caso del *De animalibus* di Pietro Ispano', in G. Guldentops and C. Steel (eds.), *Aristotle's Animals in the Middle Ages and Renaissance*. Leuven: Leuven University Press: 212–37.

Page, S. 2013. *Magic in the Cloister: Pious Motives, Illicit Interests, and Occult Approaches to the Medieval Universe*. University Park: Pennsylvania State University Press.

Pseudo-Galen. 1609. *Spurii Galeno ascripti libri*. Giunta: Venice.

Raggetti, L. ed. 2018. *ʿĪsā ibn ʿAlī's Book on the Useful Properties of Animal Parts: Edition, Translation and Study of a fluid Tradition*. Berlin: De Gruyter.

al-Rāzī (Rhazes). 1497. *Almansoris liber nonus cum expositione Syllani*. Venice: Otinum Papiensem de Luna.

Ruiz Bravo-Villasante, C. trans. 1980. *Libro de las Utilidades de los Animales*. Madrid: Fundación Universitaria Española.

Ruska, J. 1939. 'Pseudepigraphe Rasis-Schriften', *Osiris* 7: 31–94.

Saif, L. 2016. 'The Cows and the Bees: Arabic Sources and Parallels for Pseudo-Plato's *Liber vaccae* (*Kitāb al-Nawāmīs*)', *Journal of the Warburg and Courtauld Institutes* 79: 1–48.

Salmòn Muñiz, F. 2002. 'La medicina y las traducciones toledanas del siglo XII', in L. Garcia Ballester (ed.), *Historia de ciencia y de la téchnica en la Corona de Castilla*, vol. I. Valladolid: Junta de Castilla y León, Consejería de Educación y Cultura, 631–46.

Segolini, M. P. ed. 1998. *Libri medicinae Sexti Placiti Papyriensis ex animalibus pecoribus et bestiis vel avibus Concordantiae*. Hildesheim: Olms-Weidmann.

Sezgin, F. 1970. *Geschichte des arabischen Schrifttums*, vol. III. Leiden: Brill.

Stadler, H. ed. 1916–20. *Albertus Magnus. De animalibus libri XXVI.* 2 vols. Munster: Aschendorff.

Steinschneider, M. 1956. *Die hebräischen Übersetzungen des Mittelalters.* Graz: Akademische Druck- und Verlagsanstalt.

Thorndike, L. 1923. *A History of Magic and Experimental Science*, vol. II. New York: Columbia University Press.

Thorndike, L., and Kibre, P. 1963. *A Catalogue of Incipits of Medieval Scientific Writings in Latin.* Cambridge, MA: Mediaeval Academy of America.

Ventura, I. 2005. 'The *Curae ex animalibus* in the Medical Literature of the Middle Ages: The Example of the Illustrated Herbals', in B. van den Abeele (ed.), *Bestiares médiévaux: Nouvelles perspectives sur les manuscripts et les traditions textuelles.* Brepols: Louvain-la-Neuve, 213–48.

Wellmann, M. ed. 1907. *Pedanii Dioscuridis Anazarbei De materia medica libri quinque.* Berlin: Weidmann.

Zonta, M. 1996. 'Minerology, Botany and Zoology in Medieval Hebrew Encylopaedias: "Descriptive" and "Theoretical" Approach to Arabic Sources', *Arabic Sciences and Philosophy* 6(2): 263–15.

CHAPTER 4

Arabic Terms in Byzantine Materia Medica

Oral and Textual Transmission

Maria Mavroudi

For George Saliba

One of the most important and under-investigated questions in the history of Byzantine science is the degree of its contact with its contemporary science in other languages. Part of the reason for the neglect is an older negative assessment of Byzantine civilisation as introverted, exhausted in rehashing its own ancient heritage without much creative elaboration. This image is changing because the globalisation we are currently experiencing inspires scholars to identify historical phenomena of international communication. Still, until very recently, Byzantine scientific manuscripts were primarily used in order to retrieve chapters of ancient, not Byzantine, science.[1]

Beyond ideological considerations, the lack of modern scholarly interest in Byzantine medicine can partly be explained by practical obstacles: the stability of Greek technical vocabulary over several centuries makes medical and other technical texts difficult to date – a problem that a better understanding of the introduction and dissemination of foreign terms in Byzantine medical vocabulary can help address. In addition, retrieving the social and intellectual contexts in which medicine and the sciences functioned during the Byzantine millennium has hardly begun, largely because explicit information is rarely provided in the surviving Byzantine narrative sources. A solution to these problems was recently offered by scholars who paid attention to the paleographic characteristics of manuscripts and their notes in order to establish circles of users.[2]

I am grateful to Petros Bouras-Vallianatos for his generosity in sharing publications and primary source material that significantly facilitated the writing of the present chapter.

[1] A fuller discussion of this problem and how it pertains to the study of Byzantine medicine can be found in Mavroudi (2015: 42–4).

[2] See the useful articles by Degni (2012) and Mondrain (2012). Degni lists several earlier pertinent publications by Mondrain.

4.1 Limitations of the Manuscript Evidence due to Patterns of Survival

This productive approach has its chronological limitations: most of what can be gleaned from the physical appearance of Byzantine manuscripts primarily pertains to the thirteenth, fourteenth, and fifteenth centuries, simply because their survival rate is by several orders of magnitude greater for this period. To illustrate the problem with numbers that pertain to technical manuscripts, consider the larger intellectual category to which botanical and medical manuscripts belong:[3] the *Corpus Codicum Astrologorum Graecorum*, an effort to account for the totality of the Greek astrological tradition, inventoried, described, and published excerpts from a total of 600 manuscripts. Among them, only twenty-four (4 per cent) are earlier than the twelfth century.[4] Diels' two-volume catalogue of Greek medical manuscripts that appeared in 1905 and 1906 inventoried approximately 1,800.[5] Based on this catalogue, it is possible to count only 110 (6.1 per cent) that belong to the twelfth century or earlier. Among 299 manuscripts containing works on the theory of music catalogued by Thomas Mathiesen in 1988, eighteen (6 per cent) were copied between the eleventh and thirteenth centuries.[6] As for philosophy, the inventory of manuscripts with works by Aristotle and Aristotelian commentaries published in 1963, combined with its 1980 supplement, lists a total of 2,773 manuscripts.[7] Only sixty-one among them (approximately

[3] For a broader discussion of manuscript survival rates in Greek and Syriac prior to the tenth century, see Mavroudi (2014: 320–2). In summary, if we exclude the papyri and focus on Greek book manuscripts that survive in a library context, we have approximately fifty manuscripts copied in uncials prior to the ninth century, when manuscripts copied in the minuscule commence.

[4] I accept the number twenty-four as reported in Tester (1987: 95). Tester attributes this pattern of preservation to a fluctuation in the fortunes of astrology within the Byzantine Empire. In Tester's account, astrology was persecuted and went underground during the reigns of the early Christian emperors in the fourth and fifth centuries. It was repatriated to Byzantium from the East by Stephen the Philosopher and partly revived around the ninth century – the earliest surviving astrological manuscripts date to between the tenth and eleventh centuries. A true revival and license to discuss astrology in public presumably came only in the twelfth century. This history of astrology does not take into consideration the larger context of Byzantine literary production and was corrected by Magdalino (2006).

[5] My personal count from Diels extends only to those earlier than the thirteenth century. The total number of 1,800 for all manuscripts listed in Diels is given in Touwaide (1991a: 78). Touwaide (1991a: 79) mentions that his own (at the time unpublished) inventory of Greek medical manuscripts includes 2,200 (22 per cent more than Diels). I refrain from using Touwaide's numbers because I consider them unreliable. Touwaide (2016) cannot easily be used for statistical purposes; for the reasons, see Bouras-Vallianatos (2019).

[6] Count based on Mathiesen (1988).

[7] Wartelle (1963) lists a total of 2,271 manuscripts. Only fifty-nine among them (approximately 2.6 per cent of the total) were earlier than the thirteenth century. See Wartelle (1963: xvi). Wartelle (1963: xvii) specifies that the two oldest are from the ninth and tenth centuries: Parisinus gr. 1853

2.2 per cent of the total) are earlier than the thirteenth century.[8] An inventory of Plato's manuscripts earlier than the year 1600 (and omitting collections in small Balkan countries and Platonic commentaries) lists a total of 263 manuscripts, only 12 of which (4.6 per cent of the total) are earlier than the thirteenth century.[9] These numbers can certainly be refined, but a pattern is clear: surviving Greek technical manuscripts earlier than the thirteenth century represent only 5–6 per cent of the total number of Greek technical manuscripts we have.[10] They also imply that any modern understanding of ancient Greek and Byzantine technical literature is decidedly filtered through the theoretical and practical concerns, not of the entire Byzantine millennium (as is frequently asserted about modern access to the ancient classics), but of the late Byzantine and early modern period, during which 95 per cent of what was copied was excerpted, paraphrased, or otherwise organised in order to be taught and practised.

As for Arabic manuscripts (the ultimate source of our knowledge on the Arabic medical vocabulary that entered Persian, Turkish, and Greek *materia medica*), their modern study is a considerably more recent discipline and cannot yet yield as detailed and quantified data. However, scholars who work in this field are empirically aware of patterns that largely parallel those in Greek: most early surviving manuscripts in Arabic, going back to the Umayyad period and perhaps even earlier, are copies of the Qurʾān.[11] This mirrors the fact that the bulk of early Greek manuscripts that came down to us, generally dated between the fourth and the ninth centuries, are biblical. By comparison, manuscripts with technical treatises on various subjects (medicine, pharmacology, astronomy and astrology, mathematics,

(no. 1338 in Wartelle's inventory) and Vindobonensis phil. gr. 100 (no. 2196). Both belong to the group of early technical Greek manuscripts known as the 'philosophical collection'.

8 Cumulative statistics are provided in Argyropoulos and Karras (1980: 9–10). I obtained the total number of sixty-one manuscripts copied before the thirteenth century by including the six that this table dates to the twelfth and thirteenth centuries.

9 Wilson (1962: 386–95).

10 I have not been able to conduct similarly detailed counts for Latin manuscripts, but whenever I ventured into the medieval Latin manuscript tradition of technical and other treatises, I was constantly struck by the perceptibly greater survival rate of early Latin manuscripts. Obvious explanations that come to mind include the greater number of centres of production and collection of manuscripts in the medieval West (multiple royal and aristocratic courts) contrasted with the preponderance of Constantinople as a cultural centre in the later Byzantine period, and the recorded destruction of libraries and cultural patrimony during the two conquests of Constantinople, first in 1204 by the Crusaders and second in 1453 by the Ottomans.

11 For a discussion of early Qur'anic manuscripts, see Deroche (2014); in 2015 a Qur'anic fragment copied on a parchment bifolio and held at the university of Birmingham was dated, with the help of radiocarbon technology, to between 568 and 645 CE. This generated an exhilaration analogous to the one inspired by early biblical manuscripts in the late nineteenth and early twentieth centuries. See Fedeli (2018).

and philosophy) are considerably fewer and preserved in later manuscripts. Their numbers multiply exponentially as their dates progress towards the late medieval and early modern period.[12] This is expected, given that Arabic texts written on any subject earlier than the Abbasid period scarcely survive.

As is clear from the discussion thus far, neither the Greek nor the Arabic manuscript tradition yield easy answers regarding when and where oriental medicinal terms first entered Byzantine medical vocabulary, nor do they readily provide information on how these terms were eventually naturalised into Greek. Given this pattern of preservation, the survival of three Greek manuscripts with Dioscorides' herbal copied between the sixth and the ninth centuries is an exceptional event in the transmission of ancient and medieval literary culture.[13] Significantly, all three contain annotations that document the medieval and early modern transmission of *materia medica* between Greek, Latin, and Arabic. The earliest among them is the Vienna Dioscorides (Vindobonensis med. gr. 1), which was created in the early sixth century in Constantinople and contains annotations in Latin, Arabic, and Persian from later centuries.[14] Somewhat more recent is the Naples Dioscorides (Neapolitanus MS ex Vindobonensis gr. 1),[15] copied around the end of the sixth and the beginning of the seventh centuries, perhaps in Italy. It contains annotations from several different centuries in Latin that deserve detailed attention because they provide valuable information on the interaction between Byzantine and Western European science, both in antiquity and the early modern period – a chapter in the history of medieval science that is almost completely unknown.[16]

The most recent of the three manuscripts is the Paris Dioscorides (Parisinus gr. 2179).[17] Based on its paleographic characteristics, modern scholars have dated it to around the end of the eighth or perhaps the ninth century and have discussed Byzantine southern Italy, Egypt, or Palestine as

[12] For some quantification of survival patterns pertinent to Christian Arabic manuscripts, see Roisse (2004). Like for Greek manuscripts, their number rises exponentially from the thirteenth century onwards.

[13] See also the discussion in Mavroudi (2012).

[14] For a recent examination and bibliography, see Thomas (2019: 245).

[15] Description and latest bibliography in Thomas (2019: 245–6).

[16] For an important discussion on Byzantine into early modern European science, see Bouras-Vallianatos (2020: 207–14).

[17] Parisinus gr. 2179 can be viewed at https://gallica.bnf.fr/ark:/12148/btv1b525002505/f37.item.zoom (accessed 28 January 2023).

its possible place of production.[18] It is annotated in Greek, Arabic (by at least two different hands in Arabic script and a third one in Arabic written in Greek script), and Latin (by at least two different hands). Marie Cronier recently studied the Arabic terms written in Greek script on this manuscript and pointed out that the Greek-Arabic correspondences it records frequently do not occur in any of the four known Arabic translations of Dioscorides nor in any medieval Arabic botanical dictionary that includes terms from Dioscorides.[19] She also remarked that the Arabic terms written in Arabic characters on the same page do not always convey the Arabic terms written in Greek characters near them. Even when they do, the Arabic scribe seems to have occasionally found it difficult to decipher the Arabic in Greek letters.[20] The placement of the illustrations on the manuscript indicates that these were added *after* the purely Greek annotations (i.e. annotations in the Greek language written in the Greek alphabet).[21] On the basis of these observations, Cronier suggested that these three types of annotation and the illustrations of the manuscript were added within a short period of time, soon after the text of Dioscorides had been copied. Cronier briefly discussed the possibility that the Graeco-Arabic correspondences recorded on the Paris manuscript go back to the oldest known translation of Dioscorides into Arabic, fragments of which were identified by Manfred Ullmann in a unique manuscript copied in the thirteenth century.[22] Ullmann argued that this translation (*vetus translatio*) was made by Abū Yaḥyā al-Baṭrīq (d. *c.*800), who is known to have translated Galen's treatise on simple drugs and was therefore familiar with botanical vocabulary.[23] He also examined the possibility that Abū Yaḥyā relied on an earlier translation of Dioscorides from Greek into Syriac that no longer survives but dismissed the idea, concluding that the *vetus translatio* was made directly from Greek into Arabic.[24] Cronier observed that, if this were proven correct, the Paris manuscript would be indebted to a textual tradition of Dioscorides that belongs to a branch independent from the

[18] Parisinus gr. 2179 has been thought by some to be southern Italian and by others to be Palestinian. For bibliographical references to different opinions, see Rémond (1992: 345–6). The identification of this manuscript as an eighth-century Palestinian creation originated with Bernard de Montfaucon in the eighteenth century and was adopted by both palaeographers and art historians. For example, Cavallo (1977: 96, 102) and Parpulov (2015). Eminent art historians like Grabar and Weitzmann think of it as southern Italian of the ninth century. Cronier (2016) also considers it southern Italian.

[19] Cronier (2016: 250–1). [20] Cronier (2016: 255–6). [21] Cronier (2016: 256–7).

[22] Istanbul MS Süleymanye Kütüphanesi, Ayasofya 3704. Ullmann (2009).

[23] On Abū Yaḥyā al-Baṭrīq as translator of Galen's treatise on simple drugs, see Bhayro et al. (2013: 133).

[24] Ullmann (2009: 149–50). The older Syriac translation that Ullmann entertains as a possibility is the one made by Ḥunayn ibn Isḥāq.

surviving translations in Arabic. Yet the illustrations on the Paris manuscript have an obvious relationship with those copied on the manuscripts of Dioscorides' later Arabic translations. Cronier's observations challenge the clear distinctions that modern philologists sometimes adopt in order to describe the manuscript tradition of individual ancient texts through *stemmata codicum*, which implicitly imagine texts circulating among a small number of readers in limited numbers and contained geographies. An influential example on how modern scholars imagined the circulation of ancient texts is the 'Occidental', 'Alexandrian', and 'Constantinopolitan' recension of the Gospels expounded by Griesbach in the eighteenth century. In contrast, Cronier's observations indicate that both the textual and the visual information provided by the Greek and Arabic manuscripts of Dioscorides is 'contaminated' (in the technical sense that this word has in nineteenth- and twentieth-century philological vocabulary).

The degree of 'cross-contamination' of manuscript traditions can be gleaned from a rare piece of explicit information on the textual transmission of Galen's *On the Capacities of Foodstuffs* from Greek into Syriac and Arabic. Ḥunayn ibn Isḥāq (d. 873) famously explained that his Arabic rendering of this text was the result of a process of 'contamination' and compilation:[25] he first did a rendering out of a single manuscript which was 'not correct'. He later collected several Greek manuscripts of this work, which he collated and 'corrected'. In the end, out of this 'corrected' version he created a Syriac summary, enriched with details from a number of works, collecting in this way everything older authors had written on the subject. Ḥunayn later translated this enriched summary into Arabic.[26]

This means that, in order to better understand the transmission of technical texts during the medieval period, it is important to recognise the different goals of scholars who lived before and after print. The disparity can be attributed to the fact that a printed text is fixed and identical iterations of it can be disseminated to a large number of readers. Accordingly, modern critical editions aim to use as many manuscript witnesses as possible (containing different recensions of the same text) in order to arrive at a printed a text that approaches what came out of the pen

[25] See Ḥunayn ibn Isḥāq, *Risālah* (*Epistle*), ed. Bergsträsser (1925) 35 (Arabic text) and 29, no. 74 (German transl.).

[26] See also the discussion of Ḥunayn's approach to Galen's *On the Capacities of Foodstuffs* in Bhayro and Hawley (2014: 300–1): Ḥunayn enriched *On the Capacities of Foodstuffs* with passages from Galen's *On the Capacities of Simple Drugs*; for this purpose, he used the older translation of *On the Capacities of Simple Drugs* by Sergius of Resh ʿayna, sometimes adopting it almost verbatim, at other times revising it considerably.

of an ancient author as closely as possible. In contrast, for scholars before print, the inevitably Protean nature of texts in a manuscript culture was given. As copiers of manuscripts themselves, they knew that a scribe of medium competence makes, on the average, one mistake per page when copying.[27] Accordingly, their goal was to collect as many manuscript witnesses as possible in order to arrive at a text that they (and other readers) could understand and use. They recognised different recensions and the author's intent was certainly part of their deliberation, but not the only one.

The survival of these three early manuscripts of the Greek Dioscorides can be explained by their heirloom quality (enhanced by their illustrations), but especially by the fact that botanical expertise depended on accumulating information (including lexicographical information) on each plant over centuries, rather than updating by eliminating information without obvious relevance to the surroundings of each user of herbal information. Other branches of ancient and Byzantine science, such as astronomy, astrology, and dream interpretation, are also defined by the need to accumulate as much observational data as possible. Accumulation of earlier data is not a Byzantine habit. It follows a principle expressed multiple times by practising scientists since antiquity. For example, Ptolemy reiterates it a number of times in his writings, such as the proem to the *Almagest* and Book I of the *Geography*. It is reinforced in the marginal annotations found in Byzantine astronomical manuscripts.[28] Accordingly, the oldest surviving manuscript of Ptolemy's astronomical tables, which dates to the ninth century, was heavily annotated by readers who pored over its presumably outdated data for centuries. We happen to know one of these readers by name. He was Nikephoros Gregoras, one of the most competent astronomers of the fourteenth century.[29]

Paying closer attention to the accumulation of information on the technical disciplines over time, and especially the practical and theoretical goals that such an accumulation served, will help us change the modern perception of Byzantine science as little more than a fossilisation of its ancient counterpart. The annotations and interventions evident on the Byzantine manuscripts of the ancient authors indicate that the Byzantines understood their own science, not as subservient to and confined by

27 For this statistic, see Dain (1964: 46).

28 For an extensive discussion of this, see Mavroudi (2023, forthcoming).

29 The continuous use of this manuscript by readers over centuries is evident even after a superficial perusal; see Leidensis BPG 78, at https://digitalcollections.universiteitleiden.nl/view/item/1597397#page/208/mode/1up (accessed 28 January 2023).

ancient authority (as modern scholarship has frequently insisted), but as an accumulation of earlier knowledge in which they intervened by adding, summarising, explicating, and organising, in order to make it more accessible and practical. This type of intervention was also a practice in ancient science and can be viewed as characteristic of all manuscript cultures.

4.2 Medieval Manuscripts of Ancient Texts as Depositories of Old and New Knowledge

Dioscorides' herbal and Galen's works on the preparation of drugs were the two most important vehicles for the transmission of Greek pharmacology into Arabic.[30] A close connection between the two authors in the Greek pharmacological tradition was already cemented by the sixth century, because the entries on individual plants in the Vienna Dioscorides were augmented with information from Galen.[31] However, the volume of Galen's pharmacological writings, as well as the complexity of their transmission and diffusion in other languages, makes it impossible to discuss them together within the confines of the present contribution.[32]

Dioscorides was translated into Arabic multiple times from the late eighth century onwards. Consistent with the patterns in manuscript preservation outlined earlier, the earliest surviving manuscript of one of Dioscorides' multiple Arabic iterations is an illustrated copy dated to the year 1083 CE (today Leidensis or. 289).[33] More broadly, it is the earliest known Arabic manuscript with technical illustrations.[34] Significantly, it contains a number of annotations in Greek.

A series of Arabic notes on Leidensis or. 289 provide some concrete chronological and geographical context: the manuscript was copied in Samarkand. It was finished on a Monday in the middle of Ramadan in

30 The importance of Dioscorides and Galen for the development of Arabic pharmacology, alongside the incorporation of Middle Persian, Syriac, and indigenous Arabic lore, and the path of Islamicate medicine between inherited tradition and innovation, is outlined in Pormann (2011).

31 The same hand that copied Dioscorides' text on the Vienna Dioscorides also copied excerpts from Galen using uncials of a smaller size. For example, see ff. 22r–34r, 70r–76r, and elsewhere. On occasion (e.g. ff. 18r, 26r, and 27r) excerpts from Krateuas (*c.* first century BCE) are also copied.

32 On the medieval reception of Galen's pharmacology, see Ventura (2019).

33 A detailed description, with passing mention of the Greek annotations, is provided in Witkam (2007: 128–47). A study of this manuscript is provided by Sadek (1983). For a digital reproduction of Leidensis or. 289, see https://digitalcollections.universiteitleiden.nl/view/item/1578266#page/1/mode/1up (accessed 28 January 2023). In the current binding of the manuscript, the series of its folia appears to be disturbed.

34 For an overview of the Arabic reception of Dioscorides' herbal as text and illustrations, see Rogers (2007: 41–7). This overview is very broad and includes few references to concrete manuscripts. On medieval illustrated herbals, see also Gottlieb (Chapter 6) in this volume.

475 H/1082 CE which is given in the Persian solar and Muslim lunar calendar. Its model was a manuscript by the hand of al-Naṭīlī, author of an improved version (*iṣlāḥ*) of Ḥunayn ibn Isḥāq's Arabic rendering of Dioscorides. Al-Naṭīlī was an ethnic Persian. A further note in Arabic, dated to the twelfth century, informs the reader that the present manuscript served as the basis for a translation of Dioscorides' text into Persian by the very person who wrote this note. Notes in Persian can be found elsewhere in the manuscript. The one most frequently attested is a very experienced late eleventh-century hand. All of these notes are writing in Greek the names of plants that are given in the Greek language but using the Arabic alphabet within the text. The care to render them exactly in the Greek pronunciation reminds one of the care for the exact rendering of the Greek herbal terms taken by Ibn al-Bayṭar according to Ibn Abī Usaybiʿah.

The Arabic writing throughout Leidensis or. 289 is fluent but informal because it frequently omits the diacritic dots. This can be a problem for a text that includes many Greek terms, like Dioscorides. Yet the eleventh-century Greek hand is confident in its identifications. On some pages, the ink of the Greek notes is visibly in the same colour (and perhaps written with the same writing instrument) as the Arabic text of Dioscorides. An example is on f. 46v: the Arabic *mālā wa-huwa al-tufāḥ* ('*mālā*, that is, apples') is explicated with the Greek *mēla* ('μῆλα'/'apples'). The Arabic *qūdhūnīā wa-huwa al-safarjal* ('*qūdhūnīā*, that is, quince') is explained in Greek as *kydōnia* ('κυδώνια'/'quince'). The dots have been omitted from the word *safarjal* and the image of the tree is on the next page, but the Greek hand does not appear to hesitate. Likewise, on f. 45r the Arabic reads *zāā* [*sic*] *wa-huwa al-rūmān* ('*zāā*, that is, pomegranate'). In this case, *zāā* is a mistake for *rāā* (زاا instead of راا) in order to transliterate the Greek *roā*. Yet the Greek annotation confidently and correctly reads *roā* ('ῥοά'). It is possible that both the Greek and the Arabic were written by the same individual. The characteristics of the script in these words are consistent with the late eleventh century: the letters are not consistently the same size and uncial characters are used together with minuscule characters.[35] Most of these notes can be found between ff. 42b and 53b. They mostly (though not exclusively) explicate the names of edible fruit: wild pomegranate, garden myrtle, apple, quince, citron, apricots, pears, and so forth. On f. 47v (see Figure 4.1) the Greek terms *melimēla* ('μελίμηλα') and *glykymēla* ('γλυκύμηλα') are attached to the

[35] Those inexperienced in Greek palaeography who would like to confirm the eleventh-century dating of the Greek notes in Leidensis or. 289 can compare them with a dated eleventh-century manuscript in similar style, copied twenty years earlier, Vaticanus gr. 65 of the year 1063, at https://digi.vatlib.it/view/MSS_Vat.gr.65.pt.2 (accessed 28 January 2023).

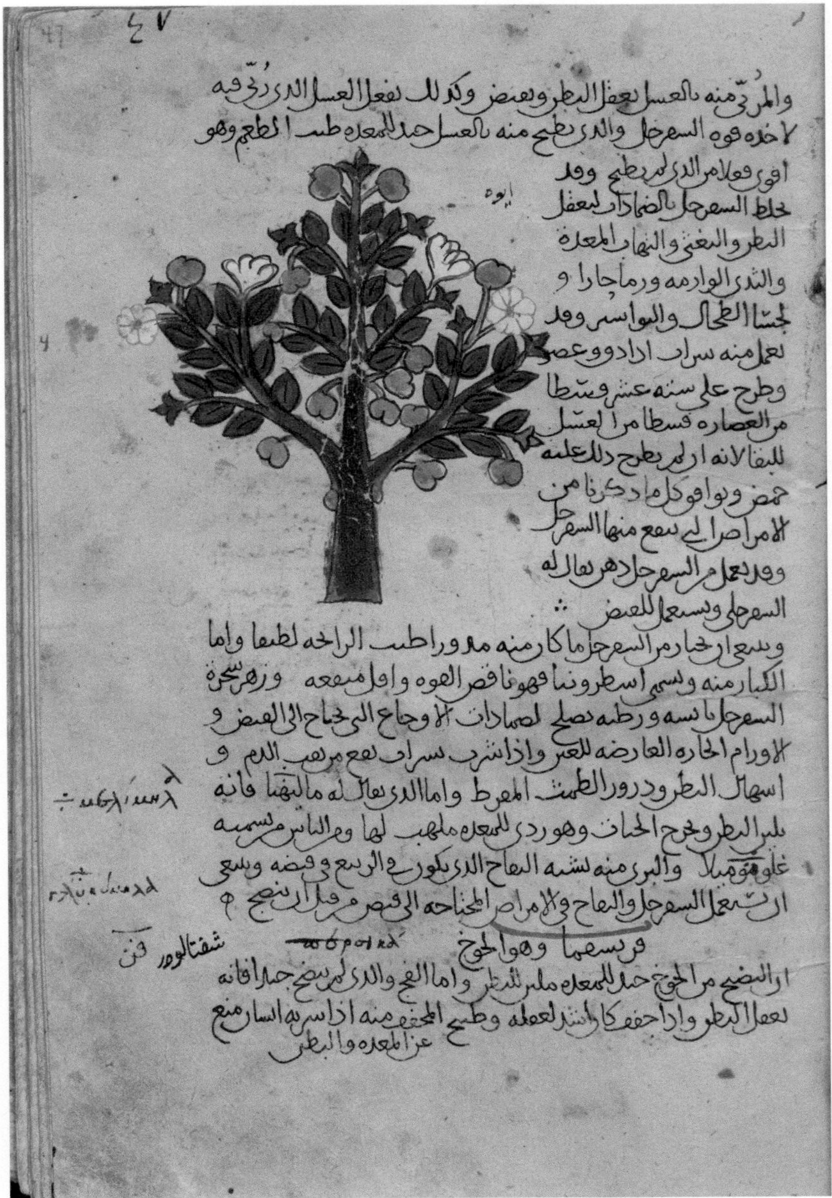

Figure 4.1 Leiden, Universiteitsbibliotheek, MS or. 289, f. 47v

(botched) Arabic transliterations *mālīhīyā* [*sic*] and *ghlūqūmīla* through reference signs of a type frequent in much earlier and contemporary Greek manuscripts. Elsewhere in the manuscript there are Greek notes in a significantly later fluent hand. Examples can be found on f. 45v ('μυρσίνη'/*myrsinē*, 'myrtle'), explicating the Arabic (*amārus* [*sic*] *wa-l-ās al-bustānī*) and on f. 156a ('μανδραγόρα'/*mandragora*, 'mandrake'). The shape of these letters is consistent with a late fifteenth- or sixteenth-century date.[36]

In addition, a handful of Greek notes were written in an awkward hand that is very difficult to date. Examples can be seen on f. 42v, 135a (in an awkward Greek hand that also wrote Arabic right next to the Greek note; both the Greek and the Arabic appear by the same hand) and f. 157a (on the verso side of the mandrake's image). It is impossible to ascertain whether it is the same hand in all three notes. The paper on f. 157 is damaged, according to Witkam's catalogue, by copper corrosion. Behind the picture of the mandrake the awkward hand that also did not know how to spell wrote to the Mother of God a Christian prayer and hymn that is frequently repeated in a liturgical context: 'την πασαν ελπηδα μου [προ]ανατηθημη μητηρ του Θ[εο]υ φηλαξον με ϋπο την σκεπην σου' (for: 'τὴν πᾶσαν ἐλπίδα μου εἰς σὲ ἀνατίθημι μῆτερ του Θεοῦ, φύλαξόν με ὑπὸ τὴν σκέπην σου', that is, 'I entrust all hope to you, Mother of God, protect me under your shelter'). These are the words of a well-known chant to the Virgin Mary. Given that accidental poisoning with mandrake is not uncommon (and copper is a known mineral poison), one wonders whether the power of the Virgin was solicited by a practitioner who was worried about his (or her) pharmaceutical competence.[37]

36 At around this period, formal hands like this are difficult to date. The reason is that the early fonts for printing Greek were modelled after the hands of famous Greek scribes, which then influenced considerably later writing fashions. The Greek hand of a sixteenth-century European scholar can be very similar to the hand of a late fifteenth-century Byzantine scholar.

37 Given the inability to date these notes, I entertain the possibility that they were added while Levinus Warner (*c*.1618–65) had this manuscript in his hands in Constantinople. Like other Western orientalists before and after him, Warner tried to convert Greek orthodox subjects of the Ottoman Empire to Protestantism. At least two people near him could have led him to native speakers of Greek: his companion (or wife) Cocone Christophorou (or de Christophe), and his scribe Niqula'us bin Butrus al-Halabi (Nicholas son of Peter from Aleppo), who was a deacon of the Greek Orthodox Church in Syria and fluent in Arabic, Turkish, and Persian. Niqula'us served as a scribe and manuscript procurer for Jacobus Golius (1596–1667) and later for Warner. He put Warner in touch with other men from Aleppo. For information on Warner's sojourn in Constantinople and his connection with Cocone and Nicholas, see Van Leeuwen and Vrolijk (2013: 43–58). Warner's will, published in Warner (1883: xi–xiii), designates her as his wife. There are notes in the manuscript that must have been added by him or at any rate after he had bought the manuscript. There is a Latino-Arabic note on f. 116b: 'v. f. ١١٨ 2' which I take to mean 'vide folium 118b'. This note must be from the time that the manuscript ended up in Warner's hands, or from later. The note is referring the reader either to the same manuscript or a different one.

Joe Glynias suggested that the Arabic Leiden Dioscorides is a product of the milieu of Melkite physicians simultaneously connected with intellectual circles in Baghdad and Byzantine Antioch around the end of the eleventh century. Antioch provided a gateway of communication between the Islamic world and Constantinople. The best recorded such figure is Ibn Buṭlān, a well-known Christian physician from Baghdad who spent considerable time in Constantinople and died in Byzantine Antioch in 1075.[38] It has recently been argued that Ibn Buṭlān taught Symeon Seth, a known physician, author, and translator from Arabic into Greek active at the court of Emperor Alexios I.[39] If Glynias is right, in the course of the eleventh century physicians competent in the Byzantine medical tradition and the spoken Greek of their time[40] were travelling not only between Baghdad, Antioch, and Constantinople, but also included Samarkand in their itineraries. These cities are on the trade routes collectively known under the name 'silk road'. The modern scholarly imagination pictures the Byzantines as confined within their empire and not travelling elsewhere, especially not somewhere as far away as Samarkand. Distant travels presumably befit only adventurous Westerners like William of Rubruck (fl. 1248–55) or Marco Polo (*c.*1254–*c.*1324). Indeed, modern scholarship has lavished its attention on Western Europeans passing through Byzantium (Dominican friars like William of Moerbeke, d. *c.*1286; merchants like Francesco Balducci Pegolotti, d. 1347; men of learning like Ciriaco d'Ancona, d. 1452). As for Byzantine figures like Gregory Chioniades (d. *c.*1320), who are known to have travelled to Tabriz in search of astronomical, astrological, and medical knowledge during the thirteenth and fourteenth centuries, they have not received comparable attention.[41] The eleventh-century information from the Arabic Leiden Dioscorides, especially as it comes from a period that we

[38] Glynias (2022). I am grateful to Joe Glynias for trusting me with his unpublished work.

[39] Pietrobelli and Cronier (2022).

[40] The importance of eleventh-century spoken Greek for the Greek annotator to Leidensis or. 289 is evident on f. 47b: ارمانياقا وهو المشمش (*armānīāqā*, that is apricots) is glossed in Greek as 'ἀρμενιακὰ ρωμαϊστὶ βρεκόκκια' (*armeniaka*, in the Roman language *brekokkia* = apricots). 'Ρωμαϊστί' is clearly the spoken Greek of the annotator's time as opposed to 'ἑλληνιστί', which extends over a longer period in the history of the Greek language. An equivalent distinction between ancient and medieval Greek is sometimes noted in the Arabic sources (*Rūmī* = Byzantine vs. *Ighrīqī* or *Yūnānī* = ancient Greek).

[41] On Chioniades and other thirteenth- and fourteenth-century Byzantine travellers to Persia, see Mavroudi (2007).

do not associate with any Byzantine world travellers, extends an invitation to rethink our own stereotypes.[42]

In order to better understand the context in which the annotations on Greek and Arabic botanical manuscripts were created, it is important to consider the evidence for the transmission of botany and pharmacology simultaneously through oral and written channels. Such a dual mode of transmission is sufficiently attested in the premodern written sources and modern ethnobotanical practice.

4.3 The Inclusion of Vernacular, Foreign, and Obsolete Botanical Terms in Medieval Manuscripts as a Result of How Botanical Texts Were Composed and Disseminated: Oral and Written Transmission

The problem of how to render technical terms from one language into another is as old as language contact itself. In botany, it is already attested in the ancient Near Eastern coexistence of Summerian with Akkadian (two languages that are not cognate but belong to different families).[43] During Graeco-Roman antiquity, from which the surviving written record is more abundant and has been studied more systematically, it is clear that the problem was not limited to *materia medica* but extended to all kinds of medical terminology, including words for medical conditions and parts of the human body.[44] The same problem is attested in the medieval Latin literary record, as current research on the thirteenth-century physician Simon of Genoa has shown.[45] Simon compiled a trilingual lexicon of Greek, Latin, and Arabic medical terms that was useful during his own time and later became the first printed dictionary of *materia medica.* He consulted both written sources and live informants. He mentions two native speakers of Greek and two of Arabic. He is explicit that three of the four were women.[46]

[42] Part of the reason we imagine the Italian but not the Byzantine merchants as travelling long distance is the survival of the Italian city archives that inform us on Italian long-distance trade. Nothing comparable survives from the Byzantine historical context.

[43] See Scurlock (2005: 302ff.), and especially the discussion on the equivalence of plants in Scurlock (2005: 309–10), where the example at hand equates plants that are clearly different, likely because they had similar pharmaceutical properties, and was probably addressed to a professional pharmacist.

[44] See Langslow (2000: 76–139).

[45] See the Simon Online project at www.simonofgenoa.org/index.php?title=Simon_Online (accessed 28 January 2023); and Zipser (2013a).

[46] See Bouras-Vallianatos (2013: 36) on the 'old woman from Crete' (*anicula Cretensis*) who taught Simon to recognise Dioscorides' plants. Simon mentions a Greek man and two Arab women, one from Aleppo and one from 'another region'. On the woman from Aleppo, see also Zipser (2013b: 150).

The earliest surviving Greek manuscripts of Dioscorides' second-century herbal indicate a sustained effort to collect and record botanical terms in languages other than Greek. In the oldest among them, the sixth-century Vienna Dioscorides (Vindobonensis med. gr. 1), the entry on each plant begins with a list of its possible names. These lists are part of the manuscript's main text and record several synonyms for the same plant in Greek, as well as its name in a wide range of other languages in Greek transcription: Latin, Tuscan, Lucanian, Tyrrhenian,[47] Egyptian, Carthaginian, Celtic, Dacian, and so forth. They also include plant names according to various learned traditions transmitted by different authors such as Pythagoras, Ostanes, Zoroaster, and 'the prophets' – an indication that strands of Neoplatonist thought had become consequential for the pursuit of botany earlier than the sixth century.[48] These terms on the Vienna Dioscorides were collected from the botanical dictionary of Pamphilus (fl. *c.*50 CE).[49]

The inclusion of foreign terms results from the hesitation to rely on written information alone and the importance of live informants in the transmission of botanical knowledge. Knowing about the appearance of a plant from a written description is not a foolproof way to recognise it for the first time in the field. It is preferable to also have it identified by someone who already knows it in real life. The problem is not unique to

[47] See Pliny, *Natural History*, 25.5, trans. Bostoc (1855), at www.perseus.tufts.edu/hopper/text?doc=Perseus:abo:phi,0978,001:25:5 (accessed 28 January 2023) with reference to a quotation of Aeschylos in Theophrastos, *Enquiry into plants* B. ix. c. 15: 'τυῤῥήνων γενεὰν φαρμακοποιὸν ἔθνος' ('The race of the Tyrrheni, a drug-preparing nation'). On the use of terms of ingredients in various languages in the same text, see also Käs (Chapter 1), Walker-Meikle (Chapter 3), and Martelli (Chapter 11) in the present volume.

[48] Much of what is known about Pythagoras is transmitted by the Neoplatonists. Further, Greek writings of the late Roman period consider Zoroaster a prophet because he was the founder of their contemporary Persian religion. For a brief outline of the Greek appropriation of Persian wisdom, see Beck (2002). The sources for the botanical lexicon found in the Vienna and Naples Dioscorides are also echoed by Pliny, *Natural History*, 25.5, trans. Bostock (1885), at www.perseus.tufts.edu/hopper/text?doc=Perseus:abo:phi,0978,001:25:5 (accessed 28 January 2023):

> In later times again, Pythagoras, that celebrated philosopher, was the first to write a treatise on the properties of plants, a work in which he attributes the origin and discovery of them to Apollo, Aesculapius, and the immortal gods in general. Democritus too composed a similar work. Both of these philosophers had visited the magicians of Persia, Arabia, Ethiopia, and Egypt, and so astounded were the ancients at their recitals, as to learn to make assertions which transcend all belief.

At the end of the fifth century, Asclepiodotos of Alexandria, credited in the *Life of Damaskios* as having an extensive knowledge of fauna and flora and being a dedicated observer of these things in their natural environment, was active as a philosopher in the Neoplatonist tradition and is known as author of a now lost commentary on Plato's *Timaeus*.

[49] The seminal essay on the topic remains Wellmann (1916).

botany. As practising physicians well know, reading on the anatomy of the human body out of an illustrated anatomical atlas is a very different experience than looking for individual organs on a cadaver. The organs do not necessarily look identical to their depiction in the atlas, nor are they consistently where the atlas promises they will be.[50] The unavoidable discrepancy between written information and lived reality necessitates both an oral and a written component in order to transmit most kinds of technical knowledge. This creates a power dynamic between teacher and student because training someone in the same discipline means creating one's own competition. Teachers may be invested in divulging or occluding specialised information, depending on their relationship with the student. In turn, this influences how a discipline is transmitted in writing. Tamsyn Barton has explored the impact of this phenomenon on ancient astrology, physiognomics, and medicine.[51] It has not yet been explored for ancient and medieval botany, although researchers may know it empirically from encountering technical manuscripts written in cryptography.[52]

A well-recorded example of simultaneous oral and written transmission of botanical knowledge is Pliny.[53] His method of compiling in writing went through oral channels: a secretary was reading to him at dinner and while being transported in a chair around Rome. He excerpted from what was read to him. If it was in Greek, he simultaneously translated it into Latin and dictated a new composition to another secretary. This procedure, oscillating between the oral and the written word, accounts for a number of errors evident in the texts produced in the end. Also, Pliny did not always summarise his source, which would have resulted in a consistently shorter text; rather, he sometimes added information or changed things to reflect his own knowledge or observation.[54] In a famous passage frequently cited in scholarship (*Natural History* 25.4–5), Pliny discussed the role of illustrated herbals in the transmission of botanical knowledge: some Greek authors appended pictures to their description of plants, and others avoided them because of the problems they presented: one needed skill and several appropriate colours to make them accurate, while their further copying was bound to introduce errors; in addition, it was difficult to convey the appearance of a plant around the year. Pliny

[50] I thank my physician father and brother for this insight.

[51] See Barton (1994).

[52] An example is Bononiensis 3632, which contains a number of botanical, medical, divinatory, and magical texts and includes parts written cryptographically.

[53] In more recent years, the study of ancient medicine has paid increased attention to the intersection between the written and the oral. See, for example, Totelin (2009).

[54] See Stannard (1965: 420–5).

himself clarifies that his acquaintance with plants was not only through books. He was able to examine in vivo almost all the plants discussed in the herbals that he read in the garden of the famous botanist Antonius Castor in Rome.[55]

The importance of personal observation and at the same time consultation of pre-existing treatises is reiterated in a number of writings from Graeco-Roman antiquity over several centuries. Dioscorides in his proem explains the same about his compilation. He acknowledges the existence of several manuals on the same topic as his own, both old and recent ones, and mentions eight of them specifically in order to point out their limitations. The names of their authors are both Greek and Latin. Still, Dioscorides argues that his own work is not superfluous because earlier manuals are either incomplete or based on hearsay, rather than practical experience and first-hand knowledge of the plants and minerals they discuss. Dioscorides gained his expertise because of his enthusiasm for knowing the *materia medica* since his youth and the fact that he led an itinerant life ('βίον στρατιωτικόν'/*bion stratiōtikon*).[56] He explains the manner of compiling his work as follows: he did not pay attention to the rhetorical elegance of

[55] Pliny, *Natural History*, 25.4–5, trans. Bostock, at www.perseus.tufts.edu/hopper/text?doc=Perseus:abo:phi,0978,001:25:5 (accessed 28 January 2023):

> In addition to these, there are some Greek writers who have treated of this subject, and who have been already mentioned on the appropriate occasions. Among them, Crateuas, Dionysius, and Metrodorus, adopted a very attractive method of description, though one which has done little more than prove the remarkable difficulties which attended it. It was their plan to delineate the various plants in colours, and then to add in writing a description of the properties which they possessed. Pictures, however, are very apt to mislead, and more particularly where such a number of tints is required, for the imitation of nature with any success; in addition to which, the diversity of copyists from the original paintings, and their comparative degrees of skill, add very considerably to the chances of losing the necessary degree of resemblance to the originals. And then, besides, it is not sufficient to delineate a plant as it appears at one period only, as it presents a different appearance at each of the four seasons of the year. Hence it is that other writers have confined themselves to a verbal description of the plants, indeed some of them have not so much as described them even, but have contented themselves for the most part with a bare recital of their names, considering it sufficient if they pointed out their virtues and properties to such as might Feel inclined to make further enquiries into the subject. Nor is this a kind of knowledge by any means difficult to obtain; at all events, so far as regards myself, with the exception of a very few, it has been my good fortune to examine them all, aided by the scientific researches of Antonius Castor, who in our time enjoyed the highest reputation for an intimate acquaintance with this branch of knowledge. I had the opportunity of visiting his garden, in which, though he had passed his hundredth year, he cultivated vast numbers of plants with the greatest care. Though he had reached this great age, he had never experienced any bodily ailment, and neither his memory nor his natural vigour had been the least impaired by the lapse of time.

On Pliny's *Natural History*, see also Doolittle (Chapter 2) in this volume.

[56] Dioscorides, *De materia medica*, pr.4, ed. Wellmann (1907) I.2.16–23.

his writing, but rather to the painstaking recording of his material with knowledge and experience.[57] He verified the information he included in his treatise either through personal experience or, when this was not possible, through comparing earlier authors and repeating what they all agreed on.

Dioscorides' method of collecting data is certainly not unique. Artemidoros reports the same regarding the composition of his own treatise on dream interpretation, written around the same time.[58] A similar attitude can be found in the writings of Ptolemy and Galen, and continued in later centuries, although we have explicit evidence for it during some periods and not others. In the late fifth century collecting knowledge from written sources, observation, and interaction with experts in the field was the method Asclepiodotos of Alexandria used to improve his knowledge of all kinds of natural science, according to Damaskios' *Philosophical History*:

> [E]ver since childhood he was declared to be the sharpest and most learned of all his contemporaries, as he never stopped occupying himself with whatever came his way, whether it was a wonder of nature or a man-made handiwork. Thus, in a short time he fully understood all the methods of mixing colours for dying and the variety of dyes prepared for clothes; also the innumerable types of wood, and the way their fibers are interwoven in straight and in complex fashion. Moreover, he would use every means to explore and find out about the manifold properties and varieties of stones and herbs, both the commonplace and the highly unusual. And he was a great nuisance to the experts in every field as he often sat with them on every point in exact detail. What he loved in particular was the natural history of plants and even more of animals; indeed, he examined closely those that he could cast his eyes on, and those which he could not find he investigated at great length through hearsay, also collecting whatever the Ancients had written about them.[59]

Two more moments in the medieval transmission of *materia medica* from Greek into Arabic, one in the early tenth century and a second in the early thirteenth, are described in the narrative sources. Both accounts make clear that written and oral transmission simultaneously contributed to developing a new botanical text. A crucial part of the task was deciding the correspondences in botanical vocabulary between Greek and Arabic.

57 Dioscorides, *De materia medica*, pr.5, ed. Wellmann (1907) I.3.4–11.

58 Some discussion can be found in Mavroudi (2002: 128).

59 Damaskios, *The Philosophical History*, ed. and trans. Athanassiadi (1999) 203–5.

The early tenth-century instance is Ibn Juljul's famous report on how a Greek manuscript of Dioscorides arrived from Constantinople to Cordoba as a diplomatic gift and was eventually translated into Arabic. In order to have it rendered into Arabic, the Umayyad caliph asked the Byzantine emperor for someone proficient in Greek and Latin who could teach (in Latin) slaves to translate the text into Arabic. He received the monk Nicholas, who not only helped with the identification of plants, but also taught a circle of pharmacologists in Spain how to prepare drugs with improved ingredients.[60]

In the early thirteenth century Ibn al-Bayṭār travelled from the western to the eastern Mediterranean, where Dioscorides had collected his information. The Damascene physician Ibn Abī Uṣaybiʿah knew him personally and mentioned him in his biographical dictionary of physicians from antiquity into the author's own time. On Ibn al-Bayṭār he includes the following:

> Ḍiyāʾ al-Dīn ibn al-Bayṭār – that is, the very illustrious, learned physician Abū Muḥammad ʿAbd Allāh ibn Aḥmad al-Mālaqī al-Nabātī – is generally known as Ibn al-Bayṭār. He was without peer in his day and was the authority of his age on the knowledge, identification, selection, and locations of plants as well as the attribution of names in terms of their differences and types. Ibn al-Bayṭār travelled to the land of the Greeks (*al-Aghāriqah*) reaching even the remotest areas of Asia Minor (*Bilād al-Rūm*) where he not only met experts in that discipline, from whom he obtained a great deal of knowledge about plants, but also observed the plants in their natural environment. In the Maghrib and elsewhere he also met with many authorities in the field of botany (*ʿilm al-nabāt*) and observed the places where the plants grew and examined their nature. Ibn al-Bayṭār had mastered the contents of the book of Dioscorides with such thoroughness that practically no one else could equal him in that regard. Indeed, I – Ibn Abī Uṣaybiʿah – found him to have an astonishing degree of insight, astuteness and knowledge about plants about what Dioscorides and Galen said concerning them. My first meeting with him was in Damascus in the year 633/1235 when I also observed his easy social qualities, the range of his honorable virtues, the excellence of his disposition, the goodness of his character and the nobleness of his soul, which were beyond description. *Indeed I witnessed with him in the outskirts of Damascus many of the plants in their native location and also read under him [i.e. under his supervision] his interpretation (tafsīr) on the names of medicines from the book of Dioscorides. And I used to find out very many things through the abundance of his knowledge, his learning and his understanding.*

[60] For an extensive discussion of this report and reference to the primary sources and secondary literature, see Mavroudi (2002: 415–17).

I used to bring with us [some] of the books authored on simple drugs, such as the book of Dioscorides, Galen, al-Ghāfiqī and the like from among the great books on this art (fann). He used to first mention what Dioscorides said in his book on the Greek pronunciation (bi-l-lafẓ al-yūnānī) according to how he had confirmed it in the land of the Byzantines (bilād al-Rūm). Then he would mention in full what Dioscorides said regarding its description, its properties and its effects. In addition, he used to mention what Galen said on the same plant regarding its description, disposition (mizāj) and effects and everything related to that. And he would mention all the accounts of the later authors and what they disagreed on, as well as the mistaken and such passages that existed in some of them regarding [a plant's] description. I used to go over these books with him and did not find him leaving out anything that was in them. I was impressed with this also because he would not mention any drugs without also specifying in which chapter from the book of Dioscorides and Galen this [drug] is [mentioned], and under which number among all the medicines mentioned in that chapter. Ibn al-Bayṭār was in the service of al-Malik al-Kāmil Muḥammad ibn Abī Bakr ibn Ayyūb, who used to rely on him for simple medicaments and herbs and appointed him the chief over the other herbalists (*raʾis ʿalā sāʾir al-ʿashshābīn*) in Egypt and master of those who cultivate plants (*aṣḥāb al-basṭāt*). He continued in al-Malik al-Kāmil's service until the ruler died in Damascus, may God have mercy upon him. He then went to Cairo, where he served al-Malik al-Ṣāliḥ Najm al-Dīn Ayyūb ibn al-Malik al-Kāmil, enjoying his favour and holding a high position during his reign. Ḍiyāʾ al-Dīn, the herbalist (*ʿashshāb*) died suddenly, may God have mercy upon him, in Damascus in the month of Shaʿbān in the year 646 [November 1248].[61]

[61] Ibn Abī Uṣaybiʿah, *ʿUyūn al-anbāʾ fī ṭabaqāt al-aṭibbāʾ* (*Sources of Information on the Classes of Physicians*), 14.58.1–3, ed. Savage-Smith et al. (2020, online version). This publication includes both an Arabic edition and an English translation. I am quoting the translation in Savage-Smith et al. (2020, online version) with the exception of the passage in italics, which offer my own rendering of the Arabic text. This publication includes both an Arabic edition and an English translation. In the passage of interest here, Savage-Smith et al. (2020, online version) offer an Arabic text identical to the one in ed. Müller (1884) II.133. The translation in Savage-Smith et al. (2020, online version) is more elegant than what I propose but renders the Arabic in a way that presupposes a primarily textual transmission between Ibn al-Bayṭār as master and Ibn Abī Uṣaybiʿah as student. However, Ibn Abī Uṣaybiʿah's narrative is clear about the oral component of the lesson and the fact that it was taking place in the field. My own, more literal translation aims to make the oral transmission visible to the modern reader. In the Brill translation, the substituted passage offers a description of Ibn al-Bayṭār's commentary. In my translation, the passage describes the oral teaching of Ibn al-Bayṭār. Ibn Abī Uṣaybiʿah marvels not at the correctness of his teacher's written commentary, but at the prodigious memory of Ibn al-Bayṭār while he was transmitting pharmacological knowledge to his student based on earlier pharmacological works as well as Ibn al-Bayṭār's own commentary on Dioscorides. It is self-evident that Ibn al-Bayṭār's oral and written presentation of the material would cover the same points and follow the same order. The translation of the italicised passage in Savage-Smith et al. (2020, online version) reads as follows:

> In his company, I inspected many plants in their native habitats on the outskirts of Damascus. Under his guidance, I also studied his commentary on the names of the medicinal

Ibn Abī Uṣaybiʿah's narrative suggests the importance attributed to the correct pronunciation of plant names as they were known in Greek. This is so because an entire strand of the Arabic pharmacological tradition had naturalised into Arabic these originally Greek terms, and constant recourse to the Greek tradition in order to secure the identity of each plant was necessary, especially given the easy corruption of foreign terms in the course of their manuscript transmission. For Ibn al-Bayṭār, the insistence on the correct Greek pronunciation of the plants may have been reinforced by his intellectual ancestry: we know that he had been taught by Abū al-ʿAbbās ibn al-Rūmiyyah, himself a traveller in search of botanical knowledge and a student of Ibn Ḥazm.[62] The epithet 'Ibn al-Rūmiyyah' indicates that he was the son of a Byzantine slave girl. Abū al-ʿAbbās did not like to be reminded of it because it negatively affected his social status and Muslim credentials. Yet one wonders whether this mother was to him both a liability and an asset – she may have been knowledgeable in Byzantine pharmacological lore in her native Greek.

Undertaking travel to the lands where pharmacological information originates was (and continues to be) an ongoing pursuit of ambitious botanists who sometimes also authored important works on pharmacology

> substances in Dioscorides' book, and so I was able to observe at first hand his vast knowledge and his understanding of a great number of subjects. For my studies with him, I had procured a number of books concerning simple drugs, such as Dioscorides' book, Galen's, the one by al-Ghāfiqī, and similar important works on that subject. Ibn al-Bayṭār's commentary begins with a reiteration of the information from Dioscorides' Greek book that he had been able to confirm in Asia Minor (*bilād al-Rūm*). It then discusses the whole of what Dioscorides says concerning the attributes, descriptions and functions of plants, and also what Galen says concerning the attributes, temperament and functions of plants and related matters. In addition, Ibn Bayṭār discusses a number of sayings of later scholars and their differences of opinion and also cites instances of error ad ambiguity that have occurred in some of their descriptions of substances. I used to analyze those books with him, and I could not find anything in them that he had got wrong. But more astounding still, he never mentioned a drug without also citing in which chapter it is to be found in the book of Dioscorides and Galen, and even under which numbered item it appears amongst all the drugs mentioned in that chapter.

Let the reader decide which translation is more appropriate to Ibn Abī Uṣaybiʿah's intended meaning on the basis of the Arabic text: ولقد شاهدت معه في ظاهر دمشق كثيراً من النبات في مواضعه وقرأت عليه أيضاً تفسيره لأسماء أدوية كتاب ديسقوريدس فكنت أجد من غزارة علمه ودرايته وفهمه شيئاً كثيراً جداً وكنت احضر لدينا عدة من الكتب المؤلفة في الأدوية المفردة مثل كتاب ديسقوريدس وجالينوس والغافقي وأمثالها من الكتب الجليلة في هذا الفن فكان يذكر أولا ما قاله ديسقوريدس في كتابه باللفظ اليوناني على ما قد صححه في بلاد الروم ثم يذكر جمل ما قاله ديسقوريدس من نعته وصفته وافعاله ويذكر أيضاً ما قاله جالينوس فيه من نعته ومزاجه وأفعاله وما يتعلق بذلك ويذكر أيضاً جملاً من اقوال المتأخرين وما اختلفوا فيه ومواضع الغلط والاشتباه الذي وقع لبعضهم في نعته فكنت اراجع تلك الكتب معه ولا أجده يغادر شيئاً مما فيها وأعجب من ذلك أيضاً أنه كان ما يذكر دواء إلا ويعين في أي مقالة هو من كتاب ديسقوريدس وجالينوس وفي أي عدد هو من جملة الأدوية المذكورة في تلك المقالة.

62 Ibn Ḥazm was a polymath who had also written on medicine. On Ibn al-Rūmiyyah, see Dietrich (2012).

throughout the centuries. The phenomenon is, of course, much better recorded for the early modern and modern periods.[63] The report of Ibn Juljul and the note on Ibn al-Bayṭār are embedded in the two famous biographical dictionaries on the lives of physicians who have survived from the Arabic Middle Ages. These, along with Ibn al-Nadīm's *Kitāb al-fihrist* (*The Catalogue*), are our most important sources of information on the transmission of Greek technical learning into Arabic. Equivalent texts do not exist in Byzantine Greek. This means that other types of sources have to be interrogated in order to yield equivalent information. Indeed, certain features of the surviving Byzantine botanical manuscripts indicate that the transmission of botanical knowledge during the Byzantine period passed through a process similar to what is described in Pliny, Simon of Genoa, Ibn Abī Uṣaybiʿah: botany was transmitted through studying texts in illustrated and unillustrated manuscripts, observing plants in real life – preferably with the help of an acknowledged expert – and composing new works by combining knowledge from written and oral sources, as well as one's own experience.

An example that illustrates some of these processes is the Lavra Dioscorides (Athous Laurae MS Ω 75), dated to the late tenth or early eleventh century on the basis of its palaeographical and codicological characteristics.[64] The manuscript is well executed but not luxurious. Its size is smaller than other manuscripts of Dioscorides, which suggests that it may have been created to be portable. A few of its marginalia indicate that its users collated its text with other manuscripts and supplemented it with information.[65]

[63] A discussion of botanists and natural scientists who travelled extensively between the European Renaissance and Darwin's travel on the *Beagle*, see Ogilvie (2006: 141–50); Ogilvie explains how individual botanists pursued a qualitatively different type of travel for the purposes of their research, but such resolution is impossible for the travelling botanists of the Middle Ages, whose names we scarcely know. Ogilvie (2006: 151ff.) also discusses the cultivation of extensive botanical gardens as a means to reduce the need for travel in order to observe plants from life. Again, this type of information hardly exists for earlier periods: for the Middle Ages, we have a vague understanding of the medicinal gardens of monasteries, while Pliny makes only a cursory mention of their existence in Roman antiquity. Our knowledge on ancient Roman gardens was in recent decades increased more through archaeology, especially through the pioneering work of Wilhelmina Feemster Jashemski (1910–2007) and less through a systematic exploration of the narrative sources from antiquity.

[64] My report here is based on the very detailed description of the manuscript by Christodoulou (1986). The same date is given in Touwaide (1991b).

[65] Examples: f. 38v: 'γράφει ἐν ἄλλῳ' ('another manuscript says . . . '); f. 106r: 'ζήτει καὶ ἕτερον . . . ' ('look for another one . . . '). These notes are reproduced in Kourilas (1935b: 33) and Kourilas (1954: 13–16). I examined a microfilm of the manuscript kept at the Patriarchal Institute for Patristic Studies in Thessaloniki in July 2015. There are frequent annotations up to f. 218v and very rare ones after that. The resolution of the microfilm at my disposal was such that the annotations were very difficult or impossible to read.

On Mount Athos, where this manuscript survives, Dioscorides' treatise was approached as the foundation of a living pharmacological tradition into the first half of the twentieth century.[66] In the 1930s, the journalist and author Sydney Loch mentioned Clement, a herbalist monk from the Athonite monastery of Dionysiou, who was covering great distances in search of herbs, 'weighted with his handwritten copy of Dioscorides, in two heavy tomes'.[67] At around the same time, an acquaintance of Loch's, the distinguished British botanist Arthur William Hill, also attests to this living tradition:

> To be a Botanist on the Holy Mountain was not regarded by the Monks as an unusual occupation, for at Karyes there is an official Botanist Monk, who occupies his time in searching for plants of real or supposed medicinal importance . . . He was a remarkable old Monk with an extensive knowledge of plants and their properties. Though fully gowned with a long black cassock he travelled very quickly, usually on foot and sometimes on a mule carrying his 'flora' with him in a large, black, bulky bag. Such a bag was necessary since his 'flora' was nothing less than four manuscript folio volumes of Dioscorides, which apparently he himself had copied out. This Flora he invariably used for determining any plant which he could not name at sight, and he could find his way in his books and identify his plants – to his own satisfaction – with remarkable rapidity. Sibthorp, it will be remembered, made his important journeys to the near East and to Athos with the object of identifying the plants recorded by Dioscordes.[68]

Hill mentions a number of other monks who were herbalists in individual monasteries, equipped with pharmacies and medicinal gardens.

The learned and indefatigable bishop Eulogios Kourilas (1880–1961) was certainly part of this active engagement with the ancient text. He was one of the best connoisseurs of the Lavra Dioscorides because he spent a considerable part of his life as monk in the very monastery where this manuscript was kept. His scholarly activities included a wide range of subjects, yet among them botany was certainly one of the most important and consistently pursued.[69] Like his ancient and medieval predecessors,

[66] The demand for 'natural' medical and alimentary products during the past few decades has certainly maintained the Athonite tradition of botany and has even expanded it into commercial applications. I have not found a way to verify whether Dioscorides continues to play a role.

[67] See Loch (195–?: 35).

[68] See Hill (1937: 197–8).

[69] Kourilas belongs to a tradition of learned church prelates in Greece and elsewhere in the Ottoman Empire during the second half of the nineteenth century and the first half of the twentieth. On his remarkable life and extensive scholarly work, both published and unpublished, see Zagkli-Boziou (2009), which provides an extensive narrative on Kourilas' life and a detailed description of his archive; see also Kosmas (2016), and Kourilas' published biobibliography (Kourilas 1935a).

Kourilas cultivated it by reading, observing from life, and consulting with experts.[70] He studied the *iatrosophia* (the collections of medical recipes preserved in Greek manuscripts of the Byzantine and post-Byzantine period) and compiled extensive lists of the plant names he encountered in these manuscripts. Most of Kourilas' research on this topic remains unpublished. In his handwritten notes, he names his manuscript sources (sometimes copied and examined by himself, other times by fellow monks at his request), as well as his informants. For botanical terms in Turkish (as well as Arabic and Persian, from which many Turkish names on *materia medica* derive) his interlocutor was the monk Pavlos Lavriotis (1885–1980), a Pontic Greek who had practised as a surgeon in the Ottoman Empire before opting for an ascetic life on Mount Athos.[71]

As Kourilas clearly understood, the collection of multiple names for the same plant is not a philological exercise but provides much-needed information, especially in a world without a standardised system of classifying and naming plants, and where doctors, herbalists, and ingredients on the marketplace were coming from faraway places. Even when an author wants to be highbrow, quoting colloquial terms is important for clarity and comprehensiveness. This fact is certainly appreciated by anyone with hands-on experience in traditional medicine and is repeatedly mentioned in both Byzantine and post-Byzantine Greek texts.[72] Even after the wide adoption of the Linnaean system of plant classification, knowledge of pre-Linnaean terms is useful in order to maximise one's access to earlier botanical knowledge.

Herbal vocabulary and other information was collected in Byzantine manuscripts containing other medical authors, as well. The currency of foreign terms, Arabic and Persian but also Latin, within the context of Byzantine (and post-Byzantine) pharmacological and medical practice is evident from the glosses added in several manuscripts of Paul of Aegina, one of

[70] Kourilas worked on botany at least since 1913 and into 1922. When Max Wellmann's critical edition of Dioscorides appeared between 1906 and 1914, Kourilas published his severe reservations on Wellmann's editorial choices in Kourilas (1935b) and Kourilas (1954). Marie Cronier recently also discussed problems with Wellmann's editorial choices; see Cronier (2006).

[71] See www.pemptousia.gr/2016/01/monachos-pavlos-lavriotis-1885-1-1-1980 (accessed 28 January 2023). He left behind an autobiography; see Pavlos [Pavlides] Monk of Lavra (1963); see also Panagiotopoulos (n.d.: 92–4) and Chrysostomos of Lavra, Bishop of Rodostolou (2000: 108–14).

[72] Langkavel (1866: xi–xii) quotes three Greek texts of various periods that make this explicit. They include the sixteenth-century correspondence of Martinus Crusius with Theodosios Zygomalas, a text on diet addressed by Michael Psellos to Emperor Constantine IX (if genuine, it would date to the eleventh century), and a text attributed to the tenth-century physician Theophanes Chrysobalantes (excerpted from old Parisinus 3502, currently Parisinus gr. 1630).

the most popular treatises of practical consultation.[73] Paul of Aegina must have been one of the early venues of Greek-Arabic (and Greek-Latin) pharmacological contact and was clearly not 'lost' in Greek during the seventh-to-ninth century 'Dark' period: during the last quarter of the eighth century, or, perhaps, the very beginning of the ninth, several scribes copied a multi-volume compendium of his *Epitome*.[74]At around the same time Paul's work was translated into Latin, while several medical authors writing in Syriac and Arabic in the course of the ninth and tenth centuries quote him in abundance.[75] Rendering this work from one language into another was certainly an exercise in medical vocabulary that modern research has not tapped yet for all it can reveal about the medieval and early modern transmission of botany.

Notes on several manuscripts of *Epitome* indicate that botanical information was imparted through oral consultation, and sometimes also suggest a multilingual environment. A securely dated and localised example is Parisinus gr. 2207. It was copied by Michael Louloudes, a scribe known from his autobiographical notes on a number of manuscripts covering the late thirteenth and early fourteenth centuries, through which he can be followed from Byzantine Ephesus to Crete.[76] In the 1370s Louloudes' manuscript was on Cyprus, and in the fifteenth century it passed to the hands of Gioan Singlitico, who had been trained as a physician at the University of Padova and served the Lusignan court of Cyprus. The manuscript has multiple annotations in Greek, Latin, and Arabic.[77]

Later notes in two eleventh-century parchment manuscripts, Parisinus gr. 2205 and Parisinus gr. 2206, are also illuminating.[78] Parisinus gr. 2206 contains a number of fourteenth-century notes in Latin, as well as Greek

[73] These manuscripts are pointed out and briefly discussed in Heiberg (1919: 272–4). I have based my remarks on the information provided by Heiberg and Omont (1888) without personally examining these manuscripts (with the exception of the Laurentianus Plut. 74.2, which is available online: http://mss.bmlonline.it/Catalogo.aspx?Shelfmark=Plut.74.2 (accessed 28 January 2023)). On the manuscripts containing Paul's work currently at the National Library of France, see Lherminier (2016).

[74] See Dobrynina (2010).

[75] See Mavroudi (2015: 43) for a discussion of Paul's Latin translation and references to bibliography on Paul's Syriac and Arabic reception.

[76] *RGK* I 281; II 385; III 464.

[77] The manuscript is available online at https://gallica.bnf.fr/ark:/12148/btv1b107237378/f17.item# (accessed 28 January 2023). The history of this manuscript is relatively well known. Details and bibliography are available at https://pinakes.irht.cnrs.fr/notices/cote/51836/ (accessed 28 January 2023).

[78] These two manuscripts are not available online and I could not examine them. I am accepting the dates given for them in Omont (1888: 214). My report on the notes relies on Heiberg (1919), which does not always provide a date for the notes it mentions.

notes in two separate hands, one of which belongs to the fifteenth century. The Greek notes include a self-reminder to 'ask the horseshoe maker about hemlock' ('ἐρότισον τὸν καλιγὰν διὰ κόνιον'). The question is crucial because hemlock is deadly and can easily be confused with other plants that are not.[79] It is not clear whether the horseshoe maker would provide botanical information or just indicate a locale where a hemlock-like plant was growing, in which case the author of the note would be responsible for deciding the plant's identity and undertake its possible eradication. In either case, the note indicates that his effort to correctly identify it included consulting this manuscript of Dioscorides. Later notes in Parisinus gr. 2205 indicate oral consultation with informants out in the fields and the natural habitat of the plants under discussion.[80] The notes are in Greek, the informant has the Muslim name Hasan, and the places mentioned indicate what is today northern Greece. The combination of information suggests a date in the Ottoman period for this note.[81] Paul's medical vocabulary is glossed with botanical terms in Greek and Arabic (written in Greek characters) on Athous Vatopedinus 535, Parisinus gr. 2292, and Marcianus gr. 292 (another manuscript copied by Louloudes).[82]

In order to better understand the mechanisms of simultaneous oral and written transmission of pharmacological knowledge it is important to briefly consider the abilities and limitations of human memory. Mary Carruthers long ago discussed that, from antiquity into the early modern period, memorising a text was understood as foundational to internalising and understanding it. This, in turn, had implications for the moral fabric of an individual and commanded considerable social respect.[83] The profound admiration Ibn Abī Uṣaybiʿah expressed for Ibn al-Bayṭār's prodigious memory and moral qualities certainly fits this pattern. The social

[79] See Koraes (1835: 176), under 'μαγκοῦνα καὶ μαγκοῦνα'; Koraes explains that these two terms must be a vernacular for 'μήκων' (pavot, opium), which various authors confuse with hemlock ('κώνειον') because they are both poisonous. Another confusion is with parsley ('πετροσέλινον'). Indeed, *conium maculatum* looks very much like parsley, but if ingested it is deadly. A further resemblance is signalled in a note from Parisinus gr. 2205 copied by Heiberg (1919: 272): 'κώνειον· κώνιον δὲ λέγεται ἡ μαγκούνα τὸ ἐοικὸς τὸν ἀμάραντον τὸ μέγα [*sic*]'. The manuscript is not available online and I could not examine it.

[80] Heiberg (1919: 273): 'πράσιον· ὅπερ με ἔδιξεν ὁ χαάσανης εἰς τὸν χάντακαν τὸ ἐοικὸς τὸ δίκταμον καὶ ἔχον μέσον τὸν φύλον ὅς σφερία κολιτζήδας τὸ λεγόμενον πισσιρίκεια'. Another note: 'σάμψυχον: τὸ ἴδον ἧς τὴν βεροίαν ἧς τοῦ χαρτοφύλακος τοῦ δρουγουβιτίας μετὰ τοῦ χασάνη τὸ ἐοικὸς τὸ δήκταμον'. Veroia is the name of a city in what is now northern Greece, but it is also the Greek name for Syrian Aleppo. The Slavic 'δρουγουβιτίας' suggests the Balkans. The office of *chartophylax* is an ecclesiastical appointment.

[81] This manuscript is not available online and I could not examine it in order to suggest a date for the notes.

[82] The notes are quoted without dates in Heiberg (1919: 272–3).

[83] Carruthers (2008).

prominence accorded to memory in this context means that educated individuals in the past possessed better exercised and more capacious memories than our own. Yet how much more capacious?

Dioscorides describes more than 550 plants, close to 80 animals or animal parts, and about 90 minerals. This number is considerable even by the standards of the sixteenth century, when acquaintance with the Americas and the first European colonial expansion in faraway geographies exposed European herbalists to a considerable number of new species.[84] It is difficult to know exactly how many plants an experienced botanist knew how to actively use as ingredients in medications. The number obviously varies by expertise. At the highest level of botanical mastery, Ibn Abī Uṣaybiʿah's narrative suggests, Ibn al-Bayṭār had memorised the properties of considerably more than the 550 species of plants Dioscorides discussed. At the same time, the student's admiration for the teacher's feat makes clear that such prodigious memory was absolutely extraordinary. Brian Ogilvie projects that, in the expanding botanical universe of the sixteenth century, practitioners grew increasingly distrustful of memory. For example, Valerius Cordus (1515–44), who composed the first known pharmacopoeia north of the Alps and is one of the most celebrated herbalists in history, could cite Dioscorides and other ancient authorities from memory, but also kept careful field notes. Indeed, many of his plant descriptions imply that they were made on site.[85] According to Ogilvie, around the year 1600 'naturalists were deeply suspicious of memory'. Ogilvie may be right regarding highly expert practitioners invested in expanding herbal knowledge by observing and describing unknown species. Yet such a practitioner has to be an apprentice before becoming expert, and for each expert there are many more who know considerably less.

Since no statistics or other such information survives from the ancient and medieval period, one has to turn to modern data. One can approach both academically trained pharmacists and traditional healers in search of answers. When asked how many plants an experienced botanist may know how to actively use as ingredients in medications, two pharmacists independently converged to approximately fifty.[86] This number seems corroborated by data collected in Israel among traditional Arab practitioners

[84] Ogilvie (2006: 52) reckons that an expert European botanist in the sixteenth century knew about 500 species (approximately Dioscorides' entire botany) but the number of plants available to European pharmacopoeia was growing exponentially. By the end of the sixteenth century, Carolus Clusius had described about 200 plants not encountered in earlier herbals.

[85] Ogilvie (2006: 181 and 147).

[86] The informants are Mrs Eleni Karagkounidou and the employee of a traditional pharmacy in Marrakesh. Both informants had pursued the study of botany in a modern university, in addition to what traditional channels brought. I interviewed Mrs Karagkounidou (b. 1958), a pharmacist at the

between the 1980s and 1998.[87] A survey from the 1980s, carried out among 60 practitioners, indicated an active use of 43 plant species; a more detailed survey in 1998 that fielded thirty-one 'significant and reliable practitioners' recorded active use of a total of 129 plant species (among the approximately 2,700 that exist in Israel). Only two among the thirty-one informants had encountered botany in the course of their academic studies.

centre of town in Thessaloniki, in December 2016. She owns what must be the oldest pharmacy in continuous operation in town. It was founded by her great-grandfather soon after he graduated from pharmacy school in Constantinople in the year 1900. She is the fourth generation of her family working there. After pharmacy, she also studied history at the University of Thessaloniki (as a hobby, never expecting to do anything with it, since she knew the pharmacy was her destiny), and she understands the value of the records of the business left by her family. She has kept pharmaceutical recipe books that definitely predate the war, which she showed me. They were handwritten, and in many respects looked like medieval and early modern pharmacological manuscripts in Greek and other languages: the format of the pages is random, a multiplicity of inks and hands is in evidence, the titles of the recipes are decided ad hoc and frequently indicate the person from whom the recipe was received and the disease it was expected to cure (worms, abortifacients, etc.). The last three generations of pharmacists in Mrs Karagkounidou's family were women: her grandmother, her mother, now herself. Given that Greek society was certainly male dominated for the better part of the twentieth century, this pattern is unusual and ought to be remembered when contemplating the three female informants of Simon of Genoa or Anicia Juliana as dedicatee of the Vienna Dioscorides.

Asked about how many ingredients a pharmacist who compounds drugs can actively use, Mrs Karagkounidou hesitated. She rightly pointed out that a lot depends on the pharmacist's expertise in the spectrum from beginner to experienced pharmacist. When asked to speculate about a very experienced practitioner, she suggested about 100 for a top expert and around 50 for an average pharmacist. She specified that this is a personal estimate based on no evidence, just an instinct about what is doable and what she understands of the previous experience in her family pharmacy. In the course of the conversation she mentioned that, during the Germans' occupation of Greece in World War II, when people both in the city and the countryside were dying of dysentery, her grandmother created a very effective drug based on garlic and toured the villages selling it, not for money (it was useless), but for food (which was scarce). This is how she kept her family alive.

During this period, her mother had eight employees in the pharmacy helping her compound this miracle drug, primarily by manually beating ingredients in mortars. This gives us an idea of what a cottage industry of drug making based on natural ingredients like the ones mentioned in Dioscorides can be like in conditions of material privation and scarcity. It may, perhaps, help us imagine the capacity of an average medieval pharmacy. It is also interesting for attesting to professional itinerancy.

In addition to Mrs Karagkounidou, I briefly interviewed the employee of a traditional pharmacy in Morocco in December 2017. The shop where he was employed was near the entrance to the Bahia palace in Marrakesh. He was around the same age as Mrs Karagkounidou and university trained like her. The conditions of the interview were not ideal and the discussion could not be extensive. The pharmacy carried several hundred specimens of *materia medica* (certainly as many as Dioscorides describes, if not more). I asked him whether anyone in the pharmacy now could actively create drugs with everything in the store. He responded that he could personally actively use about fifty and was one of the more experienced employees. His response independently corroborated the information from Mrs Karagkounidou.

87 The data discussed in Azaizeh et al. (2003).

Modern ethnobotanical practice and what is reported in the ancient sources appear consistent in other ways too: ethnobotanical research in oriental Morocco indicates that most traditional remedies are used for the digestive tract and diseases of the eyes are rarely treated, as is the case with Hippocratic pharmacology.[88] Further, modern ethnobotany suggests that a practising herbalist works with considerably less *materia medica* than what premodern botany has recorded in writing. For example, research conducted in Mauritania among 120 informants indicated that, as a group, they worked with a total of 68 plant species, which they applied to 177 different medicinal uses, only 6 of which are also recorded by Ibn al-Bayṭār. The authors of this study attribute the discrepancy to Ibn al-Bayṭār's geographic focus: he probably never travelled to Mauritania and was generally focused on the Mediterranean coast of North Africa rather than the Saharan region.[89]

It is hard to project modern numbers on the past, especially given the profound social changes during the second half of the twentieth century, which largely eradicated older material culture. In general, for antiquity and the Middle Ages it is impossible to know what part of the written tradition was actually used in practice and how the preferences (or fashions) for different medicines changed. Yet it seems safe to conclude that only part of the botanical tradition recorded in writing was actually used in practice. This is the impression conveyed by another passage from Damaskios' *Philosophical History* on Asclepiodotos of Alexandria: 'In medicine Asclepiodotus was the pupil of Iacobus [Psychrestos] and trod in his footsteps, and indeed there were areas where he surpassed him. For he re-established the long-lost use of white hellebore, which even Iacobus had not been able to recover, and through it he remedied incurable diseases against all expectation.'[90] Since Dioscorides had described white hellebore one can conclude that, back in the fifth century as now, the availability of written botanical information on a plant was not enough for someone to know how to use it medicinally. An entry on white hellebore with an

[88] On the frequency of diseases that Hippocratic pharmacology aimed to treat, see Stannard (1961). On ethnobotany in oriental Morocco, see Fakchich and Elachouri (2014).

[89] See Yebouk et al. (2020). I had no access to the fundamental ethnobotanical work by Baytop (1984). Modern ethnobotanical research generally acknowledges that several tens among the drugs used by traditional healers cannot be identified by the researchers who approached them. This closely parallels the experience of the ancient and medieval readers of Dioscorides and other treatises on *materia medica* (plants are described but their use is unknown) as is evident from the revival of hellebore's use described in the *Life of Damaskios*.

[90] Damaskios, *Philosophical History*, ed. and tr. Athanassiadi (1999: 215) fr. 85D. On Asclepiodotos, see Athanassiadi (1999: 348–9).

illustration is included in the Vienna Dioscorides, which was copied in the 510s, at around the same time that Damaskios was writing. This means that the manuscript included a plant that had recently re-entered medical practice and may have been considered a 'miracle drug' for the period.

The disappearance and reappearance of white hellebore in medical practice means that recording botanical knowledge in writing and studying from books must have had an important place in the ancient and medieval transmission of knowledge. Although Damaskios does not provide details, Asclepiodotos must have resurrected the use of white hellebore through a combination of reading and experimenting with what he read. The question that suggests itself is the following: given the importance of studying written sources in addition to oral transmission in order to become an adept herbalist, does the textual study ever become a sterile philological exercise, like modern scholarship has frequently assumed for Byzantine botanical lexicography?

The list of plant names in languages like Tuscan, Lucanian, Tyrrhenian, Egyptian, Carthaginian, Celtic, and Dacian that is recorded in the Vienna Dioscorides can be found in the Naples Dioscorides which was copied in the late sixth or early seventh century in Italy and contains the same recension of Dioscorides' text as the Vienna codex.[91] Among the manuscripts with a different recension of Dioscorides, these early botanical vocabulary lists are repeated in a single one, Marcianus gr. 273.[92] This was also copied in Italy, but considerably later, during the second half of the thirteenth century – a time by which several among the languages included in the list of plant names were presumably no longer spoken.[93] Different explanations for the preservation of obsolete medical vocabulary suggest themselves. A frequent modern explanation for such instances in Byzantine manuscripts is that scribes were overall ignorant or absent-minded, and therefore copying uncritically and mechanically. Alternatively, they were copying to preserve texts for posterity rather than to actively use them in the present. Indeed, Maria Rosa Formentin suggested that Marcianus gr. 273 was copied not for the purposes of medical instruction or practice, but in order to immortalise patrimony

[91] For a recent and brief outline of the manuscript tradition of Dioscorides' herbal, see Cronier (2015).

[92] I base this observation on multiple examples from the critical apparatus to Wellman's edition (1906–14). Marcianus gr. 273 contains the same recension as the one preserved in Parisinus gr. 2179, on which Wellmann's modern edition of Dioscorides' text is based.

[93] In Marcianus gr. 273, the work of Dioscorides is the most recent layer on palimpsest parchment. The older, erased layer was written in the eleventh and twelfth centuries and contained liturgical texts. For a description of the manuscript and the context of its production as a palimpsest, see Formentin (2005).

expressed in the Greek language, which was disappearing from the Italian peninsula. If this is so, the obsolete nature of plant names in dead languages would not have bothered readers because the manuscript was intended for few or no readers at all. However, during the past generation of scholarship, researchers have moved away from viewing the Byzantine scribes and scholars as passive and mindless 'preservers' and closer to understanding them as active and conscious users who intervene in received tradition. Accordingly, if we can imagine a practical use for the manuscript, the obsolete plant names also do not pose a problem: modern ethnobotanical practice shows respect for received tradition in writing even if it significantly departs from it.[94]

4.4 *Lexikon tōn Sarakēnōn*: An Arabic-Greek Herbal Glossary

Byzantine botanical lexicography furnishes important evidence regarding contact between Byzantine and Arabic medicine through both oral and written channels. But how Byzantine herbal dictionaries were compiled and practically consulted is little understood by contemporary scholarship. In 1971, Jerry Stannard, a leading scholar of ancient and medieval botany among an earlier generation, published an article on Byzantine botanical lexicography.[95] To the best of my knowledge, it remains the only panoramic overview of Byzantine botanical lexicography and describes it as an enterprise more relevant to philological pursuit than to medical practice:

> After Galen, compiling plant lists became a literary activity in which scholarship and editorial expertise supplanted a personal knowledge of the plant in its living state. The final state of this medico-botanical scholasticism was reached in late Byzantine times (from the thirteenth century onwards) with the rise of multilingual lexica. Often they recorded little more than synonyms and even then some of the synonymies were as questionable as their orthography.[96]

A usual problem with multilingual dictionaries is that they equate unrelated plants, which the same article interpreted as a further sign that their compilers were 'more adept at scholarship than at botany'.[97] However, close examination of an Arabic-Greek herbal glossary allows one to retrace the manner of its compilation and demonstrates that it was put together for a practical reason and not as philological exercise.

[94] See Clark (2002). [95] See the assessment of Stannard's scholarly work in Ogilvie (2003).
[96] Stannard (1971: 169). [97] Stannard (1971: 177).

The Arabic-Greek glossary in question is titled *Lexikon tōn Sarakēnōn* (*Lexicon of Saracens*) in the Greek medical manuscripts where it survives, and it gives the Arabic names of several botanical and pharmaceutical terms transliterated in Greek characters side by side with their Greek equivalents. Its edition by Margaret Thomson, based on two manuscripts, appeared in 1955.[98] The editor could not identify the source of the glossary, and in spite of her meticulous attempts to identify the Arabic equivalents of the disfigured (in the course of the Greek manuscript tradition) Arabic terms, her effort was thwarted by her inability to read Arabic.

The problems that the glossary raises were discussed (but not resolved) in a 1998 article by Nikolai Serikoff, who based his arguments on Thomson's edition.[99] Serikoff correctly observed that it contains both Arabic and Latin terms. He concluded that it was based on an Arabic herbal index, which, in its turn, was based on the medieval translations from Greek into Arabic (ninth–tenth centuries). The Latin terms included in the glossary led Serikoff to the conclusion that its Arabic source was connected with the *al-Jāmiʿ li-mufradāt al-adwiyah wa-l-aghdhiyah* (*Collector of Simple Drugs and Foodstuffs*) by Ibn al-Bayṭār (d. 1248) and the Greek translation of Ibn al-Jazzār's (fl. tenth century) *Zād al-musāfir wa-qūt al-ḥāḍir* (*Provisions for the Traveller and Nourishment for the Sedentary*), the so-called *Ephodia* (although he did not explain in any concrete terms the relationship between these two medical texts and the putative Arabic source of our herbal glossary), as well as other tenth–eleventh-century Arabic treatises on the properties of plants by al-Rāzī (d. *c*.925), al-Majūsī (fl. tenth century), and Ibn-Sīnā (d. 1037). Since these treatises are voluminous and the *Lexikon tōn Sarakēnōn* is a brief glossary of synonyms extending to twenty-two printed pages, Serikoff hypothesised that the *Lexikon tōn Sarakēnōn* is based on the table of contents of an Arabic pharmacological treatise, which was rewritten by adding the synonyms of the various terms mentioned and came to be considered an independent work. This was subsequently translated into Greek. The glossary includes phantom words that never existed either in Greek or in Arabic, as well as mistakes in translating the botanical terms from Arabic into Greek.

[98] *Lexikon tōn Sarakēnōn*, ed. Thomson (1955) 145–68. Further references to 'Thomson' accompanied by a number indicate the line of Greek text in this edition.

[99] Serikoff [Serikov] (1998). Serikoff (2013) published a botanical dictionary related to those discussed today from a Wellcome manuscript. The brief introduction to the edition repeats points from Serikoff (1998).

Serikoff went on to analyse the phantom words and mistakes included in the glossary in order to deduce to what degree its translator into Greek understood Arabic pharmacology. Although he pointed out that it is difficult to distinguish between mistakes made by the translator and by the subsequent Greek scribes who copied his work, he concluded that the Arabic text used by the translator gave herbal terms without noting the diacritical dots.[100] This, according to Serikoff, led the translator to misunderstand certain Arabic letters and resulted in many mistaken renderings of the Arabic terms. The translator also did not realise that several of the Arabic terms were borrowed from Greek, and sometimes read and translated the text in front of him word for word, without taking into account the meaning of whole phrases. Mistakes such as repetition of the same term, two or more words strung together as if they were one, and words with missing syllables should be attributed to the Greek scribes who copied the text. Serikoff concluded that the translator knew colloquial Arabic well but had not received a classical Arabic education; he seems to have read and understood correctly about 75 per cent of the Arabic terms he translated, which must be considered a remarkably high percentage, given that translating a glossary of botanical terms requires mastering a highly specialised vocabulary.

A very different interpretation of the data emerges if we take two important facts into consideration: the manner in which Byzantine herbal dictionaries were compiled in general, and the evidence furnished by a further investigation into the manuscript tradition of the *Lexikon tōn Sarakēnōn*. Besides Parisinus gr. 2180 and Parisinus gr. 2287, the two manuscripts known to Thomson, the glossary survives in at least two more, Vindobonensis med. gr. 47, and Parisinus gr. 2286.[101] Each manuscript gives a somewhat different version of the glossary, so that, at first glance, it seems that one is dealing with four different works. This impression of variety is generated by additions to the original number

[100] Serikoff (1998) is referring to the fact that several letters of the Arabic alphabet can be distinguished from one another only by the placing of one, two, or three dots above or below the shape of the letter, as in the following examples (chosen to make the phenomenon observable even to readers unfamiliar with the Arabic alphabet): possible confusion can occur between the letters ب (pronounced) ت (pronounced [t]) or ث (pronounced [th] or [s] in some of the dialects); خ ،ج، and ح.

[101] Parisinus gr. 2180 was copied by Georgios Midiates *c.*1470, as suggested by the name of the scribe and the watermarks on the paper; Parisinus gr. 2287 was copied by many hands in the second half of the fifteenth century. For the dates, see Thomson (1955: 143–4). Vindobonensis med. gr. 47 was copied around 1500. See Hunger and Kresten (1969: 98–9). Parisinus gr. 2285 is briefly described in Omont (1888: 229–30), where it is dated to the fourteenth century.

of Arabic terms listed. In Parisinus gr. 2287 the intention of the scribe to add to the terms originally constituting the dictionary is evident in the abundant spaces he left at the end of the entries under each letter, which sometimes was indeed filled in at a later time. An example of this method of compilation can be seen on Figure 4.2, Parisinus gr. 2287, f. 211r. In Vindobonensis med. gr. 47 a page of further terms was added at the very beginning of the text.

A more careful examination of the manuscripts preserving the glossary indicates that all its versions were based on the same prototype, which was compiled by someone who did not know Arabic based on a written source that gave Arabic medical terms transcribed in Greek characters. The main evidence that should be considered is the following:

1. The dictionary is arranged alphabetically, and in all three copies of it the letter *chi* (χ) begins with the entry 'χβηλχ χανδαράνα· τὸ ἀμμωνιακὸν ἅλας' (Thomson 1955: 385).[102] The Arabic word for 'ἅλας' ('salt') is not 'χβηλχ' (pronounced *hvilh*) but 'μηλχ' (*milḥ*). As the mistake 'χβηλχ' for 'μηλχ' is shared by all three manuscripts, one can deduce that all three versions of the glossary derive from the same original compilation of Arabic terms, made by somebody who did not understand Arabic and collected his terms from a written source where 'μηλχ' could be mistaken for 'χβηλχ'.
2. The same Arabic term is sometimes included more than once, even on the very same page of the dictionary. Let us consider a couple of examples. The first is the dictionary's entry on sagapenum (see Figure 4.2: Parisinus gr. 2287, f. 211r, lines 6, 18, 22, and 27; and Figure 4.3: Vindobonensis med. gr. 47, f. 429v, lines 4, 17, 21, and 25): 'σκϊβΐνη, ζασπαχένι· σαγαπηνός λέγεται. σϊκβΐνιτζ· σαγαπϊνὸς. σϊκηβήνηζ·[103] σαγάπηνος.[104] σϊκοπίτζ· σαγάπινον'. The Arabic entries all convey, with varying degrees of exactitude, the pronunciation of the Arabic *sakabīnaj*. A second example is the multiple mention of opopanax, in Arabic *jawāshır*, which is once mentioned under the letter gamma, 'γευσήρ· ὀποπάναξ' (Thomson 1955: 54), and twice under the letter tau: 'τζευουσήρ· ὀποπάναξ' (Thomson 1955: 351); 'τζεουσήρ· ὀποπάναξ' (Thomson 1955: 355). This example indicates another important fact: though the compiler of the glossary did not know Arabic, the written source from which he collected his

[102] In Arabic *milḥ andarānī*. [103] Parisinus retains 'σϊκϋβήνηζ'.
[104] Parisinus retains 'σαγάπινος'.

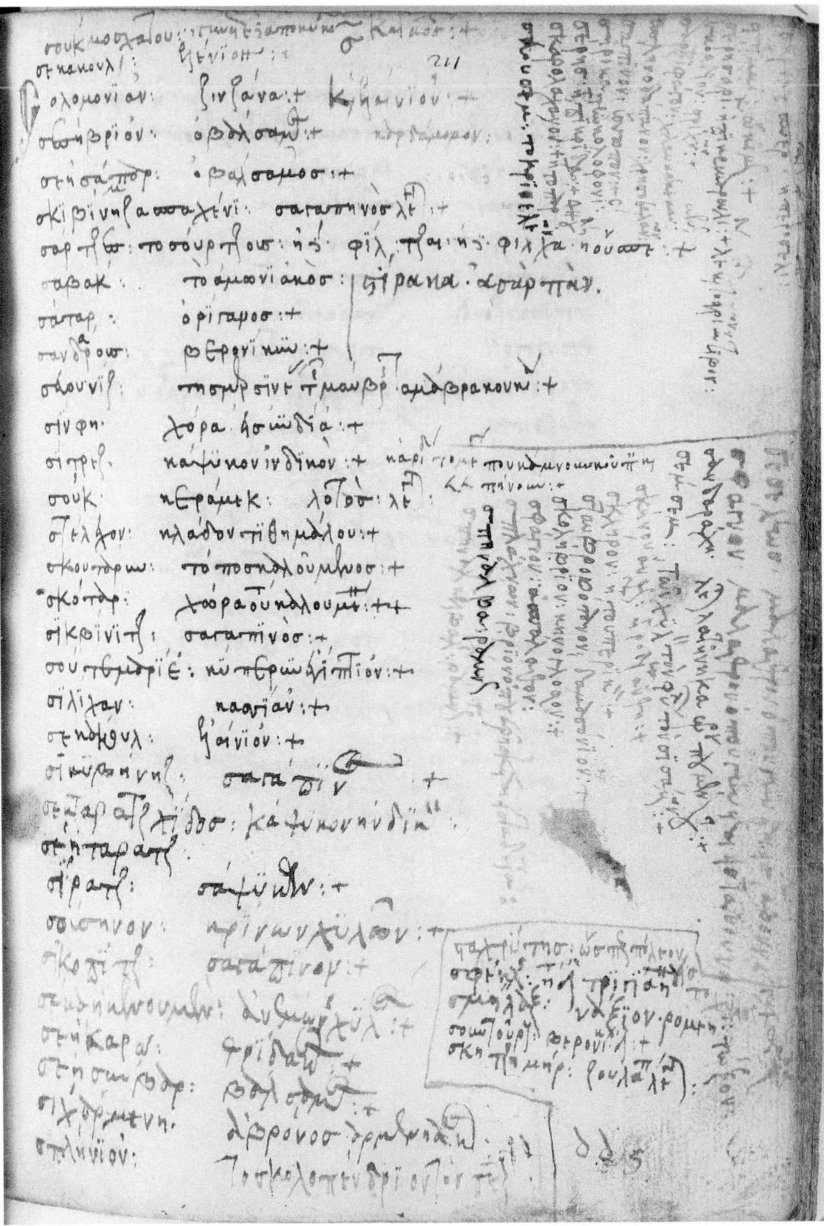

Figure 4.2 Paris, Bibliothèque nationale, MS gr. 2287, f. 211r

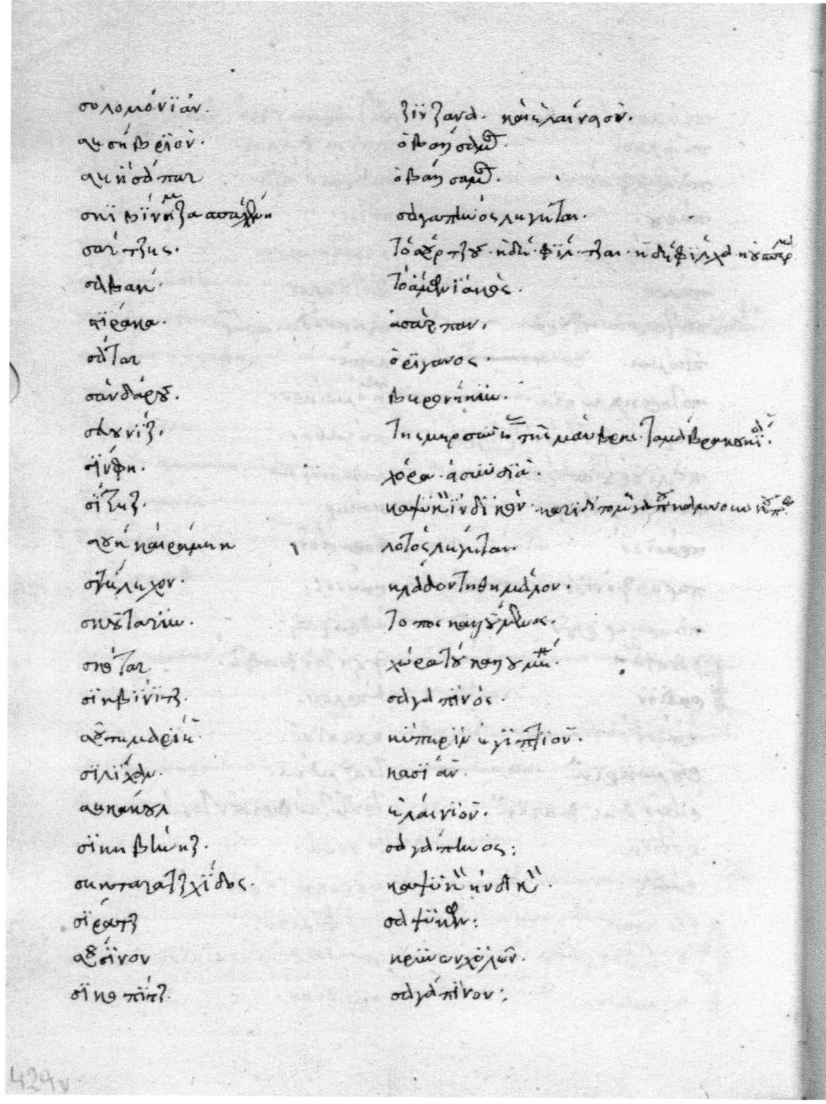

Figure 4.3 Vienna, Österreichische Nationalbibliothek, MS med. gr. 47, f. 429v

terms was written by someone proficient in Arabic whose Greek transliterations of the Arabic terms did not follow a consistent system. Both 'γ' in 'γευσὴρ' and 'τζ' in 'τζευουσὴρ' and 'τζεουσὴρ' are acceptable renderings of the sound [*dj*] written with the Arabic letter *djīm*.

Given the fact that not only the name of a plant but even its spelling are often important for its correct identification, the repetition of terms in the dictionary should not be attributed to the carelessness of its compiler, but rather to his conscientiousness. The compiler of the dictionary was collecting the Arabic terms from a written source where each of these ingredients was mentioned more than once. The spelling of each plant name was each time slightly different in his source text, not only because its prototype did not always use a consistent system for transcribing Arabic words into Greek, but also because the foreign words were later somewhat disfigured in the course of its manuscript tradition. The compiler of the dictionary was obviously using a later copy of this text, where a number of the Arabic terms were already disfigured.

So what was the written source from which the entries to our dictionary were collected? It must have been the Greek translation of an Arabic medical text, but which one? Internal evidence from the dictionary suggests the answer. The glossary includes some Arabic terms of Berber provenance, which were current in the western Arab world, including North Africa, Spain, and Arab Sicily. For example, the Arabic equivalent of the Greek 'καστόριον' ('castoreum') is given as 'φαίχισεν' from the Berber-Arabic *al-fāhisha*, and not as *jundubādastur*, which is the term current in the eastern Arab world. Assuming that the transliterated terms were found by the translator in the original, the author of the original must have been a native of the Arab west. In addition, the presence of Latin terms in the glossary (e.g. 'γλαδίολα· ἶρις' [Thomson 1955: 59] for Latin *gladiolus*; 'σανδαράχη: λέγεται λατινικὰ ωρουπουμεντου' [Thomson 1955: 329] for medieval Latin *orpimentum* from the classical Latin *auri pigmentum*, indicating the yellow sulphide of arsenic, the orpiment) implies that the translation was made in an environment where Latin was understood. The Greek translation must also have been a popular text in Byzantium, since the dictionary that rendered it more intelligible survives in as many as four manuscripts. Taking into consideration these facts, the answer to the riddle becomes obvious: the Arabic terms were collected from the immensely popular aforementioned Greek translation of the Arabic treatise *Zād al-musāfir wa-qūt al-ḥāḍir*, in Greek *Ephodia tou apodēmountos*, or *Provisions for the Traveller*,[105] whose author, Ibn al-Jazzār, was a doctor from Kairawan in North Africa. The Greek translation was made in southern Italy or Sicily by a certain Constantine of Reggio.[106] The simultaneous presence of Latin and Berbero-Arabic terms in this translation is understandable, given the trilingualism that was prevalent in Sicily and southern Italy after the gradual conquest of Sicily by the Arabs towards the end of the tenth century and the beginning of the eleventh, and the influence of the Arab west on the island's culture.

Further proof of the dictionary's provenance is furnished by examining its entries that equate unrelated terms in conjunction with the Greek text of the *Ephodia*.[107] The Greek translation usually gives the Greek and the Arabic term for a certain plant side by side, which means that, as a rule, the explanation of an Arabic term can be found in the next word, or in the next few words of the Greek text. It turns out that the entries of the dictionary that appear not to make sense are lifted word for word, or almost so, from the text, apparently because the compiler of the dictionary was expecting that the explanation for a word he did not understand would be found in the few words of the translation around the unknown term in the text he had in front of him. For example, the dictionary includes the entry: 'χάρμελ καὶ μῶλ καὶ ἀμμωνιακόν' (Thomson 1955: 405). Now the plant called in Arabic *ḥarmal abyaḍ* is indeed called in Greek *mōly*, but the plant called in Greek *ammōniakon* has nothing to do with *mōly*. The mystery is solved once we find towards the end of Book 1 of the *Ephodia* a recipe that includes these ingredients in the reverse order: 'καὶ ἀμμωνιακὸν καὶ μόλυ [*sic*] ὃ δὴ σαρακηνιστὶ χαρμέλ'.[108]

Further evidence that the *Lexikon tōn Sarakēnōn* is a collection of the Arabic terms transliterated into Greek contained in the Greek text of the *Ephodia* is the fact that the two texts were copied in the same volume in two of the three known manuscripts containing the glossary, Parisinus gr. 2287,

[105] The Greek text of the *Ephodia* remains unpublished and its considerable manuscript tradition, which comprises more than thirty manuscripts, remains largely unchartered. For the purposes of the present chapter, I rely on the text in Vindobonensis med. gr. 47. The Arabic text is somewhat more accessible. For facsimiles of two manuscripts, see Sezgin (1996). The text is also available in Suwaysī et al. (1999). Partial critical edition and English translation in ed. and transl. Bos (1997), Bos (2000), and Bos, Käs, and McVaugh (2022). The most detailed recent information on Greek translation of this text can be found in Bouras-Vallianatos (2021: 983–8).

[106] Cf. Bouras-Vallianatos (2021: 983, n. 113).

[107] See also the Introduction of the present volume by Bouras-Vallianatos, who discusses the marginal annotations of the earliest surviving witness of the *Ephodia* – that is, Vaticanus gr. 300.

[108] Vindobonensis med. gr. 47, f. 42v, lines 13–16. A similar example has been pointed out by Serikoff (1998: 103, no. 27). Serikoff realised that at least one entry of the dictionary had been lifted from the Greek *Ephodia* but did not use this information to solve the problem of the glossary's provenance.

and Vindobonensis med. gr. 47.[109] In a third manuscript, Parisinus gr. 2180, the *Lexikon tōn Sarakēnōn* appears without the *Ephodia*, on ff. 2r–4v, interjected in the midst of a recension of Dioscorides' herbal.[110] The *Lexikon tōn Sarakēnōn* is untitled and appears sandwiched between the introduction to Dioscorides' herbal and the presentation of the individual plants. A second herbal dictionary in the same manuscript, this time on ff. 86r–89r, includes some of the same botanical terms as the *Lexikon tōn Sarakēnōn*. However, some of the interpretations given for the same term are different in each of the two collections. For example, the lexicon at the beginning of the manuscript (f. 3v) gives 'ποτηροκλαυστια ἤτοι ὁ μίκον', while on f. 88r we read 'ποτηροκλάστρα, τα ἄνθη τῆς κουτζουνουδάδας'.[111] On the other hand, the two collections of words agree on 'πελίλητζ· τὸ δαμασώνιον'. This means that the foreign terms out of the *Ephodia* were collected by different botanists on at least three separate occasions: one for the *Lexikon tōn Sarakēnōn*, another one for whatever went into the second dictionary in Parisinus gr. 2180, and a third time for a collection of words titled 'Σαρακηνικὰ μεταγλωττισμένα ἐκ τῆς Εφοδίου [*sic*] βίβλου', which appears in Parisinus gr. 2286 (f. 54r).

Entries from the *Lexikon tōn Sarakēnōn* are also quoted by Du Cange in his *Glossarium ad scriptores mediae et infimae graecitatis*, first published in 1688.[112] In his list of sources for the entries of the *Glossarium*, Du Cange

109 This might also be the case with the remaining two, Parisinus gr. 2180, ff. 2r–4v and Parisinus gr. 2286, f. 54r, which do not appear to contain the *Ephodia* (or a significant portion thereof). The brief description of both manuscripts in Omont (1888: 210–11 and 229–30) does not indicate that either the *Lexikon* or the *Ephodia* are included in the manuscripts. The descriptions of Parisinus gr. 2180 and Parisinus gr. 2286 in Bourdeaux (1912: 14–16, 23–7) focus on the astrological contents of both manuscripts and omit their medical contents. For Parisinus gr. 2180, the more detailed description in https://pinakes.irht.cnrs.fr/notices/cote/51809 (accessed 28 January 2023) does not mention the *Ephodia* explicitly, although the various medical excerpts may prove to belong to the *Ephodia*. Parisinus gr. 2180 can be examined at https://gallica.bnf.fr/ark:/12148/btv1b52509195s/f1.image (accessed 28 January 2023). The dictionary of Arabic botanical terms appears on ff. 2r–4v, sandwiched between the introduction to Dioscorides' herbal and a non-alphabetical presentation of the individual plants, which are occasionally drawn next to the relevant entry. However, many blank spaces remain for illustrations of plants that were never executed. Ff. 2r–4v with the dictionary appear to have ended up as a result of a binding error. The first and second pages of Cleomedes (f. 45r–v) have interlinear annotations in Latin (usually translations of technical terms). Likewise, Parisinus gr. 2286, in its more detailed description in https://pinakes.irht.cnrs.fr/notices/cote/51916 (accessed 28 January 2023) and upon inspection in https://gallica.bnf.fr/ark:/12148/btv1b107229740/f8.image (accessed 28 January 2023), does not appear to contain the *Ephodia*, or any substantial portion thereof.

110 Coloured digital reproduction of the Parisinus gr. 2180 at https://gallica.bnf.fr/ark:/12148/btv1b52509195s/f15.item (accessed 28 January 2023).

111 This interpretation also occurs in the dictionary of Prodromenos, ed. Lundström (1903–4: 144, line 291).

112 Du Cange (1688: II.35) in the *Index Auctorum*.

included the following item: '*Glossae Graeco-Saracenicae*, ex cod. Reg. 3497 hoc titulo: Σαρακινικὰ μεταγλωττισμένα ἐκ τῆς Εφοδίου [*sic*] βίβλου. Ubi Εφοδίου βίβλος, est liber hoc lemmate scriptus à Constantino Asyncrito [*sic*] seu Asecretis, de quo suprà.'[113] The manuscript used by Du Cange for the entries from the *Lexikon tōn Sarakēnōn*, today Parisinus gr. 2286, is known to have been copied in the middle of the fourteenth century in Constantinople, at the monastery of Saint John Prodromos in Petra, by Neophytos Prodromenos, a well-known physician and intellectual.[114] Prodromenos compiled a dictionary of plants, but only one of the terms from the *Ephodia* that he copied out in Parisinus gr. 2286 also occurs in this dictionary ['ἀντζαρούτ· ἡ σαρκόκολλα' in ed. Lundström (1903–4: 134, line 46)].[115] The format of the word list in Parisinus gr. 2286 suggests a closed collection of words: the botanical terms are listed one next to the other, and the only marker to help the reader distinguish them is the red initial of each term to be interpreted. No room is left for additions. We will know more about each of these compilations of botanical and pharmaceutical vocabulary only when the *Ephodia* receives a critical edition.[116]

Once we realise the mechanism of compiling the Arabic-Greek herbal glossary in question, it is possible to understand how additions to it were made, and how other multilingual dictionaries came into being.[117] Scholars have observed that herbal glossaries in Byzantine and post-Byzantine manuscripts frequently give the impression of personal notes taken down ad hoc, as they are found in additional folia or empty pages of the codices.[118] The format of the manuscripts in which multilingual dictionaries survive suggests that they were also put together in a similar way, by enriching ad hoc a pre-existing list of words which was copied in the manuscript while leaving ample space around it for further additions over time, which means that they

113 '*Greek-Saracen glosses* from cod. Reg. 3497 by this title: "Saracen [words] transcribed from the book of the *Ephodia*," where the book of the *Ephodia* is the book in this lemma which was written by Constantine Asyncritus [*sic*] or Asecretis, on whom see above.'

114 For a discussion of this manuscript and detailed bibliography, see Touwaide (2006: 200–1). On the monastery's library, see Kakoulidi (1968).

115 Prodromenos' dictionary of plant names was published by Lundström (1903–4). For a reproduction of Parisinus gr. 2286, see https://gallica.bnf.fr/ark:/12148/btv1b107229740 (accessed 28 January 2023).

116 An edition was announced by Gerasimos Pentogalos decades ago but never materialised. See Ieraci Bio (2006). See also Miguet (2017).

117 Only some of the multilingual herbal dictionaries have been published. See Delatte (1930) and Delatte (1939 : 273–454). Unpublished ones can be found in Bononiensis 3632, ff. 364r–376r and Scorialensis gr. 284 (Y.III.14), ff. 103r–4r; it is no coincidence that the Escorial manuscript contains a collection of medical texts translated from Arabic into Greek containing Arabic terms transliterated in Greek characters, which the glossary clarifies.

118 Hunger (1978: II.272).

were compiled by collecting and explaining foreign terms from medical texts written in Greek (see, e.g. Figure 4.4, Bononiensis 3632, f. 375r). A further indication of this approach to the compilation of dictionaries is the fact that most of the terms explained in them are given not in the nominative but in the accusative case.[119] The reason is that these terms were collected from texts, where they were mentioned as ingredients for recipes and were the grammatical object of verbs such as 'λαβέ' ('take') and 'ἀνάμιξον' ('mix'). The need for dictionaries of Arabic and Persian medical terms transliterated and explained in Greek arose as the Byzantine translations from these languages became more numerous and gained wider popularity. A number of Byzantine medical translations from Arabic and Persian either give the oriental term transliterated and then explained into Greek, or give the oriental term alone.[120] The reason for this approach to translation was the pursuit of clarity and/or the lack of an exactly equivalent Greek term, though ignorance of the corresponding Greek word on the part of the translator cannot be excluded, either. However, in the southern Italian translation of Ibn al-Jazzār's *Zād al-musāfir* into Greek, from which is taken the terms of the Arabic-Greek glossary that we are focused on, it seems that the transliteration of the Arabic terms was given for two reasons: not only because it conveyed with more exactitude the name of the drug intended by the Arab author, but also because the translator himself and the readers he had in mind were familiar with the nomenclature of medical ingredients in Greek, Arabic, and Latin, possibly because they had to in order to be able to obtain them in the southern Italian and Sicilian markets.

The multilingualism of doctors in southern Italy at the end of the tenth and the beginning of the eleventh centuries, as well as the way it functioned in everyday medical practice, is reflected in Parisinus suppl. gr. 1297, a tenth-century manuscript that contains a collection of excerpts from medical texts and has long been recognised as a specimen of southern Italian book production.[121] On the margins of several folia Arabic botanical

[119] Delatte (1930: 62) also observed the frequency of this phenomenon in multilingual dictionaries (i.e. explaining a foreign term by giving its Greek equivalent not in the nominative but in the accusative case).

[120] For some remarks on the Byzantine translations of Persian medical works and some thoughts on the reasons for transcribing (instead of translating) Persian medical terms in these translations, see Kousis (1939).

[121] Reproduction of the manuscript is at https://gallica.bnf.fr/ark:/12148/btv1b110048189/f71.item (accessed 28 January 2023) on which the interested reader can check the paleographic claims made here. The present observations on Parisinus suppl. gr. 1297 repeat Mavroudi (2008: 331–3), a publication discussing the use of the Greek script in order to write the Arabic language as a broader phenomenon. In the intervening years I found out that many colleagues have difficulty accessing

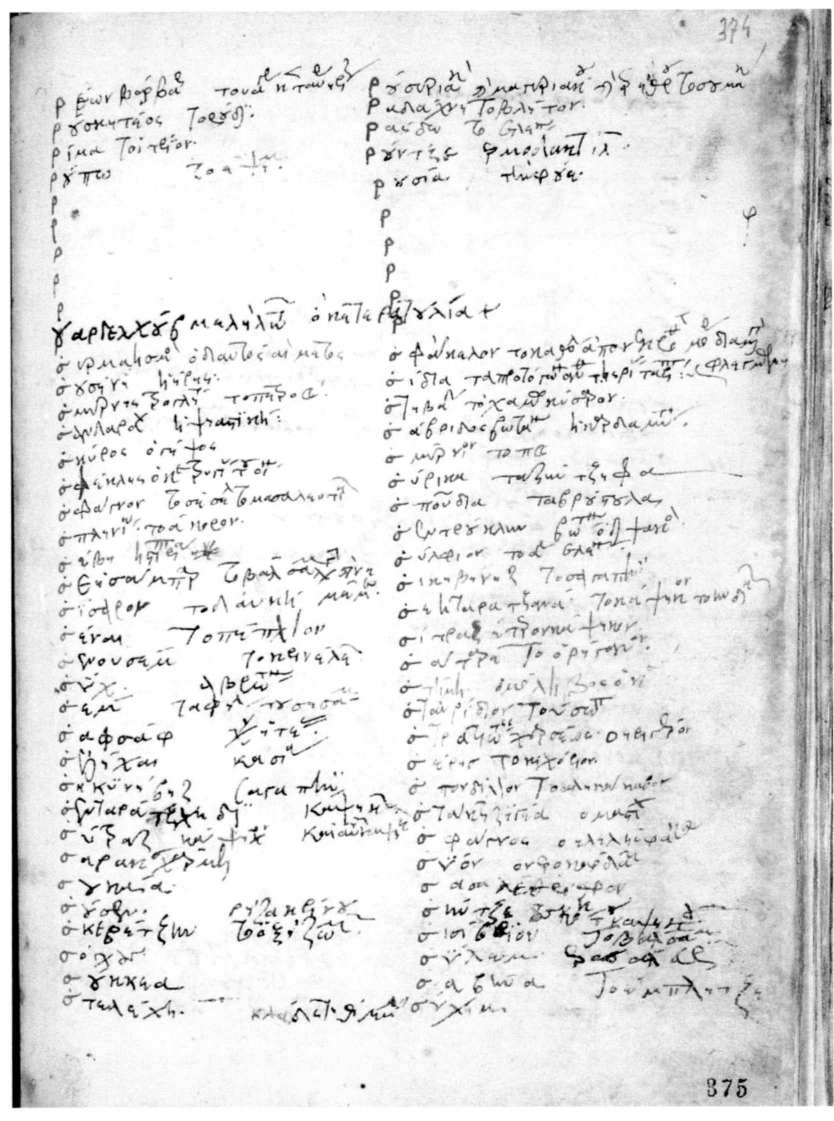

Figure 4.4 Bologna, Biblioteca Universitaria di Bologna, Alma Mater Studiorum MS 3632, f. 375r

and pharmaceutical terms are written in Arabic characters, giving the Arabic translation of Greek terms found on the same page (see Figure 4.5). In addition, a medical recipe in Arabic language is written in Greek characters on f. 121r (see Figure 4.6).[122]

The Arabic equivalents noted on the margins of the manuscript are written by an exercised hand. Occasionally the diacritical dots are omitted, which suggests a casual manner of writing.[123] The type of script presents a number of affinities with a known specimen of eleventh-century Sicilian Arabic handwriting.[124] In addition, some of the Arabic terms are those current in the west of the Arab world, which further suggests that they were written by a Sicilian or southern Italian.[125] They include several banal terms for foodstuffs, the cultivation of which is documented in the archives of southern Italy in the course of the tenth and eleventh centuries and which still constitute staples of a Mediterranean diet. Such terms include the following: التين /*al-tīn*/'figs' (f. 114r),[126] الفول/*al-fūl* /'beans' (f. 113r), العدس / *al-ʿadas* /'lentils' (f. 113r), الحمس /*al-ḥummus* /'chickpeas' (f. 113v)[127], الجوز / *al-jawz* /'walnuts' (f. 115r), and البندق /*al-bunduq* /'hazelnuts' (f. 115r).[128] This indicates that they were not written in order to help an Arabic speaker with insufficient knowledge of Greek to better understand the contents of the manuscript, since a Greek medical manuscript would have been useless to someone whose knowledge of Greek was so limited that his vocabulary

the volume in which it appeared. I deemed it practical to repeat the information here in order to make it more readily available and keep the present argument coherent.

122 Regarding this note M.-L. Concasty, in her description of Parisinus suppl. gr. 1297, remarks the following: 'Au bas du f. 121, formule de remède (?) en une langue non identifié avec certitude (arabe?), transcrite en caractères grecs (XIe s.)' ['At the bottom of f. 121, [there is a] sort of remedy (?) in a language not identified with certainty (Arabic?), transcribed in Greek characters (ninth c.)']. See Astruc and Concasty (1960: 564).

123 For example, in دقيق =ἀλεύρου=flour (f. 67v), الفول =beans (f. 113r), التين = οἱ θύνοι=tuna fish (f. 118v), and ترفاس =τὰ οἴδνα [sic for ὕδνα]=truffles (f. 116r).

124 The type of Arabic script employed presents certain characteristics that betray a kinship with western Arabic scripts, such as open ن, open loop of the س in final position, vertical stroke of the ط tilted toward the right side, and, in particular, representation of ق with only one diacritical dot above it, the way ف is usually written in eastern Arabic scripts. Cf., for example, السماف for السماق (='Rhus') on f. 68r; البندف for البندق and الفسطف for الفسطق on f. 115r.

125 For example, ترفاس 'truffle' (a word of Berber origin widely used in Maghribi Arabic) on f. 116r; جلجب instead of سمسم for 'sesame' (f. 113v).

126 For figs around Salerno, see Skinner (1997: 6, n. 14); for figs in Gaeta, see Skinner (1997: 9, n. 39); for figs in Reggio di Calabria, see Skinner (1997: 10, n. 44); for figs in Apulia, see Skinner (1997: 10, n. 45).

127 For pulses around Naples, see Skinner (1997: 8, n. 30); for red beans and pulse see (1997: 8, n. 32); around Amalfi the most frequently mentioned pulses are beans and chickpeas, according to Skinner (1997: 9, n. 35).

128 For nuts in Campania, see Skinner (1997: 9. n. 42); around Naples, see Skinner (1997: 8, n. 28); for hazelnuts in Salerno, see Skinner (1997: 6); and around Naples, see Skinner (1997: 8, n. 31).

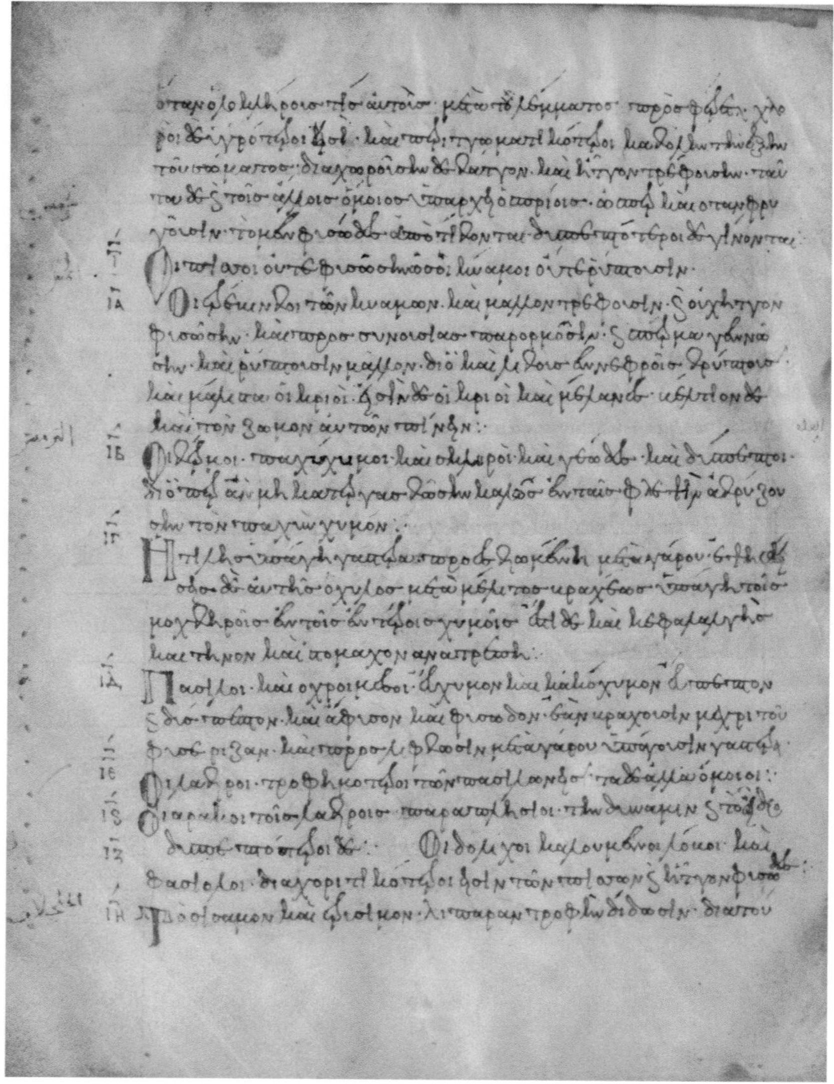

Figure 4.5 Paris, Bibliothèque nationale, MS suppl. gr. 1297, f. 113v

did not include such banal items. In several instances only the ductus of a word is written, while the diacritical dots are omitted, as, for example, in دقيق = 'ἀλεύρου' /'flour' (f. 67v), الفول =beans (f. 113r), التين = 'οἱ θύνοι'/ 'tuna fish' (f. 118v), and ترفاس = 'τὰ οἴδνα' [sic for 'ὕδνα']/'truffles' (f. 116r). The omission

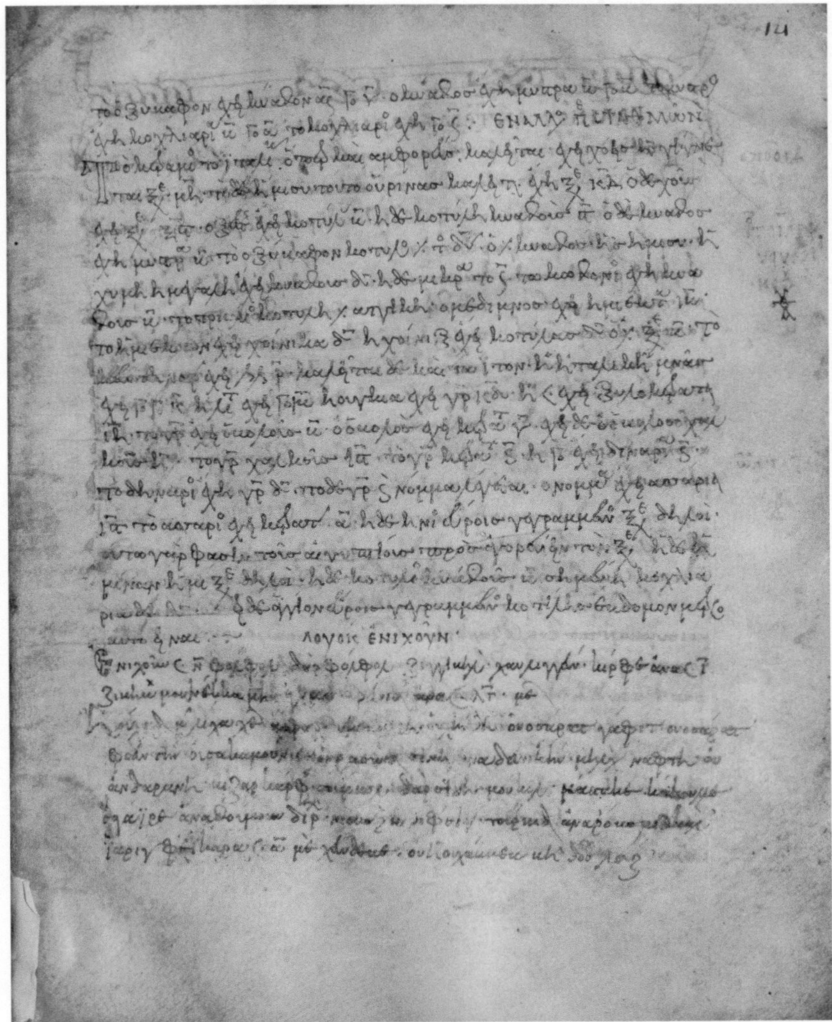

Figure 4.6 Paris, Bibliothèque nationale, MS suppl. gr. 1297, f. 121r

of the diacritical dots seems to indicate a casual attitude towards writing, as is sometimes the case in Arabic papyri, which are documents generally meant for limited private use. The kind of terms included for translation in the marginal Arabic notes, as well as the casual manner of their writing, suggests that their scribe was somebody fully fluent in both Greek and Arabic. But if the scribe is completely fluent in both languages, what was the purpose of writing these words on the margins of the manuscript? The Arabic equivalents are hardly legible on some pages. Parts thereof were cropped during subsequent bindings, as is evident in the cases where only part of a word survives while the letters at the very edge of a page are missing. But they also seem to have been erased by usage, presumably by fingers touching the edges of the pages. It is therefore certain that the number of Arabic equivalents noted on the margins of Parisinus suppl. gr. 1297 was originally greater than what is visible today and was intended not as crutches to an Arabic speaker who was not thoroughly familiar with Greek terminology but as an aid for quick reference, in other words in order to quickly locate a passage while leafing through the manuscript, an aid very much needed in view of the fact that the medical excerpts contained in the manuscript were written without any particular order. Several are concentrated on the margins of text explaining the properties of food; quick reference to such a text could help a doctor decide faster what diet to prescribe for a patient suffering from a particular kind of ailment.

The marginal notes were added at around the same time and in the same milieu as the recipe on f. 121r, which is written in the Arabic language, but in Greek characters.[129] A close comparison of the writing in the prescription with the writing in the rest of the manuscript indicates that the prescription must have been written in the same milieu and at around the same time as the main text, and at any rate no later than the first half of the eleventh century.[130] The prescription is written casually, not in classical Arabic, but in the Arabic dialect of Sicily. The scribe of the prescription used scribal conventions of both Greek and Arabic medical writings in order to convey dosage. Whole numbers (such as fifty='Ν', ten='Ι', thirty-three='ΛΓ', and one='α') are written using the letters of the Greek alphabet with a horizontal stroke above them, which indicates that they should be understood in their numerical value, according to the convention used in Greek manuscripts; these numbers are accompanied by the Greek (and Latin)

[129] The transcription and translation of the Arabic recipe written in Greek characters can be found in Mavroudi (2008: 334–5).

[130] Concasty (1953: 24) already commented on the particularity of certain letters in the main text, such as 'η' in the form of 'h' and 'ζ'. These letters appear in the same form in the Arabic note in Greek characters on f. 121r. The forms of additional letters and especially 'φ' and 'δ', the use of tremmas above 'ι' in initial position, as well as in order to separate diphthongs, the use of the same abbreviations for '-ιν', '-ις', all indicate a closeness to the principal hand. The abbreviation for 'drachma' is different (angular in the rest of the manuscript, rounded in the note), and the two abbreviations after 'χε' and 'με' in the note do not appear anywhere else in the manuscript.

abbreviation for 'drachma', in this case indicating a measure of weight which gave its name to the Arabic *dirham*. On the other hand, fractional numbers and their accompanying measures of weight are written out in full in Arabic: 'θούμουν διρχ(αμ)' ('an eighth of a *dirham*'); 'ρόβο μιθκὰλ' ('a fourth of a *mithqāl*'). In one case, writing the whole number 'two' is omitted; instead, dosage is conveyed by the grammatical form of the word for the measure of weight, which is in the dual: 'δενικὴν' ('two *daniqs*'). This practice for conveying numbers is current in Arabic medical manuscripts. Both methods of writing down numbers were simultaneously used, possibly in order to avoid confusion between whole and fractional numbers. The analogies for the ingredients are prescribed with a convention of Greek medical writings, by using the Greek preposition 'ἀνὰ' in the midst of Arabic phrases. Such a mixture of pharmacological formulae from different languages is not unparalleled, at least not in the medical writings of southern Italy. A similar use of the Greek preposition 'ἀνὰ' in the midst of Latin phrases can be found in the collection of medical prescriptions known as the *Antidotarium Nicolai*, written before the twelfth century.[131]

As the evidence of Parisinus suppl. gr. 1297 suggests, the Greek translation of the *Ephodia* was prepared in and for a trilingual environment where familiarity with medical terms in Greek, Arabic, and Latin was widespread in the medical profession and the inclusion of transliterated terms from the Arabic in a translated text added to its clarity and ease of usage. The compilation of a dictionary to include those terms became necessary once the translation gained wider popularity and circulation among readers who could scarcely, if at all, understand Arabic and Latin, yet inhabited a world in which such terms had great currency and were in the process of being naturalised as Greek medical terms.

4.5 Conclusion

The modern study of Byzantine science has cast it in two auxiliary roles: as a preserver of ancient Greek science (this is the most frequently encountered understanding of it) and as an intermediary between Islamicate and Western

[131] See the text in Lebede (1939: 37–68). The *Antidotarium* also uses the Greek preposition *dia*. See the comments in Lebede (1939: xii). The date of the *Antidotarium* is uncertain. Commentaries to it were written in the course of the twelfth century, on which, see Pasca (1994: 480). The use of *ana* seems to have become so standard in Latin medical writings that Valerius Cordus, who collected in his *Dispensatorium* (printed for the first time in 1546) much earlier medical prescriptions such as those by Nicolas of Salerno, al-Rāzī, and Ibn Sīnā (translated into Latin), did not rephrase them in order to remove it.

science (an idea with more limited circulation, but nonetheless one that has been around at least since the nineteenth century).[132] Both views are rooted in a narrative on the history of science that, in its basic form, was put together during the sixteenth century for reasons inherent to the political, social, and intellectual conditions of the time.[133] This narrative was inherited, further elaborated, and disseminated in the course of the nineteenth and early twentieth centuries in works that are still referenced in the study of the history of science. It views 'classical' Greek and 'classical' Arabic science as contributors to Western modernity and is animated by considerations attuned to the colonial environment in which it was articulated.[134]

The present contribution focused on a limited amount of botanical material in order to show that, in many respects, Byzantine science was no 'better' or 'worse' than its ancient Greek and medieval Arabic equivalents. The three shared goals, methods of research, and ways of dissemination. Presenting Byzantine science under such a light implies that the modern understanding of science as an intellectual good that is passed over as a torch from one civilisation to the next (from the ancient Near East to Graeco-Roman antiquity to the medieval Islamicate world and early modern Europe) needs to be revisited. It also leaves little room for cultural triumphalism of either the 'Western' or the 'Eastern' variety.

REFERENCES

Argyropoulos, R., and Karras, I. 1980. *Inventaire des manuscrits grecs d'Aristote et de ses commentateurs: Contribution à l'histoire du texte d'Aristote: supplément*. Paris: Les Belles Lettres.

Astruc, C., and Concasty, M.-L. 1960. *Le supplément grec: Catalogue des manuscrits grecs*, vol. III. Paris: Bibliothèque Nationale de France.

Athanassiadi, P. ed. 1999. *Damascius: The Philosophical History*. Athens: Apamea Cultural Association.

Azaizeh, H., Fulder, S., Khalil, K., and Said, O. 2003. 'Ethnobotanical Knowledge of Local Arab Practitioners in the Middle Eastern Region', *Fitoterapia* 74 (1–2): 98–108. https://doi.org/10.1016/s0367-326x(02)00285-x (accessed 28 January 2023).

[132] On Byzantine science, especially astronomy, as an intermediary between Islamicate and Western science in the early modern period, see Mavroudi (2015: 54–5). Johan Ludvig Heiberg (1854–1928), who became well acquainted with Byzantine astronomical manuscripts in the course of his editorial work on the ancient Greek mathematical sciences, was the first to draw attention to the translations of Islamicate astronomical texts into Greek during the Palaiologan period. Heiberg's research on astronomy was taken on board by Krumbacher (1897: 621–4). On Krumbacher's importance for Sarton's *Introduction to the History of Science* and how it influenced further investigation into the history of fourteenth-century Byzantine astronomy, see Mavroudi (2016: 245–6, 262–6).

[133] On the early modern debate on the importance of Greek versus Arabic science, see Hasse (2016).

[134] For a detailed discussion of this narrative and bibliography, see Mavroudi (2015).

Barton, T. 1994. *Power and Knowledge: Astrology, Physiognomics, and Medicine under the Roman Empire*. Ann Arbor: University of Michigan Press.

Baytop, T. 1984. *Türkiyede bitkiler ile tedavi: geçmişte ve bugün*. Istanbul: İstanbul Üniversitesi.

Beck, R. 2002. 'Zoroaster As Perceived by the Greeks', *Encyclopaedia Iranica*. www.iranicaonline.org/articles/zoroaster-iv-as-perceived-by-the-greeks (accessed 28 January 2023).

Bergsträsser, G. ed. 1925. *Ḥunain ibn Isḥāq: Über die syrischen und arabischen Galen-Übersetzungen*. Leipzig: F. A. Brockhaus.

Bhayro, S., and Hawley, R. 2014. 'La littérature botanique et pharmaceutique en langue syriaque', in É. Villey (ed.), *Les sciences en syriaque*. Paris: Geuthner, 285–318.

Bhayro, S., Hawley, R., Kessel, G., and Pormann, P. E. 2013. 'The Syriac Galen Palimpsest: Progress, Prospects and Problems', *Journal of Semitic Studies* 58.1: 131–48.

Bos, G. ed. and trans. 1997. *Ibn al-Jazzār on Sexual Diseases and Their Treatment: A Critical Edition, English Translation and Introduction of Book 6 of Zād al-musāfir wa-qut al-ḥāḍir (Provisions for the Traveler and the Nourishment of the Sedentary)*. New York: Kegan Paul International.

Bos, G. ed. and trans. 2000. *Ibn al-Jazzār on Fevers: A Critical Edition of Zād al-musāfir wa-qut al-ͺādir, Provisions for the Traveler and Nourishment for the Sedentary, Bk. 7, chs. 1–6*. New York: Kegan Paul International.

Bos, G., Käs, F., and McVaugh, M. R. eds. and trans. 2022. *Ibn al-Jazzār's Zād al-musāfir wa-qūt al-ḥāḍir. Provisions for the Traveller and Nourishment for the Sedentary. Books I and II: Diseases of the Head and the Face*. Leiden: Brill.

Bostoc, J. trans. 1855. *Pliny the Elder:* Natural History. London: Taylor and Francis. www.perseus.tufts.edu/hopper/text?doc=Perseus:text:1999.02.0137 (accessed 28 January 2023).

Bouras-Vallianatos, P. 2013. 'Simon of Genoa's *Clavis sanationis:* A Study of Thirteenth-Century Latin Pharmacological Lexicography', in B. Zipser (ed.), *Simon of Genoa's Medical Lexicon*. Berlin: de Gruyter, 31–48.

Bouras-Vallianatos, P. 2019. 'Rezension zu: Alain Touwaide. A Census of Greek Medical Manuscripts from Byzantium to the Renaissance. London: Routledge, 2016 (Medicine in the Medieval Mediterranean 6)', *Plekos* 21: 153–76. www.plekos.uni-muenchen.de/2019/r-touwaide.pdf (accessed 28 January 2023).

Bouras-Vallianatos, P. 2020. *Innovation in Byzantine Medicine: The Writings of John Zacharias Aktouarios (c. 1275–c. 1330)*. Oxford: Oxford University Press.

Bouras-Vallianatos, P. 2021. 'Cross-Cultural Transfer of Medical Knowledge in the Medieval Mediterranean: The Introduction and Dissemination of Sugar-Based Potions from the Islamic World to Byzantium', *Speculum* 96.4: 963–1008.

Bourdeaux, P. 1912. *Catalogus Codicum Astrologorum Graecorum*, vol. VIII.3. Brussels: H. Lamertin.

Carruthers, M. 2008. *The Book of Memory: A Study of Memory in Medieval Culture*. Cambridge: Cambridge University Press.

Cavallo, G. 1977. 'Funzione e strutture della maiuscola greca tra i secoli VIII–XI', in J. Glénisson, J. Bompaire, and J. Irigoin (eds.), *La paléographie grecque et byzantine. Colloques internationaux du Centre National de la Recherche Scientifique, no. 559 (Paris 1974)*. Paris: Éditions du CNRS, 95–137.

Christodoulou, G. A. 1986. "Ὁ Ἀθωνικὸς κώδ. Μεγ. Λαύρας Ω 75 τοῦ Διοσκορίδη. Παλαιογραφικὴ ἐπισκόπηση', in G. A. Christodoulou, *Σύμμικτα Κριτικά*. Athens: G. A. Christodoulou, 131–99.

Chrysostomos of Lavra, Bishop of Rodostolou. 2000. *Γράμματα καὶ ἅρματα στὸν Ἄθωνα*. Mount Athos: n.p.

Clark, P. 2002. 'Landscape, Memories, and Medicine: Traditional Healing in Amari, Crete', *Journal of Modern Greek Studies* 20: 339–65.

Concasty, M.-L. 1953. 'Manuscrits grecs originaires de l' Italie méridionale conservés à Paris', in *Atti dell' VIII Congresso internazionale di studi bizantini Palermo, 3-10 aprile 1951*, vol. I. Rome: Associazione nazionale per gli studi bizantini, 22–34.

Cronier, M. 2006. 'Quelques aspects de l'histoire du texte du *De materia medica* de Dioscoride: forme originelle, remaniements et revisions à Constantinople aux Xe-XIe siècles', in V. Boudon-Millot, A. Garzya, J. Jouanna, and A. Roselli (eds.), *Ecdotica e ricezione dei testi medici greci: Atti del V Convegno internazionale, Napoli, 1–2 ottobre 2004*. Naples: D'Auria, 43–65.

Cronier, M. 2015. 'The Manuscript Tradition of Dioscorides' *De Materia Medica* from Byzantium to the Arabs', in B. Pitarakis (ed.), *Life Is Short, Art Long: The Art of Healing in Byzantium*. Istanbul: Pera Museum, 34–151.

Cronier, M. 2016. 'Transcrire l'arabe en grec. À propos des annotations du *Parisinus Gr.* 2179 (Dioscoride)', in A. Boud'hors, A. Binggeli, and M. Cassin (eds.), *Manuscripta graeca et orientalia: Mélanges monastiques et patristiques en l'honneur de Paul Géhin*. Leuven: Peeters, 247–65.

Dain, A. 1964. *Les manuscrits*. 2nd edition. Paris: Les Belles Lettres.

Degni, P. 2012. 'Trascrivere la medicina a Bisanzio: Considerazioni sulle caratteristiche grafiche e materiali della produzione libraria', in G. de Gregoria and M. Galante (eds.), *La produzione scritta tecnica e scientifica nel medioevo: Libro e documento tra scuole e professioni. Atti del Covegno di studio*. Spoleto: Fondazione Centro Italiano di studi sull'alto Medioevo, 359–88.

Delatte, A. 1930. 'Le lexique de botanique du Parisinus graecus 2419', *Serta Leodensia: Bibliothèque de la faculté de philosophie et lettres de l'université de Liège* 44: 59–101.

Delatte, A. 1939. 'Glossaires de botanique', in A. Delatte, *Anecdota Atheniensia et alia*, vol. II. Liège: Faculté de Philosophie et Lettres and Paris: E. Droz, 273–454.

Deroche, F. 2014. *Qur'ans of the Umayyads: A First Overview*. Leiden: Brill.

Diels, H. 1905–6. *Die Handschriften der antiken Ärzte*. 2 vols. Berlin [*Abhandlungen der Königlich-Preussischen Akademie der Wissenschaften* 1905, *Phil.-Hist. Kl.* 3 and 1906, *Phil.-Hist. Kl.* 1].

Dietrich. A. 2012. 'Ibn al-Rūmiyya', in P. Bearman, Th. Bianquis, C. E. Bosworth, E. van Donzel, and W. P. Heinrichs (eds.), *Encyclopaedia of Islam*. 2nd edition. Leiden: E. J. Brill. http://dx.doi.org.libproxy.berkeley.edu/10.1163/1573-3912_islam_SIM_8670 (accessed 28 January 2023).

Dobrynina, E. 2010. 'Some Observations on 9th- and 10th-Century Greek Illuminated Manuscripts in Russian Collections', in A. Bravo García and I. Pérez-Martín (eds.), *The Legacy of Bernard de Montfaucon: Three Hundred Years of Studies on Greek Handwriting. Proceedings of the Seventh International Colloquium of Greek Palaeography, ed. A. Martín (Madrid-Salamanca, 15–20 September 2008)*. Turnhout: Brepols, 45–53.

Du Cange, C. 1688. *Glossarium ad scriptores mediae et infimae Graecitatis*. 2 vols. Lyon: Anisson; Posuel; Rigaud.

Fakchich, J., and Elachouri, M. 2014. 'Ethnobotanical Survey of Medicinal Plants Used by People in Oriental Morocco to Manage Various Ailments', *Journal of Ethnopharmacology* 154(1): 76–87. https://doi.org/10.1016/j.jep.2014.03.016 (accessed 28 January 2023).

Fedeli, A. 2018. 'Collective Enthusiasm and the Cautious Scholar: The Birmingham Qur'ān', *Marginalia: Los Angeles Review of Books* (3 August 3). https://marginalia.lareviewofbooks.org/collective-enthusiasm (accessed 28 January 2023).

Formentin, M. R. 2005. 'Il *Marc. gr.* 273: Stratificazione di scritture, lingue, testi', in F. Crevatin and G. Tedeschi (eds.), *Scrivere Leggere Interpretare: Studi di antichità in onore di Sergio Daris*. Trieste: EUT Edizioni Università di Trieste, 209–16.

Glynias, J. (2022). 'Baghdad on the Orontes: Between Greek and Arabic Intellectual Worlds in 11th-Century Antioch'. PhD thesis, Princeton University. http://arks.princeton.edu/ark:/88435/dsp01jw827f87j (accessed 28 January 2023).

Hasse, D. N. 2016. *Success and Suppression: Arabic Sciences and Philosophy in the Renaissance*. Cambridge, MA: Harvard University Press.

Heiberg, J. L. 1919. 'De codicibus Pauli Aeginitae observationes', *Revue des études grecques* 32: 268–77.

Hill, A. 1937. 'Introduction', in W. B. Turrill, 'A Contribution to the Botany of Athos Peninsula', *Bulletin of Miscellaneous Information, Royal Botanic Gardens, Kew* 4: 197–273.

Hunger, H. 1978. *Die hochsprachliche profane Literatur der Byzantiner*. 2 vols. Munich: C. H. Beck.

Hunger, H., Gamillscheg, E., and Harlfinger, D. eds. 1981–97. *Repertorium der griechischen Kopisten 800–1600*. 3 vols. in 9 pts. Vienna: Verlag der Österreichischen Akademie der Wissenschaften. [Cited with volume no. followed by catalogue no., e.g. RGK II 120] (RGK).

Hunger, H., and Kresten, P. 1969. *Katalog der griechischen Handscrhiften der Österreichischen Nationalbibliothek*, vol. II. Vienna: Akademie der Wissenschaften.

Ieraci Bio, A. M. 2006. 'La medicina greca dello Stretto (Filippo Xeros ed Eufemio Siculo)', in F. Burgarella and A. M. Ieraci Bio (eds.), *La cultura scientifica e technical nell'Italia meridionale bizantina*. Soveria Mannelli: Rubbettino, 109–24.

Kakoulidi, E. 1968. "Η βιβλιοθήκη τῆς μονῆς Προδρόμου Πέτρας στὴν Κωνσταντινούπολη', *Ἑλληνικά* 21.1: 3–39.

Koraes, A. 1835. *Ἄτακτα*, vol. V (μέρος πρῶτον, ἀλφάβητον τρίτον). Paris.

Kosmas, K. 2016. 'Ευλόγιος Κουρίλας, Μητροπολίτης Κορυτσάς: εθνική και εκπαιδευτική δράση.' MA thesis: Aristotle University of Thessaloniki.
Kourilas, E. 1935a. *Ἀναγραφή συγγραφῶν καὶ ἐπιστημονικῶν διατριβῶν, 1909–1935*. Athens: Typographeio Vrasdia Chalkiopoulou.
Kourilas, E. 1935b. *Διοσκορίδειοι μελέται καὶ ὁ Λαυριωτικός κῶδιξ. Μελέτη κριτική καὶ ἱστορική*. Athens: I. K. Aleuropoulos.
Kourilas, E. 1954. *Ὁ Διοσκορίδης τοῦ Wellmann καὶ ὁ Λαυριωτικὸς Κῶδιξ. Μελέτη κριτική μετ' ἀνεκδότων κειμένων. Ἐπίμετρον περὶ τῶν βοτανικῶν μελετῶν και τῶν ἀνεκδότων ἔργων μου δύο ὑπομνήματα*. Alexandria: Imprimerie du commerce.
Kousis, A. 1939. 'Quelques considérations sur les traductions en grec des oeuvres médicales orientales et principalement sur les deux manuscrits de la traduction d'un traité persan par Constantin Melitiniotis', *Πρακτικὰ Ἀκαδημίας Ἀθηνῶν* 14: 205–20.
Krumbacher, K. 1897. *Geschichte der byzantinischen Literatur: Von Justinian bis zum Ende des oströmischen Reiches, 527–1453*. Munich: Beck.
Langkavel, B. A. 1866. *Botanik der späteren griechen*. Berlin: Von F. Berggold.
Langslow, D. R. 2000. *Medical Latin in the Roman Empire*. Oxford: Oxford University Press.
Lebede, K.-H. 1939. *Das Antidotarium des Nicolaus von Salerno und sein Einfluß auf die Entwicklung des deutschen Arzneiwesens: Text und Kommentar von zwei Handschriften der Berliner Staatsbibliothek*. Inaugural-Dissertation: Mathematisch-naturwissenschaftlichen Fakultät der Friedrich-Wilhelms-Universität zu Berlin.
Leeuwen, R. van, and Vrolijk, A. 2013. *Arabic Studies in the Netherlands: A Short History in Portraits, 1580–1950*. Leiden: Brill.
Lherminier, G. 2016. 'Manuscrits de Paul d'Egine à la Bibliothèque nationale de France', *Bulletin du bibliophile* 2016.2: 229–73.
Loch, S. 195–?. *Athos, the Holy Mountain*. New York: Thomas Nelson and Sons.
Lundström, V. 1903–4. 'Neophytos *Prodromenos'* botaniska namnförteckning', *Eranos* 5: 129–55.
Magdalino, P. 2006. *L'orthodoxie des astrologues: La science entre le dogme et la divination à Byzance (VIIe–XIVe siècle)*. Paris: Lethielleux.
Mathiesen, T. 1988. *Ancient Greek Music Theory: A Catalogue Raisonné of Manuscripts*. Munich: G. Henle.
Mavroudi, M. 2002. *A Byzantine Book on Dream Interpretation: The Oneirocriticon of Achmet and Its Arabic Sources*. Leiden: Brill.
Mavroudi, M. 2007. 'Late Byzantium and Exchange with Arabic Writers', in S. T. Brooks (ed.), *Byzantium, Faith and Power (1261–1557): Perspectives on Late Byzantine Art and Culture*. The Metropolitan Museum of Art Symposia. New Haven, CT: Yale University Press, 62–75.
Mavroudi, M. 2008. 'Arabic Words in Greek Letters: The Violet Fragment and More', in J. Grand'Henry and J. Lentin (eds.), *Proceedings of the First International Symposium on Middle Arabic and Mixed Arabic Throughout History, Louvain-la-Neuve 11–14 May 2004*. Leuven: Peeters, 321–54.

Mavroudi, M. 2012. 'The Naples Dioscorides', in H. Evans with B. Ratliff (eds.) *Byzantium and Islam: Age of Transition (7th–9th Centuries): Catalogue of the Exhibition at the Metropolitan Museum of Art*. New Haven, CT: Yale University Press, 22–6.

Mavroudi, M. 2014. 'Greek Language and Education under Early Islam', in B. Sadeghi, A. Q. Ahmed, R. Hoyland, and A. Silverstein (eds.), *Islamic Cultures, Islamic Contexts: Essays in Honor of Professor Patricia Crone*. Leiden: Brill, 295–342.

Mavroudi, M. 2015. 'Translations from Greek into Arabic and Latin during the Middle Ages: Searching for the Classical Tradition', *Speculum* 90.1, 28–59.

Mavroudi, M. 2016. 'Scholars and Intellectuals in the Work of Ihor Ševčenko', *Palaeoslavica* 24.1: 245–80.

Mavroudi, M. (2023, forthcoming). 'The Byzantine Reception of Ptolemy's *Almagest* between the Seventh and the Ninth Centuries', in A. Bowen and E. Gannagé (eds.), *'In Praise of the Divine Beauty': The Philosophy of Ptolemy and Its Greek, Arabic, and Hebrew Reception*. Leiden: Brill.

Miguet, T. 2017. 'Premiers jalons pour une étude complète de l'histoire du texte grec du Viatique du Voyageur ('Εφόδια τοῦ ἀποδημοῦντος) d'Ibn al-Ǧazzār', *Revue d'Histoire des Textes* 12: 59–105.

Mondrain, B. 2012. 'La lecture et la copie de textes scientifiques à Byzance pendant l'époque paléologue', in G. de Gregoria and M. Galante (eds.), *La produzione scritta tecnica e scientifica nel medioevo: Libro e documento tra scuole e professioni. Atti del Covegno di studio*. Spoleto: Fondazione Centro Italiano di studi sull'alto Medioevo, 607–32.

Müller, A. ed. 1882–4. Muwaffaq al-Dīn Aḥmad ibn al-Qāsim ibn Abī Uṣaybiʿah: *ʿUyūn al-anbāʾ fī ṭabaqāt al-aṭibbāʾ*. 2 vols. Cairo: al-Maṭbaʿah al-Wahbiyyah.

Ogilvie, B. 2003. 'Review of Jerry Stannard', in K. E. Stannard and R. Kay (eds.), *Pristina Medicamenta: Ancient and Medieval Medical Botany*. Variorum Collected Studies Series. Brookfield, VT: Ashgate. 1999 and Jerry Stannard. *Herbs and Herbalism in the Middle Ages and Renaissance*. Edited by Katherine E. Stannard and Richard Kay. (Variorum Collected Studies Series.) Brookfield, VT: Ashgate, 1999, *Isis* 94.2: 362–4.

Ogilvie, B. 2006. *The Science of Describing: Natural History in Renaissance Europe*. Chicago, IL: University of Chicago Press.

Omont, H. 1888. *Inventaire sommaire des manuscrits grecs de la Bibliothèque Nationale*. Paris: A. Picard.

Panagiotopoulos, I. M. [n.d.]. *Τὸ περιβόλι τῆς Παναγίας. Ἁγιορειτικὰ καὶ ἄλλα ὁδοιπορικά*. Athens: Akritas.

Parpulov, G. 2015. 'The Codicology of Ninth-Century Greek Manuscripts', *Semitica et Classica* 8: 165–70.

Pasca, M. 1994. 'The Salerno School of Medicine', *American Journal of Nephrology* 14 (4–6): 478–82. https://doi.org/10.1159/000168770 (accessed 28 January 2023).

Pavlos [Pavlides], Monk of Lavra. 1963. *Αὐτοβιογραφίας δευτέρα μεσαία ἐπιτομή*. Mount Athos: n.p.

Pietrobelli, A., and Cronier, M. 2022. 'Arabic Galenism from Antioch to Byzantium: Ibn Buṭlān and Symeon Seth', *Mediterranea: International Journal on the Transfer of Knowledge* 7: 281–315.

Pormann, P. 2011. 'The Formation of Arabic Pharmacology between Tradition and Innovation', *Annals of Science* 68.4: 493–515.

Rémond, X. 1992. *Byzance: L'art byzantin dans les collections publiques françaises. Musée du Louvre, 3 novembre 1992–1er février 1993*. Paris: Réunion des musées nationaux.

Rogers, M. 2007. 'Text and Illustrations: Dioscorides and the Illustrated Herbal in the Arab Tradition', in A. Contadini (ed.), *Arab Painting: Text and Image in Illustrated Arabic Manuscripts*. Leiden: Brill, 41–7.

Roisse, P. 2004. 'La circulation du savoir des Arabes chrétiens en Méditerranée médiévale (sources manuscrites)', *Collectanea Christiana Orientalia* 1: 185–232.

Sadek, M. M. 1983. *The Arabic Materia Medica of Dioscorides*. Québec: Éditions du Sphinx.

Savage-Smith, E., Swain, S., and van Gelder, G. J. eds. 2020. *A Literary History of Medicine: The ʿUyūn al-anbāʾ fī ṭabaqāt al-aṭibbāʾ of Ibn Abī Uṣaybiʿah*. 5 vols. Leiden: Brill. https://scholarlyeditions.brill.com/reader/urn:cts:arabicLit:0668IbnAbiUsaibia.Tabaqatalatibba.lhom-ed-ara1:10.64; https://scholarlyeditions.brill.com/reader/urn:cts:arabicLit:0668IbnAbiUsaibia.Tabaqatalatibba.lhom-tr-eng1:10.64 (accessed 28 January 2023).

Scurlock, J. 2005. 'Ancient Mesopotamian Medicine', in D. C. Snell (ed.), *A Companion to the Ancient Near East*. Malden, MA: Blackwell, 302–15.

Serikoff, N. I. [=Serikov, N. I.]. 1988. 'Saracinskij Leksikon: ΦΑΚΥΝΟΝ i ΓΥΖΟΙ ΕΛΑΙΟΥ (O slovah-prizrakah v vizantijskom farmacevtiesçkom glossarii XV. v. i ih roli v izvçenii arabo-vizantijskih kontaktov v srednie veka) ['Saracen dictionary: ΦΑΚΥΝΟΝ and ΓΥΖΟΙ ΕΛΑΙΟΥ. Phantom Words in a Byzantine Pharmacological Glossary of the 15th Century and Its Role in the Study of Arabic-Byzantine Contact in the Middle Ages]', *Vizantijskij Vremmenik* 58: 84–103.

Serikoff, N. I. 2013. '"Syriac" Plant Names in a Fifteenth Century Greek Glossary', in B. Zipser (ed.), *Medical Books in the Byzantine World*. Bologna: Eikasmos, 97–121.

Sezgin, F. ed. 1996. *Ibn al-Jazzār, Zād al-musāfir wa-qut al-ḥāḍir*. 2 vols. Frankfurt: Center for the Study of Arabic and Islamic Sciences at the University of Frankfurt.

Skinner, P. 1997. *Health and Medicine in Early Medieval Southern Italy*. Leiden: Brill.

Stannard, J. 1961. 'Hippocratic Pharmacology', *Bulletin of the History of Medicine* 35.6: 497–518.

Stannard, J. 1965. 'Pliny and Roman Botany', *Isis* 56(186): 420–5.

Stannard, J. 1971. 'Byzantine Botanical Lexicography', *Episteme* 5: 168–87.

Suwaysī, M. et al. eds. 1999. *Zād al-musāfir wa-qūt al-ḥāḍir*. 2 vols. Tunis: al-Majmaʿ al-Tūnisī lil-ʿUlūm wa-l-Ādāb wa-l-Funūn, Bayt al-Ḥikmah.

Tester, J. 1987. *A History of Western Astrology*. Woodbridge: Suffolk.

Thomas, J. J. 2019. 'The Illustrated Dioskourides Codices and the Transmission of Images during Antiquity', *Journal of Roman Studies* 109: 241–73.

Thomson, M. H. ed. 1955. *Textes grecs inédits relatifs aux plantes*. Paris: Les Belles Lettres.

Totelin, L. 2009. *Hippocratic Recipes: Oral and Written Transmission of Pharmacological Knowledge in Fifth- and Fourth-Century Greece*. Leiden: Brill.

Touwaide, A. 1991a. 'The *Corpus of Greek Medical Manuscripts*: A Computerized Inventory and Catalogue', *Primary Sources & Original Works* 1: 75–92. [Reproduced: Touwaide, A. 1992. 'The *Corpus of Greek Medical Manuscripts*: A Computerized Inventory and Catalogue', in W. M. Stevens (ed.), *Bibliographic Access to Medieval and Renaissance Manuscripts: A Survey of Computerized Data Bases and Information Services*. New York & London: Haworth Press, 75–92.]

Touwaide, A. 1991b. 'Un manuscrit athonite du *Περὶ ὕλης ἰατρικῆς* de Dioscoride: l'Athous Megistis Lavras *Ω* 75', *Scriptorium* 55.1: 122–7.

Touwaide, A. 2006. 'The Development of Paleologan Renaissance', in M. Cacouros and M.-H. Congourdeau (eds.), *Philosophie et sciences à Byzance de 1204 à 1453: Les Textes, Les Doctrines Et Leur Transmission: Actes de la Table Ronde Organisée Au XXe Congrès International D'études Byzantines, Paris, 2001*. Leuven: Peeters, 189–224.

Touwaide, A. 2016. *A Census of Greek Medical Manuscripts: From Byzantium to the Renaissance*. Abingdon: Routledge.

Ullmann, M. 2009. *Untersuchungen zur arabischen Überlieferung der* Materia Medica *des Dioskurides*. Wiesbaden: Harassowitz.

Ventura, I. 2019. 'Galenic Pharmacology in the Middle Ages: Galen's *On the Capacities of Simple Drugs* and Its Reception between the Sixth and the Fourteenth Century', in P. Bouras-Vallianatos and B. Zipser (eds.), *Brill's Companion to the Reception of Galen*. Leiden: Brill, 393–433.

Warner, L. 1883. *De rebus Turcicis epistolae ineditae*. Leiden: Brill.

Wartelle, A. 1963. *Inventaires des manuscrits grecs d'Aristote et de ses commentaires*. Paris: Les Belles Lettres.

Wellman, M. ed. 1906–14. *Pedanii Dioscuridis Anazarbei De materia medica libri quinque*. 3 vols. Berlin: Weidman.

Wellmann, M. 1916. 'Pamphilos', *Hermes* 51: 1–64.

Wilson, N. 1962. 'A List of Plato Manuscripts', *Scriptorium* 16(2): 386–95.

Witkam, J. J. 2007. *Inventory of the Oriental Manuscripts of the Library of the University of Leiden*, vol. I. Leiden: Ter Lugt Press.

Yebouk, C., Redouan, F. Z., Benítez, G. et al. 2020. 'Ethnobotanical Study of Medicinal Plants in the Adrar Province, Mauritania', *Journal of Ethnopharmacology* 246: 112217. https://doi.org/10.1016/j.jep.2019.112217 (accessed 28 January 2023).

Zagkli-Boziou, M. 2009. *Ευλόγιος Κουρίλας (1880–1961). Το Αρχείο του στο Πανεπιστήμιο Ιωαννίνων*. Ioannina: University of Ioannina.

Zipser, B. ed. 2013a. *Simon of Genoa's Medical Lexicon*. Berlin: de Gruyter.

Zipser, B. 2013b. '*Simon Online*, an Alternative Approach to Research and Publishing', in B. Zipser (ed.), *Simon of Genoa's Medical Lexicon*. Berlin: de Gruyter, 149–56.

CHAPTER 5

The Theriac of Medieval al-Shām

Zohar Amar, Yaron Serri, and Efraim Lev

5.1 Introduction

Theriac is an antidote for the treatment of poisons of various kinds and origins. However, it was also used as a strong medicine for serious diseases and plagues. The production of theriac from various substances, used as an antidote for snakebites and poisons from other creatures, was known to ancient medical science. According to early Arabic sources, the name *theriac* in ancient Greek is actually a compound word made up of two words: *theria* (poisonous creatures) and *akos* (a poisonous substance).[1] This chapter focuses on the production of theriac in the medieval al-Shām.

5.2 Theriac in Early Sources

Theriac was widely described in the ancient medical literature. One kind of theriac, mithridate, was especially famous. This potion was named after Mithridates VI (132/5–63 BCE),[2] the king of Pontus in Asia Minor, and

[1] This etymology was attributed to Ḥunayn ibn Isḥāq, the greatest translator of Greek medical and scientific treatises in the Abbasid period; see al-Khaṭṭābī (1990: 237); al-Fīrūz'ābādī, *Al-Qāmūs al-muḥīṭ* (*The Surrounding Ocean*), ed. al-Buqāʿī (1995) 783. The Greek term actually derives from 'θηρίον' (venomous animals) and the suffix '-ικό-', thus 'θηριακός', 'θηριακή', 'θηριακόν'; see Boudon-Millot (2010) and Rousseau (2021).

[2] After Mithridates' father's death from poison in 120 BCE, succession struggles broke out within the royal family. It has been said that the young Mithridates was afraid that someone would poison him to prevent him from acceding to the throne. During this period he hid in the desert and swallowed toxic drugs in order to develop immunity against poisons. When he came to power, he continued this practice throughout his life and thus created the potion compatible for him. According to another version of this story, the great doctors of Mithridates' time made the formula for him. He used it regularly to protect himself from poisoning. When he was defeated by the Romans and feared falling into the hands of his enemies, he took a fatal drug, but it did not affect him due to the tolerance to theriac that he had developed. So he fell on his sword and thus ended his life. All this comes from the account of Paul of Aegina, a seventh-century Byzantine physician. See al-Khaṭṭābī (1990: 246). There are different versions of this story and of the formula for the Mithridates potion, which, according to Pliny, contained fifty-four ingredients. See Pliny, *Natural History*, 25.6–7 and 29.25, ed. Mayhoff and Jan (1897) IV.137.1–142.9 and IV.396–7. Detailed descriptions of the components of each of these

Andromachus, the physician of Emperor Nero (r. 54–68 CE) of Rome, is credited with improving the recipe.[3] Theriac was mentioned a few times in the writings of the Jewish sages, mainly in the Talmud.[4] A Jewish homily from the sixth/seventh century, written in a *midrash* from the Land of Israel, tells us about physicians who brought medicinal substances from Alexandria, from which they prepared a theriac which served as a cure.[5] Snake venom was an important component of theriac and snakes were hunted for that purpose. The Jewish religious laws (Halacha) – derived from the oral Torah and written down during the Roman period in the Land of Israel – specified that snakes were not to be hunted for medicine on Saturday (the Sabbath) unless they were dangerous to humans.[6]

From the classical period through to the medieval period dozens of books were produced dealing with antidotes for the treatment of poisons.[7] Moreover, medical encyclopaedias of the medieval and early modern periods had, in many cases, a chapter or an entry on the treatment of bites and other forms of poisoning.[8] Evidence for theriac's fame in the medieval period can be found in a Bible commentary by Nachmanides (1194–1270), who wrote:

> Theriac is not a single drug, but a compound medication in which are included sourdough and honey, flesh of insects and small reptiles, scorpions' dust and the flesh of a poisonous snake and for this reason it is called by that name, because snake venom is called in Greek 'theriac'. And so it is written in the Talmud: *theriaca ḥivya* [i.e. theriac of a snake].[9]

formulas were given by Celsus, *On Medicine*, 5.23.3, ed. Marx (1915) 210.18–211.13. Cf. Mayor (2010: 239–61). The most recent comprehensive article on Mithridates' antidote is by Totelin (2004).

3 Watson (1966); Mez-Mangold (1989: 39–43); Nutton (1997); Boudon-Millot (2010).

4 See, for example, the Babylonian Talmud, Shabbat 109b–110a; Nedarim 41b; The Talmud is a collection of rabbinic notes about the Mishnah, the Babylonian Talmud compiled in Mesopotamia during the fifth century.

5 Midrash Shir Ha-Shirim Rabbah on Song of Songs 4:5; see Dunsky (1973: 111).

6 Mishnah Eduyot 2:5. The Mishnah is a Jewish oral tradition, a compilation of rabbinical Hebrew commentaries written down in the second century.

7 Comprehensive books on theriac, written in Arabic in the Middle Ages and even earlier, were mentioned in the works of Ibn Abī ʾUṣaybiʿah, only some of which have been preserved: such essays are attributed to Ibn Juljul, Abū al-ʿAbbās al-Nabātī, al-Tamīmī, Ibn Jumayʿ, Abū Sulaymān Dāwud Abī al-Munā, Rashīd al-Dīn Abū Ḥulayqah, Muwaffaq al-Dīn ʿAbd al-Laṭīf al-Baghdādī, Sadīd al-Dīn ibn Raqīqah, ʿImād al-Dīn al-Dunaysarī, and others. In his edition of Maimonides, Muntner (1942: 35–8) lists some forty authors who wrote essays on fatal drugs and antidotes for the treatment of poisons or dedicated whole chapters to them in their books (such as al-Rāzī, Ibn Sīnā, Ibn al-Jazzār, Ibn Zuhr, Ibn Rushd); see Serri (2007: 35), Swiderski (2010: 59–94).

8 See, for example, Zahalon (1683: 23b–28b), Amar (2003: 87), and Amar and Buchman (2004: 34–5).

9 See Nachmanides, ed. Chavel (1958) on Exodus 30:34.

Other medieval Jewish Bible commentators wrote about the operating principle of theriac and its qualities; Rabbi Saadia Gaon (882–942), for example, mentions theriac as an example of the benefits that could be extracted from loathsome creatures such as snakes:

> And fats of [venomous and non-venomous snakes] are put into the theriac in order to remove the venom found in the body.[10]

Rabbi David Kimḥi (1160–1235), writing on 'And God saw that it was good' (Genesis, 1:25), explains that:

> Although they have harmful effects, they are of great benefit to many things, as the sages of experience have pointed out, the bodies of snakes and their fats are used to make theriac to remove a fatal drug from the body.[11]

Theriac also raised discussion in the Jewish tradition due to its contents; Maimonides (1138–1204) decided that, even though theriac included leaven, it could be used during Passover.[12] Other components, mainly snakes and insects that are not 'purified' according to the Jewish tradition, also raised Halachic questions.[13] For example, Rabbi David ben Zimra (1479–1573), who worked most of his life in Egypt and the Land of Israel, gave some explanations as to why eating theriac was allowed in answer to a question posed to him.[14]

5.3 Theriac from the Land of Israel and al-Shām: Its Production and Uses in the Medieval Period

The production of theriac was known in the Middle Ages in parts of the world such as Egypt,[15] Sijistan,[16] Yemen,[17] and Byzantium, and the product was even sent as a present to rulers of China.[18] One of the most famous

[10] Rabbi Saadia Gaon, *Saadya's Commentary on Genesis*, ed. Kafih (1984) 49–50.

[11] Rabbi David Kimhi, *Commentary on the Torah*, ed. Katzenellenbogen (1986) I.28. This can be seen as an expression of theodicy (the vindication of God): harmful creatures can also be useful.

[12] Maimonides, *Mishne Torah*, ed. Kafih (1984–96) Chametz U-Matzah 4.10.

[13] Shemesh (2001–2: 112–15). Shemesh (2013: 508–11) discusses in detail the response of Rabbi Shimshon Morpurgo (1680–1749) of Ancona to the physician Joseph Baruch Kasas regarding the treatment of patients suffering from *hidrokan* ('oedema' or 'ascites') by giving them the flesh of snakes to eat when no other medicine has been of any help. This was permitted because the flesh of the snakes was not considered a folk medicine but a proven drug, known for its efficacy.

[14] David ben Zimra (1882: II.470).

[15] Evliya Çelebi, *Al-Riḥlah 'ilā Miṣr wa-l-Sūdān wa-l-Ḥabashah* (*Book of Travels to Egypt, Sudan and Abyssinia*), ed. Ḥarb (2006) 342–57.

[16] Al-Jāḥiẓ, *Kitāb al-ḥayawān* (*Book of the Animals*), ed. Hārūn (1965) 168–9.

[17] Serri and Amar (2002: 51–3).

[18] Dobroruka (2016); Chen (2019). On the role of theriac as a diplomatic gift, see Durak (Chapter 13) in this volume.

centres for the production of theriac was in the Land of Israel due to the knowledge of the doctors who specialised in it and in particular to the existence of medicinal substances that are considered endemic species of flora, fauna, and minerals unique to this area. An example of this is the 'Tyre' snake, described later in this chapter.

The production of theriac was indeed a unique branch of medical production in al-Shām in the medieval period in general and in the early Muslim period (634–1099) in particular. Theriac was one of the most famous drugs for which the Land of Israel was praised, and it was exported to other countries. This is why Rabbi Saadia Gaon related the biblical word for balm to *ṣorī* (Genesis 37:25, 43:11), which was sent to Egypt with the theriac.[19] Such an identification reflects the life of his time – or the reality of it, as we might see it.[20] A lot of evidence from the tenth century indicates that Jerusalem was an important centre for the production of theriac.

5.4 The Theriac of Jerusalem

At the end of the tenth century, Rabbi Samuel ben Ḥofni Gaon (d. 1034) wrote in his commentary on the biblical word *ṣori* that 'it means the Jerusalemite theriac made out of weeds from Syria and exported to other countries, and it protects bodies from poisons'.[21] Al-Muqaddasī, a tenth-century scholar from Jerusalem who completed a geographical essay around 985, mentioned theriac as one of the products exported from the city.[22] Elsewhere he mentions the city of Jericho specifically as a source of

[19] On his Judeo-Arabic translation of the Pentateuch, see Kafih (1984: 55, 58). Rabbi Abraham Ibn Ezra, in his commentary on Genesis 37:25, says in the name of Rabbi Saadia Gaon that theriac was composed of seventy-five different components. In the biblical period, *ṣorī* was considered a clear remedy brought out of the Land of Israel to another country (Jeremiah 8:22, 46:11; Ezekiel 27:17). On the various ways proposed to identify *ṣorī*, see Amar (2012: 174–7). According to the sages' interpretive tradition of *ṣorī*, it is balsam (*Commiphora gileadensis*), which is mentioned as *balasān* in Maimonides' treatise on drugs. Apparently, there is not necessarily any contradiction between linking *ṣorī* with theriac and balsam since the latter was one of its components. Pliny, *Natural History*, 23.47, ed. Mayhoff (1897) IV.29.13–14, notes that balsam is effective against all snakebites. A tenth-century Jewish physician, Isaac Israeli ben Solomon, also mentioned balsam (*balasān*) as one of the *tiryāq al-fārūq*'s components; see Ibn al-Bayṭār *al-Jāmiʿ li-mufradāt al-adwiyah wa-l-aghdhiyah* (*Collector of Simple Drugs and Foodstuffs*), ed. Būlāq (1874) I.109.

[20] Later (in his entry on *ṣorī*), Shlomo Ben Shmuel, a fourteenth-century Persian Jewish lexicographer, cites a quotation taken – according to the editor – from a medical treatise: '*Ṣorī* – if one of its species is taken and a circle is drawn around the scorpion . . . and if a *punduq* (the word for *ṣorī* in Arabic) is tied around the arm, the scorpion will never be able to bite.' See Bacher (1900: 34).

[21] See the commentary of Rabbi Samuel ben Hofni Gaon on Genesis 43:11 in ed. Greenbaum (1978).

[22] Al-Muqaddasī, *ʾAḥsan al-taqāsīm fī maʿrifat al-ʾaqālīm* (*The Best Divisions in the Knowledge of the Regions*), ed. de Goeje (1906) 106.

snakes and scorpions (or in another version theriac snakes), which were the main ingredients in the production of theriac.[23]

A few tenth-century historical figures from Jerusalem, who were experts in the production of theriac, are mentioned in medieval literature – for example, Salāma ibn Nāhiḍ al-Maqdisī al-Tiryāqī.[24] The most famous theriac producer of tenth-century Jerusalem, however, was a physician, al-Tamīmī. Fragments of his work are found in Arabic medieval literature – Maimonides mentioned him in his medical writings many times.[25]

Al-Tamīmī was born in Jerusalem and received his medical training from a local physician, a Christian monk called Zakhariyyā ibn Thawāba. He was closely associated with the ruling elite. At first he practised in Ramle as the physician to the governor of Ikhshīdī, al-Ḥasan ibn ʿAbd Allāh ibn Ṭughj al-Mustawlī; he later moved to Egypt, staying there until 981. In Cairo he was close to the wazir, Yaʿqūb ibn Yūsuf ibn Killis (930–91). Al-Tamīmī was considered a knowledgeable physician and an expert in producing ointments and compound drugs, but he achieved fame mainly on account of his unique expertise in making the various kinds of theriac. The four texts he wrote about the production of theriac are mentioned in the medieval literature: the great treatise, the medium and the small, plus a letter (*risālah*), dedicated to his son, about the Fārūq theriac which was highly regarded by his contemporaries.[26] The physician and linguist al-Bīrūnī (973–1048) suggested two different explanations for this name: one associated with pain relief and the other with protection from poisons.[27]

Al-Fīrūzʾābādī (1329–1414) explained the term 'theriac al-Fārūq' in his dictionary *al-Qāmūs al-muḥīṭ* (*The Surrounding Ocean*) as: 'the best of all theriacs and the most esteemed of the compound drugs, since it separates sickness from health'.[28] Another famous theriac mixed by al-Tamīmī was called 'soul saver' (*mukhalliṣ al-nufūs*). It was produced in Jerusalem, considered beneficial for the treatment of various poisons, and contained the venom of poisonous snakes, scorpions, spiders, lizards, and other

[23] Al-Muqaddasī, *ʾAḥsan al-taqāsīm fī maʿrifat al-ʾaqālīm* (*The Best Divisions in the Knowledge of the Regions*), ed. de Goeje (1906) 175.

[24] Ibn al-Athīr (1994: I.214).

[25] Maimonides, *Kitāb al-fuṣūl fī al-ṭibb* (*Medical Aphorisms*), ed. Rosner and Muntner (1970) 240, see also pp. 150, 190–1, 267, 276.

[26] Amar and Serri (2004: 9–13). On al-Tamīmī's pharmacological recommendations, see also Lieberman (Chapter 8) in this volume.

[27] Al-Bīrūnī, *Kitāb al-ṣaydanah fī al-ṭibb* (*Book of the Pharmacy on Medicine*), ed. Said and Elahie (1973) 172–5.

[28] Al-Fīrūzʾābādī, *Al-Qāmūs al-muḥīṭ* (*The Surrounding Ocean*), ed. al-Buqāʿī (1995) 825.

poisonous creatures, including insects and mammals.[29] More information about the medicinal substances used for the production of the diverse kinds of theriac are found in extant passages from the lost treatises of al-Tamīmī. The most important of these treatises was *Kitāb al-murshid ʾilā jawāhir al-aghdhiyah wa-quwā al-mufradāt min al-ʾadwiyah* (*Guide to the Elements of Foodstuffs and the Qualities of Simple Drugs*), more commonly known as *al-Murshid*. Only the part on inorganic drugs survives.[30]

More information relating to drugs of vegetal origin has survived from this book thanks to quotations in Arabic medical books from the late medieval period – for example, in the works of Ibn al-Bayṭār (d. 1248).[31] One of the substances used to produce theriac was asphalt (pitch, bitumen) from the Dead Sea:

> Regarding Jewish asphalt, it is mainly one of two kinds that are produced from the sea of the Jew, that is the Dead Sea, situated in the region of Filasṭīn near Jerusalem, in between the valley of Zoar and the valley of Jericho. And it is the asphalt that is dug from the soil on the shore of the lake. And it is the better of the two kinds of Jewish asphalt, which is used in the production of the compound drug named al-Fārūq whose efficiency is guaranteed.[32]

Al-Tamīmī mentioned many wild plants that grew in al-Shām and that were known for their beneficial qualities in the treatment of snake and scorpion bites. The plants that grew in the vicinity of Jerusalem and were used in the production of theriac in his home city and the centre of his activities are of special interest. One of them, collected from the mountains of Jerusalem, is *dawqū*, identified as 'wild carrot' (*Daucus carota maximus*).[33] Other plants are *kamāfīṭūs*, identified as 'yellow bugle' or 'ground-pine' (*Ajuga chamaepytis*); and the 'seseli' (moon carrot), the so-called *sāsaliyūs* (*Seseli tortosum*).[34]

In his entry on *thūm barrī*, 'wild garlic' (*Allium* sp.), al-Tamīmī notes that it is an important plant out of which a highly effective theriac can be made, thus replacing one of its other ingredients.[35] Another plant with similar qualities that al-Tamīmī also mentioned is the *ḥazanbal*, identified

[29] See Ibn al-Qifṭī, *Tārīkh al-ḥukamāʾ* (*History of Learned Men*), ed. Lipper (1903) 105–6, 169; Ibn Abī ʾUṣaybiʿah, *ʿUyūn al-anbāʾ fī ṭabaqāt al-aṭibbāʾ* (*Sources of Information on the Classes of Physicians*), 14.14.6, ed. Savage-Smith, Swain, and van Gelder (2020).

[30] Parisinus ar. 2870. [31] Amar (1995: 49–76).

[32] Amar and Serri (2004: 101); cf. Ibn al-Bayṭār, *al-Jāmiʿ li-mufradāt al-adwiyah wa-l-aghdhiyah* (*Collector of Simple Drugs and Foodstuffs*), ed. (1874) III.26–7.

[33] Amar and Serri (2004: 30, 131–2). [34] Amar and Serri (2004: 32–3, 134, 139–40).

[35] Amar and Serri (2004: 30).

as one of the wild species of 'yarrow' (*Achillea sp.*), which grew in 'Tarsus (southern Turkey) and other locations in al-Shām as well as in Tiberias and in the mountains of Jerusalem, where it is extensively found. Its unique quality is as an antidote for the venom of scorpions'.[36]

The expertise in Jerusalem in the production of theriac and its uses was mentioned in later periods. A physician and astrologer, Abū Sulaymān Dāwud ibn abī al-Munā ibn abī al-Fānah, who was brought from Egypt to Jerusalem by the Crusader king Amalric of Jerusalem (r. 1162–74), produced the Fārūq theriac in Jerusalem for the son of the king, Baldwin IV (r. 1174–85), who was suffering from leprosy.[37] Further evidence for the use of theriac for the treatment of poisonous insects was handed down to us by Geoffrey Vinsauf, once considered by some scholars as the author of the chronicle of the Third Crusade (1191). One of his books includes a description of poisonous insects attacking the Crusaders' camp when they were on their way from Haifa to Kfar Naḥum (Capernaum). These crawling creatures, which stung at night, had very powerful venom that caused such great suffering to their victims that the affected parts of the body swelled up immediately. The wealthier Crusaders applied an ointment containing theriac to the swelling and it eased their pain.[38] It appears that the Crusaders acquired the formula for theriac from local physicians.

The Land of Israel was well known for theriac formulas produced there during the early Islamic period and also for supplying substances for its preparation during the Ayyubid period (when Maimonides was practising). Maimonides indeed wrote about a unique plant known as *ʿirq al-ḥayyah* (the root of the snakes) or *ʾiklīl al-malik*:

> [I]t came to my knowledge that the roots that are brought from al-Shām and used as theriac for the treatment of poisonous animal bites, and the roots of this kind of *ʾiklīl al-malik* are known as *ʿirq al-ḥayyah*'.[39]

[36] Ibn al-Bayṭār, *al-Jāmiʿ li-mufradāt al-adwiyah wa-l-aghdhiyah* (*Collector of Simple Drugs and Foodstuffs*), ed. (1874) II.20.

[37] Ibn Abī ʾUṣaybiʿah, *ʿUyūn al-anbāʾ fī ṭabaqāt al-aṭibbāʾ* (*Sources of Information on the Classes of Physicians*), 14.49.2, ed. Savage-Smith, Swain, and van Gelder (2020); cf. William of Tyre, *Chronicle*, ed. Huygens (1986) XXI.1. Maimonides, *Kitāb al-fuṣūl fī al-ṭibb* (*Medical Aphorisms*), ed. Rosner and Muntner (1970) 147. During this period, theriac was considered one of the most effective anti-leprosy drugs; see Maimonides, *Kitāb al-fuṣūl fī al-ṭibb* (*Medical Aphorisms*), ed. Rosner and Muntner (1970) 147.

[38] Chronicles of the Crusades (1848) 229. On drugs called *rutaylā* that provided an antidote to poisonous spider bites, see Maimonides, *Kitāb al-sumūm wa-l-mutaḥarriz min al-adwiyah al-qattālah* (*Book on Poisons and Protection against Lethal Drugs*), ed. Bos (2009) 29.

[39] Meyerhof (1940: no. 7).

In his book on poisonous drugs, he added:

> *ʿirq al-ḥayyah* – it is the root of a plant that grows in the vicinity of Jerusalem and acquired fame for itself and was proved beneficial . . . In general, every man should equip himself with it, and have it available at any moment.

This plant was identified as one of the various species of melilot (*Melilotus* sp.); however, we suggest it should be identified as the plant as a variety of fenugreek (*Trigonella kotschyi* or *Trigonella hierosolymitana*). Both species are closely related from a botanical point of view and their names have changed over the years. In any case, according to the description of the plants from medieval Arabic sources, we have identified the plant as *Trigonella hierosolymitana,* whose podlike fruit looks like horns. This species is rare in al-Shām but common in the area around Jerusalem to the present day.[40]

More information on medicinal plants used in the production of theriac in al-Shām is found in a work by ʿAlī Aḥmad ʿAbd al-ʾAthīr al-Anṣārī, *Dhikr al-tiryāq al-fārūq* (*Memoir on Antidotes for Poisons*). Al-Anṣārī was an important physician who practised medicine a few years after the death of Maimonides (1204). He was closely related to the elite of the Ayyubid dynasty and from his writings we learn the Ayyubid rulers were personally involved in the business of getting medicinal substances, mainly for the production of theriacs. Among other things he wrote about *al-ṭīn al-makhtūm*, known in English as 'sigillated earth' or *terra sigillata*:[41]

> The freight convoys of the Sultan al-Malik al-ʿĀdil Sayf al-Dīn Ibn Ayyūb [Ṣalāḥ al-Dīn (Saladin) brother ruled Egypt and Syria 1196–1218], God have mercy on him, loaded with the praised theriac of Cairo in the year 1213. And this clay was brought to him from the treasury, from what was brought earlier by the Sultan al-Darūb and it is what I have in my hand. After making the theriac, according to the formula, some leftovers were put aside; and when al-Malik al-Muʿaẓẓam ʿĪsā (r. Damascus 1218–27) the son of the above mentioned al-Malik al-ʿĀdil, God have mercy on him, produced the formula for the theriac, he used the leftovers from his father's time.[42]

Al-Anṣārī, probably active in al-Shām, cited in his work (written in 1268) earlier writers and scholars who had dealt with the production of the theriac.

[40] Maimonides, *Kitāb al-sumūm wa-l-mutaḥarriz min al-adwiyah al-qattālah* (*Book on Poisons and Protection against Lethal Drugs*), ed. Amar and Serri (2019) 16–17.

[41] Medicinal claylike earth from the island of Lemnos. It was called 'sealed' because it was sold as 'dry pressed cakes' stamped with the head of Artemis. For more details, see Meyerhof (1940: no. 172); Gunther (1959: V, no. 113).

[42] Al-Anṣārī, *Dhikr al-tiryāq al-fārūq* (*Memoir on Antidotes for Poisons*), National Library of Medicine, Bethesda, Maryland, MS 16, ff. 114b, 115a.

He gives, for example, information attributed to al-Tamīmī about medicinal plants from the Jerusalem mountains and Ashkelon, another centre of medieval theriac production. He also gives information attributed to Rashīd al-Dīn Ibn al-Ṣūrī (1178–1242), a physician from Tyre who was considered an expert in simple drugs, their names, and their benefits in his day and even wrote some books on that subject.[43] He lived in Jerusalem for two years and practised there in a hospital; he also served at the courts of Ayyubid rulers. He was known at the time as an expert on the production of theriac. Ibn Abī ʾUṣaybiʿah wrote of him that 'He also accurately formulated the ingredients of the great theriac (*al-tiryāq al-kabīr*), in which he combined such drugs as he deemed proper, with the result that its benefits became manifest and its effects powerful. He had previously prepared a great quantity of it in the days of al-Malik al-Muʿaẓẓam.'[44] Ibn al-Ṣūrī mentioned the plant *kamādriyūs*, identified as germander (thyme, wood sage, *Teucrium capitatum*):[45]

> [A]nd I saw of this plant one kind whose flowers are white, and both kinds are fragrant, and it is abundant in the mountain of Jerusalem, Nāblus and the mountains of Sidon.[46]

This plant is also mentioned by a thirteen-century Jewish pharmacist, al-Kūhīn al-ʿAṭṭār: 'the germander is a kind of wormwood (*Artemisia* sp.), and it is brought from al-Shām for the production of theriac and other things'.[47]

Many other medicinal plants from al-Shām, used to produce theriac, were mentioned in the literature of the period. At the beginning of the fourteenth century, the Muslim geographer al-Dimashqī mentioned a plant called *ḥamāmā*:

> this plant grows only in the region of Damascus on the Lebanon mountain, and it is precious and expensive, costing a *ginni* [i.e. an ancient gold coin] . . . And it is used for the production of the theriac al-Fārūq.[48]

[43] Al-Anṣārī, *Dhikr al-tiryāq al-fārūq* (*Memoir on Antidotes for Poisons*), National Library of Medicine, Bethesda, Maryland, MS 16, f. 303b.

[44] Ibn Abī ʾUṣaybiʿah, *ʿUyūn al-anbāʾ fī ṭabaqāt al-aṭibbāʾ* (*Sources of Information on the Classes of Physicians*) 15.45.2, ed. Savage-Smith, Swain, and van Gelder (2020).

[45] See Issa (1930: 179); Meyerhof (1940: no. 189); Ibn al-Bayṭār, *al-Jāmiʿ li-mufradāt al-adwiyah wa-l-aghdhiyah* (*Collector of Simple Drugs and Foodstuffs*), ed. (1874) IV.80–1.

[46] Al-Anṣārī, *Dhikr al-tiryāq al-fārūq* (*Memoir on Antidotes for Poisons*) National Library of Medicine, Bethesda, Maryland, MS 16, f. 118a–b.

[47] Al-Kūhīn al-ʿAṭṭār, *Minhāj al-dukkān* (*How to Run a Pharmacy*), ed. al-ʿĀṣī (1992) 226.

[48] Al-Dimashqī, *Nukhbat al-dahr fī ʿajāʾib al-barr wa-l-baḥr* (*Chosen Passages of Time regarding the Marvels of Land and Sea*), ed. van Mehren (1923) 199–200; the identity of this plant is not clear, but some scholars identify it as *Amomum racemosum*; see Lev (2002a: 146) and Lev and Amar (2008: 100–2).

During the same period al-ʿUthmānī, a Muslim judge from Safed, described another plant that grew in the fortress of Adchit (south of present-day Lebanon):

> it grows on the walls of the fortress, a plant with a red flower, similar to the mouth of a dog, or a snake; its consumption treats rabies and snakebite.[49]

A late testimony for the use of theriac in Jerusalem comes from an eighteenth-century document which describes the belongings of a deceased Jew[50] and from Dr Titus Tobler, who documented the condition of medicine in Jerusalem in the mid-nineteenth century. Tobler wrote it is still possible to find theriac in the pharmacy of the Jews in Jerusalem.[51] Interestingly enough, descendants of the al-Tiryāqī family, known for producing snake venom from the region of Jericho in the past, still live in East Jerusalem.

5.5 The Theriac of Ashkelon

Thanks to the medieval Muslim sources we learn that in the tenth century theriac was known and produced in the city of Ashkelon. A specialist in theriac who studied the secret of its production lived in Ashkelon and used local plants, one of which was *al-mukhalliṣa*. It was described as 'having blue flowers with long spurs, similar to the sting of the scorpion; this plant was widely grown in the fields around the city'. This description fits the violet larkspur (*Delphinium peregrinum*) or one of the varieties of the genus toadflax (*Linaria* or *Kickxia*).[52]

Judging from al-Tamīmī's description it seems that this theriac was believed to provide efficient immunity for a year. Both in Ashkelon and in Jerusalem individuals used to hold poisonous snakes in their hands to demonstrate this, probably through magic tricks and illusions. Since the risk of getting bitten was high, they needed a proven antidote. The formula for the theriac that was invented by an expert from Ashkelon was so successful that its fame quickly reached al-Tamīmī's ears. According to the sources he was considered the most important expert in the field of theriac production. From a letter sent to him from

49 Lewis (1953: 482); it is identified with Great Snapdragon (*Antirrhinum majus*); see Lev (2002a: 174–5). These uses clearly suggest the use of the doctrine of signatures; see Lev (2002b).

50 Cohen, Simon-Pikali, and Salama (1993: 482, n. 65).

51 Amar and Lev (2000b).

52 Amar (1995: 73–4); mentioned later by Ibn al-Bayṭār; see Ibn al-Bayṭār, *al-Jāmiʿ li-mufradāt al-adwiyah wa-l-aghdhiyah* (*Collector of Simple Drugs and Foodstuffs*), ed. (1874) IV.142; on the plant and its identification see Amar and Serri (2004: 37) and Amar (1995: 73–4).

Ashkelon, which included a sample of the plant, he confirmed that the plant was beneficial for the treatment of snakebites without any need for other components. It was known as a simple drug – as opposed to other kinds of theriac that were composed of several medicinal substances. Al-Tamīmī found out that the same plant grew in the vicinity of his own city of Jerusalem.[53]

5.6 The Snake Antidote of the Dead Sea Area

Theriac produced from snakes from the region of the Dead Sea was mentioned many times by pilgrims during the medieval period. The first description appeared in an account by a traveller called Antoninus of Piacenza (570): 'In the area of the shores of the river Jorden there are snakes from which the inhabitants produce theriac.'[54] From the same period comes evidence that one of the monks from the Judean desert was bitten by a snake. He was brought to the hospital by the inhabitants of the village of Lazrion (al-Eizariya) near Jerusalem.[55]

More evidence emerges from the late medieval period; we have decided to present here the case of Jacques de Vitry (mid-thirteenth century). In his book he described a snake called *ter* (adder) which lived in the desert around Jericho. According to Jacques, the flesh of this poisonous snake, together with other medicinal substances, was used to produce a theriac which was an antidote for all kinds of venoms.[56] Ernoul, a French pilgrim who completed his chronicle in 1231, also mentioned that around Jericho there was an abundance of snakes from which theriac was made. His description of the way they were hunted is of special interest: 'they used to take them to be sold in the cities, for the producers of theriac . . . the theriac that was produced from these snakes treated all kinds of poisons'.[57] Among other pilgrims from the fourteenth and fifteenth centuries who wrote about such snakes we can mention Niccolo Poggibonsi, Arnold von Harff, Francesco Suriano,[58] Adorno, and Gucci.[59] However, the most detailed description appeared in a book by a Swiss-German Dominican monk, Felix Fabri, who visited the Holy Land at the end of the fifteenth century. The local guides told him that the snake from which the theriac was made was found only in the region

[53] Serri and Amar (2002); Amar and Serri (2004: 135–9). [54] Wilkinson (1977: 82).
[55] Amar and Lev (2000a: 26). [56] Jacques de Vitry, *Historia orientalis*, ed. Bongars (1611) 1104.
[57] *Chronicle of Ernoul and Bernard the Treasurer*, ed. de Mas Latrie (1871) 76–7.
[58] Francesco Suriano, *Treatise on the Holy Land*, ed. Bellorini, Hoade, and Bagatti (1949) 145.
[59] Amar (1996–7: 22–3); Swiderski (2010: 64–5); Rubin (2014).

of the Dead Sea.[60] It was considered a very expensive drug and a monopoly of the Mamluk sultan. Due to theriac's prestige, the sultan banned the hunting of snakes; however, because of theriac's high value, many criminals ignored the decree and sold the snakes they caught to traders in Damascus, Beirut, Alexandria, and Cairo.

This is the way the venom was extracted: the snake was caught alive and put in a jar, and if it tried to escape, they then stabbed it all over with a stick until it was raging. At this point they would cut off its head and tail with a sharp knife, believing that while the snake was angry the venom would concentrate in these organs.[61] Fabri also described the snake: it was half a forearm long, and as thick as a thumb, its colour was yellowish-red, its hiss was angry and its venom lethal.[62] According to this description, the snake can be identified with an adder (*ter*) (*Echis coloratus*).

5.7 The Production of Theriac in Ayyubid Egypt

In the introduction to his book on poisonous and lethal drugs Maimonides wrote that it was impossible to find the substances for the production of theriac in Egypt, and therefore the rulers made efforts to find it in other countries. As mentioned, one of the main components was the adder from the Dead Sea region. Many contemporary sources and especially those from the Ayyubid period mention the production of theriac in Egypt as an antidote in general and for the treatment of poisonous substances in particular.

Maimonides' book *al-Maqālah al-Fāḍilīyah* (*Treatise for al-Fāḍil*) was written at the request of al-Qāḍī al-Fāḍil (d. 1200), not for personal use, but for the sake of the public at large. In the introduction Maimonides points out al-Fāḍil's concern for public affairs and his assistance for those who had been poisoned. From his words we learn that he ordered the Egyptian expert physicians to prepare the two most important theriacs (the great theriac and Mithridates' theriac) since these products were unavailable to

60 The name is probably an abbreviation of the word 'theriac' because it was an important component of the theriac formula.

61 Compare the words of Rabbi Yaakov Chagiz (1620–74), one of the great sages of Jerusalem: 'And it is also said that the snake in its head and tail is poisonous and its body is good as a medicine.' See Halachot Ketanot (1704: Orah Haim, 208).

62 Palestine Pilgrims' (1890–7) IX–X.151–3; Compare the description of Ludolf von Sochum in Palestine Pilgrims' (1890–7) XII.117, who mentioned the Tyrus snake from which the theriac was made in his description of the Dead Sea region: 'It is as thick as a finger and its colour is yellow mixed with red.' This is the description given by Arnold von Harff; see Von Groote (1860: 192). Note that the literature mentions a well-known profession of snake catchers as producing not only an antidote, but pesticides as well. See al-Qazwīnī, *ʿAjāʾib al-makhlūqāt wa-gharāʾib al-mawjūdāt* (*The Wonders of Creatures and the Marvels of Creation*), ed. Saʿd (1985) 223.

the general public. Although most of the components of these theriacs could not be obtained in Egypt (apart from the poppy), the substances required were imported into Egypt from all parts of the world, from East to West. The theriacs were supplied according to physicians' recommendations – that is, to those for whom the theriac was urgently needed. Al-Qāḍī wanted to ensure a regular supply of these expensive theriacs; however, he wished to save money and find more easily available and cheaper substitutes for those willing to accept them. Allegedly, this was the primary reason for writing this book. Later, we will see that the use of the great theriac, usually produced for the treatment of lethal and poisonous substances, involved a higher risk than that associated with the simple (and safer) substitutes which were adequate in most cases.

We cannot rule out other motives related to the tensions between the elite group of the Ayyubid authorities which backed the request of al-Qāḍī al-Fāḍil to write the book. There was a realistic fear of assassination by poisoning. This phenomenon was common throughout history, especially during the Ayyubid period, which was characterised by incessant fights and intrigues between the various rulers; therefore, the theriacs were essential to survival.[63] Fears of deliberate poisoning are hinted at in this book. Maimonides testifies that he saw the royal cooks testing the food before it was served to the rulers; he also mentions a story told about the famous physician Ibn Zuhr, who – as a highly suspicious person and because he worried about being poisoned – always carried theriac. And Ibn Abī ʾUṣaybiʿah wrote that the Jewish physician of Ṣalāḥ al-Dīn Yūsuf ibn Ayyūb (Saladin), Ibn Jumayʿ compounded the great theriac – theriac *al-Fārūq* – for his master.[64]

Ibn al-Ṣūrī wrote that in the time of al-Malik al-ʿĀdil important substances for the production of theriac in Cairo (1213), the *ṭīn al-makhtūm*, were imported; as mentioned, his son al-Malik al-Muʿaẓẓam ʿĪsā used it later.[65] Another son of Saladin, al-Kāmil Ayyūb (r. 1218–38)

[63] William of Tyre, *Chronicle*, 22.19, ed. Huygens (1986). See, for example, what the Frankish chronicler wrote about al-Afḍal's father: 'It was a well-known fact that Ṣalāḥ al-Dīn bribed the friends and servants of the prince of Mosul and caused him to receive a lethal drug, which was proven to kill within a short period of time.'

[64] Ibn Abī ʾUṣaybiʿah, *ʿUyūn al-anbāʾ fī ṭabaqāt al-aṭibbāʾ* (*Sources of Information on the Classes of Physicians*), 14.32.1, ed. Savage-Smith, Swain, and van Gelder (2020).

[65] Amar and Serri (2003: 213); Ibn Abī ʾUṣaybiʿah wrote that this physician was an expert in the production of theriac and that he formulated the great theriac at the time of al-Malik al-Muʿaẓẓam ʿĪsā; see Ibn Abī ʾUṣaybiʿah, *ʿUyūn al-anbāʾ fī ṭabaqāt al-aṭibbāʾ* (*Sources of Information on the Classes of Physicians*), 15.45.2, ed. Savage-Smith, Swain, and van Gelder (2020).

used theriac that the physician Rashīd al-Dīn Abū Ḥulayqah made for him:

> ordered him to make the theriac known as *al-Fārūq*, and Abū Ḥulayqah was occupied with its preparation for a long period of time, spending all night on it until he had determined every one of its ingredients by name according to the writings of the two masters of the medical art, Hippocrates and Galen. Meanwhile, the sultan had developed a discharge from his teeth for which he was bled.[66]

Later, when the sultan continued to suffer and no treatment eased the pain, Rashīd suggested using theriac, which he always carried with him in a small silver vessel – and it was immediately beneficial.

Another story told about Rashīd al-Dīn Abū Ḥulayqah is that:

> Because of the long time required to prepare the theriac called *al-Fārūq* and the difficulty in obtaining the correct ingredients from distant lands, he prepared a simplified theriac compounded of ingredients that are easily found everywhere. He did not intend to use it in order to obtain favours from a king or to seek money or glory in the world. Rather, he intended to seek closeness to God by aiding all of His creatures and showing compassion to all creation. He gave it freely to the sick, and with it he relieved the partially paralyzed and straightened crooked hands immediately and quickly.[67]

Another story about Rashīd and his use of theriac goes as follows:

> Al-Malik al-Kāmil (r. 1218–38) had a muezzin known as Amīn al-Dīn Jaʿfar who had a stone that was blocking his urethra. This caused him intense suffering, to the point that he was on the verge of death. He wrote to al-Malik al-Kāmil informing him of his condition and requesting authorization to go home to be treated. When he arrived at his house all the great physicians of the day were summoned, and each of them prescribed something for him, but nothing was of any benefit. But then he sent for the *ḥakīm* Abū Ḥulayqah, who gave him a dose of his theriac. In the amount of time it took for it to reach his stomach, its potency penetrated to the place of the stone and broke it up so that it came out when he urinated, stained from the colouring of the medication.[68]

According to the sources, the Ayyubid emir, Sayf al-Dīn Qalaj, wore a round yellow *bādzahr* (Bezoar stone) on his arm covered in bandages in

[66] Ibn Abī ʾUṣaybiʿah, *ʿUyūn al-anbāʾ fī ṭabaqāt al-aṭibbāʾ* (*Sources of Information on the Classes of Physicians*), 14.54.6, ed. Savage-Smith, Swain, and van Gelder (2020).

[67] Ibn Abī ʾUṣaybiʿah, *ʿUyūn al-anbāʾ fī ṭabaqāt al-aṭibbāʾ* (*Sources of Information on the Classes of physicians*), 14.54.7, ed. Savage-Smith, Swain, and van Gelder (2020).

[68] Ibn Abī ʾUṣaybiʿah, *ʿUyūn al-anbāʾ fī ṭabaqāt al-aṭibbāʾ* (*Sources of Information on the Classes of Physicians*), 14.54.8, ed. Savage-Smith, Swain, and van Gelder (2020).

order to protect himself from any attempts to poison him. He said that he received the stone from al-Malik al-Ashraf, the third son of al-ʿĀdil (r. Damascus 1229–38), who also wore one.[69]

An interesting testimony on the production of theriac in Egypt was supplied by the fifteenth-century Mamluk historiographer Ibn ʾIyās; he claims that in 1496 the Mamluk Sultan al-Ashraf Qāytbāy (r. 1468–96) ordered that the cutting up of snakes for the production of theriac at the Qalāwūn hospital should be done under his observation. Indeed the snakes were brought before him to the hall in which the basin of water was situated, and they were dissected in front of the sultan's eyes. Subsequently he granted expensive garments to the chief physician and his sons, the snake charmer, and other people involved in the process.[70]

As late as the seventeenth century a detailed description of the production of theriac from snakes is given us by Evliya Çelebi, after his visit to Cairo in 1672. Çelebi documented his impressions of the Qalāwūn hospital. His description has huge historical significance since it confirms that the production of theriac was a fully developed area of medicine, still active and flourishing at the time, thus validated his statement that some of the huge amount of theriac produced was exported to Europe. Çelebi spiced up his description with folkloric details and narratives, which in some cases, where he had heard them from his guides and companions, are exaggerated. Nevertheless, these sources are highly valuable.[71]

Conclusion

The Levant and Egypt were known in the medieval period as centres for the production of various kinds of theriac, both because they had the necessary professional know-how and because they were able to supply the various ingredients. In the tenth century many theriac specialists were active in Jerusalem, producing the antidote and exporting it to other countries. Theriac was a much-needed compound drug and the authorities took an active part in its production. This is important from an economic point of view because, as we learn from historical sources, commercial ties existed

[69] Al-Tīfāshī, *Kitāb ʾazhār al-ʾafkār fī jawāhir al-ʾaḥjār* (*Blossoms of Thoughts on Precious Stones*) ed. Ḥasan and Khafājī (1977) 121. On the Bezoar stone see Lev and Amar (2008: 358) and Amar and Lev (2017: 187–90).

[70] Ibn ʾIyās, *Badāʾiʿ al-zuhūr fī waqāʾiʿ al-duhūr* (*Flowers in the Chronicles of the Ages*), ed. Muṣṭafā (1984) III.358.

[71] Evliya Çelebi, *Al-Riḥlah ʾilā Miṣr wa-l-Sūdān wa-l-Ḥabashah* (*Book of Travels to Egypt, Sudan and Abyssinia*), ed. Ḥarb (2006) I.342–57; Leiser and Dols (1988: 49–68).

and networking took place between countries linked with the trade in the ingredients of theriac. The vast majority of these ingredients (of plant and animal origin, as well as some inorganic ones), were brought not only from the region of the Dead Sea, but also from other parts of al-Shām. During the Ayyubid and Mamluk periods, Egypt became the main centre of theriac production.

Theriac production became accredited and widespread in Europe in the late medieval and early modern periods under the influence of Greco-Arabic medicine. The theriac produced in the Middle East, especially in Egypt, became a much desired and traded drug, exported even to France and Venice.[72]

The uses of theriac were known and applied in the Middle East throughout the late medieval and early modern period[73] right through to modern times. For example, the Iraqi Jews used various kinds of theriac for the treatment of many ailments as part of their traditional (ethnic) medicine: from its external application for skin conditions to the internal treatment of poisons, epilepsy, gas, typhus, pertussis, and haemorrhoids.[74]

REFERENCES

Amar, Z. 1995. 'Ibn al-Bayṭār and the Study of the Plants of al-Shām', *Cathedra* 76: 49–76 [in Hebrew].

Amar, Z. 1996–7. 'The Export of Theriac from the Land of Israel and Its Uses in the Middle Ages', *Korot* 12: 16–29 [in Hebrew].

Amar, Z. ed. 2003. *Pri Megadim of Rabbi David de Silva*. Jerusalem: Yad Yitzhak Ben Zvi [in Hebrew].

Amar, Z. 2012. *Flora of the Bible: A New Investigation Aimed at Identifying All of the Plants of the Bible in Light of Jewish Sources and Scientific Research*. Jerusalem: Rubin Mass.

Amar, Z., and Buchman, Y. eds. 2004. *Ṣori ha-Guf by R. Nathan ben Yoel Falaquera*. Ramat Gan: Division of the History of Medicine, Bar Ilan University [in Hebrew].

Amar, Z., and Buchman, Y. 2006. *Practical Medicine of Rabbi Hayyim Vital (1543–1620)*. Ramat-Gan: Division of the History of Medicine, Bar Ilan University [in Hebrew].

72 Berman (1970: 5–12).

73 Rabbi Chaim Vital, a Kabbalist and healer (1543–1620), who lived in the Land of Israel and Syria, notes several prescriptions for the treatment of poisons. He distinguishes between snakebites and the scorpion's sting, as well as treatment methods – for example, blocking blood vessels combined with magic spells and talismans; see Amar and Buchman (2006: 79–84, 258–60, 284). An analysis of the information indicates that it is based on a compilation of material from early treatises on theriac such as those by Galen and Maimonides.

74 This term has undergone several changes throughout history; see, for example, Ben-Ya'akov (1992: I.103, 108, 204, 210, 316): among Persian Jews theriac is a synonym for opium.

Amar, Z., and Lev, E. 2000a. *Physicians, Drugs and Remedies in Jerusalem from the 10th to the 18th Centuries*. Tel-Aviv: Eretz [in Hebrew].

Amar, Z., and Lev, E. 2000b. 'Traditional Medicinal Substances in 19th Century Jerusalem According to Titus Tobler', *Harefua* 138: 604–7 [in Hebrew].

Amar, Z., and Lev, E. 2017. *Arabian Drugs in Early Medieval Mediterranean Medicine*. Edinburgh: Edinburgh University Press.

Amar, Z., and Serri, Y. 2003. 'Ibn al-Ṣūrī, Physician and Botanist of al-Shām', *Palestine Exploration Quarterly* 135: 124–30.

Amar, Z., and Serri, Y. 2004. *The Land of Israel and Syria according to al-Tamīmī's Description*. Ramat Gan: Bar Ilan University Press [in Hebrew].

Amar, Z., and Serri, Y. eds. 2019. *Maimonides, Treatise on Poisons and the Protection Against Lethal Drugs*. Kiryat Ono: Mekhon Moshe.

al-ʿĀṣī, Ḥ. ed. 1992. *al-Kūhīn al-ʿAṭṭār, Abū al-Munā Dāwud ibn Abī Naṣr al-Isrāʾīlī: Minhāj al-dukkān wa-dustūr al-aʿyān fī aʿmāl wa-tarākīb al-adwiyah al-nāfiʿah lil-abdān*. Beirut: Dār al-Manāhil.

Bacher, W. 1900. *Ein hebräisch-persisches Wörterbuch aus dem vierzehnten Jahrhundert*. Budapest: Adolf Alkalay & Sohn.

Bellorini, T., Hoade, E., and Bagatti, B. eds. 1949. *Fra Francesco Suriano Treatise on the Holy Land*. Jerusalem: Franciscan Press.

Ben Zimra, D. 1882. *Shut Haradbaz*. 2 vols. Warsaw: n.p.

Ben-Yaʿakov, A. 1992. *The Traditional Medicine of the Babylonian Jews*. 2 vols. Jerusalem: Yerid ha-Sfarim [in Hebrew].

Berman, A. 1970. 'The Persistence of Theriac in France', *Pharmacy in History* 12: 5–12.

Bongars, J. ed. 1611. *Gesta Dei per Francos*. Hanover: Apud heredes Ioan Aubrii Wechel.

Bos, G. ed. and tr. 2009. *Maimonides: On Poison and Protection against Lethal Drugs*. Provo, UT: Brigham Young University Press.

Boudon-Millot, V. 2010. 'Aux origines de la thériaque: La recette d'Andromaque', *Revue d'Histoire de la Pharmacie* 58: 261–70.

al-Buqāʿī. ed. 1995. *al-Fīrūzʾābādī, Majd al-Dīn Muḥammad Ibn Yaʿqūb: Al-Qāmūs al-muḥīṭ*. Beirut: Dār al-Kutub al-ʿIlmīyah.

Chavel, Ch. ed. 1958. *Ramban (Nachmanides): Commentary on the Torah*. Jerusalem: Mosad ha-Rav Kụk.

Chen, M. 2019. '"The Healer of All Illnesses": The Origins and Development of Rûm's Gift to the Tang Court: Theriac', *Studies in Chinese Religions* 5/1: 14–37.

Chronicles of the Crusades. 1848. London: H. G. Bohn.

Cohen, A., Simon-Pikali, E., and Salama, O. 1993. *Jews in the Moslem Religious Court: Society, Economics: Communal Organization in Ottoman Jerusalem in the XVIIIth Century*. Jerusalem: Yad Izhak Ben-Zvi [in Hebrew].

Dobroruka, V. 2016. 'Theriac and Tao: More Aspects on Byzantine Diplomatic Gifts to Tang China', *Journal of Literature and Art Studies* 6.2: 170–7.

Dunsky, S. ed. 1973. *Midrash Rabbah: Shir Hashirim*. Montreal: Northern Printing and Lithograph Company.

Goeje, M. J. de ed. 1906. *al-Muqaddasī: ʾAḥsan al-Taqāsīm fī Maʿrifat al-ʾAqālīm*. Leiden: Brill.

Greenbaum, A. ed. 1978. *The Biblical Commentary of Rav Samuel ben Hofni Gaon*. Jerusalem: Mossad Harav Kook.

Groote, E. von ed. 1860. *Die Pilgerfahrt des Ritters Arnold von Harff*. Cologne: J. M. Heberle.

Gunther, R. T. trans. 1959. *The Greek Herbal of Dioscorides*. New York: Hafner.

Halachot Ketanot. 1704. Venice: n.p.

Ḥarb, M. ed. 2006. *Evliya Çelebi: Al-Riḥlah ʾilā Miṣr wa-l-Sūdān wa-l-Ḥabashah*. Cairo: Dār al-ʾĀfāq al-ʿArabīyah.

Hārūn ʿAbd al-Salām,M. ed. 1965. *al-Jāḥiẓ, al-Baṣrī, Abū ʿUthmān ʿAmru ibn Baḥr: Kitāb al-ḥayawān*. Cairo: Muṣṭafā al-Bābī al-Ḥalabī.

Ḥasan, M. Y., and Khafājī, M. B. eds. 1977. *al-Tīfāshī, ʾAḥmad ibn Yūsuf: Kitāb ʾazhār al-ʾafkār fī jawāhir al-ʾaḥjār*. Cairo: al-Hayʾah al-Miṣrīyah al-ʿĀmmah li-l-Kitāb.

Huygens, R. B. C. ed. 1986. *Guillaume de Tyr Chronique: Corpus Christianorum Continuatio*. 2 vols. Turnhout: Brepols.

Ibn al-Athīr. 1994. *Al-Lubāb fī tahdhīb al-ansāb*. 3 vols. Beirut: Dār Ṣādir.

Ibn al-Bayṭār, Ḍiyāʾ al-Dīn ʿAbdallāh ibn Aḥmad. 1874. *Al-Jāmiʿ li-mufradāt al-adwiyah wa-l-aghdhiyah*. 4 vols. Bulaq: n.p.

Issa Bey, A. 1930. *Dictionnaires des Noms des Plantes*. Cairo: Imprimerie Nationale.

Kafih, Y. ed. 1984. *Saadya Gaon's Commentaries on the Torah*. Jerusalem: Mossad Harav Kook.

Kafih, Y. ed. 1984–96. *Moses Maimonides: Mishne Torah*. 23 vols. Jerusalem: Mekhon Moshe.

Katzenellenbogen, M. L. ed. 1986. *Rabbi David Kimhi: Commentary on the Torah in Torat Haiim*. 7 vols. Jerusalem.

al-Khaṭṭābī al-ʿArabī, M. 1990. *Al-Aghdhiyah wa-l-adwiyah ʿinda muʾallifī al-gharb al-islāmī – madkhal wa-nuṣūṣ*. Beirut: Dar al-Gharb al-Islami.

Leiser, G., and Dols, M. 1988. 'Evliya Chelebi's Description of Medicine in Seventeenth-Century Egypt', *Sudhoffs Archiv* 72: 49–68.

Lev, E. 2002a. *Medicinal Substances of the Medieval Levant*. Tel Aviv: Eretz [in Hebrew].

Lev, E. 2002b. 'The Doctrine of Signature in the Medieval and Ottoman Levant', *Vesalius* 8.1: 13–22.

Lev, E., and Amar, Z. 2008. *Practical* Materia Medica *of the Medieval Eastern Mediterranean according to the Cairo Geniza*. Leiden: Brill.

Lewis, B. 1953. 'An Arabic Account of the Province of Safad – 1', *Bulletin of the School of Oriental and African Studies* 15: 477–88.

Lippert, J. ed. 1903. *Ibn al-Qifṭī, Jamāl al-Dīn Abū al-Ḥasan ʿAlī ibn Yūsuf: Tārīkh al-ḥukamāʾ*. Leipzig: Dieterich'sche Verlagsbuchhandlung.

Marx, F. ed. 1915. *A. Cornelii Celsi quae supersunt*. Leipzig: Teubner.

Mas Latrie, L. de. ed. 1871. *Chronique D'Ernoul et de Bernard le Trésorier*. Paris: Mme Ve J. Renouard.

Mayhoff, K., and Jan, L. eds. 1875–1906. *C. Plinii Secundi Naturalis historiae libri XXXVII*. 5 vols. Leipzig: B. G. Teubner.

Mayor, A. 2010. *The Poison King: The Life and Legend of Mithradates, Rome's Deadliest Enemy*. Princeton, NJ: Princeton University Press.

Mehren, A. F. M. van ed. 1923. *al-Dimashqī, Shams al-Dīn, Muḥammad ibn Abī Ṭālib: Nukhbat al-dahr fī ʿajāʾib al-barr wa-l-baḥr*. Leipzig: Harrassowitz.

Meyerhof, M. 1940. *Un glossaire de matière médicale arabe composé par Maïmonide*. Cairo: Imprimerie de l'Institut Francais d'Archeologie Orientale.

Mez-Mangold, L. 1989. *A History of Drugs*. Basle: Editiones Roche.

Muntner, S. ed. 1942. *Moses Maimonides: Treatise on Poisons and Their Antidotes*. Jerusalem: Reuvn Mas.

Muṣṭafā, M. ed. 1984. *Ibn ʾIyās, Muḥammad ibn Aḥmad: Badāʾiʿ al-zuhūr fī waqāʾiʿ al-duhūr*. 4 vols. Cairo: Dār Iḥyāʾ al-Kutub al-ʿArabīyah.

Nutton, V. 1997. 'Galen on Theriac: Problems of Authenticity', in A. Debru (ed.), *Galen on Pharmacology: Philosophy, History and Medicine*. Leiden: Brill, 133–52.

Palestine Pilgrims' Text Society Library. 1890–7. 13 vols. London: Committee for the Palestine Exploration Fund.

Rosner, F., and Muntner, S. eds. and trans. 1970. *Moses Maimonides: The Medical Aphorisms of Moses Maimonides*. New York: Yeshiva University Press.

Rousseau, N. 2021. 'Des *Thériaques* (Θηριακά) à "la thériaque" (θηριακή): Formation et histoire du terme', in V. Boudon-Millot and F. Micheaeu (eds.), *Histoire, transmission et acculturation de la Thériaque. Actes du colloque de Paris (18 mars 2010)*. Paris: Beauchesne, 39–75.

Rubin, J. 2014. 'The Use of the "Jericho *Tyrus*" in the Theriac: A Case Study in the History of the Exchanges of Medical Knowledge between Western Europe and the Realm of Islam in the Middle Ages', *Medium Ævum* 83.2: 234–53.

Saʿd, F. ed. 1985. *al-Qazwīnī, Zakariyyā ibn Muḥammad: ʿAjāʾib al-makhlūqāt wa-gharāʾib al-mawjūdāt*. Beirut: Dār al-ʾĀfāq al-Jadīdah.

Said, H. M., and Elahie, R. E. eds. and trans. 1973. *Al-Biruni's Book on Pharmacy and* Materia Medica. Karachi: Hamdard.

Savage-Smith, E., Swain, S., and van Gelder, G. J., eds. 2020. *A Literary History of Medicine: The ʿUyūn al-anbāʾ fī ṭabaqāt al-aṭibbāʾ of Ibn Abī Uṣaybiʿah*. 5 vols. Leiden: Brill. https://scholarlyeditions.brill.com/reader/urn:cts:arabicLit:0668IbnAbiUsaibia.Tabaqatalatibba.lhom-ed-ara1:10.64; https://scholarlyeditions.brill.com/reader/urn:cts:arabicLit:0668IbnAbiUsaibia.Tabaqatalatibba.lhom-tr-eng1:10.64 (accessed 21 January 2022).

Serri, Y. 2007. 'Arabic Medical Dictionaries from the Ninth to the Thirteenth Centuries: Their Development, Components and Sources and Their Reflection in Ibn Biklārish's and Ibn Al-Suwaydī's Treatises'. Bar-Ilan University, Ramat Gan, Israel: PhD Thesis [in Hebrew].

Serri, Y., and Amar, Z. 2002. 'A letter concerning Theriac from Ashkelon', in A. Sasson, Z. Safrai, and N. Sagiv (eds.), *Ashkelon: Bride of the South*. Tel Aviv: be-aḥarayut akạdemit shel Universitạt Bar-Ilan, 49–58.

Shemesh, A. O. 2001–2. 'Use of Cures from Animals Organs according to the Halachic Literature from the Sixteenth Century till the Present', *Korot*, 15: 92–119 [in Hebrew].

Shemesh, A. O. 2013. *Medical Materials in Medieval and Modern Jewish Literature: Pharmacology, History and Halakha*. Ramat Gan: Bar Ilan University Press [in Hebrew].

Swiderski, R. 2010. *Poison Eaters: Snakes, Opium, Arsenic, and the Lethal Show*. Boca Raton, FL: Universal.

Totelin, M. V. L. 2004, 'Mithridates' Antidote: A Pharmacological Ghost', *Early Science and Medicine* 9: 1–19.

Watson, G. 1966. *Theriac and Mithridatum*. London: Wellcome Historical Medical Library.

Wilkinson, J. 1977. *Jerusalem Pilgrims before the Crusaders*. Jerusalem: Aris & Phillips.

Zahalon, J. 1683. *Otsar ha-Ḥayim*. Venice: Nella stamparia Vendramina.

Zucker, M. ed. and tr. 1984. *Saadya's Commentary on Genesis*. New York: Jewish Theological Seminary of America.

CHAPTER 6

'Already Verified'

A Hebrew Herbal between Text and Illustration

Sivan Gottlieb

Plants have been used as medicinal substances since prehistoric times.[1] According to George Lawrence, a herbal is 'a book on plants of real or alleged medicinal properties, which describes the appearance of those plants and provides information on their medicinal importance and use'.[2] Written knowledge about medicinal plants is based on folklore passed from generation to generation by word of mouth.[3] The illustrations of medicinal plants known to us from antiquity were added soon after the transmission of such texts began and have a continuous lineage.[4] The Jews, like their neighbours, preserved knowledge about medicinal plants in their writings and illustrations. In the Middle Ages, original pharmacological works were written in Hebrew,[5] or translated into Hebrew from Arabic or Latin.[6] An illuminated Hebrew manuscript about plants from northern Italy (Paris, Bibliothèque Nationale, MS hébr. 1199, hereinafter 'the Hebrew herbal'), dated to the late fifteenth century, will be the focus of this chapter. This manuscript, neither the texts nor the illustrations of which have been fully researched so far, is unique in the corpus of illuminated Hebrew medical manuscripts[7] because

I am grateful to Sarit Shalev-Eyni and Orly Lewis for their critical reading of an earlier version of this chapter and their valuable insights. I would also like to express my thanks to Petros Bouras-Vallianatos and Dionysios Stathakopoulos, the organisers of the King's College conference 'Drugs in the Medieval World' and editors of this volume, and the attendees of the conference for their useful comments. The publication of this chapter was supported by the PhD Honors program at the Jack, Joseph and Morton Mandel School for Advanced Studies in the Humanities of the Hebrew University of Jerusalem and by the Memorial Foundation for Jewish Culture.

[1] Lev and Amar (2008: 58). [2] Lawrence (1965: 3). [3] Arber (2010: XXV).

[4] Collins (2000: 25); Telesko (2001: 10).

[5] For example, the *Sefer 'Asaph* (*Book of Asaph*) or *Sefer ha-yakar* (*Precious Book*) by Shabbethai Donnolo. Hebrew became the scientific language for medical and scientific works from the twelfth century onwards, but these two works were written earlier. See Caballero-Navas (2005: 276).

[6] Caballero-Navas (2005: 275).

[7] My corpus of illuminated Hebrew medical manuscripts includes, to date, seventy-nine illuminated manuscripts from fourteenth- to sixteenth-century Europe. The manuscripts differ in the texts they contain and in the quality, number, style, and subjects of their illuminations.

of the number of its illustrations and because it is also associated with a specific group of Latin manuscripts. This group clearly demonstrates the connections between different cultures and populations and how pharmacological knowledge was shared and transmitted between them and changed accordingly.

This chapter will look at the practical use of the Hebrew herbal by its medieval readers. One of the fundamental problems in the history of medicine is bridging the gap between written theoretical works and the reality of daily practice.[8] This manuscript, with its texts and illustrations, enables us to discuss the gap between theoretical and practical medicine, as well as how multiple aspects of this discrepancy can be glimpsed in the original version of the manuscript and the comments and additions related to this subject added by subsequent owners. Aspects of the connection between pharmacology and magic, astrology, alchemy, and religion are also revealed from its texts. Before discussing this question, I will introduce the herbal tradition and the group of manuscripts called the Alchemical Herbals, in the course of which the Hebrew herbal will be analysed and another manuscript will be considered as an additional example of Jewish involvement.

6.1 A Short History of Herbals in the Latin West

The familiar source and origin of the herbal tradition, commonly known by its Latin name, *De materia medica*, was written by the Greek physician Dioscorides in the first half of the first century CE.[9] This treatise and the *Herbarium* of Pseudo-Apuleius were the two main herbal compilations used throughout the Western world and in much of the Middle East and the source of many illustrations of medical plants up until the thirteenth century.[10]

Each entry of Dioscorides' *De materia medica* contains the name or names of the plant, its description, medicinal uses, recipes with dosages, dietetic hints, and sometimes tests for false preparations.[11] There were at least three Latin translations of this treatise before the Renaissance, and in two forms – one was organised into five books, like the original Greek treatise, and the other was alphabetical. In the last centuries of the Middle Ages, Dioscorides was most frequently transmitted in the Latin West as a re-elaborated alphabetical treatise whose origin was not known with

[8] Shaw and Welch (2011: 236). [9] Stannard (1999b: 214).
[10] Collins (2000: 25); Telesko (2001: 10). [11] Stannard (1999b: 214–15).

certainty. The Latin *Alphabetical Dioscorides* was widely copied in the Middle Ages and sometimes abridged by later physicians.[12]

The second source is the Latin *Herbarium*, attributed to the fourth-century author Pseudo-Apuleius (Apuleius Platonicus). This herbal contains about 130 chapters specifying the medicinal uses of many plants. Each chapter is dedicated to one plant with its illustration and contains its name or names and medicinal uses. The text is based on Greek and Latin sources. As we can see from the large number of surviving copies (about sixty, most of them illustrated), this work became very widespread, above all in the ninth century.[13] The illustrations in these copies followed traditions of copying and 'lost' their 'truth to nature' – that is, they no longer resemble the form of the plants in nature.[14]

At the end of the thirteenth century a new illustrated herbal was compiled, called *Tractatus de herbis* (*Treatise on Herbs*). This work was a combination of the aforementioned works with other treatises. One of them, which became very popular in the Middle Ages, is known from its opening words as *Circa instans* or *Liber de simplici medicina* (*Book on Simple Drugs*). This is an alphabetic treatise on drugs and compounds, composed in twelfth-century Salerno and attributed to Matthaeus Platearius.[15] In terms of the illustrations, we see a return to the observation of nature in order to create something more scientific,[16] as well as genre scenes.[17]

According to Minta Collins, from the end of the fourteenth century to the beginning of the sixteenth century many new compilations were composed and many individual herbals were illustrated. In the fifteenth century we witness two different trends in illustrations. One is the development of plant illustrations that go back to the observation of nature. The other is the continued copying of earlier traditions of illustration. We may assume that the original plant illustrations were based on the observation of nature for practical and scientific purposes, but as they were repeatedly appropriated by others, the images of the plants became schematic and almost unrecognisable.[18] It is possible that their main purpose was to provide a decorative representation of the plant and to preserve previous

[12] Stannard (1999b: 215); Cronier (2013: 81–3). On illustrated herbals of Dioscorides, see Mavroudi (Chapter 4) in this volume.

[13] D'Imperio (1978: 73); Collins (2000: 179); Fischer (2013: 36).

[14] Collins (2000: 168, 177, 179, 186). [15] Lawrence (1965: 9–10); Ventura (2015: 255, 259).

[16] The approach to representing 'truth to nature' in scientific images has changed over the centuries. See, for example, Daston and Galison (1992).

[17] Jones (1984: 87). [18] Ragazzini (1983: 72); Collins (2000: 26, 278, 307).

illustrations according to the tradition. In later manuscripts one can see that in some cases the texts were left out and the plant illustrations were copied alone, which created 'picture books'.[19]

6.2 The Alchemical Herbals

The name Alchemical Herbals is used to describe a group of manuscripts in which alchemy is connected with medicine.[20] As we will see, the connection with alchemy was observed as far back as the sixteenth century, but this term was coined only in 2000. The name emerged from the heading of a short paragraph describing the group in Minta Collins's book on medieval herbals.[21]

This group of manuscripts belongs to the second trend discussed here, but it constitutes a specific tradition of herbal texts and illustrations. The manuscripts in the group were copied most frequently in fifteenth-century Italy.[22] In rare instances, the place of origin, date, and owner of the herbals are known. In a book published in 1983 Stefania Ragazzini identified eighteen manuscripts in this group,[23] while in 2000 Vera Segre Rutz increased the number to twenty-four. Segre Rutz divided the manuscripts into direct and indirect traditions (the Hebrew herbal is mentioned as part of the indirect tradition).[24] The direct tradition originated from the same Latin source (X) from which two different copies arose (Y and Z). None of them have survived. Three copies were created from Y and four from Z.[25]

The Alchemical Herbals are a distinctive and homogenous group which has no significant textual variations, and the images they contain vary for the most part only due to the skill of the illustrator.[26] Differences exist in the page layout. In the Y tradition the text and illustration of the plant are on the same page, whereas in the Z tradition the illustrations of the plants

[19] Collins (2000: 307, 310).

[20] The following overview is based on Ragazzini (1983), Collins (2000), and Segre Rutz (2000).

[21] Collins (2000: 279). [22] Collins (2000: 279).

[23] Ragazzini (1983). This book focuses on one manuscript from the group: Florence, Biblioteca dipartimentale di Botanica dell'Università, MS 106.

[24] Segre Rutz (2000: LXX–LXXXIX).

[25] Segre Rutz (2000: XC). Y: Paris, Bibliothèque Nationale, MS Lat. 17844; Paris, Bibliothèque Nationale, MS Lat. 17848; Vicenza, Biblioteca Bertoliana, MS G.23.2.3 (362). Z: Oxford, Bodleian Library, MS Canon. Misc. 408; Pavia, Biblioteca Universitaria, MS Aldini 211; Fermo, Biblioteca Comunale, MS 18; Florence, Biblioteca dipartimentale di Botanica dell'Università MS 106.

[26] When I use the term 'Alchemical Herbals' here, it is in reference to the direct tradition. The indirect tradition, although part of the group, has variations in the order of the plants and in the texts. The Hebrew manuscript is very close to the direct tradition.

take up a full page, with the related texts concentrated on separate pages. In these cases, the name of the plant is accompanied by a number that helps the reader find the relevant text. As we will see, in both traditions, the illustrations are given priority over the texts.

The text of the Alchemical Herbals represents a textual form typical of northern Italy, though the author is unknown.[27] It is probably an original work that is a combination of several herbal traditions and standard works from the Middle Ages presenting the medical uses of plants.[28] The little research done in this field up to now has focused on attempts to identify the plants. In Ragazzini's study only fifteen were identified with certainty.[29] More plants were identified in Segre Rutz's study, but the identification was also based on the illustrations.[30] However, the external characteristics of the plants are lacking in the texts and the illustrations. The latter are so schematic that they are hardly recognisable and the titles are helpful only in identifying several possible plants.[31]

These manuscripts are characterised by particular illustrations of plants, in which their roots, which in general contain the elements effective in healing,[32] are the focus of the illustrations. The roots usually appear in geometric, zoomorphic, or anthropomorphised forms. The aesthetic of the image does not rely on being true to nature, but on a symmetrical approach. The repetition of the same elements in the images, with their simplicity and clarity, without a doubt contributed to the popularity of these illustrated herbals and to the creation of a consistent and homogenous tradition.[33] But despite the widespread circulation of the Alchemical Herbals, it seems that this group did not, in fact, continue into the era of printing.[34] Ninety-eight chapters, one for each plant, appearing in the same consistent and specific order in all of the manuscripts, unite the Alchemical Herbals group.[35] The order is not alphabetical, as is characteristic of traditional herbals. In addition to these shared plants, every manuscript in the group includes extra plants, probably from another tradition.

Alchemy began in the first century BCE. One of its purposes was to discover how to transmute compounds into noble metals, especially gold. Another aim was to search for the elixir of immortality.[36] Few sources

[27] Ragazzini (1983: 8); Segre Rutz (2000: LXIII). [28] Bertiz (2003: 55). [29] Ragazzini (1983: 61).
[30] Segre Rutz (2000: LX). [31] Ragazzini (1983: 61); Collins (2000: 26).
[32] Segre Rutz (2000: XLIV). [33] Segre Rutz (2000: XLIV, XLVII, LXII).
[34] Segre Rutz (2000: LXV).
[35] Segre Rutz (2000: XV). For the list of ninety-eight plant names, see, for example, http://philipneal.net/voynichsources/alchemical, accessed 15 March 2020.
[36] Von Stuckrad (2006: 485).

explicitly mention which plants were in use in alchemy, and plants were used less than minerals in the alchemical process.[37] Ragazzini, and more particularly Segre Rutz in her book entitled *Il giardino magico degli alchimisti*, clearly refer to this connection, mentioning the external evidence for the association between alchemy and plants in these manuscripts that have come down to us from some sixteenth-century naturalists, who cite a few plants as being used by alchemists.[38] The naturalist and collector Ulisse Aldrovandi (1522–1605) had in his possession four manuscripts from the group in the indirect tradition.[39] In two of them the original sixteenth-century bindings contain the inscription *PIANTE DEGLI ALCHIMISTI* ('Plants of the Alchemists'), another bears the name *Plan. Luna*,[40] while in the fourth, apart from the plant names and illustrations, there are only two more words *Chimistarum* or *Alch*.[41] The assumption is that these manuscripts represent a selection of plants with desirable properties considered useful in alchemy and their function was to help physicians practise alchemy.[42] In examining one manuscript from the group,[43] Segre Rutz shows different alchemical aspects of the plants appearing in the manuscripts. For example, regarding the plant *Lunaria*, which appears four times in the list of the ninety-eight plants, alongside its medicinal uses it is also reported that alchemists believed it had the ability to transmute base metals into gold and silver. Conrad Gesner was a sixteenth-century naturalist who wrote about *Lunaria*'s value to alchemists.[44] In addition, some terms used in these texts can be read metaphorically as being related to alchemy. For example, the term 'snakebite' can be construed as meaning 'metal contamination'.[45]

Some thirteenth-century works reveal the extent to which pharmacy and alchemy were interwoven in the Middle Ages,[46] and the use of herbs was essential in both fields.[47] But from the late thirteenth century onwards the prohibition on practising alchemy expanded, and by the beginning of the fourteenth century alchemy was discussed in coded language, intended to keep outsiders in the dark. However, we must be careful not to attribute some alchemical meaning to these plants purely on the basis of

[37] Segre Rutz (2000: LXVIII). [38] Ragazzini (1983: 12); Segre Rutz (2000: XXVII).

[39] Bologna, Biblioteca Universitaria, Museo Aldrovandiano, MS 124 (151[1]; 151[2]; 152; 153).

[40] This appears to be an abbreviation of *Plant Lunaria*, but this is my speculation only.

[41] Segre Rutz (2000: XXVII–XXVIII). [42] Segre Rutz (2000: XXVII, LXVII).

[43] Pavia, Biblioteca Universitaria, MS Aldini 211. [44] Segre Rutz (2000: XXVIII).

[45] Segre Rutz (2000: XXXVII).

[46] Segre Rutz (2000: LXVI). For example, *Speculum doctrinale* (*Mirror of Doctrine*) by Vincent of Beauvais and *De erroribus medicorum* (*On Errors of Doctors*) by Roger Bacon.

[47] Henderson and Sherwood (2003: 26).

assumptions.[48] When looking at alchemical illustrations, it seems that they also depicted different instruments in different processes, some scenes and androgynous figures.[49] Those characteristic illustrations are missing from the group. The combination of different ingredients is an important element in the alchemical process and sometimes it is depicted as a mystical 'wedding' of opposed elements. Moon elements represent the female and sun elements the male. Their perfect union creates the hermaphrodite.[50]

However, to date, no alchemical manuscript has been found that could explain the connection between the manuscripts in this group. In fact, despite being labelled 'Alchemical Herbals', medicine is the predominant feature of the plants they describe. The texts focus on the healing of injuries, eye infections, liver and spleen problems, skin problems, and fertility, to list just a few examples, but they lack technical details on the preparation of the recipes.[51] Alchemy, magic, folklore, and superstition are also present.[52] Parts of some plants are used as amulets. In these cases, the plants are attributed with magical power, believed to contain hidden qualities that would be transferred to the wearer. This can also be categorised as popular belief.[53] Several types of treatment were available in the European Middle Ages, and people searched for cures by different methods, some of which were not the 'scientific' method of the time – for example, by magical means as well. Medical and what we might refer to as non- or quasi-medical methods often used the same materials for healing purposes. Thus, the line between rational and non-rational medicine is not so clear and distinct in this period.[54]

In the literature, the Alchemical Herbals are classified with manuals for physicians and pharmacists.[55] In addition to the physicians who used books in their practice, such manuals were also essential to the work of pharmacists. In antiquity it was the collectors (i.e. those who went out and gathered the herbs) who were responsible for the plants' preparation as medicine. During the Middle Ages pharmacists prepared drugs, mainly

[48] Segre Rutz (2000: XIII, XVII–XVIII, LXVII–LXVIII).

[49] One manuscript that is considered alchemical, for example, is from 1461, Milano: Pavia, Biblioteca Universitaria, MS Aldini 74. Another is München, Bayerische Staatsbibliothek Cgm 598, after 1467.

[50] http://special.lib.gla.ac.uk/exhibns/month/april2009.html, accessed 15 March 2020.

[51] Segre Rutz (2000: XX). [52] Collins (2000: 166).

[53] Telesko (2001: 21); Trachtenberg (2004: 206).

[54] Lev and Amar (2008: 54); Shoham-Steiner (2012: 42); Shemesh (2013: 35). For a discussion of the relation between medicine and magic in the Middle Ages, see, for example, Thorndike (1929–58) and Kieckhefer (1989). On the interrelationship between medicine and magic, see also Liebermann (Chapter 8) and Lewicka (Chapter 9) in the present volume.

[55] Segre Rutz (2000: LXVII).

complex compounds, while relatively simple combinations were probably made at home using basic kitchen equipment. But it was not uncommon for physicians to prepare their own medicines in the Middle Ages.[56] Whether or not these manuscripts were actually manuals for the successful gathering of plants, the group's name and the illustrations raise questions about their role and the role of the illustrations. Texts and illustrations usually work together, illustrations were added not only to glorify or to emphasise the structure of the manuscript but also to add information not included in the texts, or clarify them. In the case of the Alchemical Herbals, one possible role could be as *aides-mémoire* for a plant's uses – that is, the illustration would help a reader remember the use mentioned in the accompanying text. The people of the Middle Ages were aware of the value of visual aids.[57] Another role would be to add the visual aspect and preserve the tradition of herbals that combined texts and plant illustrations. Establishing the role of the illustrations in the manuscripts is part of a bigger discussion about the connection between text and illustrations in general.[58] The centrality of the plants, their independence from the text and the focus on the roots shows that their medical role was known at the time and the aim from the beginning was to create a format that gave pride of place to the plants.

6.3 The Hebrew Herbal (Paris, Bibliothèque Nationale, MS hébr. 1199)

The Hebrew herbal is undoubtedly part of this group and it belongs to the indirect tradition deriving from the Z group of manuscripts. Florence, Biblioteca dipartimentale di Botanica dell'Università, MS 106, may be the model for the Hebrew herbal, but it is also possible that the latter was not copied directly from it and that another manuscript that has not survived served as its model.[59] Nonetheless, small changes distinguish the Hebrew herbal from the other manuscripts in the group of the Alchemical Herbals.

56 Telesko (2001: 9); Shaw and Welch (2011: 233). 57 Evans (1980: 34).

58 For further reading, see, for example, Weitzmann (1947), Camille (1989), and Kupfer, Chajes, and Cohen (2020). For this connection specifically in the sciences, see, for example, Murdoch (1984).

59 There are several indications that the two manuscripts are connected. As regards illustrations, the Florentine manuscript is the only one to include all the illustrations that appear in the Hebrew herbal (both the seventy-two alchemical plants and the sixty-one others). There are also resemblances between the illustrations of specific plants. There are also textual similarities. In these two manuscripts the same four plants have no texts in contrast to other manuscripts in the group, where they do have texts. Moreover, the recipe for the plant *Tedorixe*, which is no. 33 according to the list, is inserted near the end of the texts in both manuscripts.

The Hebrew herbal is written on paper, 31 (blank pages) + 74 + 7 (blank pages), 199–200 × 149–50 mm, of which many pages are damaged.[60] The manuscript includes 133 plant illustrations, probably by the same illustrator, with black outlines, painted in watercolour. Here, as in the group generally, the roots are the focus of attention. They are bigger, more detailed, and creatively drawn. For example, the plant called *Lucea et de novem una* has a fish-shaped root (Figure 6.1), and the root of the plant *Illioris* has a human face. The animal or human figures are related to the magical perception of the plants and are an indication of their powers.[61]

In addition to the illustrations, there are 120 plant texts. Most of the textual information about the plants is gathered at the end of the manuscript, in seventeen written pages, starting with each plant's name (Figure 6.2). The

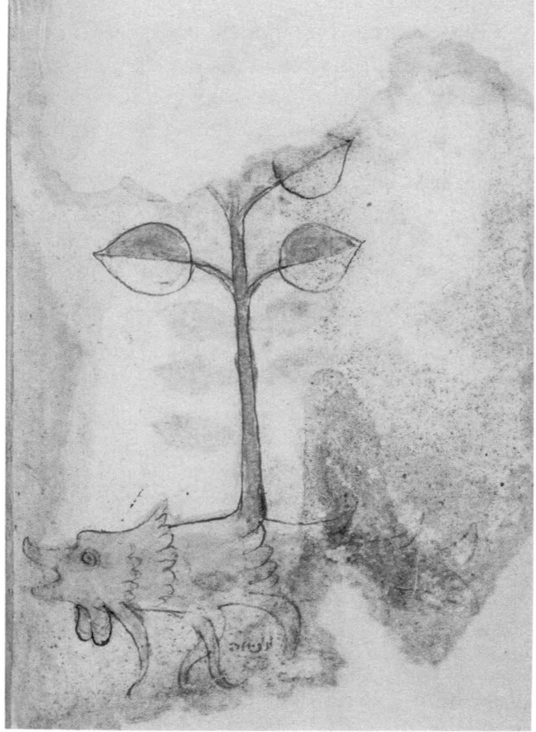

Figure 6.1 Paris, Bibliothèque nationale, MS hébr. 1199, f. 5v

60 Sed-Rajna and Fellous (1994: 306). 61 Segre Rutz (2000: LII).

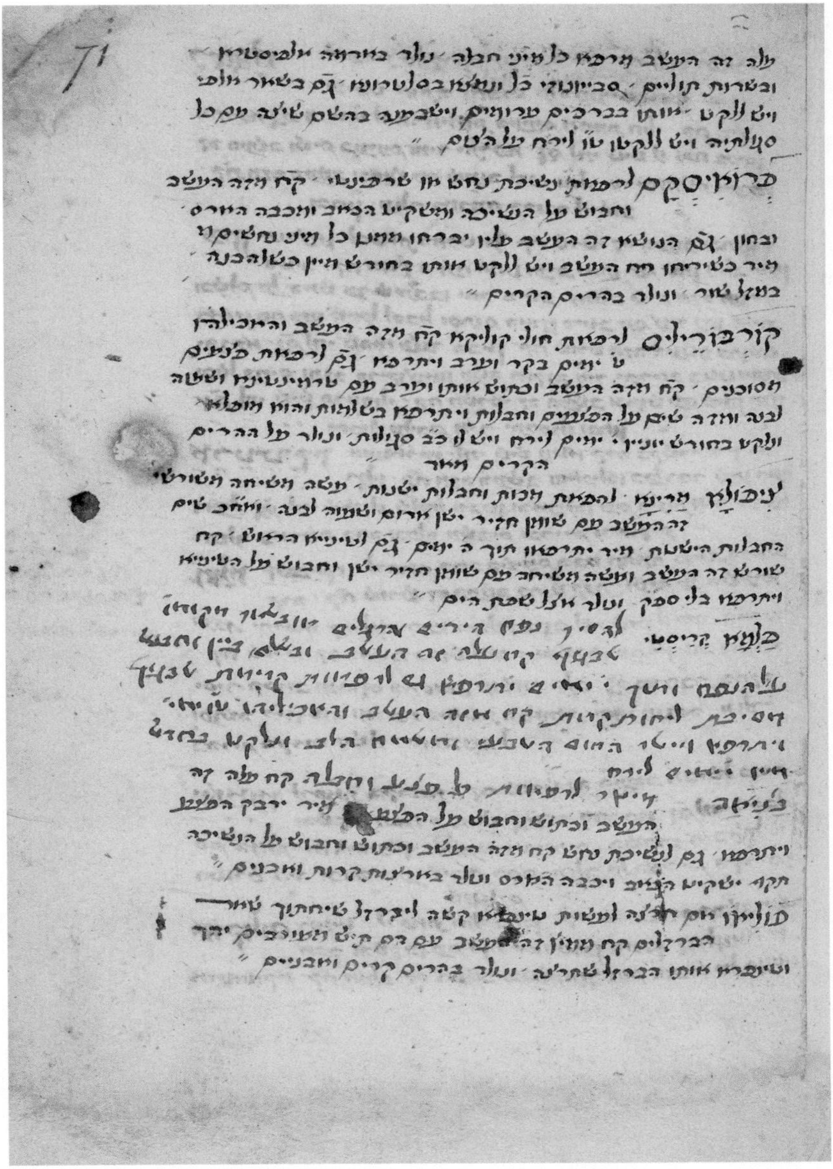

Figure 6.2 Paris, Bibliothèque nationale, MS hébr. 1199, f. 71r

texts on these pages are arranged in the same order, as in the list of the ninety-eight plants in the rest of the Alchemical Herbals group,[62] with the addition of one extra text. On the full-page illustrations, each illustration is accompanied by the corresponding plant's traditional Italian or Latin name in Hebrew letters in various places on the page (on some pages the name appears in Latin letters as well). The order of the illustrations does not follow the order of the plant texts at the end of the manuscript (i.e. the order of the other Alchemical Herbals), perhaps due to rebinding. However, there are additional texts adjacent to twenty-eight plant illustrations. It seems that these texts were added after the illustrations were already completed and thus had to be written in accordance with the plant being illustrated (Figure 6.3). These additions may confirm how the manuscript was used in practice,[63] indicating the plants that were in use at the time the text next to them was added. Some of them appear only in juxtaposition to the illustrations, and some appear twice, with the illustrations and on the relevant page of text at the end of the manuscript.

The text is written in semi-cursive script.[64] There is no colophon or any clues as to the identity of the scribes. It seems that one scribe was responsible for the texts associated with the illustrations; he may have been responsible for the names of the plants too, which are written in slightly larger script. We can identify three different hands in the textual pages at the end. In addition, comments and remarks were added in a different hand in the margins.[65]

As we will see, the texts at the end of the manuscript are translations from Latin with adaptations to Hebrew, while the texts next to the illustrations are similar to the Latin source in content but not in form.[66] The texts next to two illustrations are completely different from the Latin and their source has yet to be identified. Sometimes, the names of the Hebrew plants are different from what they should be according to the Latin, and sometimes there are differences between the names accompanying the illustrations and the names at the end. In the presentation of the texts and illustrations that follows, I will discuss the question at the heart of this research: how is the gap between theoretical medicine and medicine in practice reflected in the Hebrew herbal and the other manuscripts in the group?

[62] The Hebrew texts on these pages continue only up to plant no. 96. Five plant texts from the list are missing (no. 14 – *Toros*; no. 32 – *Amorsu serpentis*; no. 34 – *lucea et de novem una*; no. 79 – *Lunaria*; no. 86 – *Lunaria tercia*), and one is not in the place conventionally allotted to it in the list.

[63] Tomasi and Willis (2009: 11). [64] Sed-Rajna and Fellous (1994: 306).

[65] More palaeographical research on the manuscript is required. It seems that the different hands used throughout the manuscript include non-square and even cursive Ashkenazi and Italian scripts.

[66] In these manuscripts, both the Hebrew and the Latin is poor. The Hebrew herbal contains mistakes in grammar and spelling. The Latin language has been discussed in reference to two manuscripts from the Alchemical Herbals group in Bühler (1954).

6.3.1 The Texts

Toffanas – To heal lung disease. Take this herb and the herb called Istatoris, mix them together and cook them with eggs, eat this for fifteen days, and you will be healed. It has been tested and proven. Similarly, for wounded hands and legs, and throughout the body, or wounded sinews. Take this herb and pound it with the fat of a bear, and afterwards put it on the wound, the wound will be cured instantly. It grows in the cold and herb-filled Alps.[67]

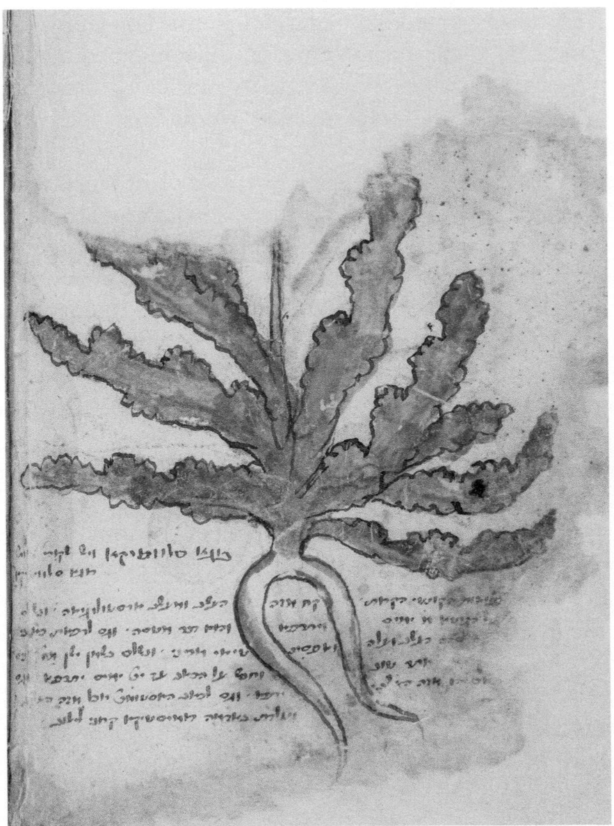

Figure 6.3 Paris, Bibliothèque nationale, MS hébr. 1199, f. 2v

[67] See the appendix for the text in Hebrew, Latin, and translations of both into English.

This is the text that appears in the manuscript for the plant *Toffanas*,[68] which is good for lung disease and wounds. It is a representative example of the texts in the manuscript. Like this passage, the other texts about plants (see the chapter's appendix for more examples) are short and focus on the essential information needed for healing. As in all the Alchemical Herbals, in the Hebrew herbal medical uses predominate and 282 medicinal uses are given for the plants, as opposed to forty-five magical ones. There is no uniformity regarding the length of the text or the information included in it. The number of cures associated with each plant also varies.[69] As we will see shortly, the text in the Hebrew herbal and in the other manuscripts of the group provides a glimpse, although it may on occasion be somewhat obscure, of different medical theories and principles according to which physicians in medieval Europe might have worked.[70] In addition, the texts include words that indicate empirical examination.

Besides the plant name, the texts begin with each plant's medicinal function. *Le-rappot*/*Le-refoʾat* ('to heal')[71] is usually the opening formula of the texts at the end of the manuscript, as in the example just provided. In the texts juxtaposed with the illustrations, the formula is different: *ze ha-ʿesev ṭov*/*ṭova* ('this herb is good [for]').[72] The most common use of the plants in the manuscript is for injuries and wounds, appearing with reference to thirty-one plants, while the second most common is for eye problems (fifteen references).

Only eight texts also mention the reasons for the patient's illness. Among them, the theory of the four humours is mentioned explicitly in relation to three plants. For example, phlegm is mentioned in relation to the plant *Sigillo de Sancta Maria* as: *ḳrirut be-gufo mi-ḥamat leḥa levana* ('coldness in his body due to phlegm').[73] This inclusion gives the manuscript a theoretical basis and connects it with the texts of the traditional herbals, which include the qualities and degrees of the substances that are missing in the Hebrew herbal.

The next part of the text is the actual recipe. The texts usually continue with the part of the plant that needs to be used. In the Hebrew texts the general rule is to use the words *ḳaḥ mi-ze ha-ʿesev* ('take this herb'),[74] without referring to a specific part of the plant. But

[68] The plant *Toffanas* is located in the twenty-eighth place in the list of ninety-eight plants and is identified as *Sanicula europaea*: Segre Rutz (2000: 88).

[69] Collins (2000: 166). [70] Shemesh (2013: 41).

[71] לרפאת/לרפואת. For example, the plants *Tortorillis*, *Trifolio*, *Ariola*, *Superna*: f. 68v.

[72] זה העשב טוב/זה העשב טובה. For example, the plants *Antolla minor*, f. 16r, and *Brotines*, f. 15v.

[73] קרירות בגופו מחמת ליחה לבנה, f. 72r.

[74] קח מזה העשב. For example, the plants *Betonega*, f. 67v, and *Triacho*, f. 68r.

when the text includes the part of the plant, it is the root that is mentioned most often (twenty-nine times), in accordance with the root's major role in pharmacology.[75] The leaf, seed, and flower also appear, but less often than the root. This part also includes instructions about the use of the plant (external or internal, powder, juice). Internal uses include eating, drinking, and inhaling the plant or its products. External uses (mainly in the form of a poultice or liniment) are more common than internal ones (sixty-six times as opposed to sixty-three). Sometimes there is also a specific recipe based on one plant or a compound. The plants are the main ingredients in the recipes, but in the process of making the drugs different products may be used. For example, in the entry for *Toffanas*, it was mixed and cooked with another herb and with eggs. The use of wine is very popular and is mentioned forty-four times;[76] animal and mineral products such as milk, honey, and salt were also used. We see the use of local names for various ingredients that still need to be deciphered. The recipes are not very detailed about the procedures involved (except in one case), and only nineteen texts have accurate measurements, including ounces and pounds (*litra*). In fact, to modern eyes, it seems that the texts do not provide enough knowledge for accurate preparation and we cannot reconstruct the recipes today according to the text alone, but the reader of the manuscript at the time was expected to have some knowledge or prior acquaintance and practical experience with the subject.[77]

The duration of use is often included as well as other practical instructions. A specific number of days is mentioned in sixty-two texts. Twelve texts state that the patient must fast before taking the drug.

Surprisingly (or perhaps not), considering the Jewish dietary rules (*kashrut*) that ban the consumption of pork, lard appears in eight Hebrew recipes. Using animal products as medicinal substances is a well-known and documented phenomenon in medieval literature. Most religious authorities tended to allow the medicinal use of unclean animal substances when necessary.[78] Dozens of recipes from the Middle Ages prove that they were used in the Jewish community for healing purposes.[79] Interestingly, throughout the Latin texts in this group (of which the Hebrew text was a translation), animals and their products that were unclean (for Jews) were used only externally.

75 Segre Rutz (2000: XLIV).

76 For example, in the plants *Lingua cornena*, f. 68v, and *llocharias*, f. 70r, the herbs need to be cooked with wine.

77 Riddle (1974: 163). 78 Lev and Amar (2008: 53). 79 Shoham-Steiner (2012: 44).

Other uses of a plant are also given in some cases. The use of plants as amulets to be worn on the body appears eighteen times. The purpose of the amulet might be medical, such as preventing injuries, or magical, such as in pursuit of love. The alchemical aspect, with direct reference to the process of transmuting compounds into noble metals, is also seen. As noted, the plant *Lunaria* appears four times in the series of ninety-eight plants, but in the Hebrew herbal this plant and its alchemical uses appear only twice (*Lunaria* for falsifying coins[80] and *Lunaria grega*[81] for making gold).

Towards the end of the entry we are told how to gather the plant. Here we see the astrological lore that constituted acceptable scientific knowledge in the Middle Ages.[82] In twenty-eight texts the optimal time for gathering the plant is included with reference to astrological influences. In six texts the signs of the zodiac are also mentioned. The months are mentioned by their Julian calendar name and not their Hebrew one, which is characteristic of the writings of Italian Jews.[83] In addition, specific, useful instructions for herb gathering are also present in ten texts. Stories about gathering and preparation are known from antiquity,[84] and we will see such a story in the next section. Most of the texts conclude with the plant's habitat. Specific places in Europe, especially the Alps, appear in thirteen texts. Segre Rutz has demonstrated that all the places mentioned by name can be identified in central and northern Italy.[85]

As mentioned, the Hebrew texts are translations from a Latin source, and the different parts of the texts described earlier in this chapter appear in the other manuscripts of the group as well. However, the Jewish scribe modified the Latin source to suit his audience with additions and omissions. In the text pages at the end of the manuscript, the addition of the common Jewish abbreviation *B'H* (*be-ʿezrat ha-shem* – 'with God's help') can be found in six texts.[86] Prayers and recitations that needed to be recited during the act of gathering were changed from the Latin and mentions of Christ were translated to Hebrew and adapted to Jewish usage and included the Hebrew words for God. The special prayers are important because, as precautionary measures, they demonstrate the powers the plants were believed to have.[87] The Hebrew text also omits parts of its Latin source. The names of six physicians who, according to the Latin text,

80 לפסול המטבע, f. 72r. The text also includes medicinal and magical use.

81 Two texts appear for this plant but only the text near the illustration includes the alchemy aspect, לעשות זהב, f. 39r. The text on f. 73r includes only magical aspects.

82 Kottek (2012: 27). On astrology in the Middle Ages, see, for example, White (1975).

83 Beit-Arié (2019: 131). 84 Randolph (1905: 489, 491). 85 Segre Rutz (2000: LXIII).

86 בע"ה. See, for example, the plant *Bonifatia*, f. 67v. 87 Segre Rutz (2000: XXV).

had verified the medicinal quality of the plant are removed from the Hebrew version. One of the physicians appears in the Latin entry for the plant *Cofflesanas* under the name and title of *Magistrum Thadeum Florentinum, Doctorem in Artibus Medicinatum*. He has been identified as Taddeo Alderotti, a thirteenth-century physician from Florence. The others are not identified but were probably active in central or northern Italy.[88] In general, Latin plant names that included the word *Sancta* ('Saint') were changed in Hebrew because of the differences in religious perception. For example, the plant called *Sigillo de Sancta Maria* in Latin was altered in Hebrew to *Sigillo Maria* because the Jews did not hold Mary sacred. Other plant names, with Christian meanings but without the word 'saint', were left as they were – for example, *Palma Christi*. Another special Jewish characteristic appears in the plant *Triacho*, when the instructions are the same as in Latin, to eat the plant on an empty stomach, but here they are written in the Talmudic Aramaic language rather than in Hebrew – *aliba reikana*.[89]

It seems that these modifications were made without changing the medical content and that they relate to the connections and conflicts between medicine and religion.[90] The scribe 'Judaises' the text through the omission of non-Jewish authorities and the addition of Jewish religious terms. However, in some cases small changes to the Latin can be crucial.[91] The various changes in these texts can be attributed to the transfer of knowledge between languages, to misunderstanding the source, to using different models of the text, or to different traditions. For example, regarding the plant *Illocharias* (see this chapter's appendix), according to the Hebrew text the plant is cooked with wine, not with eggs, as appears in the Latin. The word *ovis* was translated in this entry as wine,[92] whereas in other places in the manuscript it was translated as eggs. This may result from a misreading of *ovis* as *uvis*, a plural form of *uva*, meaning grape. Another difference may be due to an incorrect understanding of the text. The Hebrew entry for the same plant says: *ve-taḥziḳ be-piykha ḥam kama she-yukhal lisbol* ('keep it warm in your mouth as long as you can bear it')[93] but, although both texts mention the previous cooking of the herb, in

88 *Magistrum Petrum de Perposa et per Magistrum Antonium Romanum* in the entry for *Rucha savlaticha*; *Magistrum Miniatum de Florentia* in the entry for *Illioris*; *Magistrum Nicholaum de Pisiis et per magistrum Donatum de Ianua* in the entry for *Toffanas*: Segre Rutz (2000: XXI).

89 אליבא ריקנא, f. 68r. The same instructions appear also in other plants but in the Hebrew language. This inclusion of Aramaic needs further examination.

90 Shemesh (2013: 518).

91 I want to thank Noam Rytwo for his Latin translation and comments.

92 When the word 'wine' appears in other texts, we can see that it is translated from the word *vino*.

93 ותחזיק בפיך חם כמה שיוכל לסבול, f. 70r.

Latin[94] the reference is to placing the herb on the painful teeth – that is, in the Hebrew version the reference is to the patient and his mouth (in general), while in the Latin it is to the teeth, specifically to 'painful teeth'. We need to keep in mind that the texts were copied from earlier versions and written knowledge shifts over time, so errors in this process are likely. As far back as Pliny scholars were pointing out the negative results of the continuous copying of botanical sources, and he himself mentioned inaccuracies as one of them.[95] But the difference could also be due to a different medical approach. If that is the case, we see the practical nature of the Hebrew herbal here as well because the text was not only translated, but was changed according to the actual approach in use.

The effectiveness of the medical treatment is mentioned in seventy-six entries, often more than once. The words that were commonly used for this included *va-yitrape* ('will be cured').[96] The Latin equivalent is *sanabitur* and its grammatical variants are the most common in recipe texts because they can be applied to any of the remedies.[97] One of the statements that is repeated in the original text for thirty-eight plants and relates to the empirical nature of the knowledge is that the treatment has been examined and found to have worked: *baḥun* ('tested') and *menuse* ('tried')[98]. In Latin the phrase *probatum est* can be found beside medical recipes in other texts as well, like alchemy and magic spells. These words are part of the practical basis of the texts and are very important for the text being recognised as empirical. This was the 'proof' of the period – that is, the action of trying it out without the necessity of effectiveness.[99] In the Hebrew text they have even more significance, especially in light of the removal of the authorities cited in the Latin.

In the Hebrew herbal we find another empirical statement. In the margins of five entries (the entry on *Toffanas* among them), one of the owners has added (in his own handwriting, which differs from the other hands in the manuscript) a short sentence regarding its efficacy: *kvar baduḳ* ('already verified').[100] This later addition indicates that the manuscript was in practical use, especially as regards those plants that contain these

[94] *et postea sic calidam pone super dentem qui patitur dolorem*. Segre Rutz (2000: 118).

[95] Ragazzini (1983: 63); Segre Rutz (2000: XLIX).

[96] ויתרפא . This word is mentioned, for example, in the plants *Sabastrella*, f. 69v, or *Capalias*, f. 73r.

[97] Jones (1998: 202).

[98] בחון ומנוסה; and in Latin *est probatum*. See, for example, the plant *Salsifica*, f. 69v, for the word *Baḥun* or *Illioris*, f. 70v, for the word *Menuse*. The two words appear together in the plant *Toffanas*, f. 69v.

[99] Jones (1998: 199, 203). On efficacy statements, see also Doolittle (Chapter 2), Lewicka (Chapter 9), and Chipman (Chapter 10) in this volume.

[100] כבר בדוק. The other plants that receive this sentence are: *llocharias*, f. 70r, *Luza mandragola*, f.70v, *Capalarices*, f. 72v, and *Granellaria*, f. 74r.

additional words in the margins of the text. The owner has followed the recipes and returned to the manuscript to write down his findings. Whereas the empirical words in the original texts may originate from the copyist's model, meaning that those plants had not necessarily been examined when the manuscript was produced, the owner's additions in the margins confirm the effectiveness and healing properties of the plants. Here, once again, we see that for people of that time, who had some knowledge of medicine, the texts were sufficient to follow and execute the recipes. In addition to the words *kvar baduḳ*, the same owner also added in the margins of two plant entries some abbreviations – that is, key words relating to the plant's medicinal uses, together with a graphic sign. For example, the text for the plant *Mula campana* was accompanied in the margins by the words *le-ke᾿evey ḥaze ṿe-᾿isṭumakha, le-ke᾿evey shinayim* ('for pains in chest and stomach, for toothache').[101] This looks like an index for quick orientation. Another interesting note refers to the plant called in Latin *Sancta Maria*. We have already seen that the scribe 'Judaises' the text when needed. Here we see a later change to the text with the same intent. On the text page, the Hebrew name of the plant has been partially deleted, and what remains is the Hebrew letter *ṭ* and *Maria*.[102] Above the deleted word the owner added two words that are hard to make out. The first word has been deciphered as *ṿa-yis᾿ar*,[103] which might be meant to be *va-ya᾿aser* ('to be forbidden'). Next to the illustration, the name of the plant is *Ḳ-Ṭ Maria*,[104] and above that is another deleted part probably related to the denomination. The *Ḳ-Ṭ* word may be an abbreviation of *Sancta*. It is likely that the addition and deletion were made by the same owner; but even if it was done by someone else, we can still see this as evidence of things that were alien to Jewish culture.

Seven plants overall received special attention from this owner. Despite the impressive number of plants in the manuscripts, only a few were in practical medicinal use. The plants commonly used were selected because of their accessibility, affordable price, and even local medical trends, among other considerations.[105] This owner gives us access to his interests. Although in these seven plants we see different medical and magical issues, references to teeth are prominent and appear in four of these texts. We see that the medical treatment for dental problems is similar throughout, even

101 לכאבי חזה והאיסטומכא, לכאבי שיניים, f. 71v. 102 ט מריא, f. 73r.

103 ויסאר. I am grateful to Yacov Fuchs and Yael Okun from the National Library of Israel, Jerusalem, for their help in deciphering the text.

104 קט מריא, f. 39v. It could also be the letter Ḳ alone with pen decoration, or ligature.

105 Lev and Amar (2008: 21); Shaw and Welch (2011: 256).

if the plants being used are different. One needs to keep the prescribed mixture in the mouth without swallowing it. For almost any ailment there were numerous different recipes in the manuscript texts and the medical decision consisted in selecting the recipe to be used.[106] The physical signs show that this manuscript was in use as a practical medical manual. The different hands in the manuscript demonstrate that each owner added the plants that he was familiar with and used. The names of the plants written in Latin letters indicate the owner's interaction with the surrounding community.

6.3.2 *The Illustrations*

Of the ninety-eight plants included in the Alchemical Herbals, the Hebrew herbal includes seventy-two plant illustrations, as well as some additional ones that do not form part of the series. There are differences between the illustrations in the Hebrew herbal and those in the other manuscripts in the group. Some are due to the artists' skill, but some look deliberate. The practical nature of the texts makes it important to establish what the illustrations mean in this context and the significance of any changes. In what follows I examine the question of the illustrations' practical use based on the example of the plant *Luza Mandragora*, which also contains the words *kvar baduḳ* for efficacy in the margins, added by the aforementioned owner.

> Luza Mandragora – To heal wounds without any ointment. Take the leaves of this herb and pound them and apply to the wounds. After three or four hours you will be cured. And do this for every wound. It has been proven. Likewise, it is helpful for pregnancy. Take this herb and root and give it to the woman to eat as it is, with salt. Immediately after she has eaten it, her husband should be nearby to sleep with her for three nights, and she will be pregnant undoubtedly, and it is collected in the month of May, on the third day of the new moon. It should be dug out of the earth with a dog or with another animal, and see to it, when you dig it out, that you do not touch it. When you pull it, immediately tie its hands and legs with a rope and hang the rope around the dog's neck and stand far away so you will not hear the scream of the mandragora, which is so strong that the dog will die from it.[107]

This plant, known from antiquity and identified as the mandrake, had various important medicinal uses. Dioscorides mentions it and its medical

[106] Riddle (1974: 164).

[107] See the chapter appendix for the text in Hebrew, Latin, and Latin translation into English.

uses for eye problems, encouraging menstruation, causing abortion, and for the treatment of poisons and tumours.[108] It is mentioned in Genesis 30:14–17, where Rachel asks Leah to give her the mandrake Reuben has picked in order that she may conceive. This story increased the plant's reputation as an aid to fertility.[109] And, as we will see, this specific quality mentioned in the text is significant in relation to the illustration. There are twenty-one entries in this manuscript for plants that help with female medical problems such as breastfeeding and uterine issues.[110] Four other plant recipes beside the *Luza Mandragora* are useful in aiding conception.[111] As we saw with toothache, there are different medical solutions to the same problem. In order to conceive, the woman is supposed to eat the plant and having sex is mentioned in three separate entries.

The source of the anthropomorphic mandrake can be found in the writings of Dioscorides and others. Dioscorides distinguishes between two species – male and female – which both have the same medicinal qualities.[112] However, the belief that the forked root looked like the lower half of a human body was not mentioned explicitly before the Middle Ages.[113] There are depictions that represent the anthropomorphic mandrake, without specific gender, with the sex identified only in the accompanying text (Figure 6.4). This plant was also known in the medieval world for its magical uses.[114] The anthropomorphisation of this plant (and others) is connected with magical ideas and the belief in the magical powers of plants.

Dioscorides does not mention a gathering technique for this plant. The process of gathering the mandrake root, described in detail in the second part of the text in the Hebrew herbal, prevailed from the fifth century onwards and created the dominant iconography.[115] This text presents an ancient belief according to which a scream is released by the human-shaped root that causes death to any listener present when the mandrake is picked. In order to avoid a human death, a dog is tied by a chain to the root. When the dog pulls the root out of the ground, it dies instead of the human gatherer.[116]

[108] Lev and Amar (2008: 59, 212). For more on its seductive quantities, see, for example, Randolph (1905); Chidiac, Kaddoum, and Fuleihan (2012).

[109] Chidiac et al. (2012: 1438).

[110] For example, *Antolla minor*, f. 16r and f. 67r, for uterine problems, or *Tortorillis*, f. 67v, for swelling breasts.

[111] These plants are *Spigonarada*, f. 1r, *Ystatoris*, f. 37v and 73v, *Stellaria*, f. 67r, *Bonifatia*, f. 67v.

[112] Ragazzini (1983: 127). [113] Randolph (1905: 494).

[114] Gilbert (2008: 35). See also Randolph (1905). [115] Randolph (1905: 489–91).

[116] Chidiac et al. (2012: 1437).

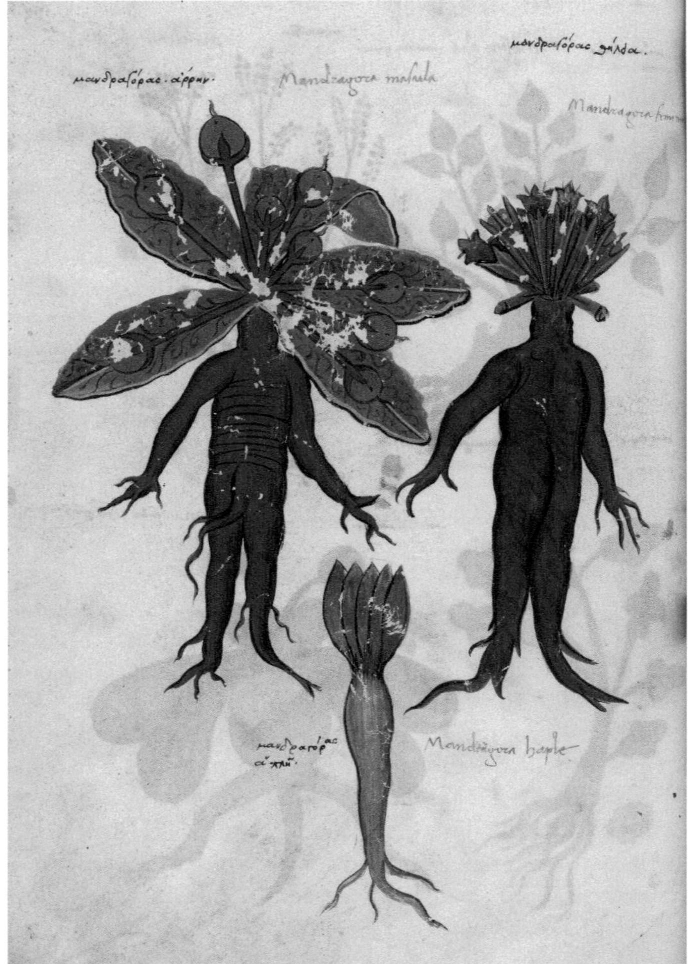

Figure 6.4 Vatican, Biblioteca Apostolica Vaticana, MS Chigi. F. VII. 159, f. 195v

The same scene, which is also the dominant iconography derived from this text, is depicted in at least seven of the Alchemical Herbals (Figure 6.5). The plant root is represented by a naked figure. Leaves and fruit flourish from its head; a leash is tied to its legs by one end and to a dog by the other. To the right, a male figure, holding a hoe, is kneeling and his hands covering his ears. However, the illustration in the Hebrew herbal differs

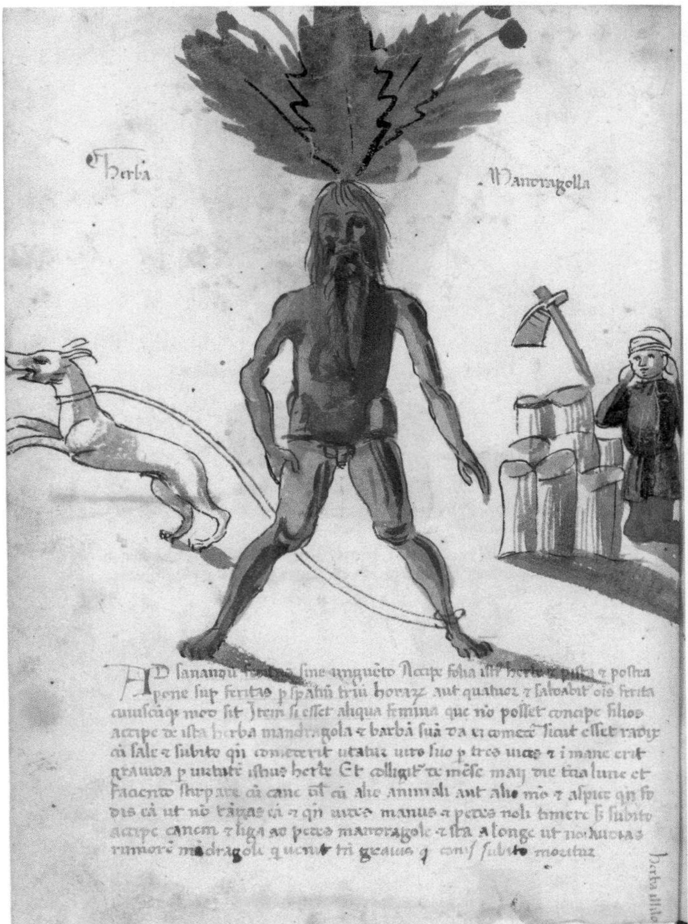

Figure 6.5 Paris, Bibliothèque nationale, MS lat. 17848, f. 20v

from this group (Figure 6.6). This is due not only to the artist's level of skill but to other considerations as well.

While in the other manuscripts in the group we can see clearly that the root-figure is a man because the penis is visible as his arms are down by his sides, in the Hebrew herbal the sex is not clear.[117] In the two Paris manuscripts in the Y tradition, this root figure is also depicted with

[117] Female mandrakes that expose their genitalia are also depicted; see Florence, Biblioteca Medicea Laurenziana, MS Plut.73.16, f. 193r.

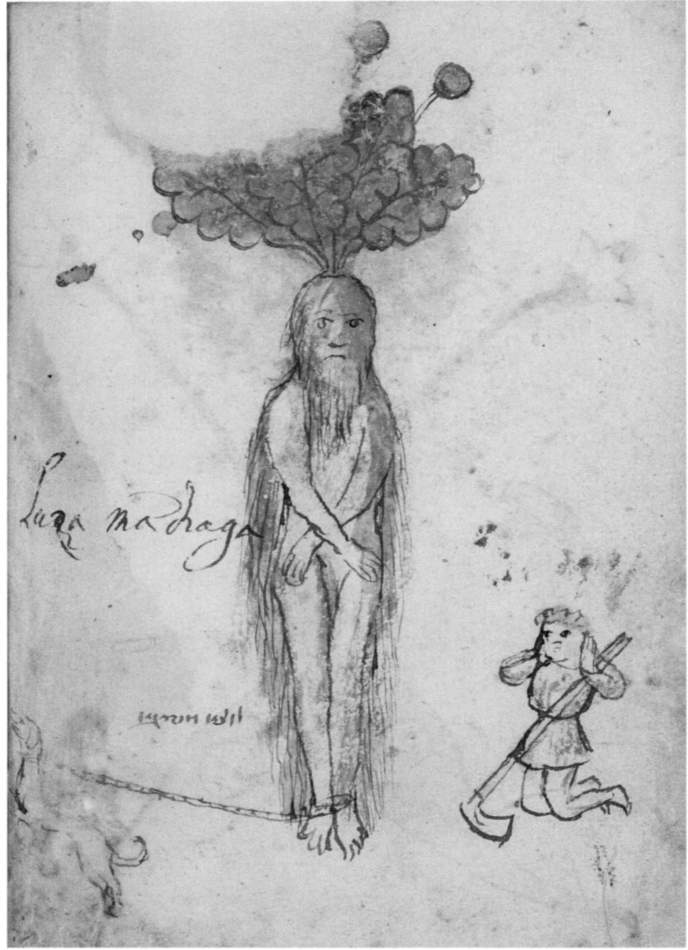

Figure 6.6 Paris, Bibliothèque nationale, MS hébr. 1199, f. 22v

a beard (see Figure 6.5). What may look like a beard in the Hebrew herbal may reasonably be assumed to be the hairs on the root. The same 'beard' appears in another manuscript that belongs to the indirect tradition (Florence, Biblioteca Medicea Laurenziana, MS Redi 165), where it is clear that the figure is a woman (Figure 6.7). The lines/hairs are depicted around the entire figure, and around the roots of other plants in the Hebrew herbal. Similar lines appear in the depictions of mandrakes in other manuscripts as well, and sometimes look like an aura. It is possible that by adding the lines

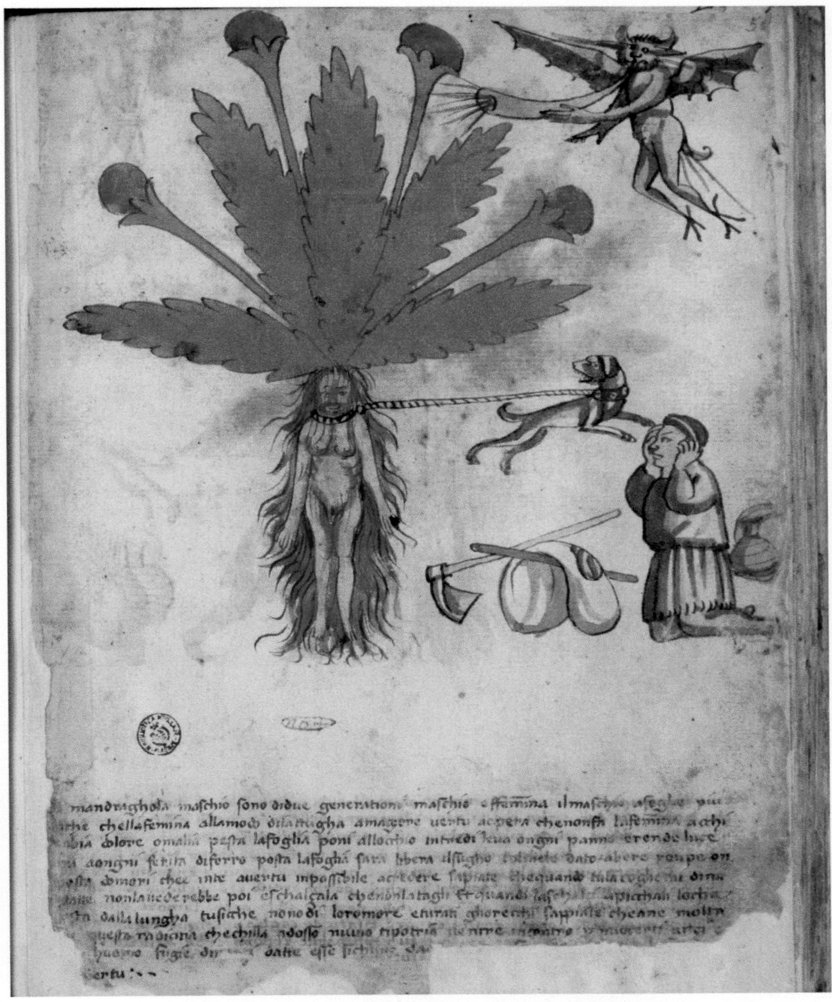

Figure 6.7 Florence, Biblioteca Medicea Laurenziana, MS Redi 165, f. 5r

there is an attempt to resemble the illustrations in other manuscripts in the group. Here it is worth mentioning that the illustrator of the Hebrew herbal knew how to draw the male body, as can be seen in the naked male demon depicted near the plant *Upercion*.[118] In the Hebrew herbal we see the female

[118] See f. 45r. This male demon also appears in the Latin manuscripts in the group.

nature of the mandrake root expressed in the gesture of the hands covering the genitalia.

This gesture is associated in Western art with the *Venus pudica*, a modesty pose, in which the right hand generally covers the breasts and the left the genitalia.[119] This pose appears in an earlier manuscript of Pseudo-Apuleius from the ninth century (Figure 6.8) where the gender is

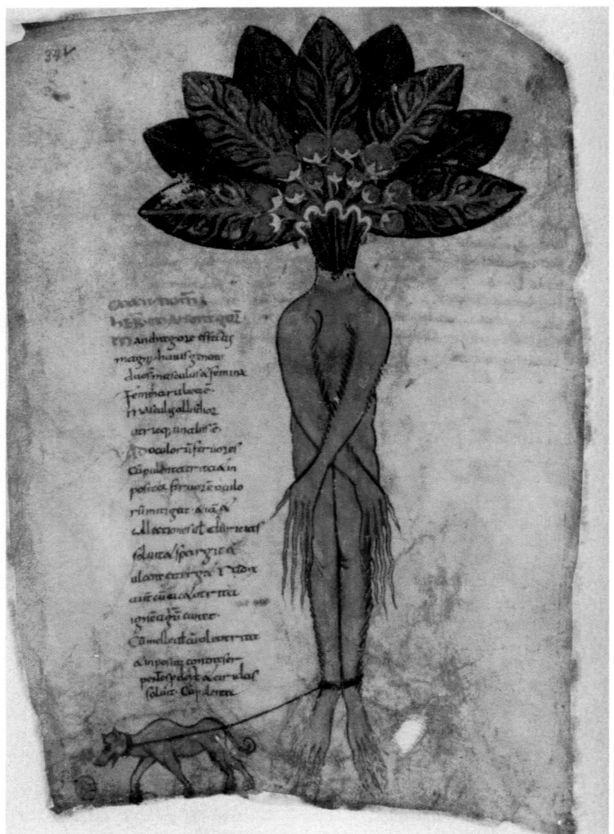

Figure 6.8 Kassel, Universitätsbibliothek Kassel, Landesbibliothek und Murhardsche Bibliothek der Stadt Kassel, 2° MS. phys. et hist. nat. 10, f. 34v

[119] Famous Renaissance examples of this pose are Masaccio's *Expulsion of Adam and Eve* (1422–6) and Sandro Botticelli's *The Birth of Venus* (1486).

also not clear. The same pose also appears in print, as in a printed encyclopaedia of natural history from 1491 (Figure 6.9), where the root is definitely a woman with long hair and breasts. In these books the male

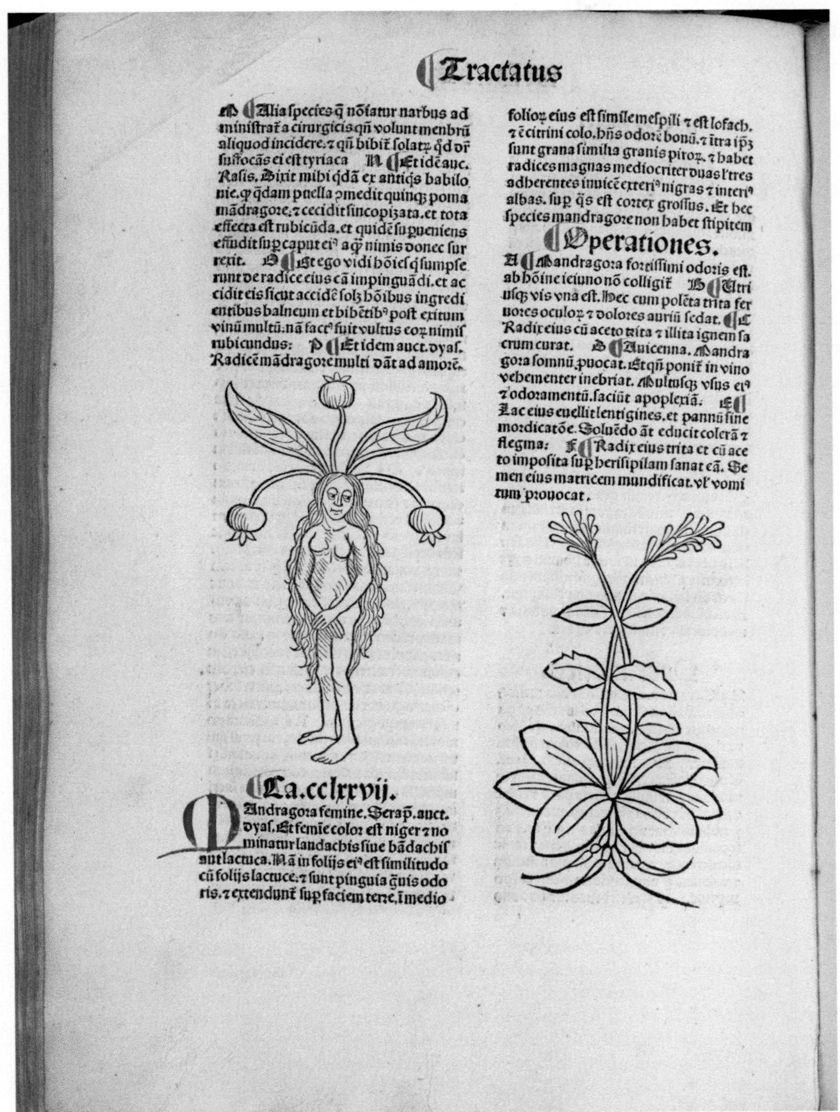

Tractatus

M Alia species q̃ nõiatur narbus ad ministrat̃ a cirurgicis qñ volunt menbrũ aliquod incidere. ⁊ qñ bibit̃ solat℞ q̃d dr̃ suffocãs ei est tyriaca N Et idẽ auc. Rasis. Dixit mihi q̃dã ex antiq̃s babilonie. q̃ q̃dam puella ꝯmedit quinq; poma mãdragore. ⁊ cecidit sincopizata. et tota effecta est rubicũda. et quidẽ supueniens effudit sup caput ei⁹ aq̃ nimis donec surrexit. O Et ego vidi hõies q̃ sumpserunt de radice eius cã impinguãdi. et accidit eis sicut accidẽ solz hõibus ingredientibus balneum et bibẽtib⁹ post exitum vinũ multũ. nã fact⁹ fuit vultus eo℞ nimis rubicundus. P Et idem auct. dyas. Radicẽ mãdragore multi dãt ad amorẽ.

Ca. cclxxvij.

Mandragora femine. Serap̃. auct. dyas. Et femĩe color est niger ⁊ nominatur landachis siue bãdachis aut lactuca. Nã in folijs ei⁹ est similitudo cũ folijs lactuce. ⁊ sunt pinguia g̃uis odoris. ⁊ extendunt̃ sup faciem terre. ĩ medio

folio℞ eius est simile mespili ⁊ est losach. ⁊ ẽ citrini colo. hñs odorẽ bonũ. ⁊ ĩtra ip̃z sunt grana similia granis piro℞. ⁊ habet radices magnas mediocriter duas l' tres adherentes inuicẽ exteri⁹ nigras ⁊ interi⁹ albas. sup q̃s est cortex grossus. Et hec species mandragore non habet stipitem

Operationes.

A Mandragora fortissimi odoris est. ab hõie ieiuno nõ colligit̃ B Utriusq; vis vna est. Hec cum polẽta trita feruores oculo℞ ⁊ dolores auriũ sedat. C Radix eius cũ aceto trita ⁊ illita ignem sacrum curat. D Auicenna. Mandragora somnũ ꝓuocat. Et qñ ponit̃ in vino vehementer inebriat. Multusq; vsus ei⁹ ⁊ odoramentũ. faciũt apoplexiã. E Lac eius euellit lentigines. et pannũ sine mordicatõe. Soluẽdo ãt educit colerã ⁊ flegma. F Radix eius trita et cũ aceto imposita sup herisipilam sanat eã. Semen eius matricem mundificat. vl' vomitum prouocat.

Figure 6.9 Moguntaie: Jacobus Meydenbach, Hortus sanitatis, 1491, p. S4v

mandrake is also presented, but in contrast to the female his hands are behind his back and the penis is exposed. From these books and others that depicted both male and female figures,[120] another possibility arose – that the intention of the artist of the Hebrew herbal was to depict in this figure male and female combined. As we have seen, the figure of the hermaphrodite is related to alchemy. If this interpretation is correct, there is a conceptual connection between the mandrake depicted in the Hebrew herbal and alchemy. The different representations of the mandrake raises questions about the modest nature of the figure in the Hebrew herbal. Was the illustrator instructed to make the figure more modest? We do not know if a similar version was available to our illustrator and whether he used that as the source of his illustration.

Ancient belief held that the plant world had its own 'signatures', according to which the very shape of medicinal herbs suggested what they should be used for or what they should be used against. This so-called theory of signatures was much admired by Paracelsus in the sixteenth century.[121] Segre Rutz notes that the figures represented by the roots are not arbitrary and are connected to the name of the plant or to the text.[122] A connection between the actual root and the name of the plant, or a connection between the text and illustration in the manuscripts, seems helpful in practical terms – for example, in remembering the use of a plant. In the mandrake illustration in the Hebrew herbal we see a change in the visual tradition that attests to the connection between a plant's illustration and its medical function. It seems that the fact that the mandrake was used for fertility and pregnancy, mentioned in the text, motivated the illustrator to depict it as a female character.

The illustrations themselves do not directly help to answer the question as to how they were useful for medical purposes, but the roots, which are the focus of the illustrations, represent the part of the plant most used as a drug for its healing virtues. The visual focus on the medicinal part of the

120 The manuscript from the indirect tradition (Florence, Biblioteca Laurenziana, MS Redi 165) also presents both female and male mandrakes on adjacent pages. Another manuscript that belongs to the indirect tradition has descriptions of both female and male mandrakes (Trento, Museo Provinciale d'Arte MS 1591). Both the female and male are depicted in this manuscript in the modesty pose, although actually the hands do not cover the private parts. The two manuscripts, written in Italian, differ from the group in the plants they contain and their order and in the texts for the plants included.

121 Telesko (2001: 21).

122 Segre Rutz (2000: LI). This phenomenon expanded in the Alchemical Herbals, and we can see it with regard to other plants too.

plant affirms the illustrator's awareness and interest in the *practica*, the function of the plant.

6.4 Another Jewish Connection in the Group of Alchemical Herbals

The distribution of these herbals in the Jewish realm is shown by another manuscript in this group, which belongs to the direct tradition. The Paris Latin manuscript (Paris, Bibliothèque Nationale, MS lat. 17844) is also written on paper and includes 279 illustrations of plants, entries on plants and an alphabetical index. The 'alchemical' plants appear on uniform pages, with the text about the plant written below its illustration. In the literature it is accepted that this manuscript is from northern Italy, but as with the Hebrew herbal, its date is attributed variously to between the fourteenth and the sixteenth centuries.[123] The catalogue of the Bibliothèque nationale de France in Paris, where this manuscript is kept, dates this codex to 1440–60.[124]

Although the text is in Latin, the manuscript is full of Hebrew. In addition to Roman numerals on the recto folios, Hebrew letters appear in black ink on the upper left side of the verso folios. The name of the plant appears in Hebrew[125] as well as in Latin and is vocalised. In the margins of the text at the end of the manuscript there are Hebrew abbreviations indicating the medicinal uses of the plants. The extensive use of Hebrew indicates that the manuscript was in Jewish ownership at some point. This is confirmed by the presence of a Hebrew inscription that includes a name and a date, which has previously gone unnoticed. This inscription is found on the last page (numbered as the first according to the Hebrew, which reads from right to left) and reads as follows: *Barṭolomiʾu Hʾ Lulyu Ḳ-TS-Ṿ* ('Barṭolomiʾu 5 July, 5196').[126] The year 5196 is the Hebrew year that starts in September 1435 and ends in September 1436. This is a specific date and it is important because it is before the assigned dating of the manuscript. We see here an interesting combination of the use of the year, in the Hebrew dating from the creation of the world, together with the day and month,

123 Ragazzini (1983: 14); Segre Rutz (2000: LXXV).

124 https://gallica.bnf.fr/ark:/12148/btv1b10032359h, accessed 31 March 2019.

125 Plant names with Christian meanings were translated in Hebrew – for example, *Palma Christi* was changed to 'Palma the Man'. The word *Sancta* was also omitted in *Sigillo de Sancta Maria* as in the Hebrew herbal.

126 ברטולומיאו ה' לוליו קצ"ו . There is also an additional abbreviation ע"ו (ע"ר) – '"Ṿ ('"R) '"Ṿ, probably an acronym of עולם ועד *ʿOlam ṿa-ʿad* ('forever and ever').

according to the Julian calendar. According to Malachi Beit-Arié, this hybrid dating is typical of Italian Jews.[127]

What is most interesting in the Hebrew additions are the annotations and instructions in Hebrew near the plants illustrations. These annotations refer to the colours that should be used to paint the plant. Interestingly, if we compare the colouring instructions with other manuscripts in the group, we see that sometimes the instructions were added even when the illustration has correct colouring. Sometimes the painter of this manuscript did not follow these colouring instructions, but the 'correct' colouring is found in other manuscripts in the group. For example, in relation to the plant *Superna*, the Hebrew instruction near the leaf that is coloured green on the outside and red on the inside is *mehopakh ḥitsoni adom ve-pnimi yarok* ('reversed, external red and internal green') (Figure 6.10).[128] The word 'reversed' highlights that the colouring already existed when the annotation was written. In other manuscripts in the group, the Hebrew herbal among them, the colours are red on the outside and green on the inside. It is reasonable to assume that the instructions were added to correct the colouring or to guide the Jewish artist of another manuscript using this one as a model, so the plants could be more easily identified.[129]

The two manuscripts are an important witness to the Jewish presence among physicians and pharmacists. Moreover, these manuscripts show the involvement of Jews in the production of manuscripts and not just in their use. Whereas the Hebrew herbal with its translations from Latin shows the transfer and adaptation of knowledge, the Latin manuscript with its Hebrew annotations offers evidence for an actual model for Hebrew manuscripts, both for copying illustrations and for the translation of texts. We have here a remarkable link between the Latin Christian world and the Hebrew Jewish world in the context of making books and transferring knowledge.

6.5 Between Theory and Practice

According to John Riddle, there was a conflict between theoretical and practical medicine in the Middle Ages. From the second half of the twelfth century, the emphasis was on theory in order to make medicine a science.

[127] Beit-Arié (2019: 131). [128] מהופך חיצוני אדום ופנימי ירוק, f. 44v.

[129] There is another example in the plant *lingua yarna* (f. 108v). If I read it correctly, the annotation is 'the "tagi" are white, but I made them black'. Probably the reference is to the black lines on the leaf, and there are none in the Hebrew herbal. This comment strengthens the fact that the colour existed before the comment. I would like to emphasise the word 'I', which may refer to a correction made in this manuscript, maybe in light of the actual plant.

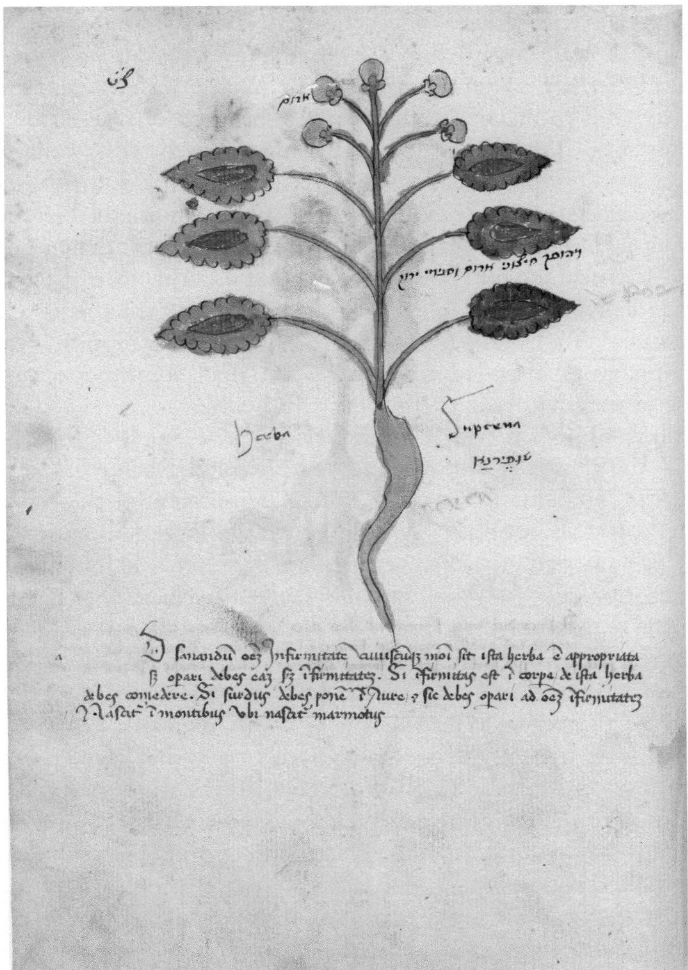

Figure 6.10 Paris, Bibliothèque nationale, MS lat. 17844, f. 44v

One effect of this was that the medical theory of pharmacy became very complex and less connected to practice.[130] It seems that the Alchemical Herbals were trying to reduce the gap between theory and practice and to function as pragmatic aids in daily medical use. The way the plants and the information about them are displayed in the Alchemical Herbals suggests

[130] Riddle (1974: 170, 175, 181).

they were concrete guides to practical medicine. Moreover, the very application of plant knowledge is in itself practical. The *practica* of the Alchemical Herbals is seen at various levels. We can see different kinds of writing styles. The texts are summarised simplifications of various well-known texts, but they do not necessarily following the strict rules for the writing of manuscripts, and the style can thus be popular and authentic. The language register is not high, and as we can see in the Hebrew herbal, the writing can be arranged in different places on the page. Even when they reflect well-known medical knowledge, such as humoral theory, we cannot call these theoretical texts. There is no elaboration on the theory and it is only mentioned for healing purposes. However, the assumption is that the manuscripts were intended for people who had some background in medicine or pharmacy and their dominant theories.

The illustrations are not 'scientific' either in as much as the aesthetic nature of the image is not related to the natural world, but relies on symmetrical, schematic shapes and two-dimensional structures. However, this does not mean that the illustrators lacked all knowledge of nature.[131] The design structure of the plant represents its essential parts: root, stem, branches, leaves, flowers.[132] Generally, the upper part of the flowers (the reproductive part) are conventional and do not receive much attention. In contrast, the underground part generally represents the part of the plant most used as a drug for its healing virtues and is more detailed. This may be the practical reason why it is the focus of attention in the illustration, with most of the anomalies occurring in that part – that is, the underground root.[133] In addition, if we take the theory of signatures into consideration or the connection between the plant's names and texts with the illustrations, we can say that the illustration may have helped the reader remember the plant's uses,[134] and this emphasises the practical purpose of the illustrations. We saw an example of this in the Hebrew herbal, where the female nature of the mandrake in the illustration was probably based on the plant's quality as an aid to fertility.

This homogeneous group of Alchemical Herbals is important for understanding the differences in language and in the transmission of knowledge between different populations. They are witnesses to the survival of multiple copyings, that produce, among other things, corrections and changes. The production of the Hebrew herbal may be a response to the distribution of other such manuscripts and it was probably commissioned by a Jewish

[131] Segre Rutz (2000: XLVII). [132] Ragazzini (1983: 45). [133] Segre Rutz (2000: XLIV).
[134] D'Imperio (1978: 15).

owner who knew this tradition, wanted one in his possession, and may even have been involved in its production. The Hebrew herbal, with its modest appearance adds to our knowledge of the practical nature of this group and confirms the actual use of this specific manuscript through its marginal confirmation of the texts 'already verified'.[135]

Throughout the texts and illustrations we encounter different methods of healing. We see that the same problem can be cured in several ways, by means of different plants, but also that the cures vary and that there are rational, empirical, and/or magical cures. Moreover, the same plant can have different powers. The alchemical nature of the manuscripts can be only partially confirmed. This connection needs to be examined further, but despite the conventional name for the group, it is hard to accept – based on the texts and illustrations – that these manuscripts were truly alchemical.

It is not known for whom the Hebrew herbal was produced. Its 'Jewishness' is more apparent in the texts than in the illustrations. After analysis and review of the multiple hands, it is possible to say that the Hebrew manuscript started with plant illustrations only and the texts were added later, by different owners, who continued to make additions when the manual was in practical use. A single illustrator followed the model of one of the manuscripts from the Alchemical Herbals group, deviating from the model intentionally in some plants, perhaps following another model. When copying the texts, the scribe followed the order of the Latin texts as they appeared in the Alchemical Herbals, but with modifications to suit a Jewish reader. Thus, non-Hebrew names were deleted, while prayers and Latin plant names were adjusted to Hebrew. The scribe who added the texts that appears next to the plant illustrations, probably had a different model for the texts. This scribe had to take the illustrations into account (because they already existed), which caused him to add the text in unusual ways, in different places on the page, at times vertically, and at times between the parts of the root. We also need to consider the person who read and used the texts, examined them, and added his own observations to the pages. In doing so, he invited us to recognise one owner of the manuscript at a specific time. This shows us that the recipes and remedies, however strange and superstitious some of them may appear to readers now,[136] were widely used among Jewish communities as well as the local population at large.

135 No examples of this marginal confirmation were found in the Latin manuscripts I have been able to examine, but further research on this is necessary.

136 Collins (2000: 307).

Appendix

Four texts with the *kvar baduḳ* in the margins.

Toffanas

Hebrew

טופנס- לרפואת חולי הריאה קח מזה העשב ומזה העשב שקורין איסטוטוריס וערבם יחד וטגנם עם ביצות ואכל טו ימי' ויתרפא ובחון ומנוסה גם לחבלות הידי' והרגלים ובכל הגוף ולחבלת הגידים קח מזה העשב וכתוש עם שומן של דוב ואח"כ חבוש על החבלה ומיד יתרפא ונולד באלפי ההרים הקרי' ומלאים עשבי'[137]

Latin

Toffanas – Ad sanadum malum pulmonis. Accipe de ista herba et de herba istatoris et insimul misce et coque cum ovis ad modum herbolate et comede per spatium XV dierum curatur et sanatur et probatum est per magistrum Nicholaum de Pisiis et per magistrum Donatum de Ianua. Item ad feritam manuum et pedum aut aliorum membrorum nervosorum. Accipe de ista herba et pistetur cum sungia ursi et postea pone super feritm: subito curatur et saldatur ferita. Nascitur in alpibus frigidis et herbatiis longis.[138]

The English translation of the Hebrew[139]	The English translation of the Latin[140]
To heal lung disease. Take this herb and the herb called Istatoris, mix them together and cook them with eggs, eat it for fifteen days, and you will be healed. It has been tested and proven. Similarly, for wounded hands and legs and throughout the body, or wounded sinews. Take this herb and pound it with the fat of a bear, and afterwards put it on the wound, the wound will be cured instantly. It grows in the cold and herb-filled Alps.	To heal lung disease. Take that herb and the Istatoris herb, and at the same time mix and cook them with eggs to a state of medical herb, eat it for fifteen days, and you would be cured and healed. It has been proved by the master **Nicholaus of Pisia** [*Nicholaus de Pisiis*] and the master **Donatus of Ianua** [*Donatus de Ianua*]. In like manner, for wounded hands and legs, or other sinewy organs. Take this herb and pound it with the **blood** of a bear, and afterwards put it on the wound: the wound would be cured and crusted instantly. It grows in the cold Alps and in vast lawns.

[137] Paris, Bibliothèque Nationale, MS hébr. 1199. f. 69v. [138] Segre Rutz (2000: 88).
[139] All translations from Hebrew are my own unless otherwise stated.
[140] All translations from Latin were made by Noam Rytwo unless otherwise stated.

Capalarices[141]

Hebrew

קפלריצים – לעשות מים שהם טובים לכל תחלואי העינים קח פרחי זה העשב ועשה באלמביקו מעופרת ומזה המים שים תוך העינים עד כ׳ ימים וידבק העינים וירפאם בשלמות ובחון גם לשים שנאה בין שניהם קח מזה העשב בליל ה׳ ושים על משקוף הבית שעוברים וישנאו זה את זה וילקט יב לירח אם תרצה לעשו ממנו רפואה[142]

Latin

Capalarices – ad faciendum aquam bonam ad omnem infirmitatem oculorum. accipe florem istius herbe et fac aquam ad campanam' et de ista aqua pone in oculis per spatium XX dierum, clarificabuntur oculi et removebitur omnis infirmitas. et hoc est probatum. item si quis vellet ponere scandalum inter duas personas per quod transibunt ille due persone et numquam se amabunt illi qui transibunt per illud hostium. et collige die duodecima lune si vis operari pro medicina.[143]

The English translation of the Hebrew	The English translation of the Latin
On a decoction that is good for every weakness of the eyes. Take the flower of that herb, make it in an alembic made from lead and put that water in the eyes for twenty days. The eyes will be cleared, and every weakness will be removed. And it has been proven. In like manner, if someone should want to put hatred between two persons. Take that herb on a Thursday night and put it on the doorframe of the house that the two persons will pass through and they will hate each other. And collect it on the twelfth day of the moon if you want to use it for healing.	To make good water for every weakness of the eyes. Take the flower of that herb, pour water in the bell [of the flower] and put that water in the eyes for twenty days. The eyes will be cleared, and every weakness will be removed. And it has been proved. In like manner, if someone would want to put a stumbling block [to provoke a quarrel] between two persons. Take that herb on one Thursday night and put it on the enemy's house, by which those two persons will pass, and those who will pass by that enemy's house will never love each other. And collect it [the herb] on the twelfth day of the moon if you want to operate by the medicine.

[141] The plant *Capalarices* is located in the seventy-fifth place in the list of ninety-eight plants, and is identified, not by name but by the illustration, as a member of the *Centaurea* family. Segre Rutz (2000: 241).

[142] Paris, Bibliothèque Nationale, MS hébr. 1199. f. 72v.

[143] Segre Rutz (2000: 241).

Illocharias[144]

Hebrew

אילוקריאה – לרפאת כאבי השיניים קח מזה העשב ובשלהו תוך חומץ חזק ותחזיק בפיך חם כמה שיוכל לסבול ויתרפא מיד ולא יכאב עוד אותם השינים ובחון. גם לרפאת הטחול קח מזה העשב ובשלהו ביין והאכיל לחולה ה' ימים ויתרפא ונולד בארצות אלפידנו זו ובשדות ובחומות[145]

Latin

Illocharias – Ad sanadum dolorem aut percussionem dentium. Accipe **radicem** istius herbe et coque in aceto forti **et postea sic calidam pone super dentem qui patitur dolorem**; subito removet dolorem et sanatur cito. Et sciendum est quod liie dens ampilius non sentiet dolorem et es probatum. Item ad sanandum malum splenis. Accipe folia istius herbe cum **ovis** cocta et da ei comedere per spatium quinque dierum curabitur et sanabitur. Nascitur in terrenis alpestribus in pratis.[146]

The English translation of the Hebrew	The English translation of the Latin
To heal toothache. Take this herb and cook it with strong vinegar and keep it warm in your mouth as long as you can bear it, and it will be cured immediately and these teeth will not feel pain anymore, and it has been proved. Likewise, to heal a disease of the spleen. Take this herb, after it has been cooked with wine, feed it to the patient for five days, and he will be cured and healed. It grows in walls, meadows and in the alpine lands.	To heal dental pain or percussion. Take the root of that herb and cook it with strong vinegar, and afterwards, when it is warm, put it on the tooth that suffers pain; it would remove the pain immediately and the tooth would be healed quickly. You should know that that tooth will not feel pain anymore, and it has been proved. Likewise, to heal a spleen disease. Take the leaves of that herb, after they had been cooked with eggs, feed them to him [the patient] for five days, and he will be cured and healed. It grows in meadows in the alpine lands.

[144] The plant *Illocharias* occupies the thirty-seventh place in the list.
[145] Paris, Bibliothèque Nationale, MS hébr. 1199. f. 70r. [146] Segre Rutz (2000: 118).

Luza Mandragora

Hebrew

לוצא מנדרגורא – לרפאת כל חבלה בלי שום משיחה קח עלה זה העשב וכתוש וחבוש על הפצע תוך ג' שעו' תתרפא או ד' וכן עושה לכל פצע ובחון גם עוזרת להריון קח מזה עשב והשורש ותאכיל לאשה כמו שהוא עם מלח ומיד כשתאכל אותו מיד יהיה מזומן אצלה בעלה לשכב עמה עד ג לילות ותהר בלי ספק ונלקט בחדש מייא ג ימי' לחדוש הירח ויש להוציאה עם א כלב או בהמה אחרת והזהר כשיחפור אותה שלא תגע בה וכשתת . . . ידיה ורגליה מיד קשור אותו עם חבל ותלה ראש החבל בצואר הכלב ותעמוד רחוק מאד כדי שלא תשמע צעקת המנדרגורא חזק מאד כי מכח הצעקה ימות הכלב.[147]

Latin

Luza Mandragora – ad sanadum feritas sine unguento. Accipe folia istius herbe et pista. Postea pone super feritas per spatium trium horarum aut quatuor saldabitur omnis ferita cuiuscumque modi sit. Item si esset aliqua femina que non posset concipere filios. Accipe de ista herba Mandragolla et barbam suam da ei comedere, sicut esset radix cum sale et subiti quando comederit utatur viro suo per tres vices et in mane erit gravida per virtutem istius herbe et colligitur e mense maii die terita lune. Et faciendo extirpare cum uno cane vel cum alio animali aut alio modo et aspice quando fodis eam ut non tanges eam. Et vides manus et pedes noli timere sed subito accipe canem et liga ad pedes mandragolle et sta alonge ut non audias rumorem mandragora qui veniet tam gravis quod canis subito moritur. [148]

The English translation of the Hebrew	The English translation of the Latin
To heal wounds without any ointment. Take the leaves of this herb and pound them and apply to the wounds. After three or four hours you will be cured. And do this for every wound. It has been proven. Likewise, it is helpful for pregnancy. Take this herb and root and give it to the woman to eat as it is, with salt. Immediately after she has eaten it, her husband should be nearby to sleep with her for three nights, and she will be pregnant undoubtedly, and it is	To heal wounds without unguent. Take the leaves of that herb and pound them. Afterwards put it on the wounds for three or four hours. Every wound, whatever state it is in, will be crusted. Likewise, if there is any woman who cannot conceive. Take that Mandragora herb and give her its wool to eat, as the root would be with salt. Immediately after she had eaten it, she should mate with her man for three times, and in the morning, she will be pregnant because of the merit of that

[147] Paris, Bibliothèque Nationale, MS hébr. 1199. f. 70v. [148] Segre Rutz (2000: 127).

(*cont.*)

The English translation of the Hebrew	The English translation of the Latin
collected in the month of May, on the third day of the new moon. It should be dug out of the earth with a dog or with another animal, and see to it, when you dig it out, that you do not touch it. When you pull it, immediately tie its hands and legs with a rope and hang the rope around the dog's neck and stand far away so you will not hear the scream of the mandragora, which is so strong that the dog will die from it.	herb, and it is collected on the third day of the moon of the month of May. The extirpate is done with a dog or with another animal or in another form, and see to it, when you dig it out, that you do not touch it. When you see the hands and legs [of the Mandragora] do not be afraid, but immediately take the dog, tie him to the Mandragora's legs and stand far away so you will not hear the shout of the Mandrake, which would come so gravely that the dog would instantly die.

REFERENCES

Arber, A. 2010. *Herbals: Their Origin and Evolution. A Chapter in the History of Botany, 1470–1670*. Cambridge: Cambridge University Press.

Beit-Arié, M. 2019. *Hebrew Codicology, Historical and Comparative Typology of Medieval Hebrew Codices based on the Documentation of the Extant Dated Manuscripts until 1540 Using a Quantitative Approach*. Preprint internet version 0.10, February (in Hebrew). www.academia.edu/en/40250708/HEBREW_CODICOLOGY_Historical_and_Comparative_Typology_of_Hebrew_Medieval_Codices_based_on_the_Documentation_of_the_Extant_Dated_Manuscripts_Using_a_Quantitative_Approach_Internet_0_3_version_27_August_2019_SEE_ABOVE_FOR_THE_FINAL_ENGLISH_VERSION_OF_THE_BOOK (accessed 20 June 2023).

Bertiz, A. A. 2003. 'Picturing Health: The Garden and Courtiers at Play in the Late Fourteenth Century Illuminated "Tacuinum Sanitatis"'. University of Southern California. PhD dissertation.

Bühler, C. F. 1954. 'An Anonymous Latin Herbal in the Pierpont Morgan Library', *Osiris* 11: 259–66.

Caballero-Navas, C. 2005. 'Medical Knowledge in Hebrew: Manuscripts and Early Printed Books', *Medicina nei Secoli* 17.2: 275–92.

Camille, M. 1989. *The Gothic Idol: Ideology and Image-Making in Medieval Art*. Cambridge: Cambridge University Press.

Chidiac, E. J., Kaddoum, R. N., and Fuleihan, S. F. 2012. 'Mandragora: Anesthetic of the Ancients', *Anesthesia and Analgesia* 115.6: 1437–41.

Collins, M. 2000. *Medieval Herbals: The Illustrative Traditions*. London: British Library.

Cronier, M. 2013. 'Dioscorides Excerpts in Simon of Genoa's *Clavis sanationis*', in B. Zipser (ed.), *Simon of Genoa's Medical Lexicon*. Berlin: De Gruyter, 79–97.

Daston, L., and Galison, P. 1992. 'The Image of Objectivity', *Representations* 40: 81–128.

D'Imperio, M. E. 1978. *The Voynich Manuscript: An Elegant Enigma*. Fort George G. Meade, MD: National Security Agency/Central Security Service.

Evans, M. 1980. 'The Geometry of the Mind', *Architectural Association Quarterly* 4.12: 32–55.

Fischer, K. D. 2013. 'Two Latin Pre-Salernitan Medical Manuals, the *Liber passionalis* and the *Tereoperica*', in B. Zipser (ed.), *Medical Books in the Byzantine World*. Bologna: Eikasmos, 35–51.

Gilbert, E. 2008. *Le piante magiche: Nell'Antichità, nel Medioevo e nel Rinascimento*. Rome: Hermes Edizioni.

Henderson, J. L., and Sherwood, D. N. 2003. *Transformation of the Psyche: The Symbolic Alchemy of the Splendor Solis*. Hove: Brunner-Routledge.

Jones, C. 1998. 'Formula and Formulation: "Efficacy Phrases" in Medieval English Medical Manuscripts', *Neuphilologische Mitteilungen* 99.2: 199–209.

Jones, P. M. 1984. *Medieval Medical Miniatures*. London: British Library in association with the Wellcome Institute for the History of Medicine.

Kieckhefer, R. 1989. *Magic in the Middle Ages*. Cambridge: Cambridge University Press

Kottek, S. 2012. 'Magical Medicine in the Talmud', *Maḥanayim* 14: 19–28 (in Hebrew).

Kupfer, M. A., Chajes, J. H., and Cohen, A. S., eds. 2020. *The Visualization of Knowledge in Medieval and Early Modern Europe*. Turnhout: Brepols.

Lawrence, G. H. M. 1965. 'Herbals: Their History and Significance', in G. H. M. Lawrence and K. F. Baker (eds.), *History of Botany: Two Papers Presented at a Symposium Held at the William Andrews Clark Memorial Library, December 7, 1963*. Los Angeles: University of California Press, 2–19.

Lev, E., and Amar, Z. 2008. *Practical Materia Medica of the Medieval Eastern Mediterranean according to the Cairo Genizah*. Leiden: Brill.

Murdoch, J. 1984. *Album of Science: Antiquity and the Middle Ages*. New York: Charles Scribner's Sons.

Ragazzini, S. 1983. *Un erbario del sec. XV: il ms. 106 della Biblioteca di Botanica dell'Università di Firenze*. Florence: Leo S. Olschki.

Randolph, C. B. 1905. 'The Mandragora of the Ancients in Folk-Lore and Medicine', *Proceedings of the American Academy of Arts and Sciences* 40.12: 487–537.

Riddle, J. 1974. 'Theory and Practice in Medieval Medicine', *Viator* 5: 157–84.

Sed-Rajna, G., and Fellous, S. 1994. *Les Manuscrits Hébreux Enluminés des Bibliothèques de France*. Leuven: Peeters.

Segre Rutz, V. 2000. *Il giardino magico degli alchimisti: Un erbario illustrato trecentesco della Biblioteca Universitaria di Pavia e la sua tradizione*. Milan: Il Polifilo.

Shaw, J., and Welch, E. 2011. *Making and Marketing Medicine in Renaissance Florence*. Amsterdam: Rodopi B.V.

Shemesh, A. O. 2013. *Medical Materials in Medieval and Modern Jewish Literature: Pharmacology, History and Halakha*. Ramat Gan: Bar Ilan University (in Hebrew).
Shoham-Steiner, E. 2012. 'A Demon, a Saint and a Crippled Jew: Jews Seeking Healing at Christian Shrines', *Zmanim: A Historical Quarterly* 118: 42–9 (in Hebrew).
Stannard, J. 1999a. 'Medieval Reception of Classical Plant Names', in K. E. Stannard and R. Kay (eds.), *Herbs and Herbalism in the Middle Ages and Renaissance*. Brookfield, VT: Ashgate Variorum, 153–62.
Stannard, J. 1999b. 'The Herbal As a Medical Document', in K. E. Stannard and R. Kay (eds.), *Herbs and Herbalism in the Middle Ages and Renaissance*. Brookfield, VT: Ashgate Variorum, 212–20.
Stuckrad, K. von ed. 2006. *The Brill Dictionary of Religion*. Leiden: Brill.
Telesko, W. 2001. *The Wisdom of Nature: The Healing Powers and Symbolism of Plants and Animals in the Middle Ages*. Munich: Prestel.
Thorndike L. 1929–58. *History of Magic and Experimental Science*. 8 vols. New York: Columbia University Press.
Tomasi, L. T., and Willis, T. 2009. *An Oak Spring Herbaria*. New Haven, CT: Yale University Press.
Trachtenberg, J. 2004. *Jewish Magic and Superstition: A Study in Folk Religion*. Philadelphia: University of Pennsylvania Press.
Ventura, I. 2015. 'Il "Circa instans" attribuito a "Platearius": Trasmissione manoscritta, redazioni, criteri di costruzione di un'edizione critica', *Revue d'Histoire des Textes* 10: 249–362.
Weitzmann, K. 1947. *Illustrations in Roll and Codex: A Study of the Origin and Method of Text Illustrations*. Princeton, NJ: Princeton University Press.
White, L. 1975. 'Medical Astrologers and Late Medieval Technology', *Viator* 6: 295–308.

PART II

The Borders of Pharmacology

CHAPTER 7

Making Magic Happen

Understanding Drugs As Therapeutic Substances in Later Byzantine Sorcery and Beyond

Richard Greenfield

A case heard before the patriarchal court in Constantinople in May 1370 nicely illustrates the complicated field into which I will be venturing in this chapter: the entanglement in later Byzantium of what we might want to term magic, medicine, and religion. It even includes an allusion to the use of a substance we would call a drug for, towards the end of this rambling trial with its ever-growing cast of characters and a plot that could have been thought up by television scriptwriters, a monk was accused of procuring an abortifacient substance for a nun he had gotten pregnant. The man who supplied him with the drug, a doctor called Syropoulos, had already been convicted by the court of performing magic and was now ratting on his clients and suppliers in hopes of reducing the severity of his sentence. He in turn claimed he had obtained his textbooks from an apparently ascetic and holy man, Gabrielopoulos, who was arrested and brought before the court with the magic books that a search of his house had turned up. These included a copy of the *Kyranides* and a notebook, found to have been compiled by an official of Hagia Sophia, Demetrios Chloros, which was 'filled with all manner of impieties including invocations of demons, spells and names'. When Chloros was himself brought to trial he claimed that his notebook was simply a collection of medical texts. But an expert panel of medical practitioners was summoned and, after hearing the content with evident horror, roundly denounced Chloros for insulting the medical art and daring to imply that Galen and Hippocrates were magicians.[1]

[1] See *Acta Patriarchatus Constantinopolitani* CCXCII, in ed. Miklosich and Muller (1860) I.541–50. See also Darrouzès (1977: 480–4, N2572). Chloros was convicted, expelled from the church, banned from teaching, and sentenced to solitary confinement in a monastery until such time as he proved properly contrite. On him, see Trapp, Walther, and Beyer (1976–96: n. 30869). The trial has received quite wide scholarly attention; see, for example, Pingree (1971: 192), Cupane (1980: 251–7), Rigo (2002: 77–9),

My contribution here, focussed as it is in the area of what we usually call magic (or sometimes miracle), hovers only on the margins of Byzantine medicine and pharmacology.[2] It looks at the use and conceptual context of substances that may be, more or less loosely, called drugs, as Byzantine people (whoever *they* may be) struggled to find alternative solutions for their medical problems as well as ways of coping with the many other pressing worries and aspirations in their lives. In doing so I do not intend to revisit ground already well studied by, for example, John Scarborough, but instead hope to build, like many others, on his important conclusions concerning the murky, muddled mixture of rational and religio-magical approaches apparent in ancient pharmacology.[3] I will also be developing some themes more recently explored by Brigitte Pitarakis to shed light specifically on the equally and typically fluid and ambiguous way in which later Byzantines (those roughly post tenth century) regarded the use of these substances.[4] Their approach was indeed very different from our own more limited conception of drugs, and I thus also add a by now happily familiar warning about reading modern categories and distinctions back into the Byzantine and wider medieval world.[5] Taken together, I hope my discussion will assist in appreciating the breadth of the Mediterranean pharmacological tradition, as well as illustrating both the considerable ambivalence that exists at the boundaries of medieval pharmacology and the importance in the daily life of that world of a diverse range of substances we might label drugs.

7.1 Medicine, Faith, and Magic: Pluralistic Approaches to Problem-Solving in the Byzantine World

Back in the early 1980s, when I was writing my own PhD thesis on Byzantine demonology, Peregrine Horden concisely summed up the relationship between early Byzantine holy men and medical doctors by saying

Copenhaver (2006: 529–31), and Mavroudi (2006: 85). Rigo (2002: 78–9) suggests that Gabrielopoulos was also a doctor. On the *Kyranides*, see later in this chapter.

2 As Bourbou (2010: 26) points out, the study of Byzantine medicine and pharmacology was once commonly dismissed, like magic (but also so much else in Byzantine culture), as pretty much worthless, an attitude neatly summarised by Scarborough (1984a: ix). On the case of therapeutics, see Touwaide (2007: 151–2).

3 See Scarborough (2010: I.1–6) and compare Scarborough (1984b). Also see, for example, Nutton's description of 'fluidity' as the dominant feature of the boundaries between the main strands of ancient medicine (2013: 278) or Nagy's phrase 'highly permeable' (2012: 71); and Faraone's brief corrective discussion (2011a: 135, 151–4).

4 Pitarakis (2015). 5 Scarborough (1991: 138, 149).

that 'competition between sources of healing could sometimes be stiff'.[6] A few years later Gary Vikan came to similar conclusions about the relationship between *miraculous* and *magical* healing:

> Our survey has revealed a continuous spectrum in early Byzantium's world of miraculous healing, between remedies and implements thoroughly Christian and those patently magical. Why? Because while one's local bishop, town doctor, and neighborhood sorceress were almost certainly at odds over how best to evict the demon that possessed one [or, I would add here, the illness that afflicted one], the possessed [i.e. sick person] did not indulge in the luxury of subtle differentiations ... Our objects ... reveal a world thoroughly and openly committed to *supernatural* healing [my italics], and one wherein, for the sake of health, Christianity and sorcery had been forced into open partnership.[7]

The emergence of the Christian faith that was to become such an important part of the identity of the new eastern Roman 'Byzantine' world was itself largely responsible for this fluidity of approach. It ushered in its own 'post-truth' age by undermining trust in the rational solutions (or debates) of the old Greco-Roman philosophical and scientific tradition, but often failed to offer immediate, tangible solutions of its own to pressing practical problems that beset people, beyond the uncertain hopes offered by prayer and supplication to God and his intermediaries.[8] This set up what Scarborough described as 'an ongoing and antagonistic free-for-all among Christians and non-Christians alike' in the world of medicine and

[6] Horden (1982: 13). Compare the clear illustration provided by Ashbrook Harvey (1984) of the complex relationship between holy man and regular medical practitioner.

[7] Vikan (1984: 86). Scarborough (1984a: ix–x) picks up and extends Vikan's point:

> although the modern physician will immediately reject any notion that magic and astrology might be useful in medical practice, many of our sources for Byzantine medicine show a strong influence of both, ranging from the religious-medical cures of pilgrims' tokens examined by Vikan ... to a continued employment of the medical astrology of the quasi-mythical Hermes Trismegistus and the firm belief in demonology.

[8] See, for example, Nutton (1984: 8–9). Scarborough (1991: 150, my italics) carefully considers the similarly ambiguous situation in antiquity. Examining the relationship between the 'rational' uses of plants in practical pharmacological botany and in traditional religious and magical practices, he stresses the '*grand and opaque jumble of opinions* characteristic of [the] "great pharmacologists" including many authors represented in the Hippocratic corpus, Theophrastus, Dioscorides, Soranus, Rufus, and Galen'. Compare his description of Galen's drug lore, the model for later Byzantine encyclopaedists, as 'a gigantic potpourri of herbs, animal products, written sources quoted verbatim, and quasi-legendary and pseudofolkloristic facts all compacted into three separate systems of organization' (1991: 154). As he says in the same paragraph, 'there was always a powerful undercurrent of folk medicine displayed in cults to the saints in the Byzantine Empire, as well as a tenacious survival of nonlearned conceptions about drugs'.

magic in the second century.[9] The complexity, if not the intensity, of this situation persisted through the Byzantine era. Regular, rational medical solutions were potentially compatible with faith-based ones since both were, necessarily, gifts of divine origin for orthodox believers in an omnipotent God. But they could also be seen as undermining or challenging the will of God who was, also necessarily, believed to have sent ill health as a punishment or test or for some other purpose. This relationship has been explored quite fully by Orthodox scholars, such as John Chirban and Demetrios Constantelos.[10] The former's assertion that in the 'psychosomatic anthropology' of Byzantine culture 'human beings were understood to have interconnected physical, mental, and spiritual components', and that this 'fostered healing that was multifaceted and itself holistic' and allowed accommodation between faith and 'scientific findings',[11] is certainly helpful in recognising and attempting to explain the fluidity of the Byzantine situation. It is, however, admittedly anachronistic in its language and certainly optimistic in its outlook, for it determinedly downplays the authority of 'hard-line' Byzantine orthodox thinkers who refused to admit any efficacy or appropriate application for rational (or magical) medicine.[12] Constantelos' claim that '[R]eligious faith and medicine were reconciled and continued to serve as an axis throughout the Byzantine centuries. Priests and physicians and churches and hospitals cooperated in the cure of illness and the restoration of health,' is likewise supportable from a *selection* of contemporary evidence but again rather rosy, given the sometimes bitter, if often posturing, depiction of doctors in hagiographical and other religious sources as incompetent at best, complete charlatans at worst.[13] The caustic commentary of the eleventh-century layman Kekaumenos should also come to mind here as a caution. 'Pray that you do not fall into the hands of a doctor, even if he has an excellent reputation, for he will prescribe things for you that are unnecessary and if your illness is minor he will

[9] Scarborough (1991: 161).

[10] Chirban (2010a, 2010b); Constantelos (2010). Also compare Constantelos (1966–7, 1991).

[11] Chirban (2010b: 38).

[12] Chirban (2010b: 52–5) describes 'monolithic', 'beclouded', 'polarized', and 'reductionist' models, but the only place he gives to magical therapies is as placebos (2010b: 43).

[13] Constantelos' claim (2010: 139). As one clear example among very many see Philotheos Kokkinos, *Vita of Gregory Palamas*, 120, in ed. Talbot (2012) 14.1–2, 344–5. On this trope, its complexities, and the dangers of taking it too seriously see Duffy (1984: 24–5); also see Talbot (2010: 162–4); Krueger (2018: 20–2; 2010: 122–3), and Lampadaridi (2018: 148–9). More generally on Byzantine attitudes to doctors see Kazhdan (1984). On the 'theology of healthcare' resulting from links between hospitals, monasteries, and healing shrines, see Crislip (2005) and Krueger (2018: 25–7).

greatly exaggerate it.'[14] The blurring between rational and orthodox religious healing is perfectly depicted in the now well-known image on f. 10v of the fourteenth-century manuscript of the *Dynameron* of Nicholas Myrepsos, now Bibliothèque nationale de France, Parisinus gr. 2243. As Stavros Lazaris has recently observed,

> These two superimposed scenes [of a *deisis* and a visit to the doctor] emphasise the link between the care of the body and that of the soul, placing the action of the doctor under the blessing of Christ. To be healed the patient must be treated by a doctor, but he is more likely to heal if he requests the Virgin and St. John the Baptist to intercede on his behalf with Christ.[15]

In illustrating the now widely accepted overlap of regular medicine with *magical* practices it is common to cite the comments of Alexander of Tralles, a doctor who was willing to allow his patients in the late sixth or early seventh century to make use of amulets in certain circumstances, but there is plenty of other evidence for the use of objects fulfilling this function in medical contexts.[16] The point is also nicely (and literally) illustrated by another manuscript familiar to students of Byzantine medicine, Bononienisis 3632. The first 260 of the 475 folios, written by a physician called John Aron in 1440, contain all sorts of medical material, including Dioscorides, Aetios of Amida, Alexander of Tralles, Paul of Aegina, and Theophilos' *On Urines*, but after that the content shifts to more obviously astrological, divinatory, and magical works, including elaborate techniques of divination related to those of the important late Byzantine sorcery handbook the so-called *Magical Treatise of Solomon*. What is important here is that the same artist illustrated both the medical material and the demonic divination rituals.[17]

[14] See Kekaumenos, *Strategikon*, 3.125, in ed. Spadaro (1998) 172–5. See also the online edition by Roueché (2013). The passage is cited in part by Bennett (2017: 155).

[15] As Lazaris (2017: 104–5) indicates, the illustration is related to a very similar one in a thirteenth-century manuscript, Bibliotheca Apostolica Vaticana, Vaticanus Palatinus gr. 199, on which see further Mondrain (1999); see also Diamantopoulos (1995: 112–13, 155) and Cavallo (2009: 165–6). Compare the depiction of Christ as physician on a sixth-century ivory medicine box in Kiraz (2015); Krueger (2018: 20).

[16] See Alexander of Tralles, *Therapeutics*, 8.2, in ed. Puschmann (1879) II.375.10–16. On him in this context see especially Duffy (1984: 26); also see, for example, Scarborough (1984a: ix–x), McCabe (2007: 16–17), and Bouras-Vallianatos (2015: 116). For a general summary on him see Scarborough (1997: 51–60). On his use of natural remedies see Bouras-Vallianatos (2016a). For a summary of the views of ancient Greek medical writers and others on amulets in the context of sickness see Faraone (2018: 21–3, 258–61).

[17] For this manuscript and its contents see Magdalino and Mavroudi (2006: 24–5); Caudano (2016). Illustrations are reproduced in, for example, Angeletti, Cavarra, and Gazzaniga (2009: cover) and Bouras-Vallianatos (2015: 110, 120). See also Marchetti (2010). Further on these, see Diamantopoulos (1995: 114–15, 159). For the magical content see Delatte (1927: 572–612); Marathakis (2011: 18–19, 115–33). A notable case, illustrating how people might turn to magical help when regular medicine was

To complete the circle, there is obviously room for considerable confusion between orthodox and unorthodox (i.e. magical) *religious* solutions as when, for example, ecclesiastical authorities suggest the substitution of orthodox images and materials for regular magical amulets. This is something to which I will return in the final section of this chapter.

What is key here is the realisation that, when faced with difficult circumstances, Byzantine people had no hesitation in pursuing a *pluralistic* approach to problem solving, be it in the field of seeking help for medical issues, in discovering what they wanted to know, or in dealing with the many practical difficulties in their lives. This is surely what Chryssi Bourbou means when she says that Byzantine medicine, and thus by implication pharmacology, should be 'viewed within the social matrix of the population it was developed to serve'.[18] Byzantines evidently opted for whatever best suited their situation, physical context, frame of mind, and individual traditions. Theoretical models that allow us to approach this culturally constructed system of competing medical resources and solutions 'flexibly, broadly and a bit sloppily', as Derek Krueger has wisely advised,[19] have been most helpfully discussed in relation to the lengthy diachronic context of Greek culture by Steven Oberhelman.[20] Following him, my thinking here is indebted to the pluralistic model of overlapping, but sometimes competing and conflicting, popular, medical, and ecclesiastical spheres previously developed for early modern Italy by David Gentilcore.[21] The approach outlined earlier in this chapter contains implicit assumptions about the nature of 'magic' and its relationship to both 'religion' and 'science'. This is obviously not the place to go into the lengthy debate concerning these issues, especially since they appear to have been largely resolved, at least at the academic level.[22] I have discussed

failing, is that of the correspondent of Michael Italikos, Tziknoglos, in the twelfth century: Duffy (1995: 92–4, 96–7); Timplalexi (2002: 269–70). Compare also the ambiguous classification of Syropoulos and Chloros in the opening example in this chapter.

18 Bourbou (2010: 26). 19 Krueger (2010: 119). 20 Oberhelman (2013: 1–12).

21 Gentilcore's (1998) model is also adapted to a Greek context by Hartnup (2004). Compare here Chirban (2010b), who adds considerable nuance to understanding how these spheres, particularly the medical and ecclesiastical, interact. Awareness of the range of options is generally now present in studies of Byzantine medicine, but understanding of the consequences of pluralism is sometimes missing. Thus, for example, Bennett (2017: 155) recognises that 'herbalists, wise women and their like' might be consulted instead of regular doctors and that 'religious faith . . . underpinned many xenon foundations', but while he notes, correctly, that patients seem willing to ascribe medical failure to the will of God, he does not consider this failure a factor in seeking alternative medical solutions by those less accepting of God's will as the final word.

22 For recent illuminating discussion see Frankfurter (2019). See also, for example, Jolly (2002); her concept of 'magic as an alternate rationality' is particularly helpful (3). MacMullen (1997: 143–4) neatly summarised this point more than twenty years ago: 'Now, the lessons of anthropology grown

my own approach to these questions elsewhere, so here the briefest possible summary will have to do.[23] For me, magic, (medical) science, and orthodox Christianity in the Byzantine world are not inherently different concepts but related ideas that lie at opposite ends of the *same* continuous spectrum of thought and behaviour. This spectrum is formed by the *attitudes* people displayed in relation to the spiritual and natural forces that were thought to control the world in which they lived. At the orthodox Christian end, at least as far as (theoretical) theology was concerned, this was all about *supplication*: given the omnipotence and omniscience of God, all that people could possibly do to affect an outcome in the everyday world was to pray to Him (or his agents) and hope that He would be encouraged, in His inscrutable wisdom, to look favourably on their behaviour and grant their requests. At the other, magical and/or rational 'scientific' end, however, it was all about *coercion* and automatic, predictable response: natural or spiritual forces could be manipulated by people with correct and sufficient knowledge and the outcome could, in theory, be guaranteed. As for what then separates magic from more rational approaches at the coercive end of the spectrum, I would suggest that it is the presence of one or more among three possible elements: the use of non-Christian spiritual or supernatural powers, the assumption of natural but occult connections, and the incorporation of ritual elaboration. We also need to be aware of a second spectrum which intersects vertically, as it were, with the first, for all these ideas also need to be plotted on an axis that captures their extensive range of *levels*. Magical, scientific (including here medical and pharmacological), and religious ideas and practices thus ranged from extreme sophistication to crude simplicity.[24] In general, the sort of 'mix-and-match' pluralism I have invoked lies in a broad grey area in the middle range of these spectrums, one where the majority of Byzantines operated.[25]

The final preliminary question, that of original sources, is again not one that may be considered at any length here. Suffice it to say that, for magical ideas and behaviours, I draw primarily on a number of Byzantine

familiar, it is common to accept the impossibility of separating magic from religion and to move on to more interesting subjects.'

23 Greenfield (2017).

24 Greenfield (1993: 79–80; 1995: 121); Russell (1995: 36); Hartnup (2004: 4–12); Schreiner (2004); Mavroudi (2006: 58). For the useful concept of 'household magic', see Maguire (1996: 118–37).

25 For a similar assessment of the situation in the medieval West, see, for example, Rider (2006: 185): 'Many people would not have had access to a university trained physician, especially in the countryside, and so would have had no need to distinguish between the medicine offered by academic physicians and the "empirical" [magical] remedies of other physicians.' For examples of the range of divination priests engaged in see Fögen (1995: 102) and Mavroudi (2006: 81–3).

'handbooks' which represent the ideas and practices of those who either saw themselves as practitioners of the magical arts or who evidently saw nothing wrong with including magical elements in the solutions they suggested. Although most of these have their origins in late antiquity or earlier (and certainly depend on traditions which stretch back far into the ancient Greek world), the manuscript tradition, references in other literature, or both, confirm that they were being accessed more or less continually over the 1,000 years of Byzantine history and were certainly available in the later period, although considerable developments had taken place in their detail and understanding.[26] I thus include here *The Testament of Solomon*,[27] the *Kyranides*,[28] and the *Geoponika*,[29] as well as the handbooks collected under the title *The Magical Treatise of Solomon* which date in their earliest form to the fifteenth century.[30] These may be supplemented by a range of scattered, and usually pejorative, references and allusions in literature, including histories, hagiographies, theological commentaries and treatises, legal documents, and correspondence. There are also medical or 'scientific' handbooks, herbals, and *iatrosophia*,[31] and some material remains.[32] Sources for miracle healings and the like are drawn principally from hagiographical literature.

7.2 The Byzantine Concept of Drugs or Therapeutic Substances: The Example of Asphodel

I now move on to look at examples of the use of substances we might consider as drugs in later Byzantine magical sources. In fact, as will become clear, 'therapeutic substance' is probably a better term to use than 'drug',

26 See Mavroudi (2006: 57), who follows here Stewart (1991).

27 McCown (1922). For English translation and commentary see Duling (1983). See also Iles Johnston (2002) and Klutz (2005).

28 Kaimakis (1976). For a partial English translation and commentary see also Waegeman (1987). More recently on the Byzantine textual history see Rigo (2002: 79–80).

29 Beckh (1895). English translation Dalby (2011). See further Rodgers (2002: 159–64).

30 Delatte (1927); English translation in Marathakis (2011). See further Greenfield (1988: 159–63; 1995: 129–30). I try to work as much as possible with evidence from the earliest and unquestionably Byzantine source, the fifteenth-century MS H (British Library, Harley MS 5596) (www.bl.uk/manuscripts/FullDisplay.aspx?ref=Harley_MS_5596, accessed 18 June 2019).

31 On *iatrosophia* see Tselikas (1995: 57–70), Touwaide (2007), Clark (2011), Oberhelman (2013: 13–21; 2015: 133–46), and Demetriades (2015). There is no comprehensive study of these sources in general; see Magdalino and Mavroudi (2006: 21–7). On the Palaiologan period, see Greenfield (1988: 154–64; 1995: 121–31). For parallels see, for example, the references and authors collected in the *Hippiatrica*: McCabe (2007).

32 Vikan (1984); Spier (1993); Maguire (1995); Russell (1995); Dauterman Maguire and Maguire (2007). On the inherited tradition see now Faraone (2018).

given the range of activity under consideration and the fact that the base meaning of the Greek verb *therapeuō* ('θεραπεύω') includes not only 'healing', but, more generally, 'assisting'. My intention is to use these examples to clarify and explore the conceptual and methodological plurality in which they must be set if we are to approach a real grasp of what 'drug' might have meant in the broad Byzantine context. By extension, this discussion will also inform consideration of the more general medieval Mediterranean pharmacological tradition. One place to start is with herbs, although for the Byzantines, as for the ancients[33] and as for modern medicine, drugs could also be derived from all manner of animal, mineral, and man-made substances. Given constraints of space, I will use the example of just one plant, asphodel. Asphodel (in modern botanical terminology *asphodelus fistulosus*, *albus*, *microcarpus*, or many other varieties found in the eastern Mediterranean and Anatolia) had a mythological connection with the underworld,[34] but evidently enjoyed a long tradition of use in 'rational' Greco-Roman medicine.[35] Galen himself, for example, in *On the Capacities of Foodstuffs*, praised its 'obstruction clearing and thinning properties',[36] and a decoction of the plant was recommended by the Latin collection known as the *Alphabetum Galieni* for kidney and urinary ailments, encouraging menstruation, and as an expectorant, while burning or crushing the bulb produced an ointment to be used on various skin conditions.[37] Pliny's *Natural History* also contains a quite substantial section on the plant's many properties and uses (taken internally, applied externally, injected into the ears, etc.), which include some related to the ailments already mentioned, but also its particular efficacy in healing the wounds caused by venomous creatures, in regenerating hair, or even as a deodorant.[38] In Pliny, however, there is a hint of somewhat less rational practice and conception. The alleged power of parts of the plant not only to cure the bites of snakes and stings of scorpions

[33] Galen, *On the Capacities of Simple Drugs*, in ed. Kühn (1821–33) XI.359–892, considers, for example, not only plants (Books 6–8), but minerals (9) and animal products (10–11).

[34] The association goes back to Homer, *Odyssey*, 11.539, 573; 24.13, where the souls of the dead are described as dwelling in a meadow of asphodel (ἀσφοδελὸν λειμῶνα). See, for example, Reece (2007).

[35] See Verpoorten (1962: 129, n. 16; 133, nn. 32 and 33) for references to its medicinal use in antiquity and in Byzantium. See also Biraud (1993).

[36] Galen, *On the Capacities of Foodstuffs*, 63, ed. Kühn (1821–33) VI.652 = ed. Wilkins (2013) 170–1. Powell (2003: 112).

[37] See Ps.-Galen, *Alphabetum Galieni*, 33, in ed. Everett (2012) 169. Everett (2012: 9) suggests the work may well have originated in its current form in a bilingual Greek and Latin environment, possibly in the fourth through sixth centuries CE. The ashes of asphodel are still recommended in a cure for migraine in an early nineteenth-century *iatrosophion*, Oberhelman (2013: 15).

[38] See Pliny the Elder, *Natural History*, 22.32, in ed. Detlefsen (1866–82) III.303–4. On Pliny's *Natural history*, see Doolittle (Chapter 2) in this volume.

but simply to act as a repellent to these creatures when scattered under the bed could be deemed rational or magical, depending on whether the mechanism involved is conceived as a physical or sympathetic reaction.[39] Other suggestions are less ambiguous: malicious magic is said to be warded off by growing the plant outside the door of a house,[40] and, it is claimed, if the root is applied to scrofulous sores and then hung in the smoke of the fireplace for four days, the sores will dry up along with the root.[41]

The Magical Treatise of Solomon, however, supplies a clear glimpse into a conceptual framework that was certainly inherited from the ancient world, but which continued to lie firmly behind the *magical* use of asphodel as a therapeutic substance in Byzantine times. In a section which describes the plants associated with the planetary powers that control the seven days of the week, asphodel is thus linked to Kronos (Saturn) and so to Saturday.[42] Here asphodel is described as possessing several apparently straightforward medical properties. For example, 'If someone has a headache, take some of the leaves, cut them up, combine them with rosewater and anoint the head and the patient will be cured,' or, 'If someone has dysentery, take half an *exagion* of the seeds and mix them with coral (this must be ground up) and let them eat this and they will be cured.' Mixed with musk and administered in liquid form, asphodel is also suggested for treating epilepsy, although ritual elaboration perhaps creeps in with the requirement to take the medicine seven times.[43] But the context here clearly indicates that the practitioner understands the medicinal properties of the plant not in terms of its physical, pharmacological characteristics as, for example, related to the inherited humorist theories of medicine, the sophisticated seventh-century 'system of degrees' of Paul of Aegina, or even the simple trial and error of traditional experience. Instead, the plant is seen to be empowered by its relationship to the planetary forces and thus its place in the vast interconnected chain of

[39] See Pliny the Elder, *Natural History*, 22.32, in ed. Detlefsen (1866–82) III.303.16–19.

[40] See Pliny the Elder, *Natural History*, 21.68, ed. Detlefsen (1866–82) III.275.32–3. The same property was long before attributed to squill by Theophrastus, *Enquiry into plants*, 8.13.4, in ed. Hort (1916) II.128–9, and see Scarborough (1991: 146–7) and Faraone (2018: 81).

[41] See Pliny the Elder, *Natural History*, 22.32, in ed. Detlefsen (1866–82) III.304.6–8. Compare the very similar prescription in Greek for the use of plantains to cure haemorrhoids in the late fourteenth-century manuscript Vatican, BAV cod. Vaticanus gr. 299, f. 410r.

[42] For the section on the planetary plants or herbs see especially Delatte (1949); see also Marathakis (2011: 81–3). Both include publication details of original texts and secondary literature. On the earlier history of this astrological tradition of planetary and zodiacal herbs see Scarborough (1991: 154–6) and Pitarakis (2015: 164).

[43] Delatte (1927: 444); the translation is my own, but compare Marathakis (2011: 198–9, 332–3). The late seventeenth-century version of this text says it is also useful in treating carbuncles and gangrenous ulcers and warding off infection (see 1.7, in ed. Delatte (1949) 162).

cosmic and, in this Christianised context, certainly spiritual, sympathy and antipathy.[44] Asphodel's properties here, then, are seen as due to its relationship to Kronos. Indeed, these properties are enhanced – may in fact only exist – if the plant is picked at the right time of day on the right day of the week (for asphodel this is on Saturday in the first hour) and when the moon is full or in conjunction with the planet appropriate to the plant. Moreover, an elaborate 'spiritual' ritual is envisaged for collecting and then preparing the plant.[45] Details vary in different versions, but essentially the practitioner, who must be free from any sexual pollution, is instructed to say a 'prayer' specific to the planet in question and then to the individual angels associated with that day and that hour. This must be done with great piety while kneeling or prostrate on the ground. In the prayer the planet (Saturn in the case of asphodel) is conjured, by the power of the Christian God and by a string of magical names, to be amenable to the activity in which the practitioner is engaged and thus to empower the plant being used. Then the specific, named angels are conjured to assist the practitioner, particularly by subduing the specific, named demons of the same hour and day who might otherwise work to inhibit the operation.[46] Once the plant has been pulled up, its roots must be censed with the specific incense appropriate to its ruling planet and it then has to be laid out in the open for a number of nights 'να ἀστρονομήσῃ' – to be empowered by the stars.[47] In other words, what makes asphodel efficacious as a therapeutic substance in this context is its cosmic relationship and a religious ritual which 'enables' it and allows its powers to function as desired by the practitioner.

44 On the theory of sympathy and antipathy in this context see Ierodiakonou (2006). On the extension of the concept of relationship between macrocosm and microcosm into contemporary medical theory, see Caudano (2016: 169).

45 On the collection of plants for use in magic in the ancient world, see the extensive treatment by Delatte (1938); on timing in particular, see chapters 1 and 24–52. See also briefly here Scarborough (1991: 144, 149–50), where he quotes Theophrastus' scepticism on the elaborate practices of the ancient 'ῥιζοτόμοι' – 'praying while cutting is perhaps reasonable, but the additions to this caution are ridiculous' – and (1991: 157–258) on collection rituals in the magical papyri. As is widely noted in the scholarship, the idea of plants and their properties being connected with particular divinities has its recorded roots as far back as Homer, notably with the herb 'μῶλυ' said to have been given by Hermes to Odysseus as protection from the potions of Circe: *Odyssey* 10.302–6. This is perpetuated in more complex ways through the persistent traditions of theurgy which saw divine agency at work in disease and its treatment; see, for example, Scarborough (1991: 139, 142). For parallel concepts and rituals in a nineteenth-century *iatrosophion* see Oberhelman (2013: 19–20).

46 See Delatte (1938: 53–148), who has separate chapters on the preparation of the practitioner, on the rites surrounding collection, on the verbal elements, on offerings to be made, and on how to collect the plant. Compare here the invocation of the sun, 'the special lord of horses', when collecting earth to be used in a treatment to prevent their being bitten by noxious animals in McCabe (2007: 179).

47 See here Delatte (1949: 154–5; 1938: 151). On treatment after collection in general see Delatte (1938: 149–56).

And, of course, when seen in this way, asphodel is not only a useful drug for treating illness, it is also believed to have all sorts of other powers. So here is an important reminder that, for the Byzantines, a 'drug' is not necessarily just something to help people resolve medical problems, but the same therapeutic substance, in this very different conceptual framework, can also be thought effective in helping to cope with all sorts of other issues that are troubling them. To think only of the *medicinal* properties of a drug, in the modern sense, is to take it out of context. For the practitioners of *The Magical Treatise of Solomon*, asphodel is thus also a 'truth serum' which when placed by the head of a sleeping person will cause them to reveal their secrets. It can be used to counter the effects of judicial corruption, it can stop dogs from barking, ward off robbers, protect against the evil eye, and expel demons. It can even help someone find hidden treasure when attached, along with houseleek and mandrake, to the neck of a white rooster.[48] In parallel sources, the *Kyranides* claims that drinking asphodel juice boiled up with ants will render someone impotent for life,[49] and the *Geoponika* recommends its use in bedding for sheep as it repels pests.[50]

7.3 Delivery of Drugs or Therapeutic Substances: Fumigation

Something else that becomes clear, even from this brief example of asphodel as a 'planetary herb', is that the Byzantines did not *only* see a drug simply as 'A medicine or other substance which has a physiological effect when *ingested or otherwise introduced* into the body' [my italics], as the *Oxford English Dictionary* definition of the term has it. Of course, drugs *were* widely administered in this fundamental way in Byzantine magical and spiritual treatments,[51] just as they were in their more rational medicine. It was thus commonly believed that harmful magic was worked through and was responsible for the effect of *ingested* poisons. Negative connotations permeate the term *pharmakon* ('φάρμακον'), which may usually be translated as 'drug', and it and its many cognates were synonymous with aspects of magic and its practitioners, although also applied to more beneficial uses and circumstances.[52] In the conceptual framework that underpins, or at least hovers vaguely in the

[48] Delatte (1927: 444–5); Marathakis (2011: 198–9, 332–3).

[49] See *Kyranides*, 2.25, in ed. Kaimakis (1976) 156.

[50] See *Geoponika*, 18.2.5, in ed. Beckh (1895) 486.19–487.1; Dalby (2011: 326).

[51] See here Pitarakis (2015: 165–76). On the use of powdered amuletic gemstones see Nagy (2012: 81).

[52] Sorcerers ('γόητες') and poisoners ('φαρμακοί') are associated with each other and linked to the demons in, for example, the *Ecloga*, 17.43, in ed. Burgmann (1983) 240–1; Humphreys (2017: 76). The same term ('φαρμακός') is also used there as a reason for disinheriting children who are poisoners or associate with them, *Ecloga*, 6.7, in ed. Burgmann (1983) 196–7; Humphreys (2017:

background of Byzantine magical, spiritual, and 'popular' practices, however, drugs as therapeutic substances did not have to be ingested in order to be seen as effective. To illustrate how these Byzantine examples may help to explain the porous boundaries of medieval Mediterranean pharmacology, I will focus on two other common methods of delivery: fumigation (in the sense of surrounding someone or something with the smoke produced by burning a substance, whether or not it is inhaled) and contagion (placing a substance in contact with or in proximity to a person or thing).

The use of fumigation to administer therapeutic substances, underpinned in part by such parallel concepts as that of 'bad air' causing sickness and the need to create a barrier against it (miasma theory), or of the attractions and aversions of sweet and unpleasant odours, is well attested in regular ancient medicine and other practice.[53] But its role in spiritual or magical healing and manipulation in the Byzantine context surely gains strong support from the biblical tradition, notably from the book of Tobit, a work which, although apocryphal in the English Bible, formed part of the canonical Byzantine Septuagint. To cut a long and complex story very short, a young man, Tobias, wants to marry a woman called Sarra, but he has a problem because the demon Asmodaeus (or, in the opinion of her maids, Sarra herself) has killed her seven previous husbands on their wedding night. Tobias, however, has the advantage of assistance from the angel Raphael, who instructs him to burn on the ashes of incense, the heart and liver of a fish he has earlier caught in the River Tigris. When this ritual is carried out in the bridal suite, the demon, as predicted, cannot stand the smell and flees to Upper Egypt, where it is bound by the angel. Tobias and Sarra live happily ever after.[54] The same story was referenced by the Testament of Solomon (5:9–10) which identified the fish in question as the sheat or *silurus* ('γλάνις', a relative of the catfish).[55] Evidence for the practical application of this legendary technique for keeping demons and evil spirits at bay comes from the *Kyranides*, which prescribes burning the

56). See further here Scarborough (1991: 139f), Timplalexi (2002: 272), and, for a more detailed sketch, Vakaloudi (2001: 280–303).

[53] Most helpful in the present context is Faraone (2011b). See also here Caseau (2001, 2007) and Pitarakis (2015: 163–4). Scarborough (1991: 153) suggests that, in antiquity, herbs like squill and the hellebores may have gained their sacred associations 'due to their heavy pungency, especially when they were bruised or cut'.

[54] Tobit 3.8, 17; 6.1–9, 14–17; 8.2–3. On the relation of the Tobit story to the antique medical and exorcistic context see Faraone (2011b: 14–16). He links this to one remedy in the *Geoponika* but does not explore the broader scope of Byzantine fumigation that I discuss later in this chapter. See also here Greenfield (1988: 148, n. 482; 227 n. 698; 264–5) and Faraone (2018: 225–6).

[55] Duling (1983) 966. For the alternative placing of this information in the 'handbook' chapter 18 of the Testament see Faraone (2011b: 15 n. 75).

bones of the same fish ('γλάνεος'),[56] but also suggests that other, presumably more easily obtainable species may be used in the same way: thus eagle fish ('ἀετός ἰχθύς') or gar ('ραφίς ἰχθύς').[57] Fumigations with other substances, such as peony root ('παιωνία' or 'γλυκισίδη'), bear hair, or wild goose dung, are said to have the same effect.[58]

The technique of fumigation is, however, certainly not reserved for dealing with evil spirits: the *Kyranides* also recommends it for all manner of conditions and situations, making use of substances that, for the most part, have to be considered magical rather than rational because of their nature and associations. Medically, for example, fumigations with vulture droppings are prescribed to treat internal female complaints or to diagnose mental illness; with wild boar dung to dispel bouts of tertian fever and hysteria; with carp liver for epilepsy; with the hoof of a brood mare to expel dead embryos or to promote quick labour; or with eagle wing to treat lethargy, hysteria, and agitation.[59] Manipulatively, fumigations with beaver dung are recommended for repelling reptiles and with peacock entrails and droppings for averting magic and other bad things.[60]

Fumigations are quite commonly prescribed for crops, gardens, and animals in the *Geoponika*. At first sight some of the substances recommended here seem quite rational: smoking fruit trees infested with caterpillars with asphalt and sulphur, for example.[61] But, whatever their chemical efficacy, these elements also have a long history in ancient fumigations for problems involving wandering wombs and demonic possession,[62] a useful warning perhaps against assuming modern rationality in the conceptions underlying these treatments. Other recommendations in the same

56 See *Kyranides*, 4.13.2–3, in ed. Kaimakis (1976) 252.

57 See *Kyranides*, 4.1.6–7, 55.4, in ed. Kaimakis (1976) 244, 283.

58 See *Kyranides*, 1.3.21–2, 2.1.13–1, 3.51.20–2, in ed. Kaimakis (1976) 36, 113, 239. See also Greenfield (1988: 264–5).

59 See *Kyranides*, 3.20, 29–33; 2.35, 11–12; 4.37, 2–3; 2.17, 12; 3.1a, 6–7 ed. Kaimakis (1976) 200, 169, 272, 144, 191. Note also here the idea in the *Hippiatrica*, present also in a number of respected Greek and Latin classical sources, that a fumigation of castor will help horses suffering from urine retention, or that the oily smoke from an extinguished lamp will produce miscarriage in mares. McCabe (2007: 168, 237).

60 See *Kyranides*, 2.19, 12; 3.42, 11–12, in ed. Kaimakis (1976) 146, 230. A fumigation with a paste made from the eyes of the *glaukos* fish, hyena bile, and various animal fats is said to make people think they are those animals or, when mixed with sea, river, or rain water, to think they see the sea, a river, or rain. *Kyranides*, 4.9, 7–12, in ed. Kaimakis (1976) 249. For repellent fumigations in antiquity, see Caseau (2001: 83).

61 Sulphur is still considered an effective insecticide as a fumigation by, for example, the US National Pesticide Information Center (http://npic.orst.edu/faq/burningsulfur.html, accessed 18 June 2019).

62 See *Geoponika*, 12.8.1, in ed. Beckh (1895) 354.8–9; Dalby (2011: 250). On the use of sulphur and asphalt/pitch in ancient traditions of fumigation see Faraone (2011b: 5, 7, 13–14, 16, 18) and in exorcistic amulets, Faraone (2018: 225–6).

section of the *Geoponika* seem more obviously magical in light of parallels in the *Kyranides* and elsewhere: using the smoke of burning bat droppings and garlic stems, for example.[63] Elsewhere, vine rust is said to be treated by a fumigation with diced catfish (a significant ingredient in light of the Tobit story) or by burning an ox's right horn and cow dung, or three crabs with cow dung and goat dung when the wind is blowing in the right direction to fumigate the entire property.[64] Other vine pests are said to be driven out by fumigations with all sorts of things; cow dung again, but also galbanum, hartshorn, goats' hoofs, ivory dust, lily root, peony, or burdock; even burning women's hair is suggested, a fumigation that is also claimed here to be an effective treatment for miscarriage or a 'risen womb'.[65] House mice are said to be repelled by burning a mixture of copper sulphate, oregano seed, celery, and love-in-the-mist, as well as hematite and green tamarisk;[66] and snakes by burning white lily root, stag's horn, goat hoof, or pellets made from chopped asafetida, love-in-the-mist, galbanum, hyssop, brimstone, pellitory-of-Spain, hog's fennel, and goat's hoofs mixed with sharp vinegar.[67] A rather different fumigation for locusts and ants, employing the smoke of some of the burnt creatures themselves, appears to rest clearly on ideas of natural magical sympathy and antipathy;[68] a similar rationale is evidently at work in the promise that smoking bugs kills leeches and smoking leeches kills bugs (as long as the couch is curtained with drapes so that they get no relief from the smell, adds the author in a nod to practicality).[69] A fumigation to catch wolves sounds riskier:

> Blennies are small sea fish; some people call them *lykoi* [wolves]. They are used as follows in the hunting of terrestrial wolves. Take a large number alive by fishing. Crush them finely on a grinding stone or in a mortar. Make a big charcoal fire on the mountain where the wolves live, and while the wind is blowing take some of the fish and throw it on the embers, and quickly mixing the fish blood with mutton flesh finely chopped, add this to the fish

[63] See *Geoponika*, 12.8.8, in ed. Beckh (1895) 355.5–7 and Dalby (2011: 250). Compare also there [*Geoponika*, 12.8.7, in ed. Beckh (1895) 355.3–5] use of the smoke produced by burning the mushrooms that grow under walnut trees.

[64] See *Geoponika*, 5.33.6; 5.33.1–2, in ed. Beckh (1895) 155.14–16, 154.17–155.2; Dalby (2011: 140–1).

[65] See *Geoponika*, 5.48.1–4, in ed. Beckh (1895) 165.9–20; Dalby (2011: 146–7). On the latter point see Faraone (2011b: 9).

[66] See *Geoponika*, 13.4.2, 13.4.8, in ed. Beckh (1895) 387.16–18, 388.14–15; Dalby (2011: 269–70).

[67] See *Geoponika*, 13.8.1–2, in ed. Beckh (1895) 391.7–14; Dalby (2011: 272).

[68] See *Geoponika*, 13.1.5–6, in ed. Beckh (1895) 386.7–15; Dalby (2011: 268). Similar remedies are suggested at *Geoponika*, 13.9.1, 13.10.1, in ed. Beckh (1895) 393.7–8, 395.2–3; Dalby (2011: 273, 274).

[69] See *Geoponika*, 13.14.7–8, in ed. Beckh (1895) 400.7–12; Dalby (2011: 278). Dried millipedes or crushed ivy leaves have the same effect. Compare *Geoponika*, 16.19, in ed. Beckh (1895) 465.6–10; Dalby (2011: 314).

> on the fire and then move away. As a strong smell develops from the fire, all the wolves in the neighbourhood will be drawn to it. As they take the meat and inhale the smoke they will be stupefied and fall asleep; approach them while they are still in this narcotic state and slaughter them.[70]

Coming back full circle to the Tobit story, another suggested way of controlling ants is by burning the root of squirting cucumber or catfish, especially mudfish (*silouros*), on a slow fire.[71]

In the more sophisticated traditions preserved in *The Magical Treatise of Solomon*, fumigations play an important part in the rituals and detailed recipes are provided for the incenses appropriate to each planet in several different versions. Staying with Kronos (Saturn) as an example, one list of ingredients is given as black incense, hoofs of a black ass, snake head, pepper, and aloe.[72] Uses vary: as mentioned already, censing the roots of a freshly pulled plant with the incense of the planet with which it is associated is thought to enhance its properties, or an amulet may require censing to operate effectively,[73] but fumigations also form part of the elaborate and important systems of protection and attraction in the rituals for summoning demons to a magic circle.[74] One set of instructions requires the practitioner to set up clay jars of hot charcoal while he is tracing his circle on the ground,[75] and to burn on them a combination of eagle-wood,[76] aromatic costus,[77] frankincense, pure musk, clove,[78] nutmeg, and saffron. It appears another practitioner has added further, less pleasant elements to this evidently sweet-smelling fragrance: sheep fodder,[79] black clove,[80]

[70] See *Geoponika*, 18.14.1–3, in ed. Beckh (1895) 493.8–21; Dalby (2011: 330), whose translation is used here.

[71] See *Geoponika*, 13.10.11, in ed. Beckh (1895) 396.3–6; Dalby (2011: 275).

[72] See ed. Delatte (1927) 404.33–405.3; Marathakis (2011: 156). See also here Pitarakis (2015: 164).

[73] For example, McCabe (2007: 148).

[74] Compare the use of a circle in a medico-religious healing recorded among the miracles of St Artemios. Pitarakis (2015: 179).

[75] See H, in ed. Delatte (1927) 417.11–18; Marathakis (2011: 168).

[76] 'Ξυλαλόη', eaglewood or aloeswood (*Aquilaria malaccensis*), a south Asian tree; compare *Kyranides*, 5.14, ed. Kaimakis (1976) 305 for its sweet-smelling properties as an incense.

[77] 'Κόστος', costus or kuth (*Saussurea lappa*), the root of an Indian thistle known for its aromatic properties, described as resembling violets when fresh but becoming more like goat when old, and for its therapeutic uses.

[78] 'Μοσχοκάρφιν', lit. 'musk nail' so probably clove, as Marathakis understands it.

[79] The texts are confused here; possibly water lily leaves. Delatte's reading of H has 'ἀπὸ τὸ χόρτον τοῦτον τῆς μυλοφαγίας' (although he appears to have misread an omicron for an omega in the last word), but the parallel passage in A, to which he refers the reader in the apparatus, has 'ἀπὸ τὸ χόρτον μηλόφαγίαν' (lit. sheep-eating) which he corrects to 'ἀπὸ τὸ χόρτον νυμφαίαν' based on the reading of B 'λουλοφανου', a term for the water lily. Delatte (1927: 24.2).

[80] H has 'καρομφίλη', which Delatte (1927: 417.16) corrects to 'καροφύλλου'. I take this as a form of the modern Greek 'γαρύφαλλο', which can mean both clove and carnation. Marathakis translates it as nigella.

asphodel root, and blood of a murdered man. The practice of fumigation in these circumstances obviously has roots in the ubiquitous ancient traditions of sacrifice and the theory of late antique theurgy, where censing served not only to communicate with and to please and attract the deities, but also to avert malign powers.[81] Here the pleasant elements are apparently propitiatory, but the use of black and unpleasant or illicit elements seeks to attract the evil spiritual powers, the demons, that the sorcerer needs to work his divinatory and manipulative magic.[82] It is perhaps worth noting that there is little to suggest that the incenses used in these sorcery rituals actually helped the practitioner to see demons in the sense that they contained psychotropic substances (the only obvious possibility is that of Zeus, which contains opium),[83] but the inclusion of asphodel root among the ingredients here again makes my point about the need to see 'drugs' as therapeutic substances in their broader Byzantine and medieval Mediterranean conceptual context.[84]

7.4 Delivery of Drugs or Therapeutic Substances: Contagion

Contagion was another way in which substances that we might think of as drugs were commonly administered in Byzantine magic. By this I mean the idea that the properties of a substance could be effective simply through contact (the precursor of the transdermal patch, perhaps), or even by proximity. Most obviously this concept underpins the ubiquitous and ancient practice of wearing amulets,[85] but it is also present in practices

[81] See, for example, the conference held at the British School at Rome and the École française de Rome in 2017 and the forthcoming publication by Bradley, Grand-Clément, Rendu-Loisel, and Vincent.

[82] As part of an elaborate and much earlier account of a dish divination, described in the Syriac records of the synod of Ephesus of 449 and clearly related to the rituals preserved in *The Magical Treatise of Solomon*, a censer is set below the table on which the divining bowl is placed. See Flemming (1917: 81.43–4), Honigmann (1944: 282), and Dickie (2003: 267). Compare also here, perhaps, the use of wicks made from mullein ('νεκύα βοτάνη' or 'φλόμος') by necromancers performing dish divination: *Kyranides*, 1.13, in ed. Kaimakis (1976) 73; Waegeman (1987) 105–6.

[83] Delatte (1927: 405.6); Marathakis (2011: 156). That of Mercury has sweet-flag root, another potential hallucinogen. Delatte (1927: 405.22); Marathakis (2011: 156).

[84] Asphodel root is also an alternative ingredient of the incense of the moon. Delatte (1927: 406.4); Marathakis (2011: 158).

[85] See now at length Faraone (2018) but also Spier (1993) and Walker (2015: 212). The first reference to the use of plants in amulets in the Greek world appears to be Pindar's third *Pythian Ode*; see Scarborough (1991: 143). For his comments on the pharmacology of amulets in the magical papyri see (1991: 158–9). Amulets were also traditionally used on animals, not just humans: for horses, see, for example, McCabe (2007: 120–1, 146–9, 166–7, 180, 272). On the use of amulets, see also Lieberman (Chapter 8) and Rinotas (Chapter 12) in the present volume, who discuss the views of Moses Maimonides and Albertus Magnus on the subject, respectively.

which saw magical materials buried or hidden in houses and other locations.

Starting, for simplicity, with asphodel again, the non-medical uses of the plant suggested in *The Magical Treatise of Solomon* and mentioned briefly earlier in this chapter, almost all involve carrying or wearing it as an amulet. One seed of the plant brought to the law court will prevent a miscarriage of justice due to a corrupt judge, and having any part of it about one's person will stop dogs from barking. More specifically, its root and seed wrapped in a piece of donkey hide and worn around the neck will keep demons away, or a piece of the root wrapped in goat skin and worn as an armband will chase off robbers.[86] The sort of complex, mixed media amulet envisaged here is most clearly represented in the surviving sources in the *Kyranides*, which is, essentially, a substantial textbook in five parts, devoted to the construction of amulets and information about their components. The first book, organised alphabetically, describes twenty-four complete amulets together with various individual properties of their components, while the other books elaborate on the properties of individual animals, birds, fish, and plants that may be used in them or employed in other ways.

Again a brief example must suffice. Under the letter epsilon in Book 1, instructions are given for making an amulet which uses the plant arugula [rocket] ('εὔζωμος'), the nightingale ('εὐβοή' or 'ἀηδών'), the sea urchin ('ἐχῖνος θαλάσσιος'), and a gemstone, probably the opal ('εὔανθος').[87] The complete amulet requires an image of Aphrodite binding up her hair to be engraved on the opal; a piece of arugula root and a nightingale's tongue are then enclosed with it. The person who wears the amulet will, it is claimed, be well liked/loved, well known, and well spoken, and, as a bonus, they will be avoided by every wild animal.[88] The epsilon section of the *Kyranides* is, however, not only concerned with the amulet, for it provides further information about the use of both arugula and nightingale as drugs, as it does in each section about all the other plant and animal ingredients. Arugula is thus said here to have the base property of producing heat (arugula in salad does indeed add a peppery quality to the flavour) but, the author explains, its green leaves actually cool sexual ardour and potency

[86] Delatte (1927: 444–5.5–7, 29–30, 23–8, 7–9); Marathakis (2011: 198–9, 332–3).

[87] See *Kyranides*, 1.5.1–8, in ed. Kaimakis (1976) 44.

[88] See *Kyranides*, 1.5.27–31, in ed. Kaimakis (1976) 45. Missing here is a description of the wrapper which, as seen in the cases already mentioned, is usually made from the skin of a particular animal. The sea urchin also gets left out of the amulet, although it is said here to relieve epilepsy when the shell is ground up and taken with honey.

and it is thus eaten by priests and other ecclesiastics to promote sexual continence. On the other hand:

> Four ounces of the seed of this [plant] and one ounce of pepper taken with honey, morning and evening, produces an erection two fingers long. If someone is of advanced age and has a drooping member, make this: sixteen ounces of arugula seed, eight ounces of cumin, four ounces of pepper, two ounces of purslane seed, ground, taken with honey. Give morning and evening; this is incomparable.[89]

Further information is also given about the properties of nightingale: if its eyes and heart are attached to a bed they will keep the person lying in it awake and 'if someone grinds these up and secretly gives them to someone to drink, that person will die from insomnia; there is no antidote'.[90]

In Book 3, swallowing the still beating heart of a nightingale with honey, or wearing the heart and tongue is said, again, to render someone well spoken and pleasant to hear, but if someone tears out its eyes while it is still alive and wears them they will never want to sleep. If a mixture of its gall and honey is spread on the eyes, it gives clear vision.[91]

Once again here, we get a glimpse into the complex and certainly sometimes confused logic behind the employment of these therapeutic substances, whatever their actual pharmacological properties may be. At some basic level they are simply linked by their names. Then there is some fairly obvious 'sympathetic magic' at work, in that the pepperiness of arugula leads to its application in conditions associated with 'heat', or the sweet song and nocturnal habits of the nightingale associate it with both dulcet tones and wakefulness.[92] There is, however, another more

[89] See *Kyranides*, 1.5.15–20, in ed. Kaimakis (1976) 44–5. For parallel uses of arugula described in a non-medical source see *Geoponika*, 12.26.1–3, in ed. Beckh (1895) 374.8–18:

> Arugula seed when drunk in wine treats the bites of a field mouse [or, possibly, weasel]. It expels intestinal worms, reduces the spleen, and, when mixed with ox-bile and vinegar, cleans black scabs. It also cures birthmarks [or moles]. Arugula mixed with honey cleans up spots on the face. Drunk with wine beforehand it lessens the pain for those being whipped. When held in the left hand, three wild arugula leaves cure jaundice . . . Arugula changes smelly armpits.

My translation; compare Dalby (2011: 275). On honey used to assist in the taking of bitter or unpleasant drugs, see, for example, Bouras-Vallianatos (2016b: 402–3).

[90] See *Kyranides*, 1.5.21–3, in ed. Kaimakis (1976) 45.

[91] See *Kyranides*, 3.4.5–10, in ed. Kaimakis (1976) 195.

[92] Compare the similar logic behind the use of bat's bile in an ointment also containing buckthorn juice and honey to promote good eyesight and remove cataracts. Even without the bat extract, buckthorn juice with honey is said to improve eyesight and to treat corneal opacity in monks. *Kyranides* 1.17.10–14, in ed. Kaimakis (1976) 83.

profound cosmic sympathy involved too, one which relates these substances to Aphrodite and thus to sex, love, and being loved.[93] Through their association with the planet Venus, the disparate substances of plant and bird are linked together and then further connected to all the other substances, animal, vegetable, and mineral, seen as appropriate to the planet; they are also woven into and empowered by the complex astrological and spiritual theory that underpins this conceptual framework. Indeed, the dangers of seeing arugula only as a drug in *our* sense of the term in the Byzantine context are also neatly underlined by a passage in Aetios' *Medical Books* which offers a close parallel to the prescription from the *Kyranides* on arugula in a cure for male impotence: 'Another [recipe] of Oribasios for erectile dysfunction, especially in old men: make up 2 drachmas of arugula seed, one ounce of cumin, and one ounce of purslane with honey, and give a spoonful morning and night'.[94] Even Aetios tacks on the advice: 'And for intercourse, he [i.e. Oribasios] says, let him start by eating a wren bird,' and 'For those bound by magic ('περιεργείας'), drink the urine of a female goat.'[95]

7.5 Drugs or Therapeutic Substances in Religious Healing

The final aspects of drugs in the Byzantine and, by extension, wider medieval Mediterranean world that I want to explore briefly here is the way concepts of their efficacy and use bleed, not only between medical and magical healing, but also into more obviously religious contexts. To start with, I continue with the idea of the amulet, something worn on the body which is thought to have an effect on the physical condition of the wearer.[96] Early church fathers inveighed against the ancient practice of wearing amulets, providing evidence, if not of specific instances of their use, then certainly of their widespread popularity in the early Byzantine period.[97] In some passages they specifically reference amulets, including

[93] See Waegeman (1987: 40–6).

[94] See Aetios of Amida, *Medical Books*, 11.35.58–60, in ed. Daremberg and Ruelle (1879) 581. For impotence, magic, and medicine in the medieval West, see especially Rider (2006).

[95] See Aetius of Amida, *Medical Books*, 11.35.60–2, in ed. Daremberg and Ruelle (1879) 581.

[96] On the parallel exchange of ideas between doctors and sorcerers in the Roman Imperial period concerning understanding and treatment of supposed uterine disorders through amulets see Faraone (2011a: 135–44). Importantly, those he discusses function on an exorcistic model of treatment, whereby a demonic cause is assumed for an apparently physical illness; compare also Faraone (2011b: 21, 25–6).

[97] On amulets and the Christian response in this period see Dickie (2003: 292–6); see also Leyerle (2013: 83–8) and Faraone (2018: 7, 22).

the sort of plant and animal material I have been describing. In the fourth century CE Athanasios of Alexandria, for example, ridicules people for 'wearing at their necks the filth of four footed animals'.[98] But the church fathers' solution was not so much to stop people using amulets altogether as to encourage instead the wearing of amulets which employed Christian materials and symbols. Athanasios thus continues his diatribe by blaming his congregation for 'setting aside the seal of the saving cross, from which not only sicknesses flee but by which the whole mass of demons is also terrified and astounded'.[99] Around 1,000 years after Athanasios, in the early fifteenth century CE, another Byzantine churchman, Joseph Bryennios, was still complaining about the same practices among his congregation, and his solution was the same, if stated even more clearly: 'The majority of people', he says:

> thus know but one cure for pain in the limbs of the body, for infertility in their fields, for sickness in their animals, and for everything which hinders them: enchantments. And so, for each limb of the body and for every concern they find, I know not where, the proper enchantment, which they also call sorcery . . . But I, who hold those who do this and who receive them equal to idolaters, instead offer the following advice to those who have not yet been caught by this passion. Do you feel pain in part of your body and wish to enchant this by an efficacious enchantment? Then seal it with the sign of the cross . . . Instead of an amulet, exalt the Virgin and fasten her about you. Instead of the root of a plant, hang the cross about your neck.[100]

The point here is that the use of drugs in the magical amulets which constituted the 'medicinal patches' of the Byzantine world also needs to be seen as part of a continuum which extends smoothly into the use of therapeutic materials in Christian amulets – holy signs and symbols, holy writing, holy images, and, closest of all to the sort of thing being discussed here, relics. Instead of pieces of plant, animal, or mineral, good Byzantine

98 See Athanasius, *Fragment on Amulets*, in ed. Migne (1857–66) XXVI.1320A.

99 See Athanasius, *Fragment on Amulets*, in ed. Migne (1857–66) XXVI.1320B. For similar suggestions by John Chrysostom on the use of scriptural amulets and, especially, the symbol of the cross see Leyerle (2013: 84–5, 87). However, as Dickie (2003: 280–3) points out in relation to Caesarius of Arles and John Chrysostom, the legitimate source and perception of the amulet's empowerment matters more than the content, even if this is outwardly Christian. On the Athanasios passage, see also Dickie (2003: 284) and Kalleres (2014: 230), although the latter's citation in note 48 there is incorrect.

100 See Joseph Bryennios, *Seventy-Seven Chapters*, 25, in ed. Voulgaris (1784) 76–7. Compare also (two centuries earlier) Kekaumenos, *Strategikon* 3.117, in ed. Spadaro (1998) 166.20–1, which basically repeats the same point: 'Do not wear an amulet unless it is the cross or a holy image or the relic of a saint.' On the mixture of Christian and magical symbols in amulets, see also, for example, Spier (1993) and Walker (2015: 212).

Christians might well carry about with them a tiny piece of a saint or of the saint's possessions, or at least something that had come into contact with their relics or sanctuary: oil from a lamp or wax from a candle made holy by burning at the shrine, water blessed there, or earth from the sacred ground itself.[101] But, in essence, the materials that composed these *enkolpia* and *eulogia* were still performing the same function as the therapeutic substances employed in magical amulets, if conceived by user or witness as having an automatic effect or result.[102] They occupied exactly the same place in the broader conceptual framework of protection from ill health, adversity, or demonic attack or of securing good health, fortune, favour, and success.

And then, only a small step further along this continuum is, surely, the use of such 'sacred' therapeutic materials as a substitute for drugs in healing miracles. Among the myriad possibilities, I will cite just two vivid examples. In the first, shortly after the sudden death, probably in the year 1001, of Athanasios of Athos, who was crushed by collapsing scaffolding in the new church he was building at his monastery of the Great Lavra on Athos, his *vita* reports that some of his monks left for Constantinople to fetch his successor. On their way they encountered a shepherd who, even though his son was close to death, choking as a result of quinsy (peritonsillar abscess), still offered them hospitality. Impressed and grateful, they went with him to attend the boy. There 'one of them, the monk Symeon, took out a handkerchief dipped in the father's [Athanasios'] blood, and placed it on the child's neck. Immediately the child slept through the whole night, and by morning was seen to be recovered well and partaking of food'.[103] More well known, but perhaps even more striking, is a story from around 500 years earlier, preserved in the sixth century *Miracles* of Kosmas and Damianos. Here a pious woman who had evidently been cured from her ailments on several occasions by the intervention of the *anargyroi*, had images of them painted all over her house in gratitude. Subsequently, when left alone while dangerously ill from a chronic and painful stomach condition:

> she dragged herself out of bed, struggled to the place where these wisest of saints were depicted, and, using her faith as a staff, hauled herself upright

[101] See, for example, Heintz (2003: 279), Krueger (2005: 302–5), Leyerle (2013: 86–7), and Pitarakis (2015: 165–76). On the *protective* function of Christian amuletic objects see especially here Pitarakis (2006).

[102] Notable here are the hematite (bloodstone) amulets which cite and/or illustrate the miracle of the Woman with the Issue of Blood; see, for example, Gansell (2003), Heintz (2003: 275–6), and Vikan (1990: 156). On the historical use of hematite amulets see Faraone (2018: 94–7, 242).

[103] See *Life of Athanasios*, 69, in ed. Talbot (2016) 338–41. The same blood-stained rag continues to function in this extraordinary way in several further incidents, some as many as ten years after Athanasios' death. *Life of Athanasios* 72, 76, in ed. Talbot (2016) 344–9, 354–7.

> and scraped away with her finger nails some of the plaster; she put what she had scraped off into some water and drank the mixture. Immediately she was healed; the pains she had inside her were ended by the visitation of the saints.[104]

These stories make the point particularly clearly, but the evidence of similar holy therapeutic substances or drugs – oil, water, wax, earth, relics, passages of holy writing, or even infusions made from the body parts of saints – being applied or ingested is almost endless.[105]

To complete this trajectory, the use of therapeutic substances in fumigations may be set on the same sort of continuum. Leaving aside the use of regular incense in most Byzantine church rituals and the role it was thought to play,[106] the idea of more elaborate incenses or 'aromata' had evidently passed into popular Christian approaches both to worship and to coping with life more generally. There is thus, for example, the now familiar account by Michael Psellos of the empress Zoe's extraordinary passion, in the mid-eleventh century, for manufacturing perfumes and using them in her devotional practices, which, he manages to insinuate, are somewhat suspect.[107] But more clearly to the point, and perhaps even more worrying for orthodox doctrinalists, is an episode recorded in the miracles of Athanasios, the late thirteenth-/early fourteenth-century patriarch of Constantinople. Here a Bithynian village priest suffering from chronic fever is cured after being told by a friend of Athanasios' posthumous reputation as a healer. The friend thus advised the priest 'to place a tiny piece of the great man's garment on coals, to deeply inhale the fumes from it, and, together with the fumigation ('θυμιάσει'), to proclaim the names of the holy man like a charm ('ἐπᾴσματος') of salvation. When the priest did

[104] See *Miracles of Saints Kosmas and Damianos*, 15, in ed. Deubner (1907) 137–8, my translation. See further Krueger (2005: 311) and Pitarakis (2015: 174). It is worth noting that there is a significant word play here in the term translated as 'plaster' ('χρίσματος') since it can also mean 'grace' or 'unction'.

[105] For discussion and many examples of these 'contact relics' see Pitarakis (2015: 165–76). Further on oil and wax see Kreuger (2018: 21) and Lampadaridi (2018: 147–8), and compare the preparation from sanctified wax of figurines to be used in sorcery or divination rituals. See ed. Delatte (1927) 410.3–5. On infusions from body parts, see *Life of Maximos the Hutburner by Niphon*, 13.1, in ed. Greenfield (2016) 398–401; also see Klein (2015: 243) and Talbot (2015: 229). For the ingestion of blessed writing in the immediate post-Byzantine period see the rituals for helping a child to learn quoted by Baun (2013: 128–9).

[106] Caseau (2007); Pitarakis (2015: 164–5).

[107] See Michael Psellos, *Chronographia*, 6.64–7, 6.159, in ed. Reinsch (2014) 1.132–4, 179. Psellos introduces into his discussion the ancient theory that perfumes, like other natural substances and rituals, can attract or drive off spiritual powers. On the satirical and contemptuous nature of this passage see Kaldellis (1999: 111–12) and further here Duffy (1995: 88–90), Schreiner (2004: 688–9), and Walker (2015: 221–2).

this . . . that lengthy and feverish affliction of his body disappeared completely so as to leave no trace'.[108] That this was not an exceptional incident is shown by the fact that, in another story, a woman called Maria Frangopoulina was held to have been cured from a potentially fatal uterine disease in much the same way. She stole a piece of the deceased patriarch's 'holy ragged garment', which she then placed in a censer over hot coals and inhaled the fumes.[109]

Conclusion

Clearly there has been limited space here in which to consider the complex and potentially sprawling subject of drugs as therapeutic substances in Byzantine magic, but hopefully enough has been said to make some basic points apparent. By looking at the role such substances played in the practices and theory of Byzantine magic and at the problems of differentiating such practices and theory from those of either more rational medicine or more spiritual religion, I think it becomes clear that the concept of a drug in the Byzantine and thence the medieval Mediterranean world was something far more fluid, far less narrowly defined than our own. Hopefully there is an indication here of important lessons to be learned about conceptualisation, as well as the dangers of cross-cultural application of terms and ideas.

REFERENCES

Angeletti, L. R, Cavarra, B., and Gazzaniga, V. 2009. *Il* de urinis *di Teofilo Protospatario centralitá di un segno clinic*. Rome: Casa Editrice Università La Sapienza.

Ashbrook Harvey, S. 1984. 'Physicians and Ascetics in John of Ephesus', *Dumbarton Oaks Papers* 38: 87–93.

Baun, J. 2013. 'Coming of Age in Byzantium: Agency and Authority in Rites of Passage from Infancy to Adulthood', in P. Armstrong (ed.), *Authority in Byzantium*. Farnham: Ashgate, 113–45.

Beckh, H. ed. 1895. *Geoponica sive Cassiani Bassi scholastici De re rustica eclogue*. Leipzig: Teubner.

Bennett, D. 2017. *Medicine and Pharmacy in Byzantine Hospitals: A Study of the Extant Formularies*. Abingdon: Routledge.

108 See Theoktistos the Studite, *Posthumous Miracles of the Patriarch Athanasios I*, 32, in ed. Talbot (1983) 84–5.

109 See Theoktistos the Studite, *Posthumous Miracles of the Patriarch Athanasios I*, 63, in ed. Talbot (1983) 112–13 with discussion on 19. A cure for eye pain recorded on f. 176v of the MS Venice, BNM cod. gr. 501, dating to the first half of the fourteenth century, requires a prayer containing orthodox, magical, and exorcistic elements to be burnt in front of the problematic eye.

Biraud, M. 1993. 'Usages de l'asphodèle et étymologies d'ἀσφόδελος', in J. Manessy-Guitton (ed.), *Actes du Colloque: Les phytonymes grecs et latins.* Nice: Centre de recherches comparatives sur les langues de la Méditerranée ancienne, 37–42.

Bouras-Vallianatos, P. 2015. 'Contextualizing the Art of Healing by Byzantine Physicians', in B. Pittarakis (ed.), *'Life Is Short, Art Long': The Art of Healing in Byzantium.* Istanbul: Pera Museum Publications, 104–22.

Bouras-Vallianatos, P. 2016a. 'Modelled on Archigenes *Theiotatos*: Alexander of Tralles and His Use of Natural Remedies (*Physika*)', *Mnemosyne* 69: 382–96.

Bouras-Vallianatos, P. 2016b. 'Case Histories in Late Byzantium: Reading the Patient in John Aktouarios' *On Urines*', in G. Petridou and C. Thumiger (eds.), *Homo Patiens: Approaches to the Patient in the Ancient World.* Leiden: Brill, 390–412.

Bourbou, C. 2010. *Health and Disease in Byzantine Crete (7th–12th centuries AD).* Aldershot: Ashgate.

Bradley, M., Grand-Clément, A., Rendu-Loisel, A.-C., and Vincent, A. eds. (forthcoming). *Sensing Divinity: Incense, Religion and the Ancient Sensorium.*

Burgmann, L. ed. 1983. *Ecloga: Das Gesetzbuch Leons III und Konstantinos V.* Frankfurt: Löwenklau Gesellschaft E.V.

Caseau, B. 2001. 'Les usages médicaux de l'encens et des parfums : Un aspect de la médecine populaire antique et de sa christianisation', in S. Bazin-Tacchela, D. Quéruel, and Ė. Samama (eds.), *Air, Miasmes et Contagion : Les épidémies dans l'Antiquité et au Moyen Age.* Langres: Dominique Guéniot, 75–85.

Caseau, B. 2007. 'Incense and Fragrances from House to Church', in M. Grünbart, E. Kislinger, A. Muthesius, and D. Stathakopoulos (eds.), *Material Culture and Well-Being in Byzantium (400–1453).* Vienna: Verlages der Österreichischen Akademie der Wissenschaften, 75–92.

Caudano, A.-L. 2016. '"These Are the Only Four Seas": The World Map of Bologna, University Library, Codex 3632', *Dumbarton Oaks Papers* 70: 167–90.

Cavallo, G. 2009. 'Note', in L. R. Angeletti, B. Cavarra, and V. Gazzaniga (eds.), *Il* de urinis *di Teofilo Protospatario centralitá di un segno clinic.* Rome: Casa Editrice Università La Sapienza, 164–9.

Chirban, J. T. 2010a. 'Holistic Healing in Byzantium: Historical Perspectives on Byzantine Healing', in J. T. Chirban (ed.), *Holistic Healing in Byzantium.* Brookline, MA: Holy Cross Orthodox Press, 3–36.

Chirban, J. T. 2010b. 'Holistic Healing in Byzantium: Understanding the Importance of Epistemologies and Methodologies', in J. T. Chirban (ed.), *Holistic Healing in Byzantium.* Brookline, MA: Holy Cross Orthodox Press, 37–69.

Clark, P. A. 2011. *A Cretan Healer's Handbook in the Byzantine Tradition.* Farnham: Ashgate.

Constantelos, D. 1966–7. 'Physician-Priests in the Medieval Greek Church', *Greek Orthodox Theological Review* 12: 141–53.

Constantelos, D. 1991. 'The Interface of Medicine and Religion in the Greek and Christian Greek Orthodox Tradition', in J. T. Chirban (ed.), *Health and*

Faith: Medical, Psychological and Religious Dimensions. Lanham, MD: University Press of America, 13–24.

Constantelos, D. 2010. 'Faith and Healing in Sacramental Life: The Byzantine and Modern Greek Orthodox Experience', in J. T. Chirban (ed.), *Holistic Healing in Byzantium*. Brookline, MA: Holy Cross Orthodox Press, 131–48.

Copenhaver, B. P. 2006. 'Magic', in K. Park and L. Daston (eds.), *The Cambridge History of Science*, vol. III. Cambridge: Cambridge University Press, 518–40.

Crislip, A. 2005. *From Monastery to Hospital: Christian Monasticism and the Transformation of Health Care in Late Antiquity*. Ann Arbor: University of Michigan Press.

Cupane, C. 1980. 'La magia a Bisanzio nel secolo XIV: Azione e reazione', *Jahrbuch der Österricheischen Byzantinistik* 29: 237–62.

Dalby, A. trans. 2011. *Geoponika: Farm Work*. Totnes, Devon: Prospect Books.

Daremberg, C., and C. É. Ruelle, C. É. eds. 1879. *Oeuvres de Rufus d'Éphèse*. Paris: Imprimerie Nationale.

Darrouzès, J. 1977. *Regestes des actes du patriarcat de Constantinople : Fasc. 5. Les regestes de 1310 à 1376*. Paris: Institut Français d'Études Byzantines.

Dauterman Maguire, E. H., and Maguire, H. 2007. *Other Icons: Art and Power in Byzantine Secular Culture*. Princeton, NJ: Princeton University Press.

Delatte, A. ed. 1927. *Anecdota Atheniensia I: Textes Grecs inédits relatifs à l'histoire des religions*. Liège: Champion.

Delatte, A. 1938. *Herbarius: Recherches sur le cérémonial usité chez les anciens pour la cueillette des simples et des plantes magiques*, 2nd ed. Liège: Bibliothèque de la Faculté de Philosophie et Lettres de l'Université de Liège, Fasc. LXXXI.

Delatte, A. 1949. 'Le traité des plantes planétaires d'un manuscrit de Léningrad', *Mélanges H. Gregoire : Annuaire de l'Institut de philologie et d'histoire orientales et Slaves* 9: 145–77.

Demetriades, A. K. 2015. *Iatrosophikón: Folklore Remedies from a Cyprus Monastery. Original Text and Parallel Translation of Codex Machairas A.18*. Nicosia: Foundation A. G. Leventis.

Detlefsen, D. ed. 1866–82. *C. Plinii Secundi Naturalis Historia*. 3 vols. Berlin: Weidmann.

Deubner, L. ed. 1907. *Kosmas und Damian: Texte*. Leipzig: Teubner.

Diamantopoulos, Th. 1995. 'Εἰκονογραφήσεις βυζαντινῶν ἰατρικῶν χειρογράφων', in E. Glykatze-Arveler, Th. Diamantopoulos, A. Hohlweg, and A. Tselikas (eds.), *Ἰατρικὰ Βυζαντινὰ Χειρόγραφα*. Athens: Domos, 71–168.

Dickie, M. W. 2003. *Magic and Magicians in the Greco-Roman World*. Abingdon: Routledge.

Duffy, J. 1984. 'Byzantine Medicine in the Sixth and Seventh Centuries: Aspects of Teaching and Practice', *Dumbarton Oaks Papers*, 38: 21–7.

Duffy, J. 1995. 'Reactions of Two Byzantine Intellectuals to the Theory and Practice of Magic: Michael Psellos and Michael Italikos', in H. Maguire (ed.), *Byzantine Magic*. Washington, DC: Dumbarton Oaks, 83–97.

Duling, D. C. 1983. 'The Testament of Solomon', in J. H. Charlesworth (ed.), *The Old Testament Pseudepigrapha. I.* Garden City, NJ: Doubleday, 935–87.

Everett, E. ed. 2012. *The Alphabet of Galen*. Toronto: University of Toronto Press.

Faraone, C. A. 2011a. 'Magic and Medicine in the Roman Imperial Period: Two Case Studies', in G. Bohak, Y. Harari, and S. Shaked (eds.), *Continuity and Innovation in the Magical Tradition*. Leiden: Brill, 135–57.

Faraone, C. A. 2011b. 'Magical and Medical Approaches to the Wandering Womb in the Ancient Greek World', *Classical Antiquity*, 30.1: 1–32.

Faraone, C. A. 2018. *The Transformation of Greek Amulets in Roman Imperial Times*. Philadelphia: University of Pennsylvania Press.

Flemming, J. ed. 1917. *Akten der ephesinischen Synode vom Jahre 449*. Abhandlungen der Königlichen Gesellschaft der Wissenschaften zu Göttingen. Philologisch-historische Klasse. Neu Folge XV. Berlin: Weidmannsche Buchhandlung.

Fögen, M. T. 1995. 'Balsamon on Magic: From Roman Secular Law to Byzantine Canon Law', in H. Maguire (ed.), *Byzantine Magic*. Washington, DC: Dumbarton Oaks, 99–115.

Frankfurter, D. 2019. 'Ancient Magic in a New Key: Refining an Exotic Discipline in the History of Religions', in D. Frankfurter (ed.), *Guide to the Study of Ancient Magic*. Leiden: Brill, 3–20.

Gansell, A. R. 2003. 'Amulet Portraying the Woman with the Issue of Blood', in I. Kalavrezou (ed.), *Byzantine Women and Their World*. New Haven, CT: Yale University Press, 283–4.

Gentilcore, D. 1998. *Healers and Healing in Early Modern Italy*. Manchester: Manchester University Press.

Greenfield, R. P. H. 1988. *Traditions of Belief in Late Byzantine Demonology*. Amsterdam: Hakkert.

Greenfield, R. P. H. 1993. 'Sorcery and Politics at the Byzantine Court in the Twelfth Century: Interpretations of History', in R. Beaton and C. Roueché (eds.), *The Making of Byzantine History: Studies Dedicated to Donald M. Nicol*. Aldershot: Variorum, 73–85.

Greenfield, R. P. H. 1995. 'A Contribution to the Study of Palaeologan Magic', in H. Maguire (ed.), *Byzantine Magic*. Washington, DC: Dumbarton Oaks, 117–53.

Greenfield, R. P. H. ed. 2016 'Life of Maximos the Hutburner by Niphon', in R. P. H. Greenfield and A.-M. Talbot (eds.), *Holy Men of Mount Athos*. Cambridge, MA: Harvard University Press, 369–439.

Greenfield, R. P. H. 2017. 'Magic and the Occult Sciences', in A. Kaldellis and N. Siniossoglou (eds.), *The Cambridge Intellectual History of Byzantium*. Cambridge: Cambridge University Press, 215–33.

Hartnup, K. 2004. *'On the Beliefs of the Greeks': Leo Allatios and Popular Orthodoxy*. Leiden: Brill.

Heintz, M. H. 2003. 'Magic, Medicine, and Prayer', in I. Kalavrezou (ed.), *Byzantine Women and Their World*. New Haven, CT: Yale University Press, 274–81.

Honigmann, E. 1944 'A Trial for Sorcery on August 22, A.D. 449', *Isis* 35.4: 281–4.

Horden, P. 1982. 'The Case of Theodore of Sykeon', in W. J. Shiels (ed.), *The Church and Healing: Studies in Church History*, vol. XIX. Oxford: Blackwell, 1–13.

Hort, A. F. ed. 1916. *Theophrastus: Enquiry into Plants*. Cambridge, MA: Harvard University Press.

Humphreys, M. trans. 2017. *The Laws of the Isaurian Era: The Ecloga and Its Appendices*. Liverpool: Liverpool University Press.

Ierodiakonou, K. 2006. 'The Greek Concept of *Sympatheia* and Its Byzantine Appropriation in Michael Psellos', in P. Magdalino and M. Mavroudi (eds.), *The Occult Sciences in Byzantium*. Geneva: la Pomme d'Or, 97–117.

Iles Johnston, S. 2002. 'The *Testament of Solomon* from Late Antiquity to the Renaissance', in J. Bremmer and J. Veenstra (eds.), *The Metamorphosis of Magic from Late Antiquity to the Early Modern Period*. Leuven: Peeters, 35–49.

Jolly, K. L. 2002. 'Medieval Magic: Definitions, Beliefs, Practices', in K. Jolly, C. Raudvere, and E. Peters (eds.), *Witchcraft and Magic in Europe: The Middle Ages*. London: Athlone Press, 3–71.

Kaimakis, D. ed. 1976. *Die Kyraniden*. Meisenheim am Glam: Hain.

Kaldellis, A. 1999. *The Argument of Psellos'* Chronographia. Leiden: Brill.

Kalleres, D. 2014. 'Drunken Hags with Amulets and Prostitutes with Erotic Spells: The Re-feminization of Magic in Late Antique Christian Homilies', in K. B. Stratton and D. S. Kalleres (eds.), *Daughters of Hecate: Women and Magic in the Ancient* World. Oxford: Oxford University Press, 119–251.

Kazhdan, A. 1984. 'The Medical Doctor in Byzantine Literature of the Tenth to Twelfth Centuries', *Dumbarton Oaks Papers*, 38: 43–51.

Kiraz, M. 2015. 'Catalogue 12', in B. Pitarakis (ed.), *'Life Is Short, Art Long': The Art of Healing in Byzantium*. Istanbul: Pera Museum Publications, 212–13.

Klein, H. 2015. 'Materiality and the Sacred: Byzantine Reliquaries and the Rhetoric of Enshrinement', in C. Hahn and H. A. Klein (eds.), *Saints and Sacred Matter: The Cult of Relics in Byzantium and Beyond*. Washington, DC: Dumbarton Oaks, 231–52.

Klutz, T. 2005. *Rewriting the Testament of Solomon: Tradition, Conflict and Identity in a Late Antique Pseudepigraphon*. London: T&T Clark.

Krueger, D. 2005. 'Christian Piety and Practice in the Sixth Century', in M. Maas (ed.), *The Cambridge Companion to the Age of Justinian*. Cambridge: Cambridge University Press, 291–315.

Krueger, D. 2010. 'Healing and the Scope of Religion in Byzantium: A Response to Miller and Crislip', in J. T. Chirban (ed.), *Holistic Healing in Byzantium*. Brookline, MA: Holy Cross Orthodox Press, 119–28.

Krueger, D. 2018. 'Healing and Salvation in Byzantium', in B. Pitarakis and G. Tanman (eds.), *Life Is Short, Art Long: The Art of Healing in Byzantium, New Perspectives*. Istanbul: Istanbul Research Institute, 15–40.

Kühn, C. G. ed. 1821–33. *Claudii Galeni Opera omnia*. Lipsiae: C. Cnobloch.

Lampadaridi, A. 2018. 'Sick and Cured: St. Eugenios of Trebizond and His Miraculous Healings', in B. Pitarakis and G. Tanman (eds.), *Life Is Short, Art Long: The Art of Healing in Byzantium, New Perspectives*. Istanbul: Istanbul Research Institute, 139–49.

Lazaris, S. 2017. 'Scientific, Medical and Technical Manuscripts', in V. Tsamakda (ed.), *A Companion to Byzantine Illustrated Manuscripts*. Leiden: Brill, 55–113.

Leyerle, B. 2013. '"Keep Me, Lord, As the Apple of Your Eyes": An Early Christian Child's Amulet', *Journal of Early Christian History* 3.2: 73–93.
MacMullen, R. 1997. *Christianity and Paganism in the Fourth to Eighth Centuries*. New Haven, CT: Yale University Press.
Magdalino, P., and Mavroudi, M. 2006. 'Introduction', in P. Magdalino and M. Mavroudi (eds.), *The Occult Sciences in Byzantium*. Geneva: la Pomme d'Or, 11–37.
Maguire, H. 1995. 'Magic and the Christian Image', in H. Maguire (ed.), *Byzantine Magic*. Washington, DC: Dumbarton Oaks, 51–71.
Maguire, H. 1996. *The Icons of Their Bodies: Saints and Their Images in Byzantium*. Princeton, NJ: Princeton University Press.
Marathakis, I. 2011. *The Magical Treatise of Solomon or* Hygromanteia. Singapore: Golden Hoard Press.
Marchetti, F. 2010. 'Un manoscritto "senza pari": Le illustrazioni', in B. Antonino with P. Moscatelli (eds.), *BUB: Ricerche e cataloghi sui fondi della Biblioteca Universitaria di Bologna*. Bologna: BUB, 41–64.
Mavroudi, M. 2006. 'Occult Science and Society in Byzantium: Considerations for Future Research', in P. Magdalino and M. Mavroudi (eds.), *The Occult Sciences in Byzantium*. Geneva: la Pomme d'Or, 39–95.
McCabe, A. 2007. *A Byzantine Encyclopaedia of Horse Medicine: The Sources, Compilation, and Transmission of the* Hippiatrica. Oxford: Oxford University Press.
McCown, C. C. ed. 1922. *The Testament of Solomon: Edited from Manuscripts at Mount Athos, Bologna, Holkham Hall, Jerusalem, London, Milan, Paris and Vienna*. Leipzig: J. C. Hinrichs.
Migne, J.-P. ed. 1857–66. *Patrologiae cursus completus . . . Series Graeca*. 161 vols. Paris: J.-P. Migne.
Miklosich, F., and Muller, I. eds. 1860–90. *Acta et diplomata Graeca medii aevi sacra et profana collecta*. 6 vols. Vienna: Carolus Gerold.
Mondrain, B. 1999. 'Nicolas Myrepse et une collection de manuscrits médicaux dans la première moitié du XIVe siècle: A propos d'une miniature célèbre du Parisinus gr. 2243', in A. Garzya and J. Jouanna (eds.), *I testi medici greci: Tradizione e ecdotica. Atti del III Convegno Internazionale, Napoli 15–18 ottobre 1997*, Collectanea 17. Naples: D'Auria, 403–18.
Nagy, Á. M. 2012. '*Daktylios Pharmakites*: Magical Healing Gems and Rings in the Graeco-Roman World', in I. Csepregi and C. Burnett (eds.), *Ritual Healing: Magic, Ritual and Medical Therapy from Antiquity until the Early Modern Period*. Florence: Sismel, 71–106.
Nutton, V. 1984. 'From Galen to Alexander: Aspects of Medicine and Medical Practice in Late Antiquity', *Dumbarton Oaks Papers* 38: 1–14.
Nutton, V. 2013. *Ancient Medicine*. 2nd ed. London: Routledge.
Oberhelman, S. 2013. 'Introduction: Medical Pluralism, Healing, and Dreams in Greek Culture', in S. Oberhelman (ed.), *Dreams, Healing, and Medicine in Greece: From Antiquity to the Present*. Farnham: Ashgate, 1–30.
Oberhelman, S. 2015. 'Towards a Typology of Byzantine and Post-Byzantine Healing Texts', *Athens Journal of Health* 2.2: 133–46.

Pingree, D. 1971. 'The Astrological School of John Abramius', *Dumbarton Oaks Papers* 25: 189–215.

Pitarakis, B. 2006. 'Objects of Devotion and Protection', in D. Krueger (ed.), *Byzantine Christianity*. Minneapolis, MN: Fortress Press, 164–81.

Pitarakis, B. 2015. 'Empowering Healing: Substances, Senses and Rituals', in B. Pitarakis (ed.), *'Life Is Short, Art Long': The Art of Healing in Byzantium*. Istanbul: Pera Museum Publications, 162–79.

Powell, O. trans. 2003. *Galen: On the Properties of Foodstuffs*. Cambridge: Cambridge University Press.

Puschmann, T. ed. 1878–9. *Alexander von Tralles: Original-Text und Übersetzung nebst einer einleitenden Abhandlung; ein Beitrag zur Geschichte der Medicin*. 2 vols. Vienna: Wilhelm Braumüller.

Reece, S. 2007. 'Homer's Asphodel Meadow', *Greek, Roman, and Byzantine Studies* 47, 389–400.

Reinsch, D. R. ed. 2014. *Michaelis Pselli Chronographia*. 2 vols. Berlin: De Gruyter.

Rider, C. 2006. *Magic and Impotence in the Middle Ages*. Oxford: Oxford University Press.

Rigo, A. 2002. 'From Constantinople to the Library of Venice: The Hermetic Books of Late Byzantine Doctors, Astrologers and Magicians', in C. Gilly and C. van Heertum (eds.), *Magia, alchimia, scienza dal '400 al '700: L'Influsso di Ermete Trismegisto*, vol. I. Venice: Centro Di, 77–84.

Rodgers, R. 2002. '*Kêpopoiïa*: Garden-Making and Garden Culture in the Greek *Geoponika*', in A. Littlewood, H. Maguire, and J. Wolschke-Bulmahn (eds.), *Byzantine Garden Culture*. Washington, DC: Dumbarton Oaks, 159–75.

Roueché, C. ed. 2013. *Kekaumenos, Consilia et Narrationes*. London: SAWS Edition. https://ancientwisdoms.ac.uk/library/kekaumenos-consilia-et-narrationes/index.html, accessed 15 March 2020.

Russell, J. 1995. 'The Archaeological Context of Magic in the Early Byzantine Period', in H. Maguire (ed.), *Byzantine Magic*. Washington, DC: Dumbarton Oaks, 35–50.

Scarborough, J. 1984a. 'Introduction', *Dumbarton Oaks Papers* 38: ix–xvi.

Scarborough, J. 1984b. 'Early Byzantine Pharmacology', *Dumbarton Oaks Papers* 38: 213–32.

Scarborough, J. 1991. 'The Pharmacology of Sacred Plants, Herbs, and Roots', in C. A. Faraone and D. Obbink (eds.), *Magika Hiera: Ancient Greek Magic and Religion*. Oxford: Oxford University Press, 138–74.

Scarborough, J. 1997. 'The Life and Times of Alexander of Tralles', *Expedition* 39.2: 51–60.

Scarborough, J. 2010. 'The Pharmacology of Sacred Plants, Herbs, and Roots', reprinted with addenda and corrigenda in J. Scarborough, *Pharmacy and Drug Lore in Antiquity: Greece, Rome, Byzantium*, vol. I. Farnham: Ashgate, 1–6.

Schreiner, P. 2004. 'A la recherché d'un folklore à Byzance', in J. Hamesse (ed.), *Bilan et perspectives des études médiévales (1993–1998)*. Turnhout: Brepols, 685–94.

Spadaro, M. D. ed. 1998. *Raccomandazioni e consigli di un galantuomo (Στρατηγικόν)*. Alessandria: Edizioni dell'Orso.

Spier, J. 1993. 'Medieval Byzantine Magical Amulets and Their Tradition', *Journal of the Warburg and Courtauld Institutes* 56: 25–62.

Stewart, C. 1991. *Demons and the Devil: Moral Imagination in Modern Greek Culture*. Princeton, NJ: Princeton University Press.

Talbot, A.-M. 1983. *Faith Healing in Late Byzantium: The Posthumous Miracles of the Patriarch Athanasios I of Constantinople by Theoktistos the Stoudite*. Brookline, MA: Hellenic College Press.

Talbot, A.-M. 2010. 'Faith Healing in Byzantium', in J. T. Chirban (ed.), *Holistic Healing in Byzantium*. Brookline, MA: Holy Cross Orthodox Press, 151–72.

Talbot, A.-M. ed. 2012. 'Miracles of Gregory Palamas', in A.-M. Talbot and S. F. Johnson (eds.), *Miracle Tales from Byzantium*. Cambridge, MA: Harvard University Press, 299–405.

Talbot, A.-M. 2015. 'The Relics of New Saints: Deposition, Translation, and Veneration in Middle and Late Byzantium', in C. Hahn and H. A. Klein (eds.), *Saints and Sacred Matter: The Cult of Relics in Byzantium and Beyond*. Washington, DC: Dumbarton Oaks, 215–30.

Talbot, A.-M. ed. 2016. 'Life of Athanasios of Athos, Version B', in R. P. H. Greenfield and A.-M. Talbot (eds.), *Holy Men of Mount Athos*. Cambridge, MA: Harvard University Press, 127–367.

Timplalexi, P. 2002. *Medizinisches in der byzantinischen Epistolographie (1100–1453)*. Frankfurt: Peter Lang.

Touwaide, A. 2007. 'Byzantine Hospital Manuals (*Iatrosophia*) As a Source for the Study of Therapeutics', in B. S. Bowers (ed.), *The Medieval Hospital and Medical Practice*. Aldershot: Ashgate, 147–73.

Trapp, E, Walther, R., and Beyer, H.-V. eds. 1976–96. *Prosopographisches Lexikon der Palaiologenzeit*. 12 vols. Vienna: Verlag der Österreichischen Akademie der Wissenschaften.

Tselikas, A. 1995. 'Τὰ Ἑλληνικὰ γιατροσόφια: Μία περιφρονημένη κατηγορία χειρογράφων', in E. Glykatze-Arveler, Th. Diamantopoulos, A. Hohlweg, and A. Tselikas (eds.), *Ἰατρικὰ Βυζαντινὰ Χειρόγραφα*. Athens: Domos, 57–70.

Vakaloudi, A.D. 2001. *Η μαγεία ως κοινωνικό φαινόμενο στο πρώιμο Βυζάντιο (4ος-7ος μ.Χ. αι.)*. Athens: Enalios.

Verpoorten, J.-M. 1962. 'Les noms grecs et latins de l'asphodèle', *L'Antiquité Classique Année* 31: 111–29.

Vikan, G. 1984. 'Art, Medicine and Magic in Early Byzantium', *Dumbarton Oaks Papers* 38: 65–86.

Vikan, G. 1990. 'Art and Marriage in Early Byzantium', *Dumbarton Oaks Papers* 44: 145–63.

Voulgaris, E. ed. 1784. *Ἰωσὴφ Μοναχοῦ τοῦ Βρυεννίου τὰ Εὑρεθέντα, vol. III τὰ Παραλειπόμενα*. Leipzig: Vreitkopph.

Waegeman, M. trans. 1987. *Amulet and Alphabet: Magical Amulets in the First Book of Cyranides*. Amsterdam: J.C. Gieben.

Walker, A. 2015. 'Magic in Medieval Byzantium', in D. J. Collins (ed.), *The Cambridge History of Magic and Witchcraft in the West*. Cambridge: Cambridge University Press, 209–34.

Wilkins, J. ed. 2013. *Galien: Sur les facultés des aliments*. Paris: Les Belles Lettres.

CHAPTER 8

Remedies or Superstitions
Maimonides on Mishnah Shabbat 6:10

Phillip I. Lieberman

Do magical recipes work? I begin with a story. A number of years ago I gave a graduate seminar in Islamic law at New York University. One of my students was earning her master's degree part time and worked the rest of the time as an editor for *Glamour* magazine, a publication whose articles provide advice in the areas of fashion and beauty. I proposed to her that I write an article for *Glamour* on magical recipes from the Cairo Genizah. Magic focuses on harnessing superhuman powers and transcending the laws of nature for one's own ends; since *Glamour* was devoted to harnessing extraordinary powers to find one's 'soulmate', I thought the perpetual nature of the magazine's concerns would be of interest to its readers. Gideon Bohak, scholar of ancient Jewish magic, identifies a number of domains in which Jewish magic has sought to intervene across the millennia – 'to heal the sick, harm the healthy, make a woman love a man, make a newly wed man impotent or release him from such impotence, and perform other real changes in the world around them'[1] – and some of these very areas are regularly the subject of articles in *Glamour*. So I thought the magazine might like an article on medieval magical recipes for doing the same.

Ultimately the editors at *Glamour* did not like my suggestion, perhaps because in the article I wished to focus on what happens when 'magical' remedies *do not work*. Magazines whose advertisers sell products designed to help 'make a woman love a man' or the reverse probably do not even want to consider the possibility that such products might not work. However, just because a product is ineffective in a particular instance does not mean that it 'does not work'. Humans and their relationships are extremely complex, and as the saying goes, 'your mileage may vary'.

[1] Bohak (2008: 359).

I had long wondered how robust belief in magical recipes might be even when those recipes seemed not to work for a particular individual. Of course, where the predictions of a recipe are unfalsifiable, an individual's belief need not be challenged and no cognitive dissonance need arise if the recipe fails to deliver. But where those predictions are more precise, the system of magic faces a more challenging problem: how to prevent an aspirant losing faith in the magical system when desired outcomes do not obtain. However, Bohak reassures us that the failure to perform does not weaken the integrity of the magical system one iota:

> We may also note that if an amulet failed to alleviate the affliction, it was assumed that something was wrong with this specific amulet, and perhaps also with the person who produced it, so that one could simply turn to another amulet-writer, who may have a more accurate knowledge of what needed to be in the amulet.[2]

That is to say, even if the amulet itself were faulty, the system of producing such amulets would not lose credibility. The error would certainly have been with the product or the manufacturer – not the recipe. Additionally, if there was any possibility that the 'end user' of the amulet might have failed to follow proper instructions, believers in the magical system could turn to this too as the reason for the amulet's failure to perform.

All this suggests that systems of magic had more than ample means to parry a challenge that magical recipes themselves are ineffective. Of course, when desired consequences *do* follow when a magical recipe is implemented, the 'producer' of the magic and the 'end user' could both rely on the psychologists' 'confirmation bias' to identify the magical recipe as the source of the desired consequences.[3] Thus, magical recipes may be difficult to reject where users ignore or downplay disconfirming evidence, leaving even a society which eschews the use of magic great difficulty extirpating belief therein and its practice.[4]

The connection between amulets and drugs may be obvious, but it bears mention here: both provide us with recipes to be followed precisely in order to produce specific results. Both magic and medicine might be subject to the scepticism of end users who have carefully followed the instructions of experts yet whose efforts did not achieve the desired result. Indeed, the boundary between these two disciplines is flimsy at best, particularly where the antique and medieval worlds are concerned.

[2] Bohak (2008: 375). [3] For a discussion of confirmation bias, see Koslowski and Maqueda (1993).

[4] On the interrelationship between magic and medicine with a focus on the use of drugs as therapeutic substances in later Byzantium, see Greenfield (Chapter 7) in this volume.

The work of Jacques Jouanna on the use of amulets by physicians in the Graeco-Roman world highlights the permeability of this boundary in the Mediterranean.[5] In this chapter I wish to place the approach of the Mediterranean thinker Moses Maimonides (1138–1204) to the permeable boundary between medicine and magic in line with rabbinic literature and the Islamicate medical tradition alike. I aim to explore Maimonides' approach to the perennial problem of how the authority of formal prescriptions interacts with (at times contradictory) human experience.[6]

In his *Dalālat al-ḥā'irīn* (*The Guide to the Perplexed*), Maimonides sheds much ink squaring both biblical and rabbinic literature with rational thought and the sciences, arguing that biblical law was itself designed to combat false beliefs and superstitions. Thus, for example, the sacrifices in the Temple in Jerusalem were enjoined on the Israelites to snuff out popular cult sacrifice in local idolatrous sanctuaries throughout the land of Israel.[7] Likewise, the Torah's prohibitions on magic point to the folly of witchcraft and the like and to return the individual to trust in the divine order governed by natural law.

However, humanity's natural tendency towards the confirmation bias is powerful, and probably impossible to uproot despite the Torah's attempts to discredit magic and witchcraft by proscribing acts that suggest superstition and indeed outlawing magical practices generally. In this vein, Maimonides writes: 'To set all their magical practices at a remove, the Torah bans any pagan act, even those linked with agriculture, animal husbandry, and such – anything supposedly helpful but not prescribed by natural science rather than the supposed occult properties of things.'[8] But as scholars of operant conditioning have pointed out, behaviours rewarded with intermittent reinforcement are in fact highly resistant to extinction.[9] That is to say, when some sort of action garners a desired response *intermittently*, greater effort will have to be expended to unhitch the perceived connection between the behaviour and the response.

[5] See Jouanna (2011).

[6] Indeed, I hope to examine this question in greater depth in a future book-length project in which I contextualise commercial manuals running from antiquity to the high Middle Ages in light of commercial practice, asking how the end users of those commercial manuals viewed their literary sources when they were challenged by empirical experience.

[7] Cf. Moses Maimonides, *Dalālat al-ḥā'irīn* (*The Guide to the Perplexed*), 3.32, ed. Munk (1856–66) III.30. All translations of the *Guide* in this chapter come from my forthcoming translation (with Lenn Goodman), to be published by Stanford University Press in 2024. Translations of other primary sources in the chapter are my own.

[8] Moses Maimonides, *Dalālat al-ḥā'irīn* (*The Guide to the Perplexed*), 3.37, ed. Munk (1856–66) III.37.

[9] See Skinner's (1957) work on *variable ratio schedules*.

This, according to the behavioural psychologist B. F. Skinner, is what leads to the development of superstitions. Noting in an experiment that pigeons ascribed consequences to the delivery of food that in fact came according to a regular schedule, Skinner noted that:

> A few accidental connections between a ritual and favorable consequences suffice to set up and maintain the behavior in spite of many unreinforced instances. The bowler who has released a ball down the alley but continues to behave as if he were controlling it by twisting and turning his arm and shoulder is another case in point. These behaviors have, of course, no real effect upon one's luck or upon a ball half way down an alley, just as in the present case the food would appear as often if the pigeon did nothing – or, more strictly speaking, did something else.[10]

Skinner identified ways superstitions are formed in the mind – by intuiting a connection between one's action and the desired reaction, even when that connection is not really there. As a student of experimental medicine, Maimonides too was very interested in the formation of mental connections between cause and effect. Seeing the Torah's interest in extinguishing false beliefs, Maimonides – also known as the Great Eagle – was concerned with what happens when magical recipes seem to work. As we shall see, Maimonides militates against simply relying on one's experience – after all, Skinner's pigeons relied on their experiences, and that led them to superstition – but at the same time, he cannot shut the door to experience. Having been trained in medicine, Maimonides was well familiar with the Galenic experimental method.

Furthermore, in the *Guide* but also certainly in his legal *magnum opus*, the *Mishneh Torah*, Maimonides is loyal to the rabbinic tradition.[11] Thus, despite his claim in the *Guide* that the Torah eschews magical performances which are justified neither by logic (Judeo-Arabic, *qiyās*) or reason (Judeo-Arabic, *ʿaql*), Maimonides is well familiar with the fact that Talmudic literature actually seems to open the door to a number of remedies that smack of magic, unsupported by either logic *or* reason. The Mishnah, the third-century compilation of statements of the early rabbinic sages (Tannaim) that underpins the Talmud, explains in Shabbat 6:10 that:

> One may go out with a locust egg, or with a fox's tooth, or with the nail of one who has been hanged, for the sake of remedies, these are the words of

10 Skinner (1948).

11 That is to say, the focus of *The Guide to the Perplexed* is often biblical law and language rather than rabbinic law, which is the province of the *Mishneh Torah*.

> Rabbi Meir. But the Sages say: This is forbidden even on a weekday because it imitates the ways of the Amorites.[12]

As with much of the Mishnah's material on the Sabbath, one concern in this text could be that carrying such items into the public domain could be considered a type of work and therefore prohibited – however, 'remedies' are exempt from this general prohibition. Thus, the Mishnah generally prohibits 'amulets' from being carried in the public domain on the Sabbath 'if they are not from an expert'.[13] Presumably, the end-user of an amulet *not* produced by an expert could not be assured of its effectiveness, in which case carrying such an amulet would not be subject to the exemption for 'remedies' and would amount to (prohibited) carrying in the public domain.[14] But as for an amulet produced by an expert, or a locust egg, and so forth – these items are *understood* to be effective.

Yet the effectiveness of these remedies is not the Mishnah's only concern. The opinion of the Sages that these remedies are forbidden even on days other than the Sabbath points not to the prohibition on carrying in the public domain (which applies only on the Sabbath) but to 'imitating the ways of the Amorites' – perhaps ultimately drawing on the Bible's directive not to 'walk in their ways' (Leviticus 18:3).[15] The Mishnah also alludes to the 'ways of the Amorites' in Ḥullin 4:7,[16] including their burying an aborted animal fetus at a crossroads or hanging it in a tree; and the Babylonian Talmud lists a number of such practices in Shabbat 67b, attributed to the Amorites, which are used in divination. These include, say, dancing in front of a pot of *kutaḥ*, a milk and bread-based dish – but they do not include placing a chip from a berry bush or broken pieces of glass in a pot so it will boil more quickly.

Thus, had Maimonides wished to prohibit such remedies entirely, he could have relied on the opinion of the Sages. Surprisingly, he takes a different tactic. He begins by explaining in the *Guide* that the practices the Mishnah mentions are acceptable, but goes a step farther in arguing that other, similar, practices are permitted – even pinning a peony on an epileptic, using dog droppings for a sore throat, and treating hard, swollen tendons by fumigation with vinegar and marcasite is acceptable. As we

[12] Mishnah, ed. Albeck (1951–8). Note that there are variant texts of this Mishnah; in Kafiḥ's edition (1963–8) II.42, of Maimonides' commentary on the Mishnah, the opinion of Rabbi Meir is given as that of Rabbi Yose, and that of the Sages is given by Rabbi Meir.

[13] Mishnah Shabbat 6:2. [14] See Albeck's (1951–8) commentary.

[15] Note that the biblical verse itself prohibits only the ways of 'the land of Egypt' and of 'the land of Canaan', but the Mishnah nonetheless alludes to the prohibition of Amorite ways as well.

[16] They are also detailed in Tosefta Shabbat, 7–8, ed. Zuckermandel (1970).

shall see, Maimonides leaves open the possibility that one may engage in those practices which – like those permitted by Rabbi Meir in the Mishnah – are understood to be effective.

It is worthwhile pointing out that in allowing certain remedies, Maimonides is not only channelling rabbinic literature here, but also medical practices that appear in the literature of the time such as the tenth-century *Kitāb al-murshid* (*The Guide*) by the physician al-Tamīmī.[17] Resonances of Ibn Sīnā too may be found here – the latter mentions marcasite (when combined with pine resin, not vinegar) as a treatment for hard swellings.[18] Thus, Maimonides has subtly brought together what might seem to us as magical remedies found in rabbinic literature along with medical treatments from the Arabic medical literature which we might think are on more solid ground. The common ground through which he does this is his statement in the *Guide* that 'Any such empirically confirmed remedy is permitted therapeutically' (Judeo-Arabic: *kulla mā ṣaḥḥat tajrubatuhu mithla hādhi*).[19] This gives Maimonides a way out of his problem in the *Guide* squaring Athens with Jerusalem, reason with revelation: the fox's tooth and the nail of one who has been hanged are legitimate treatments because experience in the Talmudic period led Rabbi Meir's constituents to believe that these were not simply the 'ways of the Amorites' but had actually passed the test of experience – just as peonies, dog droppings, and the like had purchase on Maimonides' own contemporaries as popular remedies that were believed to be effective.

Surprisingly, Maimonides allows these remedies 'even if not prescribed by reason' (*wa-in lam yaqtaḍhu qiyās*)[20] – which seems to mean here that one could not demonstrate the effectiveness of the remedy from first principles, that its empirical success is sufficient to incline us towards accepting its legitimacy. Of course, it *is* possible that the line between cause and effect is illusory – think back to our pigeons in Skinner's experiment. Looking at Maimonides' own discussion of the rabbinic

[17] Al-Tamīmī, *Kitāb al-murshid* (*The Guide*), 14, ed. and trans. Schönfeld (1976). See also Maimonides' *Kitāb al-fuṣūl fī al-ṭibb* (*Medical Aphorisms*), 22.17–20, ed. Bos (2015) 5–6, for some of these remedies. On pharmacological material in al-Tamīmī's see also Amar, Serri, and Lev (Chapter 5) in this volume.

[18] Ibn Sīnā, *Qānūn fī al-ṭibb* (*Canon of Medicine*), ed. Būlāq (1877) I.366. Thanks are due to Gerrit Bos for this citation.

[19] Moses Maimonides, *Dalālat al-ḥāʾirīn* (*The Guide to the Perplexed*), 3.37, ed. Munk (1856–66) III.37. Note also the eleventh century *Dispensatory* of Ibn al-Tilmīdh, which includes several remedies verified 'by experience' (*mujarrab*) – cf. Kahl (2007: 33). On Ibn al-Tilmīdh, see also Käs (Chapter 1) in this volume.

[20] Moses Maimonides, *Dalālat al-ḥāʾirīn* (*The Guide to the Perplexed*), 3.37, ed. Munk (1856–66) III.37.

remedies in his *Commentary on the Mishnah* will give us a clearer idea of how Maimonides sees the experimental method generally, as well as the relationship between experimental success and derivation from first principles.

Commentary on the Mishnah finds Maimonides explaining that locust eggs were used as a talisman – *khāṣṣiyah* in Judeo-Arabic – for weakness in the sinews of the hip. This is in itself worthy of note because the Babylonian Talmud explains[21] (Shabbat 67a) that the locust egg is actually used for a different reason: 'for the benefit of a fetus'. This would seem to be an apotropaic usage, a principle Giuseppe Veltri describes as *similia similibus* ('like cures like').[22] Veltri describes this as a 'typical empirical principle', perhaps not known directly from Marcellus Empiricus, where it can also be found, but 'nevertheless . . . from the Latin Greco-Roman world' of the Talmud. Rashi actually explains the Talmud differently, glossing the strange word *shiḥla* as 'a pain in the ear',[23] though the medieval Aramaic dictionary *ʿArukh ha-shalem* does support the translation of the text as fetus – which Veltri seems to accept.[24] Since the Palestinian Talmud explains that the locust's egg is good for the ear (Aramaic: *ṭav le-udna*),[25] Rashi may be reading the Babylonian Talmud in light of the Palestinian, as *shiḥla* can also mean flux from the ear.[26] Further, the word is known to have had this same sense in the literature of the post-Talmudic Babylonian geonim since it is used in a responsum of Naṭronay Gaʾon (r. 857–65) in this sense.[27]

Yet the ills that the locust's egg is understood to treat are not limited to the fetus or an earache: drawing on a tannaitic source cited in the Babylonian Talmud (Bekhorot 40a), Maimonides' eleventh-century predecessor Isaac al-Fāsī explains in his Talmudic digest *Halakhot rabbati* that the word *shiḥla* refers to the thigh.[28] This clarifies Maimonides' understanding of the Mishnah – he relies on neither of the Talmuds but instead turns to al-Fāsī.

But aside from what it is that the locust's egg is supposed to heal, does it work? That is to say, does Maimonides believe that the locust's egg is effective in treating weakness of the thigh? Here, as I have said, in his

[21] Talmud Bavli Shabbat 67a. [22] Veltri (1998a). [23] Rashi to Talmud Bavli Shabbat 67a.

[24] See Veltri's translation of the Talmudic passage at Veltri (1998b).

[25] See Palestinian Talmud Shabbat 6:9 [8c], translated by Veltri (1998b).

[26] Cf. Sokoloff (2002) s.v. שיחלא.

[27] Cf. *Teshuvot of Naṭronay* (*Responsa of Naṭronay Gaʾon*), ed. Brody (1994) 470, cited in Sokoloff (2002), s.v. שיחלא.

[28] See al-Fāsī, *Halakhot Rabbati* (*The Great Laws*) to Talmud Bavli Shabbat 30b (1974).

Commentary on the Mishnah, Maimonides is explicit that this is *khāṣṣiyah*, magic or a talisman. It may be significant, then, that when he recounts the remedies mentioned in the Mishnah, he leaves this one off and mentions only the fox's tooth and the nail of a hanged man. Rather, he sees it as a talisman and not as an effective remedy per se.

Of further note is the fact that when he mentions the fox's tooth and a nail from a hanged man, he does not bring them in the order presented in the Mishnah itself. Somewhat out of line with how he usually brings rabbinic sources, he reorders the text of the Mishnah and cites it only selectively: first he mentions the nail and then the fox's tooth, and (as I said) he lets the locust's egg drop from the Mishnah, as though he were mentioning these remedies casually and not bringing forward the tannaitic statement in the Mishnah as the very pillar of rabbinic literature. This approach to the text of the Mishnah seems causal, but in fact it may be read as very deliberate and careful. Seeing the locust's egg as a talisman, he would have been eager to cast it off, but not so the other two. The fox's tooth, as he explains in his *Commentary on the Mishnah*, is used to treat either insomnia or what a somnologist would call 'excessive daytime sleepiness' – a live fox to quell the former, a dead fox to treat the latter. In his commentary, he does not call the fox's tooth a talisman but simply says that 'people use it for sleep' (Judeo-Arabic: *yastaʿamalū lil-nawmi*).[29] One might say that he even leaves open the possibility that this cure is effective. However, in the case of a nail from a hanged man, Maimonides is much more circumspect, even sceptical: 'Likewise, magicians claim that if one takes a spike from the wood of a hanged man and hang it on upon one who has a persistent fever, he will benefit from it.'[30] Here, he does not describe the wooden nail or spike as a talisman, but he does describe this idea as what the 'magicians claim' (Judeo-Arabic: *yazʿamu aṣḥāb al-khawāṣṣ*).[31] By dropping off from the Mishnah the locust's egg which he describes in *Commentary on the Mishnah* as a talisman, Maimonides leaves us in the *Guide* with the two remedies that he does not describe as a talisman. The wooden nail may be the province of magicians, but Maimonides seems not to think of it as a talisman.

Maimonides is helped here in that Greek and Roman medicine reveals parallels with the ideas in the Talmud: Pliny's *Natural History* includes both a wolf's tooth and a nail from a cross or pieces from the gallows of an executed convict as items with healing powers.[32] The remedies they provide

29 Moses Maimonides, *Commentary on the Mishnah*, ed. Kafiḥ (1963–8) II.42.

30 Moses Maimonides, *Commentary on the Mishnah*, ed. Kafiḥ (1963–8) II.42.

31 On *khawāṣṣ*, see also Walker-Meikle (Chapter 3) and Lewicka (Chapter 9) in the present volume.

32 On Pliny's *Natural History*, see Doolittle (Chapter 2) in this volume.

ameliorate conditions slightly different from those mentioned in the Talmuds and in Maimonides' *Commentary on the Mishnah* – as Veltri explains, the former treats childish terrors and ailments due to teething and the latter a fever recurring every third day. Pliny's application of the wooden nail to recurring fever sheds some light on Maimonides' *Commentary on the Mishnah* because the Babylonian Talmud actually prescribes the nail for a spider's bite and the Palestinian Talmud (Shabbat 6:9 [8c]) prescribes it for inflammation. And whereas Maimonides' attachment of the locust's egg to a weakness in the thighs may be traced back to al-Fāsī, al-Fāsī gives us no such precedent for Maimonides here – rather, he says (channelling the Babylonian Talmud) that the wooden nail is used to relieve inflammation, giving us in *Halakhot rabbati* the Judeo-Arabic *iḥtaraqan*.[33] Nor can we find a precedent for Maimonides in the Palestinian Talmud, which explains that the wooden nail is a remedy for a spider bite. Here we have more than what Veltri calls a 'deep similarity' between Jewish and Roman minds: we have a precedent upon which Maimonides could have relied indirectly (since he did not read Pliny himself) in turning away from the various voices in rabbinic literature to find an application for this particular remedy – the wooden nail – in Greek science.

In *Commentary on the Mishnah*, Maimonides is in some way forced to explain all three remedies Rabbi Meir presents, but not so in the *Guide*. Likewise, he includes all three remedies mentioned in the Mishnah in his so-called *magnum opus*, the *Mishneh Torah* (*Laws of the Shabbath* 19:13), and he even includes there a fourth remedy for corns mentioned earlier in the Mishnah, which he describes in *Commentary* as a talisman. But his seemingly disorganised inclusion in the *Guide* of the wooden nail and the fox's tooth and the omission of the locust's egg are intentional or at least convenient: he has left in the two remedies that he does *not* describe as talismans, and the wooden spike which he describes as capturing the interest of magicians (even if it is itself not called a talisman) is backed up by support from Pliny's *Natural History*.

Indeed, this section of the *Guide* is anything but a lesson in the history of talismans. Maimonides vindicates the two of the three items from the Mishnah by explaining that these items are permissible even though one might not think so *because they were considered in their time to derive from experience and accordingly pertained to medicine*. That is to say, magicians might or might not believe these remedies to be talismans, but the belief garnered through experience that they were effective is sufficient in Maimonides' mind for them not to be included the category of talismans,

[33] Al-Fāsī, *Halakhot Rabbati* (*The Great Laws*), Shabbat 30b (1974).

themselves understood by rabbinic literature to have been the province of the Israelites' evil Amorite neighbours. Instead, Maimonides sees them as effective medical treatments. Concerning these items he explains that 'in their time, practical experience excluded them (from the category of Amorite practices) and they fell into the category of medical practices'.[34] Having identified these remedies which might otherwise be considered to be talismans found in the Mishnah, Maimonides makes a subtle move, likening to this category a few other things: 'hanging a peony on an epileptic and the giving of a dog's excrement in cases of swelling of the throat and fumigation with vinegar and marcasite in cases of hard swellings of the tendons'. Yet these additions are not remedies mentioned in the Talmud, and Maimonides does not repeat the allusion he made to an earlier time when those remedies were believed to be effective. That is to say, the peony, dog dung, vinegar, and marcasite might have been remedies *from Maimonides' own time*. The peony, for instance, is known from the writings of Galen, who mentions it as a treatment for epilepsy as well.[35] Gerrit Bos informs us that marcasite features in the *Kitāb al-murshid* of al-Tamīmī, as I have mentioned, as it does in Dioscorides, Pliny, and Galen. Maimonides' Andalusian contemporary Ibn al-Bayṭār even mentions its application with vinegar for skin affections – just as Maimonides has it in the *Guide*.[36] All this kind of advice calls to mind the *physika* (natural remedies) of ancient and late antique authors.[37] We may therefore see the intellectual underpinnings of this brief passage in the *Guide* as beginning with the Mishnaic period and continuing all the way up to the twelfth century, vindicating remedies that were rendered therapeutic rather than magical by virtue of the common experience of being effective.

Indeed, as Maimonides explains elsewhere in his *Commentary on the Mishnah* (Yoma 8:4), urging one to disregard the fast of Yom Kippur in order to administer medicine:

> The Sages only disregard a commandment for a treatment justified by logical reasoning (*qiyās*) and common experience (*wa-l-tajribah al-qarībah*), whereas magical treatments are not allowed, since they are weak

[34] Moses Maimonides, *Dalālat al-ḥā'irīn* (*The Guide to the Perplexed*), 3.37, ed. Munk (1856–66) III.37, p. 80b.

[35] Galen, *On the Capacities of Simple Drugs*, 6.3, ed. Kühn (1821–33) XI.859–60. I thank Petros Bouras-Vallianatos for this reference. This work is, of course, known in Syriac and Arabic.

[36] Cf. Ibn al-Bayṭār, *al-Jāmi' li-mufradāt al-adwiyah wa-l-aghdhiyah* (*Collector of Simple Drugs and Foodstuffs*), trans. Leclerc (1877–83) II.312, no. 2116.

[37] On the *physika*, see Bouras-Vallianatos (2014: 348–52) and (2016). For the use of amulets by physicians in the Graeco-Roman world, as discussed by Galen, see Jouanna (2011).

> and not supported by logic, infrequently supported by experience, and they are false claims – know this great rule![38]

Now, it would seem that here Maimonides is requiring recourse *both* to logical reasoning and to experience, but it is equally possible that the conjunctive *wāw* is disjunctive in this case – that *either* logical reasoning or experience would be sufficient to ascribe validity to the treatment – a reading supported by the fact that, in the *Guide*, Maimonides measures remedies only by their perceived effectiveness tested through experience. Indeed, in the *Guide*, he is explicit – even if reason does not prescribe a particular remedy, it may be used and does not fall into the category of Amorite practices if experience supports it. Here, Maimonides stands clearly in the rabbinic tradition – as Bohak explains, the rabbis limited the category of Amorite practices and 'opened a wide door for the entry of numerous foreign customs, as long as they were deemed by knowledgeable experts, or by the rabbis themselves, to have real medical value'.[39]

And what of situations in which experience seems to go against logical reasoning? As Maimonides says, following our passage, 'Any such empirically confirmed remedy is permitted therapeutically, on the analogy of laxatives, even if not prescribed by reason.'[40] With this in mind, we might indeed read the *wāw* in Maimonides' *Commentary on the Mishnah* disjunctively – that is, *either* logic *or* experience is sufficient – because, as he says in the *Guide*, experience is sufficient even in the absence of reason.[41]

The ancient debate on medical empiricism is well known, as is Galen's own position in it tending towards the empiricist position, basing itself entirely on experience.[42] Maimonides' own respect for Galen is also well known, as is his appreciation of empiricism generally, which leads Maimonides to praise his predecessor the physician Ibn Zuhr of Seville, whose son apparently told Maimonides of the seemingly anomalous remedies he recommended.[43] Yet as attractive as the experimental method might have been to Galen and by extension to Maimonides, it could

[38] Moses Maimonides, *Commentary on the Mishnah*, ed. Kafiḥ (1963–8) II.265.

[39] Bohak (2008: 384–5).

[40] Moses Maimonides, *Dalālat al-ḥā'irīn* (*The Guide to the Perplexed*), 3.37, ed. Munk (1856–66) III.37.

[41] On the role of experience in the use of amulets, see also Rinotas (Chapter 12), who examines the case of Albertus Magnus.

[42] For Galen's position on empiricism generally, see Matthen (1988).

[43] See Maimonides' *Kitāb al-fuṣūl fī al-ṭibb* (*Medical Aphorisms*), 22.35–70, ed. Bos (2015) 11–22 and Bos' introduction (2015: xx–xxii).

sometimes lead to uncomfortable results, including sometimes endorsing practices that smack of magic, superstition, or at least of pigeons. And while Maimonides might have felt at least a general commitment to supporting the Mishnah and rabbinic literature – while nonetheless subtly excluding elements he might find problematic – we find a similar discourse regarding magical remedies in the *Kitāb filāhah al-nabaṭiyah* (*The Nabatean Agriculture*), a controversial work ascribed to the tenth century which may or may not preserve earlier literary traditions but which was certainly in Maimonides' library and to which he refers regularly in the *Guide*. As Jaakko Hämeen-Anttila explains in his volume on *The Nabatean Agriculture*, 'The relations between magicians and sages is also far from unambiguous . . . one sees how the traditions of prophets, magicians and sages intersect.'[44] Hämeen-Anttila quotes a section of the book referring to an individual named Jaryānā whose general tendency was to denigrate magicians, but at times he would praise some of their talismans: 'He mentions that he deduced them through analogy and then experimented with them, saying: "Experiment with them so that you know whether they are valid or not."'[45] Reminiscent of Maimonides' commentary to Mishnah Yoma 8:4, Jaryānā relies on both analogy and experimentation – but like the *Guide*, Jaryānā holds that experimentation alone can vindicate a remedy. Although Maimonides often rails against the magical practices described in *The Nabatean Agriculture* – as Hämeen-Anttila explains, 'Magic, even though it is in general abhorred by the author, is still a source of national pride to the Nabateans, who are magicians par excellence'[46] – he seems to agree in the *Guide* that experimentation, at least in this case, is a sufficient condition for accepting what might at first blush look like a magical recipe passed down through traditional means, from teacher to student.

Maimonides' approach to experimentation versus logical reasoning (*qiyās*) or reason itself (*ʿaql*) is particularly important when we look at his approach to one of the central questions of the *Guide*, *creation ex nihilo*, and examining his approach to this question allows us to trace out the broader implications of his opening the door to the fox's tooth or wooden nail that are mentioned in the Mishnah and Talmud despite their apparent magical roots. For it is well known that Maimonides has no demonstrative proof for *creation ex nihilo* in the *Guide* just as

[44] Hämeen-Anttila (2006: 189). [45] Hämeen-Anttila (2006: 190).
[46] Hämeen-Anttila (2006: 189).

Aristotle has no demonstrative proof for the theory of eternity – in Maimonides' own words, 'There are no proofs at all of thoughts as deep and sublime as these – not from our point of view as adherents of Scripture, nor from that of the Philosophers, with their conflicting opinions on this.'[47] Such matters, to his mind, can be resolved only by recourse to a dialectical proof. We might, therefore, see a parallel between the recourse to first principles or *qiyās* in the magical remedies of Jaryānā mentioned in *The Nabatean Agriculture* and Maimonides' initial attempts to vindicate *creation ex nihilo* through some sort of demonstrative proof. And while we might hope that logic and first principles would get us far enough, Jaryānā demands more – that he experiment with those remedies – in order to prove whether they are valid. So too Maimonides admits the limits of logic in furthering the case for creation, and yet nonetheless encourages us to look to experience to make sense of the world:

> But they saw no difference between God's determining that this plant be red rather than white, or sweet rather than bitter, and His determining that the heavens have the shape they have rather than being square or triangular. They based their doctrine of determination on the premises you now know. But I'll ground it properly, using philosophical premises based on the nature of things.[48]

His recourse to the contingency of the world in the case of creation versus eternalism – that is, in metaphysics – should be seen as of a piece with his recourse to empirical knowledge in the study of creation itself – that is, in physics. In praising the anomalous recipes of Ibn Zuhr or permitting the pinning on a peony to treat an epileptic or marcasite for swollen tendons, we may find Maimonides admitting that first principles cannot dictate to us, say, whether the sun should arise in the east or the west, a question that experience alone can reveal. And while logic cannot dictate whether hanging a fox's tooth around a particular individual's neck will meaningfully treat insomnia or daytime sleepiness, experience can. And as research into the placebo effect continues into our own time, Maimonides' permitting these seemingly magical remedies makes more and more sense for a populace that is predictably irrational.

[47] Moses Maimonides, *Dalālat al-ḥāʾirīn* (*The Guide to the Perplexed*), 3.21, ed. Munk (1856–66) III.21, 44b.

[48] Moses Maimonides, *Dalālat al-ḥāʾirīn* (*The Guide to the Perplexed*), 2.19, ed. Munk (1856–66) II.19, 40a.

REFERENCES

Albeck, H. 1951–8. *Mishnah*. 6 vols. Tel Aviv: n.p.

Bohak, G. 2008. *Ancient Jewish Magic: A History*. Cambridge: Cambridge University Press.

Bos, G. ed. 2015. *Maimonides: Medical Aphorisms, Treatises 22–25*. Provo, UT: Brigham Young University Press.

Bouras-Vallianatos, P. 2014. 'Clinical Experience in Late Antiquity: Alexander of Tralles and the Therapy of Epilepsy', *Medical History* 58.3: 337–53.

Bouras-Vallianatos, P. 2016. 'Modelled on Archigenes *Theiotatos*: Alexander of Tralles and His Use of Natural Remedies (*physika*)', *Mnemosyne* 69: 382–96.

Brody, R. ed. 1994. *Responsa of Naṭronay Ga'on*. Jerusalem: Makhon Ofeq.

al-Fāsī, I. 1974. *Halakhot rabbati*. 2 vols. Jerusalem: n.p.

Hämeen-Anttila, J. 2006. *The Last Pagans of Iraq: Ibn Waḥshiyya and His Nabatean Agriculture*. Leiden: Brill.

Ibn Sīnā. 1877. *Qānūn fī al-ṭibb*. 3 vols. Bulaq: n.p.

Jouanna, J. 2011. 'Médecine rationnelle et magie: Le statut des amulettes et des incantations chez Galien', *Revue des Études Grecques* 124: 47–77.

Kafiḥ, J. ed. 1963–8. *Mishnah im Perush R. Moshe Ben Maimon: Makor we-Targum*. 6 pts. in 7 vols. Jerusalem: n.p.

Kahl, O. ed. and trans. 2007. *The Dispensatory of Ibn at-Tilmīd*. Leiden: Brill.

Koslowski, B., and Maqueda, M. 1993. 'What Is Confirmation Bias and When Do People Actually Have It?' *Merrill-Palmer Quarterly* 39.1: 104–30.

Kühn, C. G. ed. 1821–33. *Claudii Galeni opera omnia*. 20 vols. Leipzig: Knobloch.

Leclerc, L. trans. 1877–83. *Traite des simples*. 3 vols. Paris: National Printing Office.

Matthen, M. 1988. 'Empiricism and Ontology in Ancient Medicine', *Apeiron* 21.2: 99–122.

Munk, S. trans. 1856–66. *Le Guide des Égarés*. 3 vols. Paris: Franck.

Schönfeld, J. 1976. *Über die Steine das 14. Kapitel aus dem 'Kitab al-Muršid' des Muḥammad Ibn Aḥmad al-Tamīmī*. Freiburg: Klaus Schwarz.

Skinner, B. F. 1948. 'Superstition in the Pigeon', *Journal of Experimental Psychology* 38: 168–72.

Skinner, B. F. 1957. 'The Experimental Analysis of Behavior', *American Scientist* 45.4: 343–71.

Sokoloff, M. 2002. *A Dictionary of Jewish Babylonian Aramaic of the Talmudic and Geonic Periods*. Ramat Gan: Bar Ilan University Press.

Veltri, G. 1998a. 'On the Influence of "Greek Wisdom": Theoretical and Empirical Sciences in Rabbinic Judaism', *Jewish Studies Quarterly* 5.4: 300–17.

Veltri, G. 1998b. 'The Rabbis and Pliny the Elder: Jewish and Greco-Roman Attitudes toward Magic and Empirical Knowledge', *Poetics Today* 19.1: 63–89.

Zuckermandel, M. 1970. *Tosefta*. Reprint. Jerusalem: n.p.

CHAPTER 9

When the Doctor Is Not Around

Arabic-Islamic Self-Treatment Manuals As Cultured People's Guides to Medico-pharmacological Knowledge. The Mamluk Period (1250–1517)

Paulina B. Lewicka

Writings produced by the Arabic-speaking authors of the Islamic Middle Period[1] in the field of medicine and pharmacology constitute a voluminous corpus covering a whole range of issues pertaining to health, illness, and therapy. Among them one can find a number of books which, while dealing with preventative measures and cures for various health disorders, were addressed to those who, unable or reluctant to consult a physician, tended to care for their health themselves.

Modest in size and meant for domestic use by educated non-specialists, the self-treatment compendia instructed how to treat diverse illnesses with food and substances which, according to some of the authors, could be prepared from well-known, widely available, and not-very-expensive ingredients. Apart from that, they did not differ much from general treatment manuals which, more comprehensive, were apparently chiefly intended as reference books for qualified medical practitioners and other more skilled or competent readers. Typical of the medico-pharmacological culture they represented, both kinds of manuals involved the same syncretic approach to questions of health, disease, and therapy. Rooted in assorted kinds of

This research has been supported by the National Science Centre, Poland (Research Project: 'Medycyna bez lekarzy. Edycja krytyczna domowego poradnika medycznego z czternastowiecznego Kairu, z wprowadzeniem, tłumaczeniem i komentarzami', no UMO-2018/31/B/HS3/00145). All translations are my own unless otherwise stated.

[1] The term 'Islamic Middle Period' is used here as a replacement for the ever-convenient term 'Middle Ages' which, when employed to cover the specific period of the history of the Arabic-Islamic world, is often rather vague and may sometimes prove misleading. The term 'Islamic Middle Period' is applied here to the time frame defined by two events – the rise of the Umayyads in 661 (i.e. following the formative period of Islam) and the beginning of the Ottoman occupation of the Arab domains in 1517.

knowledge and systems of belief, this approach manifested in a multiplicity of therapeutic methods, ideas for healing, modes of drug application, explanatory models, practices, and cures from multiple sources. Authors merged these elements in different ways in their compilations; consequently, each book formed a separate, unique assemblage of pieces taken to varying extent from Galenic, Hermetic, Ayurvedic, Christian, Islamic, and other writings. Full of therapeutic recommendations and advice regarding preventive medicine and treatment of various ailments, both the self-treatment compendia and the general treatment manuals constitute very attractive source material for the study of the Arabo-Islamic medical, medico-dietary, and pharmacological culture of the premodern period. Of the two, however, the self-treatment compendia seem to possess a special value in this respect. Meant for domestic use by non-specialist, 'ordinary' readers, they involve written information which circulated among literate, Arabic-speaking urbanites (and in their milieus) and which quite probably contributed to their thinking about health, illness, and therapy. As such, the compendia offer insights into otherwise understudied and rarely accessible issues related to the sphere of household medicine as recognised by historical populations in the cities of the Near East, their confessional affiliation notwithstanding.

Prescriptive rather than descriptive, such texts cannot be used as sources of information regarding actual, true-life daily household medical or pharmacological practices. They can reveal, however, clues to the knowledge about disease management and medicinal substances that was available for ordinary literate people, who had never been trained as physicians or scholars. At the same time, an analysis of the therapeutic choices which such people, as target readers of these texts, were recommended should shed some light on the intellectual tradition which informed their potential convictions in this respect.

While constituting an attempt to address these issues, the present chapter is focused on two compendia of this kind. Both were written in the Arabic language and within Egyptian-Mamluk/early post-Mamluk space-time and, as such, reflected aspects of the medico-pharmacological culture of 'a Mediterranean society'. At the same time, however, both were a part of a broader, Mediterranean-wide tradition, within which the health-related concerns, beliefs, habits, traditions, ideas, and timeless medico-dietary expertise were transmitted, 'absorbed, rearranged and emitted in increments over and over'[2] across time, space, and politico-linguistic boundaries. Available in Greek, Latin, Arabic, Judeo-Arabic, and Hebrew, the body

[2] Silla (1996: 614).

of specialised, text-based knowledge which emerged from this process contributed to the coherence of the medico-pharmacological and medico-dietary discourse of the literate Mediterranean world of the medieval period. As a part of this discourse, the two compendia and the knowledge they promoted can be indicative regarding the processes of transfer and assimilation of medical ideas, drugs, and drug-related concepts as occurred within the Mediterranean as well as between the Mediterranean and the Indo-Persian world. As a subgenre of the Arabic medical literature of the Islamic Middle Period, the self-treatment compendia – of which no fewer than eleven survive – seem to have escaped the notice of contemporary scholarship. Studies dealing with the history of Arabo-Islamic medicine appear to contain no references to any of these texts. Moreover, the very few comments in the secondary literature that refer to self-treatment compendia actually confuse them with *ṭibb al-fuqarāʾ*, or the 'medicine for the poor', a similar, but different subgenre of medical writing.[3] Although comparable as far as content is concerned, the self-treatment manuals and the books of the medicine for the poor differ with regard to the idea behind them: while the former were addressed directly to the sick (or their caregivers) who belonged to the literate, middle-upper, or upper echelons of society, the latter were meant for physicians who treated (or were intending to treat) the destitute and poor.

Compiled by different authors who belonged to diverse groups of educated professionals, the Arabic-language self-treatment compendia differed considerably from one another in their contents and did not offer a uniform set of knowledge. This should not be surprising: after all, their authors came from various social, political, ethnic, and religious environments and lived in different epochs and geographical locations. But the diversity within the genre also reflects the general heterogeneity and pluralism of the medico-pharmacological culture of the Islamic Middle Period as well as the complexity of the literary-intellectual tradition, all of which shaped the character of the Arabic medical-pharmacological texts written at that time. Based on Graeco-Roman medical lore and elaborated with elements taken from the Indo-Persian heritage, this tradition was, moreover, interlaced with ideas and items derived from popular knowledge as well as from the Arabo-Christian and Arabo-Islamic environment in which it developed.

Greek medical thought, on which this hybrid collection was founded, predominated from the very beginning, from the moment when – in the

[3] See Bos (1998: 366–70).

course of the ninth/tenth centuries – the ancient Greek legacy was translated into Arabic. The process resulted in the emergence of so-called Graeco-Arabic medicine,[4] which, having been assimilated into the multicultural Islamicate world, became a prevailing medical theory, at least among cultured city dwellers. The bulk of the Graeco-Arabic medical writings was based on or related to the Galenic doctrine of humoral pathology, a medical system established upon the ancient concept that all things are composed of four elements, which in the human body are transformed into four 'humours' or bodily fluids.[5]

The humoral theory, which dominated the learned medical discourse of the medieval Islamicate world, was not the only kind of medical knowledge adopted from the Graeco-Roman intellectual tradition that adapted well to the Islamic setting of the eastern Mediterranean. In fact, apart from the Hippocratic-Galenic concepts, the local culture also acquired insight into ancient medical magic,[6] the origins of which were traced back to great sages of undisputed authority such as Hermes Trismegistos, a mythical author of occult works. It should not be surprising, therefore, that the Arabic-language authors, being heirs to the Greek medical tradition, referred to the name of Hermes, if much less frequently, yet in the same manner as they did to the names of Hippocrates, Galen, Paul of Aegina, or Rufus of Ephesus. It should not be surprising either that the majority of the Arabic-language medical manuals (the self-treatment compendia included), although deeply rooted in the spirit of Hippocratic-Galenic thought, often pointed to the therapeutic effectiveness of occult-magical formulae.[7] The concept of magical medicine was based on the idea of

[4] Somewhat misleadingly, Graeco-Arabic medicine, which was based on ancient Greek foundations or, more precisely, on the Hippocratic-Galenic doctrine of humoral pathology, is also referred to as 'Arabo-Islamic', 'Islamic', and 'Graeco-Islamic'. 'Graeco-Arabic' would seem to be the most appropriate designation, if only because the medicine in question was an exemplary product of the fusion of Greek thought and Arabic language with all its cultural potential. And, no less important, it was devoid of religious elements. 'Graeco-Islamic', on the other hand, seems to be correct only in reference to the *ṭibb al-nabī*, or the 'medicine of the Prophet', which was indeed a combination of Greek and Islamic medical teachings.

[5] For a more detailed discussion of the Greek foundations of Graeco-Arabic medicine see, for example, Ullmann (1970, 1978), Conrad (1995), Attewell (2003), and Pormann and Savage-Smith (2007: 6–143).

[6] In the present chapter the term 'magic' applies to the whole of beliefs and practices which are based on the conviction that within animate and inanimate nature exist invisible and unobservable forces which can be activated by appropriate actions and employed so as to influence aspects of tangible reality. Such forces can be associated with aspects of nature, man-made objects, graphic signs, texts, sounds, and so forth.

[7] For a discussion of the tradition of medical magic in the Arabo-Islamic world see, for example, Ullmann (1978: 107–14), Dols (1992, 2004), and Pormann and Savage-Smith (2007: 144–61). On Hermes and the Hermetic tradition see Peters (2004).

khawāṣṣ – special, inexplicable, esoteric properties ascribed to animate and inanimate nature that could be activated by appropriate actions and used both for treating ailments and protecting against them.[8]

As time passed, elements of Greek thought started to mingle more and more freely with spiritual-religious perspectives and medical folklore. Humours, temperaments, qualities, and Hermetic substances became more and more frequently combined with quotations from the Qurʾān, the Sunna, and the works of Islamic theologians. The authority of legendary *awāʾil* – Greek sages such as Plato, Hippocrates, Hermes, and Galen – coexisted with the legendary wisdom of the Prophet or his companions. This phenomenon intensified from approximately the thirteenth century onward, when religio-medical texts known as the Medicine of the Prophet permeated Arabic-Islamic medical culture.

At the same time, another tendency could be observed in medico-pharmaceutical literature. Due to their voluminousness and complexity the use of learned medical works was in fact limited to well-educated doctors and other members of the intellectual elite. To address the needs of more ordinary readers, some authors simplified medical, pharmacological, and dietetic knowledge. The manuals they produced were either shortened versions of more difficult and voluminous works or new, multi-topic compilations dealing with hygiene (meaning a healthy way of life and preventative practices), as well as curative and preventive therapies and pharmacology. The self-treatment compendia belonged to the second group.

It seems that the pioneer of the genre was ʿĪsā Ibn Māssa (d. *c.*888), a Baghdadi physician and author of a number of medical works. One of them was a manual entitled *Man lā yaḥḍuruhu al-ṭabīb* (*For the One Who Is Not Attended to by a Doctor*).[9] However, the text seems not to have survived. The oldest Arabic-language compendium of this kind available today is an identically titled manual written by Abū Bakr al-Rāzī (d. 925), an erudite Persian physician and philosopher. As al-Rāzī explained in the introduction to his book, his intention was to 'help those who cannot afford the elaborate and hard-to-reach medicaments, which prevail in the advice proposed by well-known doctors and which can only be found in

[8] On the concept of *khawāṣṣ* see also Walker-Meikle (Chapter 3) in the present volume.

[9] See Ibn al-Nadīm, *Kitāb al-fihrist* (*The Catalogue*), ed. Flügel (1871) I. 296; Ibn ʿAlī al-Ruhāwī, *Adab al-ṭabīb* (*Ethics of the Physician*), ed. Levey (1967) 73; al-Ṣafadī, *Al-Wāfī bi-l-wafayāt* (*The Complete Book on Eminent Persons*), ed. Arnāʾūṭ and Muṣṭafā (1998) XXIII.159.

the royal medicine cabinets'.[10] In the manual, which has more than 100 sections, al-Rāzī explains how to cure ailments with foods and medicaments prepared according to his prescriptions, using well-known and widely available ingredients.

ʿĪsā Ibn Māssa and al-Rāzī, who were the earliest Arabic-speaking authors to compose self-treatment manuals, were not, however, the inventors of the genre. As is usually the case with Arabic medical literature, the evidence leads back to Greece. Most probably, at least one of these authors, if not both, was inspired by Rufus of Ephesus (first century CE), the second most frequently quoted Greek author after Galen, whose contribution to the field of medical literature included what seems to be a self-treatment compendium. The Arabic-speaking scholars of the period known as the Renaissance of Islam[11] apparently heard of Rufus' book, and some of them had a chance to read it. What exactly they read, however, is not obvious, as the information regarding this work is rather confusing. According to the *Fihrist*, or Ibn al-Nadīm's (tenth century) authoritative encyclopaedia of authors and works, Rufus' compendium was titled *Kitāb tadbīr man lā yaḥḍuruhu ṭabīb* (*Book of Regimen for the One Who Is Not Attended to by a Doctor*).[12] The same version of the title was later repeated by, for example, Ibn Sīnā (d. 1037) in his *Qānūn fī al-ṭibb* (*Canon of Medicine*) and, still later, by Ibn Abī Uṣaybiʿah (thirteenth century) in *ʿUyūn al-anbāʾ fī ṭabaqāt al-aṭibbāʾ* (*Sources of Information on the Classes of Physicians*).[13]

Intriguingly, the title *Kitāb tadbīr man lā yaḥḍuruhu ṭabīb* was never mentioned by al-Rāzī, who knew the works of Rufus and quoted from them extensively. However, while referring to what seems to be Rufus' self-

10 Al-Rāzī, *Man lā yaḥḍuruhu al-ṭabīb* (*For the One Who Is Not Attended to by a Doctor*), ed. al-Ḍannāwī (1999) 9.

11 The Renaissance of Islam, sometimes called the Islamic Golden Age, was a period characterised by a surge of interest in Greek scholarship, the progress of the Graeco-Arabic translation movement, and cultural and scientific flourishing that lasted from the second half of the eighth century (foundation of Baghdad) to circa the thirteenth (Mongol invasions and the siege of Baghdad in 1258, but also the progressing radicalisation of Islam).

12 Ibn al-Nadīm, *Kitāb al-fihrist* (*The Catalogue*), ed. Flügel (1871) I.291. Some scholars interpret Arabic *tadbīr* ('regimen') as 'diet' and identify diet with regimen, which further complicates attempts to properly classify some of Rufus' works. See Abou-Aly (1992: passim) and Ullmann (1994: 1339).

13 Ibn Abī Uṣaybiʿah, *ʿUyūn al-anbāʾ fī ṭabaqāt al-aṭibbāʾ* (*Sources of Information on the Classes of Physicians*), 4, ed. Riḍā (1965) 57; see also the recent edition by Savage-Smith, Swain, and van Gelder (2020). See also Sezgin (1996: III.65, no. 2). Authors writing in Arabic could also have known similar compendia written by Filagrios (third century) and Oribasios (fourth century); see Sezgin (1996: III.156, no. 154) and Bos (1998: 366). According to Ibn al-Nadīm, who claimed to have seen an Arabic copy, Filagrios' compendium was titled *Kitāb man lā yaḥḍuruhum ṭabīb*, or *Book for Those Who Are Not Attended to by a Doctor*, which title was later repeated by Ibn Abī Uṣaybi'ah; Ibn al-Nadīm, *Kitāb al-fihrist* (*The Catalogue*), ed. Flügel (1871) I.292; Ibn Abī Uṣaybi'ah, *ʿUyūn al-anbāʾ fī ṭabaqāt al-aṭibbāʾ* (*Sources of Information on the Classes of Physicians*), 5, ed. Riḍā (1965) 150.

treatment compendium, al-Rāzī used the title *Ilā man lā yajidu ṭabīban* (*To the One Who Cannot Find a Doctor*), which phrasing differs from the version of the title provided some decades later by Ibn al-Nadīm. In fact, the three fragments of this work that al-Rāzī included in *Kitāb al-ḥāwī* (*Comprehensive Book*) are probably the only identifiable surviving parts of the self-treatment compendium written by Rufus.[14]

Contemporary scholars such as Manfred Ullmann and Amal Abou-Aly tend to allow for the possibility that *To the One Who Cannot Find a Doctor/ Book of Regimen for the One Who Is Not Attended to by a Doctor* are alternative titles of Rufus' *To the Laymen* (*Ilā al-ʿAwāmm*),[15] which al-Rāzī quotes some thirty times in *Kitāb al-ḥāwī*.[16] Consequently, a self-treatment compendium and a comprehensive volume which reportedly 'encapsulated all Rufus' teachings'[17] are in contemporary scholarship either confused with each other or treated as one and the same work.[18]

Whatever inspired the idea that the three titles refer to one book and that the two books are one item, there are reasons to doubt the correctness of such a reasoning. There is a fragment in Rufus' *To the Laymen* that, quoted by al-Rāzī, informs the reader that 'whoever urinates with black urine without a disease or pain, a stone will be created shortly in his kidney, especially if he is an old man'. Then the author recommends that 'the *doctor* [italics P. L.] should hasten to give him either a softener/laxative or diuretics and order him to relax, as much effort causes stones in the kidneys'.[19] In fact, a self-treatment manual could not include suggestions regarding treatment offered by a physician if only because this kind of manual was, as a rule, addressed to persons who were not able to consult a professional medical practitioner. This implies that a book which recommended the kind of therapy which a physician should provide could not be a self-help medical compendium. Rather, it could be a kind of general handbook of medicine addressed to persons who were not medical practitioners, which seems to have been the case of Rufus' *To the Laymen*.

[14] The fragments of Rufus' works preserved in al-Rāzī's *Kitāb al-ḥāwī* (*Comprehensive Book*) were published in Latin by Daremberg and Ruelle (1879: 453–548). See also Ullmann (1970: 71–6).

[15] Ullmann (1970: 74); Abou-Aly (1992: 45).

[16] Like *Book of Regimen for the One Who Is Not Attended to by a Doctor* and *To the One Who Cannot Find a Doctor*, *To the Laymen* survives only in al-Rāzī's quotations.

[17] Nutton (2008a: 17).

[18] For example, Nutton (2008a: 17, 2008b: 154, 2013: 215, 388 n. 67); Draycott (2016: 435). At the same time, some of the authors who discuss the self-help medical literature of antiquity mention Rufus' *To the Laymen*, but never speak of his *To the One Who Cannot Find a Doctor/Book of Regimen for the One Who Is Not Attended to by a Doctor*; see, for example, Ferngren (2016: 38).

[19] Al-Rāzī, *Kitāb al-ḥāwī* (*Comprehensive Book*), 6, ed. Ismāʿīl (2000) II.66.

In other words, if ʿĪsā Ibn Māssa's or/and al-Rāzī's self-treatment compendia were inspired by a book written by Rufus of Ephesus, it must have been *Book of Regimen for the One Who Is Not Attended to by a Doctor/ To the One Who Cannot Find a Doctor* and not *To the Laymen*.

9.1 *Ghunyat al-labīb* by Ibn al-Akfānī

For several centuries after al-Rāzī's time, between the tenth and sixteenth centuries, a number of other manuals of this kind were compiled. In the context of the medico-pharmaceutical culture of the eastern Mediterranean of the Mamluk period (1250–1517), two of them appear to be more useful than the rest. One was written in fourteenth-century Cairo by an Iraqi-Egyptian physician named Muḥammad Ibn al-Akfānī and is entitled *Ghunyat al-labīb fī mā yustaʾmal ʿinda ghaybat al-ṭabīb* (*Wealth of Information for the Intelligent Man When the Doctor Is Not Around*).[20] In order to avoid confusion with other works, the compendium will be referred to here as *Ghunyat al-labīb (I)*. The other manual, written by a certain Abū al-Ḥasan ʿAlī Ibn ʿAbd Allah Muḥammad al-Qurashī,[21] has an almost identical title to that of Ibn al-Akfānī's work: *Ghunyat al-labīb ḥaythu lā yūjad al-ṭabīb* (*The Richness of Information for the Intelligent Man When the Doctor Is Not Around*). In the present chapter it will be referred to as *Ghunyat al-labīb (II)*.

The author of *Ghunyat al-labīb (I)*, Shams al-Dīn Muḥammad Ibn Ibrāhīm Ibn Saʾīd al-Anṣārī Ibn al-Akfānī al-Sinjārī (d. 1349), was a well-educated physician who, having left his home in provincial Iraq, moved to Mamluk Cairo. Employed as a doctor and supply manager in the Cairene hospital known as al-Bīmāristān al-Manṣūrī, he found time to write books dealing with topics from fields of science, including medicine. Ibn al-Akfānī died during the Great Plague, which decimated the city population.[22] *Ghunyat al-labīb (I)* survived in at least fifteen copies, two of which are preserved in Sarajevo Library, six in archives in Turkey, one each in the libraries of Baghdad, Beirut, Cambridge, Gotha, Cairo, Los Angeles, and Dublin, and, quite possibly, in other places yet to be

[20] The phrasing of the title and the form of the name of the author may differ depending on the manuscript. For example, the manuscripts from the collection of Gazi Husrev-begova biblioteka in Sarajevo and a number of copies preserved in Turkish archives are entitled *Risāla fī ḥifẓi al-ṣiḥḥah* – that is, *Treatise on the Prevention of Health.* Their content is not identical with the Paris, Beirut, Baghdad, and other copies, but the modifications are not significant.

[21] See below, pp. 307ff.

[22] The most detailed biography of Ibn al-Akfānī is to be found in al-Ṣafadī, *Al-Wāfī bi-l-wafayāt* (*The Complete Book on Eminent Persons*), ed. Arnāʾūṭ and Muṣṭafā (2000) II.20–1.

identified. Obviously, such a large number of surviving copies suggests that the manual enjoyed relative popularity.[23]

As Ibn al-Akfānī writes in the introduction to *Ghunyat al-labīb (I)*:

> [This treatise], small in size but rich in knowledge, includes what is essential for medical issues related to health care, disease prevention, and treatment of ailments when the doctor is not around or when he is not trustworthy. One can also find in it useful information on hidden properties of things – both those which we tested, and those which we trustfully borrowed from the most outstanding physicians.[24]

The manual is composed of four chapters, three of which reflect a Hippocratic-Galenic perspective, while one reveals Ibn al-Akfānī's inclination towards occult-magical approach to medicine. The chapters' titles are as follows: 1. 'On the Advisability of Caring for Health in General and on the Benefits It Yields'; 2. 'On How to Deal with an Illness When the Doctor Is Not Around or When the One Who Is Available Is Not Trustworthy'; 3. 'On Useful Advice in These Two Cases (i.e. Caring for Health and Cure of Illnesses)'; 4. 'On Substances Having Special Properties (Mostly Medical) That Have Been Tested'.

As is often the case with Arabic-language medico-pharmacological compendia, *Ghunyat al-labīb (I)* starts with a chapter presenting basic aspects of preventive care seen from the perspective of humoral medicine. This chapter does not mention any drugs at all – according to the Hippocratic-Galenic concept of health, effective prevention was determined exclusively by a healthy lifestyle; consequently, any pharmacological therapy would be irrelevant. Typically, the chapter is focused on questions related to proper nourishment.[25]

[23] In the 1980s an edition of *Ghunyat al-labīb fī mā yusta'mal 'inda ghaybat al-ṭabīb* (*Wealth of Information for the Intelligent Man When the Doctor Is Not Around*) based on the Baghdad and Beirut manuscripts was published by Ṣāliḥ Mahdī 'Abbās (1989) in Baghdad. Muḥammad Mihrān'far (2015) published a Persian translation of Ibn al-Akfānī's work in Tehran. All references to *Ghunyat al-labīb (I)* pertain to the printed version of the work (Baghdad 1989).

[24] Ibn al-Akfānī, *Ghunyat al-labīb fī mā yusta'mal 'inda ghaybat al-ṭabīb* (*Wealth of Information for the Intelligent Man When the Doctor Is Not Around*), ed. 'Abbās (1989) 27.

[25] The issues of preventive medicine and hygiene as seen from the perspective of humoral medicine were also discussed in separate treatises, usually called *Fī ḥifẓ al-ṣiḥḥah* (*On the Prevention of Health*) or something similar, which were inspired by Galen's *On the Preservation of Health*. For *On the Preservation of Health* see Green (1951) and Wilkins (2016). *On the Preservation of Health* was also important for medieval European authors who, inspired by Galen's work, compiled their own compendia on hygiene, such as that ascribed to Peter of Spain (sometimes identified with Pope John XXI, 1276–7); see dos Santos and da Conceição Fagundes (2010). On the healthy way of life as presented in the Greek, Roman, Arabo-Islamic, and medieval European writings see Sotres (1998: 291–318).

Chapter 2 is devoted to the topic announced in the title of the manual – that is, ways of dealing with the disease when the sick person cannot or does not want to consult a physician. Offering a variety of cures and remedies, the text also warns against thoughtless reliance on drugs and suggests – in line with the Hippocratic-Galenic tradition – that the administration of drugs, especially powerful ones, should be a last resort rather than the first-choice therapeutic option. As Ibn al-Akfānī maintains, 'the doctors agreed that whenever possible, a disease should be countered by embarking on a proper diet rather than by administration of drugs. And if there is a need to administer drugs, let nutritional medicaments be used, if possible. And if drugs have to be administered, let them be mild and simple rather than compound'.[26]

Such an approach suggests the implementation of a mild therapy which may involve procedures such as: 1. delicate bloodletting by means of scarification; 2. relaxation of the stomach with the use of *shīrkhashak*[27] and Persian manna,[28] violets and quince jam, cold rose syrup, plum jam, and so forth; 3. administration of a mild enema; 4. inducing vomiting with a drink of barley water and oxymel;[29] 5. feeding with the so-called *muzawwarāt*, or 'fake' dishes – that is, non-meat dishes which simulate meat content;[30] 6. cooling the temperament with tamarind, cherry, and apricot solution; 7. warming the temperament with bitter ginger and grape syrup. In addition to this preferred approach, Ibn al-Akfānī presents two other therapeutic alternatives. One of them assumes that the fight against the disease can be left to the forces of nature,[31] while the other involves reliance on drugs – that is, implementing an intensive therapy,

[26] Ibn al-Akfānī, *Ghunyat al-labīb fī mā yusta'mal 'inda ghaybat al-ṭabīb* (*Wealth of Information for the Intelligent Man When the Doctor Is Not Around*), ed. 'Abbās (1989) 67. For a discussion of food used for medicinal purposes cf. Waines (1995: 556–7).

[27] The name rarely appears in Arabic-language sources. According to a Persian dictionary of traditional medicine, *shīrkhashak* is a sweet-sour fruit which grows in the Alborz mountains and is used as a laxative (https://sites.google.com/site/traditionalmedicinedictionary, accessed 15 March 2020).

[28] Persian manna (Ar. *taranjabīn*) is an edible, sweet, semi-solid resinous substance which appears on the leaves and branches of the camel's thorn shrub (*Alhagi mannifera*, *Alhagi persarum*). These shrubs are native to the steppes of western Asia and to Egypt. For details see Ramezany, Khademizadeh, and Kiyani (2013).

[29] Borrowed from Graeco-Roman culture, oxymel (Ar. *sakanjabīn*) was a medicinal drink or syrup made up of vinegar and honey, sometimes mixed with other ingredients (such as quince or pomegranate juice, celery, endive, and parsley water, etc.), generally used as an expectorant.

[30] The dishes are discussed in detail in Waines and Marín (2002: 303–15) and Lewicka (2011: 261–2). On 'counterfeit' dishes see also Chipman (Chapter 10) in the present volume.

[31] By which Ibn al-Akfānī means 'refraining from forcing the sick person to do something or from forbidding him another thing, and allowing him to eat moderately if he wishes'. Ibn al-Akfānī, *Ghunyat al-labīb fī mā yusta'mal 'inda ghaybat al-ṭabīb* (*Wealth of Information for the Intelligent Man When the Doctor Is Not Around*), ed. 'Abbās (1989) 64–5.

which includes bloodletting procedures, paracentesis, application of laxatives or a powerful enema, and using strong medicaments to provoke vomiting and strong compound drugs such as theriac (i.e. an antidote).

Ibn al-Akfānī's presentation of cures for specific ailments[32] is rather sketchy and generally follows the Hippocratic-Galenic principle of avoiding unnecessary reliance on drugs and implementing a mild therapy instead. Most of these recipes are very like what was transmitted in the much earlier medical works written in Arabic, such as al-Rāzī's *Kitāb al-ḥāwī* or Ibn Sīnā's *Qanūn fī al-ṭibb*. These works might also have been the main source of the Persian influences apparent in *Ghunyat al-labīb (I)*, of which ingredients such as *shīrkhashak* and Persian manna are probably the most obvious examples. Apart from the imports from Persian culture, Ibn al-Akfānī's manual also includes the so-called *muzawwarāt*, or non-meat dishes originally meant for 'the sick, and monks, and Christians during Lent',[33] which constituted a Christian contribution to the Graeco-Arabic medico-culinary culture. Other elements added to the Graeco-Roman base of the manual were, like *sawīq*,[34] taken from the traditional Arab cuisine or came from the local environment and included ingredients such as nenuphar or Egyptian rosewater:

> Anyone who suffers from excessive diarrhoea should cool his body and be treated with jams that are effective in the treatment of diarrhoea, such as apple jam ... or Egyptian rosewater or pomegranate juice with *sawīq* ... Non-meat dishes (*muzawwarāt*) that are effective in the treatment of diarrhoea, such as *rummāniyyah* [with pomegranate seeds], *summāqiyyah* [with sumac] and *zarkashiyyah* with purslane branches and sorrel are also useful. And anyone who suffers from vomiting should be treated with sour grape jam with mint or sour grape syrup with mint or *sawīq* with quince jam.[35]

According to the humoral theory of medicine, in addition to food mild therapies included a variety of compresses, fluids, and aromas, made of leaves, flowers, or bits of fruit, which were applied directly on the body, introduced into it or, depending on their form, placed or sprinkled in the room of the ailing person.

32 Ibn al-Akfānī, *Ghunyat al-labīb fī mā yusta'mal 'inda ghaybat al-ṭabīb* (*Wealth of Information for the Intelligent Man When the Doctor Is Not Around*), ed. 'Abbās (1989) 71–5.

33 See Lewicka (2011: 256–62).

34 A meal of parched grain made into a kind of gruel, to which water, butter, or fat from sheep's tails were added.

35 Ibn al-Akfānī, *Ghunyat al-labīb fī mā yusta'mal 'inda ghaybat al-ṭabīb* (*Wealth of Information for the Intelligent Man When the Doctor Is Not Around*), ed. 'Abbās (1989) 73.

> And whoever suffers from nosebleed should have his face washed with very cold water and be given camphor with rosewater or fresh squeezed donkey dung to smell. He should also have his forehead fomented with nenuphar leaves or cucumber skin or watermelon skin or sandalwood with Egyptian rosewater ... He can also have pulverised acorns blown into his nose; alternatively, a pledget made of spider's web, soaked in ink and covered with aloes, can be used ... He should be given a lot of skimmed milk to drink. He should not look on red things, especially gleaming ones.[36]

And further on:

> When someone suffers a lot from sciatica, he should apply a compress of dried pulverised myrtle or rose leaves ... He should wear clothes made of linen saturated with sandal [aroma] and camphor ... The air should be cooled by sprinkling cold water and the bedding coated with leaves of willow, wild olive, wet myrtle and henna flowers.[37]

But the Graeco-Roman Galenic perspective, interspersed with a number of imports from Christian, Persian, and Egyptian traditions, only partly characterises Ibn al-Akfānī's attitude to medicaments and curative therapy in general. Chapter 4[38] of *Ghunyat al-labīb (I)*, entitled 'On substances having special properties (mostly medical) that have been tested', differs significantly from the preceding chapters. The Arabic title includes the term *khawāṣṣ*, which pertains to special, inexplicable, esoteric properties, associated with aspects of animate or inanimate natural elements, which could be activated by appropriate action and used both in the treatment of ailments and as a means of protecting oneself from them. In the Arabic-speaking world of the Islamic Middle Period, very much like in the Mediterranean of Antiquity, the existence of hidden properties of objects, creatures, and graphic signs was a natural part of general knowledge and the local belief system. So much so that both al-Rāzī and Ibn Sīnā promoted therapeutics based on such properties too and their efficacy was said to be 'proved'. The recipes for remedies that included substances with such properties were often described as *mujarrabāt*, or 'tested', which term corresponds to *pepeiratai*, a remark frequently used in

[36] Ibn al-Akfānī, *Ghunyat al-labīb fī mā yusta'mal 'inda ghaybat al-ṭabīb* (*Wealth of Information for the Intelligent Man When the Doctor Is Not Around*), ed. 'Abbās (1989) 75.

[37] Ibn al-Akfānī, *Ghunyat al-labīb fī mā yusta'mal 'inda ghaybat al-ṭabīb* (*Wealth of Information for the Intelligent Man When the Doctor Is Not Around*), ed. 'Abbās (1989) 74–5.

[38] Chapter 3 of *Ghunyat al-labīb fī mā yusta'mal 'inda ghaybat al-ṭabīb* (*Wealth of Information for the Intelligent Man When the Doctor Is Not Around*), entitled 'Useful advice regarding the issues presented pertaining to caring for health and treating disease', is very short and consists of brief repetitions of basic rules discussed earlier in Chapters 1 and 2; see (Ibn al-Akfānī, *Ghunyat al-labīb fī mā yusta'mal 'inda ghaybat al-ṭabīb* (*Wealth of Information for the Intelligent Man When the Doctor Is Not Around*), ed. 'Abbās (1989) 76–7.

Greek medical writings to characterise medicaments both simple and compound.[39] In the case of Ibn al-Akfānī's book *khawāṣṣ* involved substances which, he says, 'we tested as well as those, which we trustingly borrowed from most outstanding doctors'.[40]

Different medical manuals presented occult medical knowledge in different ways. In some cases, especially when the book was arranged according to the parts of the body and their respective disorders, the magical formulae were woven into the text of each chapter among other therapeutics and cures recommended for a given ailment.[41] However, some authors, having recognised the distinctness of occult-magical approach to medicine, devoted separate treatises to it[42] or collected medico-magical recommendations in a separate chapter of a manual. Having chosen the latter method, Ibn al-Akfānī divided his chapter into two sections. One introduced a list of names of the most important substances with occult properties together with short notices as to what each of them was effective for and how to apply them. Thus, for example, myrtle (like frankincense, wax, or tar) – when inhaled – was good in epidemics. Ruby – when hung [around the neck?] – was good against plague. The same was true of a drink made from Armenian clay and medicinal clay (Ar. *ṭīn makhtūm*; Lat. *terra sigillata*). Coconut, when hung around [the neck (?)] of the sick person was effective against malarial fevers. The same was true of the horns of a horned viper, bone of a frog, bone from a dead person, or bone with an aperture, such as could be found in the wings of a cock. Likewise, hair cut from the beard of a billy goat and then wrapped in a cloth was helpful against quartan fever if hung around the neck of a person suffering from it.[43] A sick person was also

39 See Totelin (2011: 75, 84–6). See also the use of brief efficacy statements in medieval Latin and Hebrew recipes discussed by Doolittle (Chapter 2), Gottlieb (Chapter 6), and Chipman (Chapter 10) in this volume.

40 Ibn al-Akfānī, *Ghunyat al-labīb fī mā yusta'mal 'inda ghaybat al-ṭabīb* (*Wealth of Information for the Intelligent Man When the Doctor Is Not Around*), ed. 'Abbās (1989) 27.

41 As is the case, for example, of al-Rāzī's *Kitāb al-ḥāwī* (*Comprehensive Book*) and a thirteenth-century medical compendium compiled by the Damascene physician Ibn Ṭarkhān al-Suwaydī and entitled *Tadhkirat al-Suwaydī fī al-ṭibb* (*Al-Suwaydī's Treatise on Medicine*).

42 Such treatises, entitled *Kitāb al-khawāṣṣ*, or *Book on Substances Having Special Properties*, were reportedly written by al-Rāzī, a Persian physician; Ibn Jazzār (tenth century), a physician from Kairouan; and Abū al-'Alā' Ibn Zuhr (eleventh–twelfth centuries), a physician from al-Andalus. The most famous Arab author who specialised in the knowledge of 'secret properties' was Abū Mūsā Jābir Ibn Ḥayyān (ninth century), an erudite scholar and alchemist who presumably compiled *Kitāb al-khawāṣṣ al-kabīr* (*Big Book of Substances with Special Properties*).

43 Ibn al-Akfānī, *Ghunyat al-labīb fī mā yusta'mal 'inda ghaybat al-ṭabīb* (*Wealth of Information for the Intelligent Man When the Doctor Is Not Around*), ed. 'Abbās (1989) 81–2. According to Greek medical lore, quartan fever belonged to the group of hectic fevers which developed as a consequence of corruption in principal organs. Quartan fever appeared every fourth day (seventy-two-hour cycle).

recommended to wear the unwashed shirt of a woman who had given birth.[44]

Typically for Arabic (and Greek) medical compendia, the list of therapeutic substances is followed by a catalogue of ailments arranged according to the parts of the body – that is, from head to toe – with each entry introducing suggestions for remedies effective for a given disorder. For example, the section entitled 'Head' includes a recommendation for a remedy for persons suffering from headache and migraine: 'sever the horns of a live ram and make a comb out of each of them, then comb the hair of the ailing person with them – the right side with the comb made from the right horn, the left with the one made of the left horn'.[45] This section also covers health problems such as sleeplessness, good and bad dreams, forgetfulness, epilepsy, chills and love, for according to the Arabo-Islamic (and Greek) way of thinking, love was an ailment which had to be medically treated. Next come the eye and its diseases, such as inflammation of the eye or weakened sight; then the ear and its diseases, such as pain or an insect which has gotten into the ear. Then come the nose, mouth, teeth, and throat with their diseases,[46] followed by the chest, heart, and spleen. In the case of the latter it is recommended that the ailment called 'rigidity of the spleen' is to be cured by 'urinating backwards, like a camel, many times, so that the rigidness will pass'.[47] The recommendation is addressed specifically to men and includes a description of how to perform such an operation.

One of the last parts of the body mentioned in the list is the seat (*maqʾada*). Of the three recommendations included in this entry two deal with haemorrhoids, of which one involves a kind of remote therapy:

> Whoever comes to the caper plant at sunset and says: 'you are the haemorrhoid of this and that person', and then comes to it at dawn and says the same thing, then comes to it at sunset and says the same thing, and after that pulls the plant out, then in the same way the haemorrhoids of this sick person will be pulled out. The plant should not be pulled out with anything made of iron.[48]

[44] Ibn al-Akfānī, *Ghunyat al-labīb fī mā yustaʾmal ʿinda ghaybat al-ṭabīb* (*Wealth of Information for the Intelligent Man When the Doctor Is Not Around*), ed. ʿAbbās (1989) 80. Cf. Ullmann (1978: 109).

[45] Ibn al-Akfānī, *Ghunyat al-labīb fī mā yustaʾmal ʿinda ghaybat al-ṭabīb* (*Wealth of Information for the Intelligent Man When the Doctor Is Not Around*), ed. ʿAbbās (1989) 105.

[46] Ibn al-Akfānī, *Ghunyat al-labīb fī mā yustaʾmal ʿinda ghaybat al-ṭabīb* (*Wealth of Information for the Intelligent Man When the Doctor Is Not Around*), ed. ʿAbbās (1989) 118.

[47] Ibn al-Akfānī, *Ghunyat al-labīb fī mā yustaʾmal ʿinda ghaybat al-ṭabīb* (*Wealth of Information for the Intelligent Man When the Doctor Is Not Around*), ed. ʿAbbās (1989) 127.

[48] Ibn al-Akfānī, *Ghunyat al-labīb fī mā yustaʾmal ʿinda ghaybat al-ṭabīb* (*Wealth of Information for the Intelligent Man When the Doctor Is Not Around*), ed. ʿAbbās (1989) 132. The taboo on iron seems to date back to the beginnings of the Iron Age, when people might have been reluctant to replace traditional bronze with a new and unknown material. The objection to iron was adopted later by the

As the recommendation can also be found in a number of other medical compendia,[49] it makes one wonder whether it in any way testifies to its popularity, especially given how common haemorrhoids supposedly were in the eastern Mediterranean. Intriguingly enough, the third remedy included in the entry refers to passive pederasty (*ubna*): 'If hair from the right leg of a male hyena is burnt and a catamite [i.e. passive partner in homosexual anal intercourse] carries it with him, his pederasty will be eliminated. Hair from the left leg of a female hyena works the other way around [*sic*].'[50]

In some cases the occult-medical power of flora, fauna, or minerals had to be activated by the influence of astral bodies. Performing certain operations in favourable astral circumstances or at an appropriate time of night or day was required, above all, in the case of protective procedures: 'If someone drinks half a *mithqāl*[51] of the gall of the mountain goat with a decoction of wild lettuce on the day when the sun enters the sign of Aries, he will be protected against poisons and stings.'[52] 'If someone looks on al-Suhā – which is a little planet in the constellation of Ursa Maior that people spot in order to check their sight – neither a viper, nor a scorpion will bite him that night.'[53] 'When someone says: "I've sworn to God the Highest that I would not eat chicory or meat" while looking at the new moon at the beginning of the month, he will not suffer from pain in the wisdom teeth that month.'[54] 'Whoever wears an emerald when the Moon enters the sign of Libra will sleep well and will have sweet dreams.'[55] The list of body parts and their ailments ends with diseases typically associated with the surface of the body, such as smallpox, measles, ulcer, tumour, leprosy, papilla, and

Graeco-Roman world – the bans on using it in the medical-pharmacological context can be detected, for example, in *Natural History* by Pliny the Elder and in Ptolemy's *Centiloquium*; see Frazer (1922: 224–6), Richardson (1934: 561), and Brévart (2008: 4, n. 6; 10).

[49] Such as, for example, Ibn Ṭarkhān al-Suwaydī's *Tadhkirat al-Suwaydī fī al-ṭibb* (*Al-Suwaydī's Treatise on Medicine*). See al-Sha'rānī, *Mukhtaṣar tadhkirat al-Suwaydī fī al-ṭibb* (*Abridgement of al-Suwaydī's Treatise on Medicine*), ed. Shāhīn (1289/1872) 68.

[50] Ibn al-Akfānī, *Ghunyat al-labīb fī mā yusta'mal 'inda ghaybat al-ṭabīb* (*Wealth of Information for the Intelligent Man When the Doctor Is Not Around*), ed. 'Abbās (1989) 132.

[51] Circa 4.25 grams.

[52] Ibn al-Akfānī, *Ghunyat al-labīb fī mā yusta'mal 'inda ghaybat al-ṭabīb* (*Wealth of Information for the Intelligent Man When the Doctor Is Not Around*), ed. 'Abbās (1989) 85.

[53] Ibn al-Akfānī, *Ghunyat al-labīb fī mā yusta'mal 'inda ghaybat al-ṭabīb* (*Wealth of Information for the Intelligent Man When the Doctor Is Not Around*), ed. 'Abbās (1989) 86. Al-Suhā, a little planet hidden in the constellation of Ursa Maior, was also mentioned by other authors writing in Arabic; see Ideler (1809: 25).

[54] Ibn al-Akfānī, *Ghunyat al-labīb fī mā yusta'mal 'inda ghaybat al-ṭabīb* (*Wealth of Information for the Intelligent Man When the Doctor Is Not Around*), ed. 'Abbās (1989) 118.

[55] Ibn al-Akfānī, *Ghunyat al-labīb fī mā yusta'mal 'inda ghaybat al-ṭabīb* (*Wealth of Information for the Intelligent Man When the Doctor Is Not Around*), ed. 'Abbās (1989) 107.

whitlow. The chapter ends with a remark about the properties of a number of substances, considered effective for a good mood and successful social relations, the attainment of which in some manuals is featured among health problems:[56]

> Anyone who wears an obsidian ring or hangs a piece of it on him, will move away the evil coming from someone's evil glance. The same result is achieved with a feather of the peacock and a stone known as al-Karak.[57]
>
> Anyone who wears a ruby will be respected by people.[58]

The spectrum of substances which could be used in magical medicaments was extremely broad. In fact, it had no limits as far as authors' inventiveness was concerned. Ibn al-Akfānī mentions dozens of cures, from coconut and citron seeds to human teeth reduced to ashes, hair soaked in vinegar, the right eye of a ferret, wolf or rooster, to emerald, petrol, and sulphur. In order to prepare compound antidotes (theriac) for snake and particularly viper bites one had to get the dried liver of a wolf, meat of the hedgehog, gall of the rooster, urine, and an excretion from the human ear, river crayfish cooked in goat's milk, root of the colocynth (desert gourd), the dried testicle of a deer as well as its penis.[59] The range of practices required for activating the healing powers hidden in these kinds of substances was also extensive and involved procedures which were sometimes quite challenging – such as severing the horns of a live ram in order to make combs effective against headache from them or urinating like a camel. Interestingly, Ibn al-Akfānī's therapeutic recommendations pertaining to occult-magical medicine do not include graphics of any kind – there are no magic squares, charts, combinations of letters, signs, fragments of the Quran, spells, or any other sort of inscriptions which can sometimes be found in medical literature of that period.[60]

[56] Ibn al-Akfānī, *Ghunyat al-labīb fī mā yusta'mal 'inda ghaybat al-ṭabīb* (*Wealth of Information for the Intelligent Man When the Doctor Is Not Around*), ed. 'Abbās (1989) 137.

[57] Ibn al-Akfānī, *Ghunyat al-labīb fī mā yusta'mal 'inda ghaybat al-ṭabīb* (*Wealth of Information for the Intelligent Man When the Doctor Is Not Around*), ed. 'Abbās (1989) 138.

[58] Ibn al-Akfānī, *Ghunyat al-labīb fī mā yusta'mal 'inda ghaybat al-ṭabīb* (*Wealth of Information for the Intelligent Man When the Doctor Is Not Around*), ed. 'Abbās (1989) 138.

[59] Ibn al-Akfānī, *Ghunyat al-labīb fī mā yusta'mal 'inda ghaybat al-ṭabīb* (*Wealth of Information for the Intelligent Man When the Doctor Is Not Around*), ed. 'Abbās (1989) 86–8. On theriac see also Amar, Serri, and Lev (Chapter 5) in this volume.

[60] Cf. natural remedies, or *physika* in Greek medical writing; see, for example, Bouras-Vallianatos (2014: 348–52) and Bouras-Vallianatos (2016: 389–94), where the case of Alexander of Tralles is discussed. See also Lieberman (Chapter 8) in the present volume, who discusses magical recipes in Moses Maimonides, and Gottlieb (Chapter 6), who refers to the interrelationship between medicine and magic with a focus on the uses of plants in the so-called alchemical herbals.

9.2 *Ghunyat al-labīb* by al-Qurashī

In addition to Ibn al-Akfānī's *Ghunyat al-labīb (I)* another extant self-treatment manual seems pertinent to the issue of the household medicines as recorded in the discourse of the Mamluk period. Due to the problematic character of its author's identification, the time and place of its creation cannot be confirmed. With an almost identical title to that of Ibn al-Akfānī's work: *Ghunyat al-labīb ḥaythu lā yūjad al-ṭabīb* (*An Abundance of Information for the Intelligent Man When the Doctor Is Not Around*), it has survived in at least nine manuscripts, two of which are preserved in the Bibliothèque Nationale, Paris,[61] one in Hasan Pasha Library, Çorum, one in Süleymaniye Library, Istanbul, one in Beyazit Library, Istanbul, one in the Bibliothèque Royale, Rabat,[62] one in the King Saʾūd University Library, Riyadh,[63] one in the Forschungsbibliothek, Gotha[64] and one in the Dār al-Kutub archives in Cairo.[65] It will be referred to as *Ghunyat al-labīb (II)* in the present chapter.

At least two of the nine copies – that is, the Cairene copy and one of the Parisian copies – mention a certain Abū al-Ḥasan ʿAlī Ibn ʿAbd Allah Muḥammad al-Qurashī as the author of the book and there is no obvious reason to question the reliability of this information. However, at least for the time being, there is no way of knowing who this person was. In fact, the text of *Ghunyat al-labīb (II)* includes a number of clues which point to the author's Egyptian connections. At the same time, a remark in another book of his *Kitāb al-ḥikma fī al-ṭibb (Book of Wisdom in Medicine)*, suggests that the author could have lived in the second half of the fifteenth century and the beginning of the sixteenth.[66] But until his identity can be confirmed, any speculation regarding the Egyptian-Mamluk provenance of the manual has to be acknowledged as just that – pure speculation.

Apart from the Dār al-Kutub copy, which is much longer than the other eight, the manuscripts of *Ghunyat al-labīb (II)* contain a relatively short text (*c.* twenty folios) the contents of which differ in many respects from the manual written by Ibn al-Akfānī. Composed of fragments taken from multiple partly unnamed sources, the compilation lacks the traditional division into chapters

[61] MS BNF arabe 5718; MS BNF arabe 3039.

[62] For technical reasons, the copies from Hasan Pasha, Süleymaniye, Beyazit and Bibliothèque Royale could not be used in the present study.

[63] King Saʾūd University, MS 5980.

[64] Gotha, MS 2014 (arab.765; Stz. Kah. 537).

[65] Dār al-Kutub MS 699, ff. 32a–75; see *Fihris al-makhṭūṭāt* (*Catalogue of Manuscripts*) (2011) III.484.

[66] See Abū al-Ḥasan ʿAlī ibn ʿAbd Allah Muḥammad Al-Qurashī, *Kitāb al-ḥikma fī al-ṭibb (Book of Wisdom in Medicine)*, British Library, Oriental Manuscripts, MS Add 6026, 112; digital version available at Qatar Digital Library, http://www.qdl.qa/en/archive/81055/vdc_100044433795.0x000001, accessed 3 August 2023.

or thematic sections arranged according to the parts of the body or therapeutic substances. The absence of such an arrangement – otherwise typical of medical books compiled by professional physicians or medically trained scholars – may suggest that al-Qurashī had not had much classical medical education and, therefore, had not had the opportunity to familiarise himself with the Graeco-Arabic medical literature. That was probably why he was unable to comprehend the Graeco-Arabic ordering of the subject matter and to include theoretical aspects of the Hippocratic-Galenic doctrine, discussion of which is lacking in his manual.

Furthermore, unlike Ibn al-Akfānī, al-Qurashī does not distinguish between occult-magical and humoral remedies and freely mixes both categories, interspersing them with cures belonging to folk medicine and with the health-related traditions belonging to the Sunna of the Prophet. But whereas blending magical and non-magical remedies in one text was not unusual, even in the case of professional physicians and other authors trained in classical medicine,[67] dotting the medical manual with hadiths was not typical of this kind of writing. However, this was, in fact, practised in the so-called Medicine of the Prophet, a subgenre of religious literature elaborated and promoted by Islamic theologians interested in medicine, who during the Mamluk period used it as a means to accomplish their ideological and social aims.[68]

However, al-Qurashī's *Ghunyat al-labīb (II)* is not an example of this kind of writing, if only because the Prophet's tradition does not constitute a fundamental or prerequisite element of it. Unlike the theologians of the Mamluk period, al-Qurashī refers to the hadiths only occasionally, as if to inform the reader of the Prophet's experience with this or that ingredient or with this or that ailment. In other words, he uses hadiths for devotional-thematic reasons and not as a pretext for producing an ideologically biased, quasi-medical book.

Furthermore, al-Qurashī does not refer exclusively to religious authorities. Apart from pious transmitters of the Prophetic traditions he quotes Ibn Sīnā and takes some eye medicaments from *Ṭibb al-fuqarāʾ* (*Medicine*

[67] Such as, for example, Abū Bakr al-Rāzī, Ibn Ṭarkhān al-Suwaydī, Ibrāhīm Ibn ʿAbd al-Raḥmān Ibn al-Azraq, or Dāwud al-Anṭākī.

[68] For a more detailed discussion of the Mamluk period books on Prophetic medicine, see Lewicka (2014: passim). Interestingly enough, in one case al-Qurashī admits that the hadith he quotes was taken from Abū Nuʿaym al-Iṣfahānī's (tenth–eleventh centuries) *Al-Ṭibb al-nabawī* (*Medicine of the Prophet*) which, while being one of the earliest specialised collections of 'medical' hadiths, was also the most extensive one. As such, the book became a valuable source for later compilers of medico-religious texts; see Perho (1995: 54).

for the Poor) by an unknown author.[69] He also quotes what he calls *Hippocrates' Memorandum for His Son*, an odd, longish text which incidentally merits a separate analysis. And, above all, throughout the manual he mentions unnamed 'sages' and 'learned men' (*ḥukamāʾ* and *arbāb al-kutub*) as his sources. Intriguingly enough, unlike other authors of medical books, he never speaks of *aṭibbāʾ* or 'physicians' in this context.

Al-Qurashī's unbiased approach to medical knowledge notwithstanding, the significance of his religio-spiritual perspective should not be underestimated, all the more so given that it is strongly emphasised by the *bi-idhn Allāh taʿālā* or 'God willing' added at the end of almost every recipe. Intended to stress that a given medicament would heal the sick only if God wished it, the phrase rarely occurs in medical books compiled by authors educated in the spirit of the Hippocratic-Galenic, so-called rational medicine. In fact, al-Qurashī's piety and his commitment to the God-fearing aspect of healing constitute yet another way in which his work is different from that of Ibn al-Akfānī whose manual, almost entirely free of religious references, is in fact devoid of the spiritual dimension.

Unsystematic as it is, the text of *Ghunyat al-labīb (II)* is divided into approximately twenty irregular sections.[70] They refer, for example, to topics such as: the medical benefits of various rinds and shells; cures for worms; the medical benefits of garlic, onions, and rue; cures for nosebleed; cures for overeating; explanation of the need for medical treatment; powders for problems with the digestive system; a remedy against worms; a cure for bleeding made from the lung of a horse or a wild donkey; Hippocrates' memorandum to his son; a prescription for a beneficial drug; cures for headache; and cures for eye problems.

Al-Qurashī declares in the introduction – very much like al-Rāzī had done some centuries earlier[71] – that his intention in composing the manual was to recommend ways of curing health disorders with foods and medicaments prepared from 'well-known and easily available ingredients'.[72] And, indeed, it seems he did his best to follow his guidelines. In this context the opening fragment of the manual is probably the most distinctive. In it al-Qurashī stresses the medical usefulness of otherwise worthless

[69] The recipes for eye medicaments al-Qurashī quotes are not included in *Ṭibb al-fuqarāʾ wa-l-masākīn* (*Medicine for the Poor and the Destitute*) by Ibn al-Jazzār; Ibn al-Jazzār, *Ṭibb al-fuqarāʾ wa-l-masākīn* (*Medicine for the Poor and the Destitute*), ed. Āl Ṭaʿma (1996) 63–6.

[70] The headings of these sections differ slightly depending on the manuscript.

[71] See above, pp. 295–6.

[72] Al-Qurashī, *Ghunyat al-labīb ḥaythu lā yūjad al-ṭabīb* (*An Abundance of Information for the Intelligent Man When the Doctor Is Not Around*), King Saʿūd MS 5980, f. 1b; MS BNF arabe 5718, f. 27b; MS BNF arabe 3039, f. 82a.

rinds and shells and encourages people not to throw them away, but rather to use them to treat their ailments. In this respect al-Qurashī quotes unnamed sages and learned men, according to whom 'there are nine[73] kinds of rinds/shells [*qushūr*], which people in Egypt throw away and which could be utilised. These include bitter orange rinds, pomegranate rinds, eggshells, poppy head shells, green banana rinds, river mussel shells, green and yellow melon rinds and hazelnut shells'.[74]

Some of these items were very easy to use. Others, however, required additional ingredients and extra effort if their curative properties were to be activated. In the case of the river mussel shells, for example, it was enough to burn and then pound them to get a hair growth remedy for anyone who had had his hair shaved in the *hammam*. The powder was supposed to work when sprinkled on a bald head. The juice extracted from pounded banana skin was said to heal a wound if simply dripped on it. As for the bitter orange rind, it was even more simple to use, and its curative quality was universal. It was enough to eat half a dirham of dried rinds to become safe from colic, gripes, winds, swelling, stomach rumbling from under the ribs, and corruption of the stomach. It was also useful for the digestion.[75]

In order to stop bleeding, however, more work was necessary: burned river mussel shells were to be kneaded with bee's honey and then squeezed in a woollen cloth made of camel hair. If a woman carried the product to someone who was bleeding, the blood would stop flowing. At the same time, three dirhams of pulverised eggshells with half an *ūqiyyah*[76] of white sugar taken for three consecutive days on an empty stomach were said to stop dysuria, while a remedy composed of one *mithqāl* of pulverised and sieved poppy head shells, a *mithqāl* of Aswanian clay, and a *mithqāl* of white cumin, if taken for three days, would stop diarrhoea, among other ailments.

The remedies based on shells and rinds were not only cheap, but also relatively easy to get and prepare. Many other recipes from al-Qurashī's collection called for simple and seemingly easily available ingredients too. Of the several recipes for remedies against intestinal worms, for example, one called for substances such as the root of sour and sweet pomegranate, another for the leaves of the peach tree, and yet another for bitter lupins

[73] Depending on the manuscript, the list covers seven or nine items.

[74] Al-Qurashī, *Ghunyat al-labīb ḥaythu lā yūjad al-ṭabīb* (*An Abundance of Information for the Intelligent Man When the Doctor Is Not Around*), King Saʾūd MS 5980, f. 1b; MS BNF arabe 5718, f. 27b; MS BNF arabe 3039, f. 82a.

[75] Al-Qurashī, *Ghunyat al-labīb ḥaythu lā yūjad al-ṭabīb* (*An Abundance of Information for the Intelligent Man When the Doctor Is Not Around*), King Saʾūd MS 5980, f. 2a.

[76] Circa 75 grams.

which, when pounded, should be licked [*sic*] with molasses and vinegar. Another remedy against worms consisted of two seeds of wheat which, when chewed, were to be washed down, after an hour's sleep, with a drink made from mint. What must have been an even cheaper remedy was based on pigeon droppings, the smell of which, when held under a bleeding nose, was supposed to stop the blood flow.[77]

Apart from a number of otherwise inedible items, most of the ingredients used in al-Qurashī's pharmacology were known from everyday cooking. Those particularly frequently mentioned included garlic (usually burnt), onions, honey, vinegar, salt, eggs, nigella, rue, and so forth. It should be borne in mind that the medicine of the premodern eastern Mediterranean, like probably all medical systems and cultures, depended heavily on edibles and was strongly linked to local foodways and nutritional traditions. This is normal, as humans instinctively tend to care for their health by eating what their habitat provides. In the cities of Mamluk Egypt and Syria, however, very much like in other parts of the Mediterranean, this innate motivation was rationalised by the theses of the Galenic doctrine of humours which, among other things, assumed that food had medicinal properties and that foodstuffs were fundamental to both curative and preventive treatments.

Consequently, the difference between food and medicament was not always obvious. Probably the only way to define the difference between the two categories is to note that, while food (both simple and sophisticated) was often used as a medicament[78] – that is, a therapeutic substance serving different medicinal purposes – medicaments were generally not used as food. A good illustration of such a situation is the case of all the medicinal pastes (*maʿājin*), pastilles (*aqrāṣ*), syrups (*ashriba*), tonics, electuaries (*jawarīshāt*), potions, digestive beverages (*hāḍimāt*), and so forth, which, although composed of edible substances and sometimes even described in cookery books, were generally not used as nourishment or treats. This is also the case with one of al-Qurashī's remedies for back pain which, while resembling a regular dish, seems to have been atypical enough to discourage anyone from using it as an ordinary meal.

> If you suffer from back pain take garlic, nigella, licorice, caraway, sesame seed oil, three dirhams of each, three eggs and an *ūqiyyah* of [olive?] oil. Then peel the garlic, clean the nigella and caraway, mix them in the

[77] Al-Qurashī, *Ghunyat al-labīb ḥaythu lā yūjad al-ṭabīb* (*An Abundance of Information for the Intelligent Man When the Doctor Is Not Around*), King Saʿūd MS 5980, f. 4a.

[78] On the aspects of the food-drug continuum in Greece of the fifth and fourth centuries BCE, see Totelin (2015).

> [*ṭājin*-type of] pan and throw in some oil and sesame seed oil, and fry them until the garlic burns and becomes like black coal. Then throw the garlic away from the pan [into another pan?], break three eggs into it and leave them until they soft-boil. Then take the preparation off the fire, sprinkle powdered licorice on it, and eat it for breakfast with an *ūqiyyah* of bread. Do not eat any cold snacks with it and refrain from drinking water for a sidereal hour. Wise men have said that whoever eats this preparation will be safe from back pain for a whole year, God willing.[79]

Of course, as in every medical manual, in al-Qurashī's recipes one can also find odd substances. Blood of hoopoe for example, if dried, pounded, sieved through a piece of silk, and smeared on the edges of the eyelids, was supposed to remove leukoma from the eye.[80] Blood of cow and dog ticks which, mixed with tar, could ensure that an eyelash, once torn out, would not appear again.[81] Two *mithqāls* of the right lung of a wild donkey or a horse, burnt in the oven, pounded, and mixed with three *mithqāls* of bee's honey or pomegranate syrup and taken for three days on an empty stomach, were said to stop a heavy cough for good.[82]

In fact, recipes which involved peculiar ingredients were typical of occult-magical medicine, or the sphere in which increased weirdness and secrecy were supposed to result in the increased power of the *khawāṣṣ* and thus enhance therapeutic effectiveness. Quite often, such ingredients went hand in hand with strange procedures. In some cases, however, no ingredients were necessary, as the procedures themselves sufficed as a cure:

> When anybody whose nose is bleeding ties together the little finger and ring finger of both hands and opens the palms of his hands, the bleeding will stop, God willing.[83]
>
> When anybody whose nose is bleeding writes [something] in blood on his hand and looks at what is written, the bleeding will stop, God willing.[84]

[79] Al-Qurashī, *Ghunyat al-labīb ḥaythu lā yūjad al-ṭabīb* (*An Abundance of Information for the Intelligent Man When the Doctor Is Not Around*), King Saʾūd MS 5980, ff. 3b–4a.

[80] Al-Qurashī, *Ghunyat al-labīb ḥaythu lā yūjad al-ṭabīb* (*An Abundance of Information for the Intelligent Man When the Doctor Is Not Around*), King Saʾūd MS 5980, f. 7b; Dār al-Kutub MS 699, ff. 38b-39a; MS BNF arabe 5718, f. 39a; Ghota MS 2014, f. 6b.

[81] Al-Qurashī, *Ghunyat al-labīb ḥaythu lā yūjad al-ṭabīb* (*An Abundance of Information for the Intelligent Man When the Doctor Is Not Around*), King Saʾūd MS 5980, f. 7b.

[82] Al-Qurashī, *Ghunyat al-labīb ḥaythu lā yūjad al-ṭabīb* (*An Abundance of Information for the Intelligent Man When the Doctor Is Not Around*), King Saʾūd MS 5980, f. 5a.

[83] Al-Qurashī, *Ghunyat al-labīb ḥaythu lā yūjad al-ṭabīb* (*An Abundance of Information for the Intelligent Man When the Doctor Is Not Around*), King Saʾūd MS 5980, f. 4a.

[84] Al-Qurashī, *Ghunyat al-labīb ḥaythu lā yūjad al-ṭabīb* (*An Abundance of Information for the Intelligent Man When the Doctor Is Not Around*), King Saʾūd MS 5980, f. 4a.

The belief in *khawāṣṣ*, or the occultic properties of things, has often been referred to by modern scholars as 'irrational'. Misleadingly enough, this term was intended as a contrast with the 'rationality' and accuracy of the Galenic doctrine of humours and, in a way, to confirm it. True, as a product of deductive reasoning, humoral medicine was extremely logical and, in that sense, 'rational' – unlike the belief in inexplicable occult properties. However, the literate urbanites of the Islamic Middle Period, both the learned and the common man, did not evaluate medical knowledge in this way. The two approaches to healing represented equal constituents of the general standard of knowledge and system of ideas and there was no obvious reason to reject or discredit either of them – all the more so given that it was quite often simply impossible to distinguish what was an occult property and what was something else, and what theoretical category a given recipe was supposed to belong to:

> Anyone who is afflicted with vitiligo [otherwise an incurable skin condition] should take garlic and burn it until it turns into ash, then put it into bee's honey and spatter it on the white vitiligo patches; then they will go away, God willing.[85]

And even if a recommendation was ascribed to Hippocrates himself, it did not make the classification any easier:

> Anyone who entered the *hammam* after he had eaten his fill and then became semi-paralysed, should only blame himself . . . Anyone who had sexual intercourse with a menstruating woman and whose son contracted leprosy should only blame himself.[86]

In fact, the only clear means of identifying a formula as an example of Hippocratic-Galenic therapy was to check whether it included any terms specifically associated with the humoral doctrine. As is typical of medical manuals written in the Islamic Middle Period, the humoral terminology incorporated into al-Qurashī's eclectic collection is limited to a number of basic notions, such as the four humours, or bodily fluids – yellow bile (*ṣafrāʾ*), phlegm (*balgham*), blood (*dam*), and black bile (*sawdāʾ*); the qualities – coldness, hotness, moisture and dryness; and temperament – that is, manifestation of the dominating humour (*mazāj*). Like most of his

[85] Al-Qurashī, *Ghunyat al-labīb ḥaythu lā yūjad al-ṭabīb* (*An Abundance of Information for the Intelligent Man When the Doctor Is Not Around*), King Saʿūd MS 5980, f. 2b; Ghota MS 2014, f. 3a.

[86] Al-Qurashī, *Ghunyat al-labīb ḥaythu lā yūjad al-ṭabīb* (*An Abundance of Information for the Intelligent Man When the Doctor Is Not Around*), King Saʿūd MS 5980, f. 5b.

contemporaries, al-Qurashī likely accepted any means of healing and, like them – but unlike Ibn al-Akfānī – he did not apparently much care what label was put on a given formula or according to what criteria it was assigned. Characteristically, al-Qurashī freely puts Galenic ideas into the same category as magic and often insists on the pious, spiritual dimension of healing.

> Take two *mithqāls* of roasted garlic and mix it with half an *ūqiyyah* of bee's honey. If you lick it on an empty stomach it will get rid of the *phlegm* and kill stomach worms, God willing.[87]
>
> The dangerous aspects of garlic are that it produces headache, is bad for the brain, weakens the sight, disturbs *yellow bile*, and makes the breath stink.[88]
>
> If you fill your ear with green rue, it will push out both *hotness* and *coldness*, God willing.[89]
>
> Too much food and excessive eating changes one's *temperament* and produces silliness and blurred vision.[90]
>
> Black kohl[91] from Isfahan is the best . . . its nature is *cold* and *dry* and it is beneficial for the eyes, it makes them stronger, keeps them healthy, removes excessive redness.[92]

But even if one could recognise 'scholarly' terminology in a recipe, it would not necessarily mean he perceived the difference between the humoral and the magical. For an average man, the green rue that expels *hotness* and *coldness* when placed in someone's ear was probably no more comprehensible than the cure for bleeding that required the right lung of a wild donkey. Moreover, it must have mattered very little to a suffering patient whether a remedy which was supposed to bring him/her relief belonged to this or that theoretical category. In this respect, the tenets of the humoral doctrine were as good as the idea of activating the

87 Al-Qurashī, *Ghunyat al-labīb ḥaythu lā yūjad al-ṭabīb* (*An Abundance of Information for the Intelligent Man When the Doctor Is Not Around*), King Saʾūd MS 5980, f. 2b.

88 Al-Qurashī, *Ghunyat al-labīb ḥaythu lā yūjad al-ṭabīb* (*An Abundance of Information for the Intelligent Man When the Doctor Is Not Around*), King Saʾūd MS 5980, f. 3a.

89 Al-Qurashī, *Ghunyat al-labīb ḥaythu lā yūjad al-ṭabīb* (*An Abundance of Information for the Intelligent Man When the Doctor Is Not Around*), King Saʾūd MS 5980, f. 4a.

90 Al-Qurashī, *Ghunyat al-labīb ḥaythu lā yūjad al-ṭabīb* (*An Abundance of Information for the Intelligent Man When the Doctor Is Not Around*), Ms BN arabe 5718, f. 39a; Ghota MS 2014, f. 6a.

91 Made by grinding antimony trisulfide, kohl (*kuḥl*) has been used since antiquity as protection against eye ailments and an eye cosmetic in the Near and Middle East, North and West Africa, the Red Sea basin, and South Asia.

92 Al-Qurashī, *Ghunyat al-labīb ḥaythu lā yūjad al-ṭabīb* (*An Abundance of Information for the Intelligent Man When the Doctor Is Not Around*), King Saʾūd MS 5980, f. 7b.

occult therapeutic powers allegedly hidden in things and procedures according to some unknown key.[93]

Conclusion

Written by different authors, who intended their works for slightly different audiences, Ibn al-Akfānī's *Ghunyat al-labīb (I)* and al-Qurashī's *Ghunyat al-labīb (II)* diverge in a number of aspects. However, while each of these works constitutes a distinctive collection of multiple therapeutic approaches, curative ideas, practices, and cures of various origins, brought together in one narrative of healing, both represent one and the same medico-pharmaceutical culture of the Mediterranean. And, as such, both testify to its hybrid or pluralistic character. However, Ibn al-Akfānī's preoccupation with the Hippocratic-Galenic concept of health and his perception of occult-magical approach as a separate subcategory of medicine might incline us to think of medical pluralism as the coexistence of different medical systems. At the same time, al-Qurashī's spontaneous mixture of diverse healing ideas and curative approaches in an agglomeration of medical knowledge points to therapeutic eclecticism.

Different as the two manuals are, together they provide a new insight into the theoretical dimension of literate urbanites' health concerns. However, *Ghunyat al-labīb (II)* or, more properly, its author's presumably amateur medical status, may prove particularly valuable in this context. Non-professional as it was, al-Qurashī's manual shows that basic terminology pertaining to Hippocratic-Galenic thought, even if it was not always entirely understood, was commonly present in the medical discourse of ordinary literate people, and not only in the specialised language of physicians, scholars, or other well-educated persons. At the same time, by revealing which elements of humoral doctrine were circulating among fifteenth-century urbanites, al-Qurashī's text shows the place this doctrine held in literate people's thinking about medicaments and healing. Once the prevailing medical theory of the urban elites, over time Galenic medicine became more popular while, at the same time, having increasingly to give

[93] While insisting that all things were composed of the four elements, which embodied the qualities of hot, cold, dry, and wet, and which transformed in human bodies into four substances called humours, the doctrine implied a peculiar style of therapy. Based on the principle of allopathic contraries, or the conviction that a contrary drives away a contrary (*contraria contrariis curantur*), it involved treating a diagnosed disease with therapeutics whose alleged qualities were supposed to be contrary to the proclaimed qualities of this disease. Consequently, the doctrine promoted treatments which, according to the state of knowledge that we have today were absurd, except in accidental cases.

way to other kinds of medical knowledge and compete with an increasing number of elements coming from religious, magical, and folk approaches. Simplified and recombined, in the end it became no more than one component of a complex medico-pharmaceutical culture. The latter, reshaped by the transfer and assimilation of non-humoral medicaments and healing ideas, became a neo-Galenic hybrid. Judging by Ibn al-Akfānī's manual, however, in more demanding circles humoral theory could still enjoy the reputation of an indisputable axiom.

It is true that both *Ghunyat al-labīb (I)* and *Ghunyat al-labīb (II)* are theoretical, prescriptive texts and that, in analysing their content one cannot seek answers to the most intriguing questions – for example, what the most frequent health problems were of people living in the Egyptian and Syrian cities of the Mamluk period, and what they did or took in order to cure this or that ailment. Nevertheless, while comparing the two self-treatment manuals one can hardly refrain from asking how faithfully – if at all – these theoretical narratives reflect the daily experience of their authors and readers. One wonders what is more promising as far as the documentary value of such a text is concerned: is it the methodical accuracy, erudition, and expertise of Ibn al-Akfānī, who, working as a physician and a supply manager for the Cairene hospital, must have had quite good knowledge of the pharmacological market and, more particularly, of the medicinal substances used in the treatment of the hospital's patients? Or is it al-Qurashī's spontaneity which, seemingly untainted by medical education, may suggest his more down-to-earth perspective and, consequently, more authentic reflection of day-to-day household medical practice?

All we have, for the time being at least, are certain clues to the health problems from which Near Eastern urbanites may have suffered, the therapeutic options ordinary, literate people had, the medical substances which may have been available in the food and pharmaceutical markets, as well as practices which may have been used to restore health. However, in order to properly read the clues included in the two compendia, it is necessary to construct a broad, Mediterranean-wide contextualisation of their texts and to situate them in relation to other historical writings of the time. As this is a work in progress, the present chapter provides only preliminary remarks on the subject, which requires further investigation.

REFERENCES

ʿAbbās, Ṣ. M. ed. 1989. *Ibn al-Akfānī, Muḥammad Ibn Ibrāhīm, Ghunyat al-labīb ʿinda ghaybat al-ṭabīb*. Baghdad: Wizārat al-Taʾlīm al-ʿAlī wa-al-Baḥth al-ʾIlmī, Jāmiʾat Baghdād.

Abou-Aly, A. M. 1992. 'The Medical Writings of Rufus of Ephesus'. University College London: PhD thesis (http://discovery.ucl.ac.uk/1317541/1/246073.pdf, accessed 15 March 2020).

Āl Ṭaʾma, W. K. ed. 1996. *Ibn al-Jazzār, Ṭibb al-fuqarāʾ wa-l-masākīn*. Tehran: n.p.

Amarante dos Santos, D. O., and da Conceição Fagundes, M. D. 2010. 'Health and Dietetics in Medieval Preventive Medicine: The Health Regimen of Peter of Spain (Thirteenth Century)', *História, Ciências, Saúde-Manguinhos* 17.2: 333–42. (www.scielo.br, accessed 25 July 2018).

Arnāʾūṭ, A., and Muṣṭafà, T. eds. 1998, 2000. Al-Ṣafadī, Khalīl Ibn Aybak: *Al-Wāfī bi-l-wafayāt*, vols. XXIII, II. Beirut: Dār al-Iḥyāʾ al-Turāth al-ʿArabī.

Attewell, G. 2003. 'Islamic Medicines: Perspectives on the Greek Legacy in the History of Islamic Medical Traditions in West Asia', in H. Selin and H. Shapiro (eds.), *Medicine across Cultures: History and Practice of Medicine in Non-Western Cultures*. Dordrecht: Kluwer Academic, 325–50.

Bos, G. 1998. 'Ibn al-Jazzār on Medicine for the Poor and the Destitute', *Journal of the American Oriental Society* 118: 365–75.

Bouras-Vallianatos, P. 2014. 'Clinical Experience in Late Antiquity: Alexander of Tralles and the Therapy of Epilepsy', *Medical History* 58: 337–53.

Bouras-Vallianatos, P. 2016. 'Modelled on Archigenes *Theiotatos*: Alexander of Tralles and His Use of Natural Remedies (*Physika*)', *Mnemosyne* 69.3: 382–96.

Brévart, F. B. 2008. 'Between Medicine, Magic, and Religion: Wonder Drugs in German Medico-Pharmaceutical Treatises of the Thirteenth to the Sixteenth Centuries', *Speculum* 83.1: 1–57.

Conrad, L. 1995. 'The Arab-Islamic Medical Tradition', in L. Conrad, M. Neve, V. Nutton, R. Porter, and A. Wear (eds.), *The Western Medical Tradition 800 BC to AD 1800*. Cambridge: Cambridge University Press, 93–138.

Al-Ḍannāwī, M. A. ed. 1999. *Al-Rāzī, Abū Bakr Muḥammad Zakariyāʾ, Man lā yaḥduruhu al-ṭabīb*. Beirut: Dār al-Kutub al-ʿIlmiyya.

Daremberg, Ch. , and Ruelle, Ch.-É. eds. 1879. *Oeuvres de Rufus d'Ephèse: Texte collationné sur les manuscrits, traduit pour la première fois en français, avec une introduction*. Paris: Imprimerie nationale.

Dols, M. W. 1992. 'The Practice of Magic in Healing', in M. W. Dols (ed.), *Majnūn: The Madman in Medieval Islamic Society*. Oxford: Oxford University Press, 274–310.

Dols, M. W. 2004. 'The Theory of Magic in Healing', in E. Savage-Smith (ed.), *Magic and Divination in Early Islam*. Aldershot: Ashgate, 87–102.

Draycott, J. 2016. 'Literary and Documentary Evidence for Lay Medical Practice in the Roman Republic and Empire', in G. Petridou and C. Thumiger (eds.), *Homo Patiens: Approaches to the Patient in the Ancient World*. Brill: Leiden, 432–50.

Ferngren, G. B. 2016. *Medicine and Health Care in Early Christianity*. Baltimore, MD: Johns Hopkins University Press.

Fihris al-makhṭūṭāt al-ʿarabiyyah bi-Dār al-Kutub al-Miṣriyya. Al-Majāmiʾ, vol. III. 2011. Cairo.

Flügel, G. ed. 1871–2. *Kitâb al-Fihrist, mit Anmerkungen hrsg. von Gustav Flügel, nach dessen Tode besorgt von Johannes Roediger und August Mueller. Erster Band, den Text enthaltend, von Dr. Johannes Roediger*. 2 vols. Leipzig: F. C. W. Vogel.

Frazer, J. F. 1922. *The Golden Bough: A Study in Magic and Religion*. New York: Macmillan.

Green, R. M. trans. 1951. *A Translation of Galen's Hygiene (De Sanitate Tuenda)*. Springfield, IL: Charles C. Thomas.

Ideler, L. 1809. *Untersuchungen über den Ursprung und die Bedeutung der Sternnamen*. Berlin: J. F. Weiss.

Ismāʾīl, M. M. ed. 2000. *Al-Rāzī, Abū Bakr Muḥammad Zakariyāʾ, Al-Ḥāwī fī al-Ṭibb (Continens Liber)*, vol. II. Beirut: Dār al-Kutub al-ʿIlmiyya.

Levey, M. ed. 1967. 'Medical Ethics of Medieval Islam, with Special Reference to al-Ruhāwī's "Practical Ethics of the Physician"', *Transactions of the American Philosophical Society* 57.3: 1–100.

Lewicka, P. B. 2011. *Food and Foodways of Medieval Cairenes: Aspects of Life in an Islamic Metropolis of the Eastern Mediterranean*. Leiden: Brill.

Lewicka, P. B. 2014. 'Medicine for Muslims? Islamic Theologians, Non-Muslim Physicians, and the Medical Culture of the Mamluk Near East', in S. Conermann (ed.), *History and Society during the Mamluk Period (1250–1517)*. Bonn: Bonn University Press at V&R Unipress, 83–106; 2012. *ASK Working Paper 03*, Bonn (www.mamluk.uni-bonn.de/publications/working-paper/ask-working-paper-03-22.11.2012.pdf, accessed 17 September 2019).

Mihrānʾfar, M. trans. 2015. *Muḥammad Ibn Ibrāhīm Ibn Sāʿid al-Anṣārī maʿrūf bi-Ibn al-Akfānī, Tarjumah-ʾi kitāb-i Ghunyat al-labīb ʿinda ghaybat al-ṭabīb, yā, Tarfand darmānī-i khiradmand dar nabūd-i pizishk, tarjumah va taḥshīh-i Muḥammad Mihrānʾfar*. Tehran.

Nutton, V. 2008a. 'Healers in the Medical Market Place: Towards a Social History of Graeco-Roman Medicine', in A. Wear (ed.), *Medicine in Society: Historical Essays*. Cambridge: Cambridge University Press, 15–58.

Nutton, V. 2008b. 'Rufus of Ephesus in the Medical Context of His Time', in P. E. Pormann (ed.), *On Melancholy: Rufus of Ephesus*. Tubingen: Mohr Siebeck, 139–58.

Nutton, V. 2013. *Ancient Medicine*. 2nd ed. London: Routledge.

Perho, I. 1995. *Prophet's Medicine: A Creation of the Muslim Traditionalist Scholars*. Helsinki: Finnish Oriental Society.

Peters, F. E. 2004. 'Hermes and Harran: The Roots of Arabic-Islamic Occultism', in E. Savage-Smith (eds.), *Magic and Divination in Early Islam*. Aldershot: Ashgate, 55–86.

Pormann, P. E., and Savage-Smith, E. 2007. *Medieval Islamic Medicine.* Edinburgh: Edinburgh University Press.

Ramezany, F., Khademizadeh, M., and Kiyani, N. 2013. 'Persian Manna in the Past and the Present: An Overview', *American Journal of Pharmacological Sciences* 1.3: 35–7 (http://pubs.sciepub.com/ajps/1/3/1, accessed 16 September 2019).

Richardson, H. C. 1934. 'Iron, Prehistoric and Ancient', *American Journal of Archaeology* 38.4: 561.

Riḍā, N. ed. 1965. Ibn Abī Uṣaybiʿah: *ʿUyūn al-anbāʾ fī ṭabaqāt al-aṭibbāʾ*. Beirut: Dār Maktabat al-Ḥayāh.

Savage-Smith, E., Swain, S., and van Gelder, G. J. eds. 2020. *A Literary History of Medicine: The ʿUyūn al-anbāʾ fī ṭabaqāt al-aṭibbāʾ of Ibn Abī Uṣaybiʿah*. 5 vols. Leiden: Brill (https://scholarlyeditions.brill.com/reader/urn:cts:arabicLit:0668IbnAbiUsaibia.Tabaqatalatibba.lhom-ed-ara1:10.64; https://scholarlyeditions.brill.com/reader/urn:cts:arabicLit:0668IbnAbiUsaibia.Tabaqatalatibba.lhom-tr-eng1:10.64, accessed 21 January 2022).

Sezgin, F. 1996. *Geschichte des arabischen Schrifttums*, vol. III. Leiden: Brill.

Shāhīn, M. ed. 1289/1872. *Ash-Shaʿrānī, ʿAbd al-Wahhāb, Mukhtaṣar Tadhkirat al-Suwaydī fī al-ṭibb*. Cairo.

Silla, E. 1996. '"After Fish, Milk Do Not Wish": Recurring Ideas in a Global Culture', *Cahiers d'études africaines* 36.144: 613–24.

Sotres, P. G. 1998. 'The Regimens of Health', in M. D. Grmek (ed.), *Western Medical Thought from Antiquity to the Middle Ages*. Cambridge, MA: Harvard University Press, 291–318.

Totelin, L. 2011. 'Old Recipes, New Practice? The Latin Adaptations of the Hippocratic Gynaecological Treatises', *Social History of Medicine* 24.1: 74–91.

Totelin, L. 2015. 'When Foods Become Remedies in Ancient Greece: The Curious Case of Garlic and Other Substances', *Journal of Ethnopharmacology* 167: 30–7.

Ullmann, M. 1970. *Die Medizin im Islam*. Leiden: Brill.

Ullmann, M. 1978. *Islamic Medicine*. Edinburgh: Edinburgh University Press.

Ullmann, M. 1994. 'Die arabische Überlieferung der Schriften des Rufus von Ephesos', *ANRW* 2.37: 1293–1349.

Waines, D. 1995. 'Medicinal Nutriments As Home Remedies: A Case of Convergence between the Medieval Islamic Culinary and Medical Traditions', in M. C. Vázquez de Benito and M. Á. Manzano Rodríguez (eds.), *Actas XVI Congreso UEAI*. Salamanca: Agencia Española de Cooperación Internacional: Consejo Superior de Investigaciones Científica, 551–8.

Waines, D., and Marín, M. 2002. 'Muzawwar: Counterfeit Fare for Fasts and Fevers', in D. Waines (ed.), *Patterns of Everyday Life*. Aldershot: Ashgate, 303–16.

Wilkins, J. 2016. 'Treatment of the Man: Galen's Preventive Medicine in the *De Sanitate Tuenda*', in G. Petridou and C. Thumiger (eds.), *Approaches to the Patient in the Ancient World*. Leiden: Brill, 413–31.

CHAPTER 10

Digestive Syrups and After-Dinner Drinks
Food or Medicine?

Leigh Chipman

Dietetics formed an important part of regime and therapy in Galenic medicine, and indeed the rise of superfoods shows that the interest in foods as more than nourishment is still going strong.[1] Where does the line between food and medicine lie? Drawing this line, or studying where it has been drawn historically, has received increased attention in recent years, as shown not only by books but also by special issues devoted to the joint histories of food and medicine.[2] However, the emphasis in these works is usually on modern or early modern experiences in European or European-influenced cultures. Even when premodern societies are studied, the Islamicate world tends to remain the preserve of specialists and is only mentioned briefly in more general works. This is not to say that the interface between food and medicine in the Islamicate world has not been examined at all. Indeed, this chapter would not have been possible without the trailblazing writings of A. J. Arberry, David Waines, Manuela Marín, and, more recently, Nawal Nasrallah and Paulina Lewicka.[3] This chapter is an attempt to look at the topic of dietetics of the medieval Middle East through comparing two kinds of recipe collections: the cookbook and the pharmacopoeia. Their connection can be seen in the way David Waines ends his 1999 article 'Dietetics in Medieval Islamic Culture' by citing an Arabic saying: 'the stomach is the abode of disease, and abstaining from injurious foods is the principal part of medicine'.[4] In this chapter I will be looking mainly at the other end of the Mediterranean,

[1] For example, Etkin (2006); Chen (2009).
[2] Pennell and Rich (2016); Adelman and Haushofer (2018).
[3] Arberry (1939); Marín and Waines (1989, 1993); Waines (1999); Nasrallah (2007, 2018); Lewicka (2011).
[4] Waines (1999: 240). Waines calls this 'a popular Arabic saying of eleventh-century al-Andalus'; for the more common ascription to the Prophet or to al-Ḥārith ibn Kalādah, see, for example, Perho (1995: 101).

at Egypt in the Fatimid to Mamluk periods (eleventh to fifteenth centuries), examining the way certain kinds of foods were also understood as medicines, and the way this is expressed in a number of written genres.

In the medieval Islamicate world, foodstuffs and drugs were part of a continuum that ran from poisons through drugs through medicinal nutriments to foodstuffs, with occasional debates as to which side of the dividing line a particular simple might lie, as can be seen by the genre of books of *adwiyah wa-aghdhiyah*, drugs and nutriments. My focus, however, will rather be on compounds – both pharmaceutical and culinary. This is because most of what is ingested as food or medicine has more than one ingredient. Even the simplest syrup contains some form of plant together with a sweetener. What do these compounds have in common, and what differences are there? How and where is the line between food and medicine drawn? This chapter will begin by comparing recipes appearing in two books composed in Mamluk Cairo: *Minhāj al-dukkān* (*How to Run a Pharmacy*), a pharmacopoeia composed in 1260 by an otherwise unknown Jewish pharmacist,[5] and *Kanz al-fawāʾid fī tanwīʿ al-mawāʾid* (*Treasure Trove of Benefits and Variety at the Table*), an anonymous cookbook dated by the editors and translator to fourteenth-century Cairo.[6] It will then turn to another aspect of diet and medicine: the mostly vegetarian foods prescribed for invalids, comparing the instructions appearing on prescriptions from the Cairo Genizah to the recipes appearing in the relevant chapter of *Kanz al-fawāʾid*. Finally, I will look at an important forerunner of *Kanz al-fawāʾid*, the tenth-century Baghdadi cookbook *Kitāb al-ṭabīkh* (*Book of Dishes*), which explicitly states its dependence on medical sources in its subtitle.[7]

10.1 Digestive Syrups and Sweets in Mamluk Cairo

Even if culinary and medical compounds constitute a continuum, can we – or should we – differentiate between a pharmacopoeia and a cookbook? Both are collections of recipes for preparing compounds, and the topic of recipes and recipe collections has been the subject of great interest among scholars of European history for the past few years, especially among early

[5] Abū al-Mūnā Dawūd ibn Abī Naṣr al-Kūhīn al-ʿAṭṭār, *Minhāj al-dukkān* (*How to Run a Pharmacy*). See ed. al-ʿĀṣī (1997).

[6] See ed. Marín and Waines (1993) and trans. Nasrallah (2018). All English versions of recipes from *Kanz al-fawāʾid fī tanwīʿ al-mawāʾid* (*Treasure Trove of Benefits and Variety at the Table*) in this chapter are adapted from Nawal Nasrallah's amazing translation.

[7] Nasrallah (2007: 65).

modernists.[8] My own understanding of recipes owes a great deal to William Eamon's magisterial *Science and the Secrets of Nature: Books of Secrets in Medieval and Modern Cultures*.[9] Admittedly, neither *Minhāj al-dukkān* nor *Kanz al-fawāʾid* can be thought of as books of secrets in the European sense; perhaps the physicians' notebooks found in the Genizah can be considered as such.[10] However, recipes are recipes, whether written in Latin, English, or Arabic, and, according to Eamon,

> a recipe implies a contract between the reader and the text. It is a prescription for taking action ... no less significant are the differences between recipes and oral instructions, such as those an apprentice artisan learns. Unlike oral instructions, recipes exist independently of the teacher. Once they are recorded in a book, they become depersonalised and acquire a more general, universal quality.[11]

At the same time, though, recipes often assume practical knowledge, as anyone quickly finds out who has tried to make sense of the difference between soft and stiff peaks by looking at pictures rather than actually beating egg whites.

With this in mind, let us look at a particular class of foods/medicines: digestives, or perhaps *digestifs*, rather, since most of the recipes I looked at were for liquids rather than solids. As mentioned, I am comparing an anonymous fourteenth-century cookbook of Egyptian provenance and a thirteenth-century pharmacopoeia written in Cairo by a certain al-Kūhīn al-ʿAṭṭār. On one hand, we have chapter 11 of *Kanz al-fawāʾid*, whose title is *fī al-juwārishāt wa-al-maʿājin wa-al-ashribah* – in English, 'digestive stomachics, electuaries and drinks offered before and after the meal' – with a total of forty-four recipes. On the other hand, we have three chapters of *Minhāj al-dukkān* – chapter 2, *fī al-ashribah* 'on drinks/syrups'; chapter 5, *fī al-maʿājin* 'on electuaries'; and chapter 6, *fī al-juwārishāt* 'on stomachics' – with more than double the number of recipes in the chapter on syrups alone. The first stage of my comparison was to see how many of the recipes appeared under the same name in both books. Several of the syrups appeared both in *Kanz al-fawāʾid* and in *Minhāj al-dukkān*, but if they had no indications in the former, the same was true in the latter, making it rather difficult to judge them actually medicinal rather than merely soothing. None of the recipes called *maʿjūn* in *Kanz al-fawāʾid*

[8] See, for example, the Recipes Project: https://recipes.hypotheses.org, accessed 5 August 2019. For a discussion of the development of culinary recipes as a specific type of text in English, see Görlach (1992).

[9] Eamon (1994). [10] On such notebooks, see Lev (2013). [11] Eamon (1994: 131).

appear in *Minhāj al-dukkān* – and it is interesting, and perhaps significant, that none of the *Kanz* recipes have indications. Apart from their location in a chapter dealing with preserving or improving digestion, we do not know – from the text – that they have any medicinal function. This is often true of recipes throughout *Minhāj al-dukkān*, as well – while most recipes do state their purpose and provide indication, a large minority do not, especially in the chapters on syrups and robs.[12] This is of course highly frustrating to the researcher, who must guess at the use of the medicine from the combined properties of its ingredients.

As my interest is in the medicinal aspects of these recipes, my next step was to look at all the recipes in these chapters of *Kanz al-fawāʾid* that did have indications and try to identify their parallels in *Minhāj al-dukkān*. Very few of the *juwārishāt* in *Kanz al-fawāʾid* appear in *Minhāj al-dukkān* – yet they all have indications except for the digestive stomachic of aloeswood (*juwārish al-ʿūd*), for which there are several recipes in *Minhāj al-dukkān*, none identical to this one (see more on this later in this chapter). Systematic examination revealed several cases of almost identical recipes. For example, here are two recipes for types of *naql*, sweets intended to aid digestion during drinking parties. Recipe 370 in *Kanz al-fawāʾid* reads as follows:

> Recipe for lemon-flavoured hard candy drops, only good as food nibbled while imbibing alcoholic drinks.
>
> For each *raṭl* [i.e. pound] of sugar syrup, which you leave to boil until it thickens, use [the juice of] a medium-size lemon, neither big nor small. [When the syrup boils down to a thick syrup,] beat it with a *dakshāb* [i.e. wooden paddle-like stirring utensil] until it looks white and then pour it into moulds.[13]

The version appearing in *Minhāj al-dukkān* specifies that the moulds should be of wood, and adds another line: *wa-al-darbah fī ʿamal hādhā khuṣūṣan muʿayyanah dūn al-khabar* – 'and the dosage when making this by itself is a diamond-shaped lozenge without the report'.[14] The final phrase is meaningless in this context, and since we are talking about something intended to be eaten while drinking alcohol, I suggest that the final letter

[12] See the many cases of indications listed as 'none' in Chipman (2010: 185–270), Appendix 2.

[13] Anonymus, *Kanz al-fawāʾid fī tanwīʿ al-mawāʾid* (*Treasure Trove of Benefits and Variety at the Table*), 370, ed. Marín and Waines (1993) 138; and trans. Nasrallah (2018: 260). The additions in parentheses are taken from Nasrallah's glossary of technical terms. British spellings have replaced the American spellings used by Nasrallah throughout, and the transliteration has been made consistent with that used in this volume.

[14] See al-ʿĀṣī (1997: 19). All translations are my own unless otherwise stated.

may be a *zāʾ* whose dot has fallen rather than a *ray*, thus reading *dūn al-khubz*, 'without bread'. In other words, if you have no bread, eat a single piece of hard candy.

Another such recipe follows immediately as recipe 371 in *Kanz al-fawāʾid*, this time without any indication:

> Recipe for chewy tamarind candy.
>
> Take 1 *ūqīyyah* [i.e. ounce] tamarind, soak it in water and strain the liquid. Add to it 2 *ūqīyyahs* sugar and put it in a soapstone pot on a low fire, that is, on smouldering embers. Continue stirring it until it reaches the consistency of chewy candy; this is the brittle state. Store it in a marble bowl that has been greased with almond oil.[15]

In the version in *Minhāj al-dukkān*,[16] the practical portion of the recipe is identical, up to and including the explanation of a low fire as smouldering embers. However, al-Kūhīn al-ʿAṭṭār, the author of *Minhāj al-dukkān*, adds his source: the *qāḍī* Fatḥ al-Dīn – an Islamic judge whose name is unfortunately too common for him to be identified, but is suggestive of connections between the Jewish and the larger Muslim communities. Al-Kūhīn al-ʿAṭṭār ends the recipe with an evaluation: 'I made it several times and it came out well'. Such evaluations appear from time to time in *Minhāj al-dukkān*, and I think they are more meaningful than the laconic *mujarrab* – 'tried and tested' – that appears in pharmacological literature generally, since they are not quite as formulaic.[17] In most cases al-Kūhīn al-ʿAṭṭār cites a written source and the term *mujarrab* may be derived from there rather than his own experience.

While these recipes seem clearly to be for foods, at the beginning of chapter 11 of *Kanz al-fawāʾid* we have another recipe (numbered 349) for hard lemon drops, of which it is said 'these excite the appetite and strengthen digestion'.[18] Looking at these two recipes, they appear to be much the same – the main difference is that the second recipe has the sugar and lemon juice mixture dropped straight from a spoon, while the first one has an intermediate stage of beating and moulding. There seems to be no obvious reason why one should be merely a snack for eating with alcoholic drinks, while the other is stated specifically as strengthening digestion. And

[15] Anonymus, *Kanz al-fawāʾid fī tanwīʿ al-mawāʾid* (*Treasure Trove of Benefits and Variety at the Table*), 371, ed. Marín and Waines (1993) 138. Trans. by Nasrallah (2018: 260).

[16] Al-Kūhīn al-ʿAṭṭār, *Minhāj al-dukkān* (*How to Run a Pharmacy*), ed. al-ʿĀṣī (1997) 23.

[17] On efficacy statements, see also Doolittle (Chapter 2), Gottlieb (Chapter 6) and Lewicka (Chapter 9), in this volume.

[18] Anonymus, *Kanz al-fawāʾid fī tanwīʿ al-mawāʾid* (*Treasure Trove of Benefits and Variety at the Table*), 349, ed. Marín and Waines (1993) 123. Trans. by Nasrallah (2018: 251).

it is particularly fascinating that only the first recipe, the one with no explicit medical purpose, appears in *Minhāj al-dukkān*.

Yet another example of a recipe for a *naql* with no medical indications in which al-Kūhīn al-ʿAṭṭār provides his opinion[19] bears the title *sakanjabīn ʿaqīd* ('thick oxymel').[20] Al-Kūhīn al-ʿAṭṭār begins by giving the recipe used, as he says, in the market, for this oxymel: for each *raṭl* of sugar – one *ūqīyyah* of sugar and a lemon. Most use nothing more than this because otherwise the colour changes and the sugar burns. This recipe in fact reads very much like the ones for lemon drops – and includes no vinegar, which is almost compulsory in oxymel recipes. However, al-Kūhīn al-ʿAṭṭār himself has a different recipe, which he considers both easier and superior: for each *raṭl* of sugar, he uses four *ūqīyyahs* of wine vinegar (*khall khamr*). The combination is cooked on a soapstone pot over a low fire until it reaches the consistency of *ʿaqīd* (i.e. congeals). The result is spread on a marble slab oiled with almond oil and left to cool. 'This reaches the correct sourness', al-Kūhīn al-ʿAṭṭār declares, 'and neither its colour nor its taste changes'.[21] Compare recipe 348 in *Kanz al-fawāʾid*:

> Oxymel of chewy candy.
>
> This is the best *naql* to be had with alcoholic drinks for people whose humours are naturally prone to heat.
>
> It is made by boiling sugar syrup (*jullāb*) until it thickens, and then throwing in pure, clear very sour vinegar – for each *raṭl* [i.e. pound] of *jullāb* use 3 *ūqīyyahs* [i.e. ounces] vinegar. Continue boiling until it thickens to a brittle stage of consistency. Spread it on a marble slab after you oil its surface, and use [as needed].[22]

Based on other recipes for similar sweets in other chapters of *Kanz al-fawāʾid*, Nasrallah adds that the candy mass should be shaped into a disc and cut into triangles.[23] This recipe is more 'medical' than the previous two, with an actual reference to Galenic humoral theory – which is more than appears in *Minhāj al-dukkān*! What indeed is the difference between a cookbook and a pharmacopoeia on this occasion? Not very much, it would seem. The difference seems to be the context of each recipe, on the one hand, and the cumulative purpose of all the recipes in a collection, on

19 Al-Kūhīn al-ʿAṭṭār, *Minhāj al-dukkān* (*How to Run a Pharmacy*), ed. al-ʿĀṣī (1997) 22–3.

20 'Oxymel of chewy-candy' in Nasrallah's translation of a similar recipe in *Kanz al-fawāʾid fī tanwīʿ al-mawāʾid*; see later in this chapter.

21 Al-Kūhīn al-ʿAṭṭār, *Minhāj al-dukkān* (*How to Run a Pharmacy*), ed. al-ʿĀṣī (1997) 23.

22 Anonymus, *Kanz al-fawāʾid fī tanwīʿ al-mawāʾid* (*Treasure Trove of Benefits and Variety at the Table*), 348, ed. Marín and Waines (1993) 123. Trans. by Nasrallah (2018: 250–1).

23 Nasrallah (2018: 251, n. 5).

the other. The same recipe, when appearing in the midst of recipes that are clearly nutritional, is part of a cookbook (*Kanz al-fawāʾid*) yet forms part of a pharmacopoeia (*Minhāj al-dukkān*) when surrounded by recipes whose purpose is to heal, not to nourish.

I return now to the digestive stomachic of aloeswood I mentioned earlier, number 378 in *Kanz al-fawāʾid*. This reads as follows:

> Recipe for digestive stomachic of aloeswood.
>
> Take 2 *mithqāls* [i.e. 9 grams] rosebuds with their hypanthia removed. Also, take Indian spikenard, cloves, green cardamom, and nutmeg, 1 *mithqāl* [i.e. 4½ grams] of each; mastic gum, Indian aloeswood – 2 dirhams [i.e. 6 grams] of each. Also add black cardamom and ṭabāshīr – 1 *mithqāl* [i.e. 4½ grams] of each; as well as wild nard and Ceylon sandalwood – 1 dirham of each [i.e. 3 grams].
>
> Finely pound all of these spices and knead them with honey, which has been boiled and its froth skimmed; and sugar syrup, use an equal amount of each. Add enough [honey and sugar] to give the mix the consistency of *juwārish* [i.e. a thick and chewy texture]. Store it away, and [when needed] use ½ dirham [i.e. ¼ teaspoon] to 1 dirham of it.[24]

A very similar recipe appears in *Minhāj al-dukkān* and is stated there to be 'from Ibn al-Mudawwar',[25] a Karaite court physician of the last Fatimid and first Ayyubid rulers. According to the biobibliographer Ibn Abī Uṣaybiʿah, Ibn al-Mudawwar wrote books, but none appear to have survived.[26] The wording in this case is not identical, but it is certainly the same recipe, with the same ingredients and the same quantities prepared in the same manner. The only differences appear at the end: at the stage of adding honey and sugar, where *Kanz al-fawāʾid* has equal amounts of honey and sugar syrup, sufficient to give the mixture a thick and chewy consistency, *Minhāj al-dukkān* merely has the spices kneaded with three times their weight in sugar and honey. Interestingly, in this case it is the cookbook, rather than the pharmacopoeia, that provides a dosage. There are no indications in either place. Some of the recipes bearing the title *juwārish al-ʿūd* (aloeswood stomachic) in *Minhāj al-dukkān* are recommended as 'strengthening cold liver and stomach, good for palpitations and excessively cold temperaments, improving digestion and purging,

[24] Anonymus, *Kanz al-fawāʾid fī tanwīʿ al-mawāʾid* (*Treasure Trove of Benefits and Variety at the Table*), 378, ed. Marín and Waines (1993) 142. Trans. by Nasrallah (2018: 264).

[25] Al-Kūhīn al-ʿAṭṭār, *Minhāj al-dukkān* (*How to Run a Pharmacy*), ed. al-ʿĀṣī (1997) 85.

[26] Ibn Abī Uṣaybiʿah, *ʿUyūn al-anbāʾ fī ṭabaqāt al-aṭibbāʾ* (*Sources of Information on the Classes of Physicians*), ed. Riḍā (1965) 259–60; see also the recent edition by Savage-Smith, Swain, and van Gelder (2020).

reviving and strengthening for the old',[27] but others again bear no indications.[28] Clearly, the line between medicines and nutriments was very fine indeed.

10.2 Dietary Advice in Prescriptions

The preceding examples come from Cairo, one of the two places in the Mashriq (the Middle East, east of Libya) from which both cookbooks and pharmacopoeias have survived from the medieval period to the present day – the other being Baghdad.[29] It is interesting, and possibly of importance, that both cities were in their day major metropolises and cultural centres in many fields. From Paulina Lewicka's work, it is clear that the culinary tradition of Cairo differed from the earlier one of Baghdad, and from the later Ottoman tradition too[30] – it is not so clear whether this is true of pharmacopoeias as well, as to the best of my knowledge, such research has not yet been conducted. Nonetheless, there is another reason for choosing to examine Cairo's traditions: the existence of the documentary material of the famous Cairo Genizah, which provides a unique glimpse of actual practice in several spheres of life. One such sphere is medicine, which is illuminated by the surviving prescriptions, a selection of which were published a few years ago.[31] For the purposes of this chapter, what is important is the dietary advice that appears at the end of several prescriptions, recommending that the patient eat particular foods as well as – and sometimes together with – taking his or her medicine.

For example, T-S Ar. 30.305 is a prescription for an electuary containing endive, liquorice, berberry, and more. As is common in Genizah prescriptions, no indications appear – since the prescribing physician and the patient or his or her representative knew what was being treated – but the last lines are as follows: 'take with a dish of pullet [cooked] in sour grape-juice and pickled almonds'.[32] Another prescription, T-S AS 155.277, this time for a syrup whose ingredients indicate that it is likely to have been a purgative or a cough medicine, ends with the instructions: 'Diet: young meat with lemon and almond syrup and also pumpkin with lemon and sugar'.[33] Several prescriptions recommend chicken, spinach,

[27] Al-Kūhīn al-ʿAṭṭār, *Minhāj al-dukkān* (*How to Run a Pharmacy*), ed. al-ʿĀṣī (1997) 80.

[28] Al-Kūhīn al-ʿAṭṭār, *Minhāj al-dukkān* (*How to Run a Pharmacy*), ed. al-ʿĀṣī (1997) 81, 82, 85.

[29] Pharmacopoeias: Kahl (2003; 2007). Cookbooks: Arberry (1939), Nasrallah (2007).

[30] Lewicka (2011). [31] Lev and Chipman (2012). [32] Lev and Chipman (2012: 30).

[33] Lev and Chipman (2012: 86).

or both as an appropriate diet,[34] and T-S Ar. 41.72, a prescription for a purgative, requires a dish known as *zīrbāj* (a kind of stew; see further later in this chapter) as the patient's diet.[35]

These foods, especially the vegetarian ones, belong to a class known as *muzawwarāt*, literally 'fakes'. Apparently deriving at least partly from the Nestorian Christian custom of meatless fast days, such dishes replaced the meat of ordinary foods with vegetables, most usually pumpkins, onions, and taro.[36] As Lewicka puts it,

> such meatless dishes, while constituting a rightful part of the Arabic-Islamic medico-culinary tradition, never became a rightful part of the Arabic-Islamic cuisine. Considered a therapy for invalids, they were, in fact, nothing more than that. Nothing can probably reveal their position better than the Arabic term designating them, *muzawwarāt*. As *muzawwarāt*, or "counterfeit dishes", they only simulated or imitated those which contained meat.[37]

Not surprisingly, chapter 8 of *Kanz al-fawāʾid*, which is devoted to 'vegetarian dishes for the nourishment of the sick' (*fīmā yataghadhdhā bihi al-ʿalīl min muzawwarāt al-buqūl*),[38] includes recipes for all the foods mentioned in the Genizah prescriptions, and many more. Equally interestingly, in the same way that the directions appearing in the prescriptions are very similar but not identical to the recipes appearing in pharmacopoeias, the dietary advice there is not precisely the same as the recipes in *Kanz*. A recipe explicitly based on young chicken (no. 219)[39] – as well as a recipe for pumpkin (no. 214),[40] which suggests that young chicken can replace the gourd – cook it with pomegranate seeds and cassia (*dār ṣīnī*)[41] rather than sour grape juice and pickled almonds. The spinach-based dishes are slightly more detailed than the simple directive 'diet: spinach' appearing in the prescriptions. In one case (recipe no. 215), the spinach is simply boiled, drained, and then seasoned with sesame oil and coriander.[42] In the other (recipe no. 221), the seasoning is more elaborate: after boiling, the spinach is

[34] Lev and Chipman (2012: 60, 68). [35] Lev and Chipman (2012: 62).

[36] Marín and Waines (1993).

[37] Lewicka (2011: 262). See also Lewicka (Chapter 9) in this volume.

[38] Anonymus, *Kanz al-fawāʾid fī tanwīʿ al-mawāʾid* (*Treasure Trove of Benefits and Variety at the Table*), ch. 8, ed. Marín and Waines (1993) 81–9. Trans. by Nasrallah (2018: 184–92).

[39] Anonymus, *Kanz al-fawāʾid fī tanwīʿ al-mawāʾid* (*Treasure Trove of Benefits and Variety at the Table*), 219, ed. Marín and Waines (1993) 86. Trans. by Nasrallah (2018: 189).

[40] Anonymus, *Kanz al-fawāʾid fī tanwīʿ al-mawāʾid* (*Treasure Trove of Benefits and Variety at the Table*), 214, ed. Marín and Waines (1993) 85. Trans. by Nasrallah (2018: 188).

[41] This is Nasrallah's translation. For a discussion of the identification and uses of *Cinnamomum zeylanicum* and *Cinnamomum cassia*, see Lev and Amar (2008: 143–6).

[42] Anonymus, *Kanz al-fawāʾid fī tanwīʿ al-mawāʾid* (*Treasure Trove of Benefits and Variety at the Table*), 215, ed. Marín and Waines (1993) 85. Trans. by Nasrallah (2018: 189).

dressed with pomegranate juice, sugar, mastic, and cassia, rather like the chicken recipes.[43] As for *zīrbāj* (savoury stew), *Kanz al-fawāʾid* contains no fewer than ten recipes for this 'delicately sour golden stew' as Nasrallah calls it, three meatless versions in chapter 2, one with fish, and six with meat (of which four are made with chicken).[44] The recipes have certain elements in common, principally the use of saffron, which gives the stew its golden colour, and of vinegar, for sourness. Other recurrent ingredients are almonds (for thickening), sugar or sugar syrup, and a spice blend called *aṭrāf al-ṭīb*,[45] whose components would be ground separately, then mixed and stored. Of the three vegetarian recipes, one (no. 226) is said to be for people with excess yellow bile, the second has no indications, and the third, most elaborate recipe – the one most similar to the first 'ordinary' *zīrbāj* recipe – has a full explanation of its benefits:

> Its properties are almost perfectly balanced. It benefits people whose dominant humour is yellow bile, and those with inflamed livers and weak stomachs. It is also good for jaundice, blockages in the liver and spleen, and ascites.
>
> Take some onion, chop the amount you need, and throw it into a small pot placed on low fire. Add almond oil, sesame oil, or olive oil, depending on the temperament [of the person who will eat the dish].[46]

The first sentence, stating that this is a food that is almost perfectly balanced, explains just why *zīrbāj* is considered particularly appropriate for convalescents. As we see, not only medicines, but also foods, are meant to be individualised and adapted to the patient's temperament.

Almost all the recipes appearing in the *muzawwarāt* chapter have indications, which is not surprising, and even to be expected, assuming that such foods indeed functioned, as David Waines suggests, as home remedies as well as nourishment.[47] Additional recipes for food for invalids, or at least with medical benefits, appear scattered throughout *Kanz al-fawāʾid*. One is a savoury condiment meant to replace anchovies (no. 259), called *ṣaḥna kadhdhāba* or 'false fishpaste',[48] which appears in

[43] Anonymus, *Kanz al-fawāʾid fī tanwīʿ al-mawāʾid* (*Treasure Trove of Benefits and Variety at the Table*), 221, ed. Marín and Waines (1993) 87. Trans. by Nasrallah (2018: 190).

[44] Nasrallah (2018), index, *s.v.*

[45] According to Nasrallah (2018: 531), this was a mixture of spikenard, betel leaf, bay leaves, nutmeg, mace, green cardamom, cloves, rosebuds, fruit of Syrian ash tree (*lisān al-ʿuṣfur*), long pepper, ginger, and black pepper.

[46] Anonymus, *Kanz al-fawāʾid fī tanwīʿ al-mawāʾid* (*Treasure Trove of Benefits and Variety at the Table*), 226, ed. Marín and Waines (1993) 88. Trans. by Nasrallah (2018: 191).

[47] Waines (1999: 238–9).

[48] Anonymus, *Kanz al-fawāʾid fī tanwīʿ al-mawāʾid* (*Treasure Trove of Benefits and Variety at the Table*), 259, ed. Marín and Waines (1993) 101. Trans. by Nasrallah (2018: 206–7).

the chapter containing 'all kinds of dishes made with different varieties of fish'. This mixture of sumac, parsley, mint, and rue with toasted walnut paste and tahini, flavoured with garlic and zaʾtar, is said to be 'beneficial for people whose dominant humour is yellow bile. It refreshes the stomach'. Several more appear in the chapter on sweet dishes, such as a 'thick gourd pudding' (*qarʿīya*, no. 314), said to be good for 'moistening dry humoral properties and for breaking up dense humours',[49] and a 'confection made with melon' (*ḥalāwat biṭṭīkh ʿAbdulī*, no. 336), of which it is said, 'This is truly delicious, and it is beneficial for sicknesses related to black bile disorders.'[50]

Perhaps the medical advice that seems most unlikely to our modern ears is that appearing in a recipe for 'thick jujube pudding' (*khabīs al-ʿunnāb*, no. 288):

> This is recommended for weight gain. Its properties are moderately hot and high in moisture. It nourishes the thin and the weak, provides the bodily system with the needed moisture. It induces euphoria, lightens the skin colour, softens the complexion and gives it lustre. It strengthens a hot stomach, and helps soften the bowels, and deflates winds. It is diuretic, and beneficial to the kidneys and bladder. It helps women gain weight quickly, which is something they care a lot about. It also helps reduce the density of their humours. However, it is harmful for phlegmatics and the old [who suffer from excessive cold and wet humours].[51]

This amazing dessert contains kernels of the seeds of a range of cucurbits, pistachios, hazelnuts, almonds, poppy-seeds, and purslane seeds, to mention only the first part of a long list of ingredients that are each pounded and sifted separately, then mixed with half their total weight of toasted white breadcrumbs. The same quantity of jujubes and of white sugar are boiled together with five times the amount of water, and the froth is removed. Then the spice-breadcrumb mixture is added, together with sufficient fat – almond oil, sesame oil, or ghee from cow milk – to combine everything. This is all cooked together until thickened, then removed from the fire.

To sum up, it is not surprising that the recipes for *muzawwarāt* in *Kanz al-fawāʾid* are more detailed than the dietary recommendations appearing

[49] Anonymus, *Kanz al-fawāʾid fī tanwīʿ al-mawāʾid* (*Treasure Trove of Benefits and Variety at the Table*), 314, ed. Marín and Waines (1993) 119. Trans. by Nasrallah (2018: 235).

[50] Anonymus, *Kanz al-fawāʾid fī tanwīʿ al-mawāʾid* (*Treasure Trove of Benefits and Variety at the Table*), 336, ed. Marín and Waines (1993) 127–8. Trans. by Nasrallah (2018: 244–5).

[51] Anonymus, *Kanz al-fawāʾid fī tanwīʿ al-mawāʾid* (*Treasure Trove of Benefits and Variety at the Table*), 288, ed. Marín and Waines (1993) 110–11. Trans. by Nasrallah (2018: 222–3).

in the Genizah prescriptions. It might even be said that this is only to be expected, given the different genres. The fact that the same ingredients and even the same names of dishes appear in both is not, however, something that should necessarily be taken for granted. This is particularly so in light of the range of recipes with medicinal value found in *Kanz al-fawāʾid*, which is much more extensive than that of the prescriptions.

10.3 A Baghdadi Cookbook

The discrepancies between *Kanz al-fawāʾid* and *Minhāj al-dukkān* are surprising; I expected more of an overlap there, with the same recipes appearing in both, especially those from *Kanz al-fawāʾid* with indications. My conclusion at this point was that additional sources are necessary since we do not know exactly where all the recipes in *Kanz al-fawāʾid* come from. Further comparisons with earlier cookbooks and pharmacopoeias – from both Cairo and Baghdad – would no doubt be enlightening. And indeed, comparison with the Baghdadi tradition in pharmacy as exemplified by the pharmacopoeias of Sābūr ibn Sahl and Ibn al-Tilmīdh revealed that these works, major sources of *Minhāj al-dukkān*, have almost no overlap with *Kanz al-fawāʾid*. The only exceptions appear to be recipes for a digestive stomachics of quince (*juwārish al-safarjal*) and of cumin (*juwārish al-kammūn*), versions of which appear in Sābūr ibn Sahl's *al-Aqrābādhīn al-ṣaghīr* (*Small Dispensatory*). Even here, the similarities are in the indications and method and the ingredients are not identical. For example, the quince stomachic (recipe no. 242) is 'useful against abdominal disorder, gastric debility, vomiting, poor digestion and it embellishes the complexion', according to Sābūr ibn Sahl,[52] and it is 'temperate in properties, it fortifies the stomach, stimulates the appetite, strengthens the nerves, and aids good digestion. It enhances the complexion, and curbs bowel movements', according to *Kanz al-fawāʾid* (recipe no. 374).[53] Both recipes call for peeling quinces and cooking them in wine or grape juice until the liquid evaporates, adding an equal quantity of honey and cooking that together, then sprinkling the quince-honey mixture with various spices (the list differs between the two recipes) and beating all together until completely absorbed. The final stage has the mixture rolled out onto a marble slab (possibly oiled), then cut into pieces, wrapped in citron

[52] Sābūr ibn Sahl, *al-Aqrābādhīn al-ṣaghīr* (*Small Dispensatory*), 242, trans. Kahl (2003: 125–6).

[53] Anonymus, *Kanz al-fawāʾid fī tanwīʿ al-mawāʾid* (*Treasure Trove of Benefits and Variety at the Table*), 374, ed. Marín and Waines (1993) 139–40. Trans. by Nasrallah (2018: 261).

leaves and stored in jars. Throughout, Sābūr ibn Sahl gives more precise quantities, recommends alternative ingredients, and his instructions are more detailed – very much what I was expecting from a pharmacopoeia as compared to a cookbook.

On the other hand, as noted, the famous tenth-century Baghdadi cookbook, *Kitāb al-ṭabīkh*, has as its subtitle 'Preparing salubrious foods and delectable dishes extracted from medical books and told by proficient cooks and the wise'.[54] Entire chapters are devoted to the humoral theory and the appropriate foods for each human temperament, as well as to the humoral properties of various foods. In fact, of the 131 chapters of the book, chapters 6–20, 22, 24–30, 125–9, and 131 deal with health-related aspects of food. This is different not only from *Kanz al-fawāʾid*, but also from *Minhāj al-dukkān*, neither of which include a theoretical discussion of the humours and their influence on human well-being.[55] However, it does help explain why recipes for *naql* might be found in both books and even include more medical information in the cookbook versions.

Should we therefore expect to find parallels to *Kitāb al-ṭabīkh* in pharmacopoeias? In her magisterial translations, Nawal Nasrallah has looked for Ibn Sayyār al-Warrāq's source material, as well as that of *Kanz al-fawāʾid*, and found that many of them are medical men, particularly Abū Bakr al-Rāzī's *Kitāb al-manṣūrī fī al-ṭibb* (*Book on Medicine for al-Manṣūr*), the short book on food for monks and invalids by Ibn ʿAbdūn (i.e. the physician Ibn Buṭlān), and works by Yuḥannā Ibn Māsawayh and Isḥāq ibn Yaʿqūb al-Kīndī.[56] Comparing *Kitāb al-ṭabīkh* to *Minhāj al-dukkān* and the later Baghdadi pharmacopoeias revealed syrups (*ashribah*) and stomachics (*juwārishāt*) with the same name, but these were never the same recipe. Since all three authors of pharmacopoeias are relatively punctilious about citing their sources, this was not a surprise. I am not sure what to make of the fact that no recipe named a *maʿjūn* appears in the explicitly medical chapters of *Kitāb al-ṭabīkh*, although they are mentioned in passing in the introduction.[57]

Finally, Nawal Nasrallah, the translator of both cookbooks, conducted an extensive comparison between the two, pointing out individual recipes and entire chapters that were more or less identical.[58] However, the connection between the two books remains uncertain: it is perhaps more likely that both borrowed from the same sources than *Kanz al-fawāʾid* borrowed from *Kitāb al-ṭabīkh*. In the case of *muzawwarāt*, of the six

[54] Nasrallah (2007: 65). [55] See Chipman (2010: 18).
[56] Nasrallah (2007: 15–22; 2018: 13–19). [57] Nasrallah (2007: 68). [58] Nasrallah (2018: 15–16).

recipes that appear in both books, the first – a *muzawwarah* for people with fevers – is explicitly noted as coming from Ibn Māsawayh and the chapter's title and contents clearly derive from him. As Nasrallah says: 'the picture we get is rather that of works drawing on common culinary sources and independently concocted'.[59] And my suggestion, in an earlier work, that *Kanz al-fawā'id* quotes *Minhāj al-dukkān* rather than vice versa,[60] would appear to be reinforced by the fact that *Kitāb al-ṭabīkh* quotes medical books and authors, but its own recipes are not cited in Baghdadi pharmacopoeias. This may be because unlike *Minhāj al-dukkān*, written by and for the community pharmacist, Sābūr ibn Sahl and Ibn al-Tilmīdh were physicians writing for hospital pharmacists – where diet was the business of a different functionary,[61] a cook likewise receiving instructions from a physician.

Conclusion

Minhāj al-dukkān and *Kanz al-fawā'id* come from more or less the same medical/culinary environment. My working hypothesis was that *Minhāj al-dukkān*, as a pharmacopoeia, would contain more medical information than *Kanz al-fawā'id*, but at the same time, that those recipes in *Kanz al-fawā'id* that contained such information would be likely to appear in *Minhāj al-dukkan*. This proved, with a few exceptions, not to be the case. In contrast, comparison between *Kanz al-fawā'id* and dietary advice in prescriptions revealed many parallels and similarities in the food recommended for invalids – exactly what I had indeed hoped to find. Comparison with the earlier Baghdadi tradition revealed the cookbook studied to be far more medically inclined than *Kanz al-fawā'id*, but parallels there are largely from books written by physicians on the harms and benefits of various foods, and not to books calling themselves pharmacopoeias (Ar.: *aqrābādhīn*). Later pharmacopoeias from Baghdad had almost no parallels to *Kitāb al-ṭabīkh*.

In another premodern medical tradition, that of China, we find certain similarities in practice to the medieval Arabic one. This is a case of convergence rather than influence, as far as I know: Ignoring developments of the Yuan and post-Mongol periods (mid-thirteenth century and onwards), when we might expect and indeed do find parallels between

[59] Nasrallah (2018: 18). [60] Chipman (2010: 105).

[61] Cf. the discussion of hospital functionaries and functions in Chipman (2010: 135–42) and Ragab (2015: 176–222). On Sābūr ibn Sahl's and Ibn al-Tilmīdh's dispensatories, see Käs (Chapter 1) in the present volume.

Islamicate and Chinese pharmacy, already in the Tang period (618–907 CE) and more prominently in the Song (960–1279 CE), a range of years within which almost all the Arabic material mentioned in this chapter was composed, we find interest in food as medicine in the Chinese tradition. A fairly recent article on this topic sums it up: 'The overlap between drugs and foods in Chinese medicine is epitomized by the category of dual-purpose substances. But this does not mean that drugs and foods can ever be entirely equivalent, or that there is no need to distinguish between them.'[62]

The same things might be said of the Islamicate world, for the overlap between food and medicine in Chinese medicine operates in many similar ways to those found in Islamicate medicine. While diet as such was an important element of the preservation or restoration of health in the Islamicate world, many pharmaceutical ingredients were also used – and indeed, today may be far more familiar – as culinary ones. Pepper, ginger, and cinnamon probably head this list. While I would not go so far as to say that the line between pharmaceutical recipes and culinary ones was in fact be so fine as to be non-existent, I argue that, in very many cases, it was invisible.

REFERENCES

Adelman, J., and Haushofer, A. 2018. 'Introduction: Food As Medicine, Medicine As Food', *Journal of the History of Medicine and Allied Sciences* 73.2: 127–34.

Arberry, A. J. trans. 1939. 'A Baghdad Cookery Book', *Islamic Culture* 13: 21–47, 189–214.

al-ʿĀṣī, Ḥ. ed. 1992. al-Kūhīn al-ʿAṭṭār, Abū al-Munā Dāwud ibn Abī Naṣr al-Isrāʾīlī: *Minhāj al-dukkān wa-dustūr al-aʿyān fi aʿmāl wa-tarākīb al-adwiyah al-nāfiʿah lil-abdān*. Beirut: Dār al-Manāhil.

Chen, N. 2009. *Food, Medicine, and the Quest for Good Health: Nutrition, Medicine, and Culture*. New York: Columbia University Press.

Chipman, L. 2010. *The World of Pharmacy and Pharmacists in Mamlūk Cairo*. Leiden: Brill.

Eamon, W. 1994. *Science and the Secrets of Nature: Books of Secrets in Medieval and Early Modern Culture*. Princeton, NJ: Princeton University Press.

Etkin, N. 2006. *Edible Medicines: An Ethnopharmacology of Food*. Tucson: University of Arizona Press.

Görlach, M. 1992. 'Text Types and Language History: The Cookery Recipe', in M. Rissanen, O. Ihalainen, T. Nevalainen, and I. Taavitsainen (eds.), *History of Englishes: New Methods and Interpretations in Historical Linguistics*. Berlin: De Gruyter, 736–61.

62 Zheng (2006: 55).

Kahl, O. trans. 2003. *Sābūr ibn Sahl: The Small Dispensatory. Translated from the Arabic together with a Study and Glossaries*. Leiden: Brill.

Kahl, O. ed. 2007. *The Dispensatory of Ibn at-Tilmīḏ: Arabic Text, English Translation, Study and Glossaries*. Leiden: Brill.

Lev, E. 2013. 'Mediators between Theoretical and Practical Medieval Knowledge: Medical Notebooks from the Cairo Genizah and Their Significance', *Medical History* 57.4: 487–515.

Lev, E., and Amar, Z. 2008. *Practical* Materia Medica *of the Eastern Mediterranean According to the Cairo Genizah*. Leiden: Brill.

Lev, E., and Chipman, L. 2012. *Medical Prescriptions in the Cambridge Genizah Collections: Practical Medicine and Pharmacology in Medieval Egypt*. Leiden: Brill.

Lewicka, P. 2011. *Food and Foodways of Medieval Cairenes: Aspects of Life in an Islamic Metropolis of the Eastern Mediterranean*. Leiden: Brill.

Marín, M., and Waines, D. 1989. 'The Balanced Way: Food for Pleasure and Health in Medieval Islam', *Manuscripts of the Middle East* 4: 123–32.

Marín, M., and Waines, D. eds. 1993. *Kanz al-fawāʾid fī tanwīʿ al-mawāʾid*. Beirut: Franz Steiner.

Nasrallah, N. trans. 2007. *Annals of the Caliphs' Kitchens: Ibn Sayyār al-Warrāq's Tenth-Century Baghdadi Cookbook*. Leiden: Brill.

Nasrallah, N. trans. 2018. *Treasure Trove of Benefits and Variety at the Table: A Fourteenth-Century Egyptian Cookbook*. Leiden: Brill.

Pennell, S., and Rich, R. 2016. 'Food, Feast and Famine', *Virtual Issue: Social History of Medicine*. June. https://academic.oup.com/shm/pages/virtual_issue_, accessed 15 March 2020.

Perho, I. 1995. *Prophetic Medicine: A Creation of the Muslim Traditionalist Scholars*. Helsinki: Finnish Oriental Society.

Ragab, A. 2015. *The Medieval Islamic Hospital: Medicine, Religion and Charity*. Cambridge: Cambridge University Press.

Riḍā, N. ed. 1965. Ibn Abī Uṣaybiʿah: *ʿUyūn al-anbāʾ fī ṭabaqāt al-aṭibbāʾ*. Beirut: Dār Maktabat al-Ḥayāh.

Savage-Smith, E., Swain, S., and van Gelder, G. J. eds. 2020. *A Literary History of Medicine: The ʿUyūn al-anbāʾ fī ṭabaqāt al-aṭibbāʾ of Ibn Abī Uṣaybiʿah*. 5 vols. Leiden: Brill. https://scholarlyeditions.brill.com/reader/urn:cts:arabicLit:0668IbnAbiUsaibia.Tabaqatalatibba.lhom-ed-ara1:10.64; https://scholarlyeditions.brill.com/reader/urn:cts:arabicLit:0668IbnAbiUsaibia.Tabaqatalatibba.lhom-tr-eng1:10.64 (accessed 21 January 2022).

Waines, D. 1999. 'Dietetics in Medieval Islamic Culture', *Medical History* 43: 228–40.

Zheng, J. [Barrett, P. trans.]. 2006. 'The Vogue for "Medicine As Food" in the Song Period (960–1279 CE)', *Asian Medicine* 2.1: 38–58.

CHAPTER 11

Late Byzantine Alchemical Recipe Books
Metallurgy, Pharmacology, and Cuisine

Matteo Martelli

11.1 Introduction: Alchemy and the Circulation of Recipes in Byzantium

Like shifting atoms of knowledge, recipes have been disseminated in a variety of alchemical treatises of different genres (e.g. technical essays, commentaries, dialogues) or simply piled into collections of variable length, as either lists or more structured compilations. Byzantine alchemical anthologies are the main sources for these types of text, which share similarities with recipes pertaining to contiguous areas of expertise. Indeed, comparable sets of ingredients, tools, and operations appear in procedural texts that describe how to prepare a medicine, how to make a dyeing *pharmakon*, and, as we shall see, how to cook a cake. Moreover, a similar tension between tradition and innovation is detectable in both the medical and the alchemical traditions. Byzantine compendia of remedies include recipes ascribed to a wide array of authorities, from famous Graeco-Roman physicians, such as Archigenes and Galen, to Christian saints. Likewise, alchemical anthologies collect Graeco-Egyptian recipes along with later compilations.[1] The vernacular vocabulary of these compilations, which also include Arabic and Latin loanwords as the result of cross-cultural influences, did not prevent their compilers from relying on the authority of ancient and mythical authors, such as Isis or Cleopatra (see Section 11.2).

This publication is part of the research project *Alchemy in the Making: From Ancient Babylonia via Graeco-Roman Egypt into the Byzantine, Syriac, and Arabic Traditions*, acronym *AlchemEast*. The *AlchemEast* project has received funding from the European Research Council (ERC) under the European Union's Horizon 2020 research and innovation programme (G.A. 724914). I warmly thank Petros Bouras-Vallianatos for his invaluable help and precious suggestions. All translations are my own unless otherwise stated.

[1] For Aetios' *Medical Books*, for instance, see Ejik, Geller, Lehmhaus, Martelli, and Salazar (2015: 198–204).

Moreover, the lines of transmission of medical and alchemical recipes overlap at times. Medical manuscripts can also include technical recipes: for instance, MS Angelicus gr. 17 (fourteenth–fifteenth century), which transmits medical treatises by both ancient (Hippocrates and Galen) and Byzantine authors (e.g. Oribasios, Paul of Aegina, and John the Physician), also features recipes on the making of golden inks and purple dyes.[2] Conversely, alchemical manuscripts can incorporate medical prescriptions, as we shall see by analysing MS Vaticanus gr. 1174 (see 11.3).

Technical recipes are included in the earliest manuscript on alchemy that has come down to us: MS Marcianus gr. 299 (tenth–eleventh century). Kept at the Marciana National Library in Venice, where it belonged to the personal collection of Cardinal Bessarion (1403–72), this manuscript transmits a rich collection of Graeco-Egyptian, late antique, and early-middle Byzantine alchemical works, often in epitomised forms, which testifies to a 1,000-year-old written tradition.[3] Along with the works attributed to the founders of alchemy, such as Pseudo-Democritus (first century AD) or Zosimus of Panopolis (third–fourth century), and the writings of more recent authors, such as Stephanos of Alexandria (seventh century) and the so-called philosopher Anepigraphos (eighth–ninth century),[4] the Marcianus manuscript also includes clusters of recipes, often grouped according to their technical topics. One finds formulas transmitted under the names of mythical figures (e.g. Moses or Agathodaimon) as well as anonymous recipes that can be tentatively dated only on the basis of internal elements, such as linguistic marks, loanwords, and scanty historical references. A few Arabic names of ingredients, for instance, occur in two recipes on how to dye copper and quench iron (f. 108r–v):[5] these loanwords have been read as evidence of an early influence of Arabic on Byzantine alchemical texts prior to the tenth century.[6] At f. 106 r, a group of three recipes deals with the making of silver:[7] the first describes how to whiten lead by treating the melted metal with a substance called

[2] Technical recipes edited in Schreiner and Oltrogge (2011: 51–2, 55, 57, 61–2, 64, 73); see also *CMAG* II.209. On the medical section see Sonderkamp (1987: 197–8) and Zipser (2009: 26–7).

[3] The manuscript has been described in *CMAG* II.1–22 and Mioni (1981: 427–33); see also Mertens (1995: XXII–XXIX), Saffrey (1995), and, more recently, Roberts (2020), who emphasises the role of MS Marcianus as an important source for middle Byzantine intellectual history.

[4] For an introduction to Graeco-Egyptian and early Byzantine alchemical authors see Letrouit (1995), Merianos (2017), Viano (2018), and Martelli (2019a: 45–118).

[5] See ed. Berthelot and Ruelle (1887–8) II.346.10–11, which mentions a 'red pastille' ('φοινοκοπάστιλλος') called *natēph* ('νατήφ') by the Arabs; II.347.10–11, that mentions the date palm ('φοινικοβάλανος'), called *elileg* ('ἐλιλέγ'; also spelled 'βελιλέγ') in Arabic.

[6] See Mavroudi (2002: 400–3); Roberts (2022: 568–70).

[7] See ed. Berthelot and Ruelle (1887–8) II.36.19–37.16.

'Cleopatra's glass' (*hyelos kleopatrinon*), an otherwise unknown ingredient whose name points to the famous Egyptian queen (see later in this chapter); the second recipe explains how to dye tin with bitumen and salt in order to make silver and use it in the church (*eis ergon ekklēsias*); the last one, which only specifies how much lead is necessary to produce ten librae of silver, is said to have been inscribed 'on the upper column' (*eis anōteran stēlēn*), in lines with the late Hellenistic *topos* of alchemical formulas hidden in Egyptian temples.[8] Different historical layers seem to be detectable in these recipes, even though it is difficult to interpret them in isolation, detached from the fluid textual tradition that hands down these types of texts. A recipe might have been copied countless times over centuries: single elements could be easily inserted or left aside in the course of their transmission, and their language could be easily readjusted or updated in terms of grammar, syntax, or technical nomenclature.

Moreover, recipes were often collected and organised in different compendia, which could include texts coming from a variety of earlier sources. The number of these compendia dramatically increase in manuscripts dating between the thirteenth century and the fifteenth. For instance, MSS Parisini gr. 2325 (thirteenth century) and 2327 (copied in Crete by Theodoros Pelekanos in 1478) systematically expand the collection of alchemical writings already included in the Marcianus gr. 299, by adding a great variety of 'new' technical texts. We find recipes on how to make artificial gemstones and pearls, which feature various references to the Arabs along with Arabic loanwords.[9] The description of a complex procedure to produce a round pearl (*chalaza*)[10] is explicitly attributed to the 'famous Arab Salmanas', tentatively identified with Sālim al-Ḥarrānī, credited with alchemical works in Arabic sources.[11]

[8] See, for example, Pseudo-Democritus, *On Natural Secrets* (*Physika kai mystika*), 3, in ed. Martelli (2013) 82–5; Zosimus, *Final Account*, 5, in ed. Berthelot and Ruelle (1887–8) II.242–3. Festugière (1950: 275–81, 362–8) published a more reliable edition and translation of Zosimus' text and also discussed (1950: 319–24) late Hellenistic accounts on the discovery of hidden books.

[9] See the recipe book *Deep Tincture of Stones, Emeralds, Rubies and Jacinths from the Bool Taken from the Sancta Sanctorum of Temples*, in ed. Berthelot and Ruelle (1887–8) II.350–64 and the various recipes on the making of pearls in ed. Berthelot and Ruelle (1887–8) II.364–71. The earliest witness of these collections is MS Parisinus gr. 2325 (ff. 152r–173v).

[10] On this particular meaning of the term *chalaza* ('χάλαζα', 'hailstone, pebble') see Du Cange (1688: II.1724–5).

[11] Greek text in Berthelot and Ruelle (1887–8) II.364–7; see Kraus (1942: 39, n. 3) and Roberts (2022: 570–1). Kraus (1933: 11) identified our alchemist with Salm, director of the 'House of Wisdom' (*ṣāḥib bayt al-ḥikma*) under the Abbasid caliph al-Maʾmūn, who would have translated Aristotle's books into Arabic. Ullmann (1972: 216–17), however, has questioned this hypothesis.

Metallurgy is certainly the most prominent field of expertise that emerges from the recipes included in alchemical manuscripts. In fact, metallurgical procedures – that is, a great variety of techniques aiming at dyeing metals and producing alloys that look like gold and silver – are described in voluminous compendia, such as the anonymous collection entitled *With God's Help, Explanation of the Most Noble and Illustrious Art of Goldsmiths*, which is preserved in two slightly different versions by MS Parisinus gr. 2327 (ff. 280r–289v) and MS 97 of the Saint Stephen's Monastery at Meteora (ff. 180v–202v).[12] Other collections are attributed to specific authors: the enigmatic figure of Cosmas the *hieromonachos* (lit. 'priestmonk') is credited with a collection of recipes *On Chrysopoiia* (i.e. the making of gold), which includes formulas said to have been copied from the works of the ancients (in particular Zosimus of Panopolis) along with four recipes tacitly taken from Psellos' *Letter on the Making of Gold* (on Psellos see later in this chapter);[13] the philosopher and physician Nikephoros Blemmydes (1197–1272) is presented as the author of a short recipe book entitled *On Egg-chrysopoiia* (*ōochrysopoiia*, i.e. making of gold through egg-based dyeing drugs) that focuses on the distillation of eggs.[14]

The earliest witness of Blemmydes' alchemical work is MS Parisinus gr. 2509 (ff. 137r–140v; fifteenth century), which mainly hands down astrological works.[15] As already pointed out, collections of alchemical recipes, in fact, are also included in multi-text manuscripts that combine writings pertaining to different fields. Particularly rich in this respect are MSS Parisinus gr. 2419 and Holkhamicus gr. 109, both dating to the fifteenth century, which combine medical, astrological, and magical texts with two collections of alchemical recipes that partially overlap.[16] These collections are all the more interesting since they feature recipes that depend on Latin

[12] Greek text edited in Berthelot and Ruelle (1887–8) II.321–37. On the two versions of this recipe book see Martelli (2018: 109–17).

[13] The title reads: 'ἑρμηνεία τῆς ἐπιστήμης τῆς χρυσοποιίας ἱερομονάχου τοῦ Κοσμᾶ' ('Explanation of the science of the making of gold, by the *hieromonachos* Cosmas'), ed. Colinet (2010) 66–76.

[14] Text edited in Steiner (2022) 436–41. Blemmydes is also credited with a collection of alchemical excerpts attributed to Hermes, Democritus, Aristotle, and Cleopatra. However, only the title of this work is transmitted by MS Atheniensis EBE 1070, f. 224r (thirteenth–fourteenth century; see *CMAG* V.149): 'τοῦ σοφωτάτου καὶ πολυμαθεστά[του] Βλιμμίδ[ου] παρεκβο[λαὶ] ἐκ τῶν Ἑρμοῦ καὶ Δημοκρίτου. Ἀριστοτέ[λους] τε καὶ Κλεοπάτρας χρυσουργιῶν. σαφήν[ει]α καλλίστη καὶ θαυμασία'. I warmly thank Vangelis Koutalis for providing me with a digital copy of the manuscript.

[15] *CMAG* I.131–2.

[16] The two recipe books are edited in Colinet (2010) 1–64. For a description of the two manuscripts see ibid.

sources, which were probably translated into Greek during the Palaiologan period.[17]

All these manuscripts are witnesses to a widespread interest towards a rich array of technical texts: despite their different origins and multilingual sources, these formulas and procedures were considered pieces of a long-lasting tradition that could accommodate recent collectors of recipes along with the mythical fathers of alchemy.

11.2 Isis, Orpheus, and Cleopatra: Late Byzantine Alchemy in Disguise

Parisinus gr. 2314 manuscript is a composite codex assembled by joining formerly independent codicological units – that is, a quire or a discrete number of quires written by different copyists which originally were not meant to be bound together. Texts of different genres are collected in the manuscript, such as a long monolingual lexicon of Greek words (ff. 167r–269v),[18] commentaries on the works of Church Fathers (ff. 289r–317v), and an anonymous treatise, *On the Mystery of the Alphabet* (ff. 323r–343v).[19] The first part (ff. 1r–166v; fourteenth–fifteenth century) is mainly medical and preserves extended excerpts from a large therapeutic book in at least eight tomes,[20] which includes a rich selection of recipes (at f. 1r the first formula recorded is for an eye salve attributed to a certain Maximianos). In this part we also find the third *recensio* of the Byzantine handbook on regimen usually referred to as Hierophilus' *Dietary Calendar* (ff. 87r–93v, line 10)[21] along with an anonymous synopsis on pulses (ff. 93v, line 10–97r). More importantly for our inquiry, folia 274r–278v – an

[17] See Colinet (2010: XLVII–CIV).

[18] We must note that f. 199 (written by another hand who copied medical recipes) does not belong to this unit and that many folia in this section are misplaced. The Parisinus MS also preserves two medical lexica of plants at ff. 280r, line 10–281v, line 33 and ff. 283r, line 1–288r, line 12, respectively edited in Delatte (1927–39) II.450–4 and 331–9.

[19] This last text is edited in Bandt (2007) 101–205. On this Parisinus MS see pages 90–1; the codex was described by Omont (1888: 235).

[20] At f. 11r, line 10 the incipit of the third tome is recorded ('Ἀρχὴ τοῦ τρίτου τόμου'), followed by its table of contents (with 35 chapters); at ff. 45r, line 16–50v, line 5, we find a detailed table of contents of the sixth tome ('κεφάλαια τοῦ ἕκτου τόμου', including 155 chapters), whose incipit is recorded at f. 50v, line 6 ('ἀρχὴ τοῦ ϛ´ τόμου'); at f. 123v, line 10 we read 'Beginning of the second tome' ('ἀρχὴ τοῦ δευτέρου τόμου'), but at f. 127r, line 10 we have 'End of the third tome' ('τέλος τοῦ γ´ τόμου'), followed by the incipit 'Chapter(s) of the fourth tome' ('κεφάλαιον τοῦ τετάρτου τόμου'). The last folium of this part (166r–v) lists the chapters of the eighth tome ('κεφάλαια τοῦ ὀγδόου τόμου'). Some folia are clearly missing or misplaced.

[21] See ed. Romano (1999). The third recension of this Byzantine calendar on regimen was edited by Delatte (1927–39) II.455–66. On this text see also Delacenserie (2014).

independent codicological unit dating to the fourteenth–fifteenth century – preserves a remarkable alchemical recipe book that, though known to seventeenth-century scholars, has not attracted the interest of modern philologists or historians of Byzantine science.[22] This short collection of recipes is here edited and translated for the first time (see the chapter's appendix).

The recipe book was mentioned by the French philologist Charles du Fresne du Cange (1610–88) in his lexicon of medieval Greek, where it is referred to as 'Orpheus' and Cleopatra's (al)chemical book' (*Liber chymicus Orphei & Cleopatrae*).[23] Du Cange's Latin description clearly mirrors the heading that introduces the alchemical text in the Paris manuscript (f. 274r, lines 1–2): 'Findings from the alchemical book on the making of gold by Isis (?), Orpheus and Cleopatra'. However, in Du Cange's scanty references to our text, only Orpheus and Cleopatra are mentioned, while the name of Isis is left aside. Indeed, the presence of the Egyptian goddess in the title is uncertain since, instead of her name (*Isis*/'Ἶσις' or *Isidos*/'Ἴσιδος' at the genitive), we read the rather obscure form *khryth* ('χρύθ') in the manuscript. The term is a *hapax* which does not occur in other classical or Byzantine texts. Perhaps in order to cope with this difficulty, the copyist wrote *mouth* ('μοῦθ') in the margin, which might be interpreted as an attempt to explain or correct the otherwise unintelligible term occurring in the title. The form *mouth*, in fact, surprisingly corresponds to one of the Egyptian names that Plutarch attributed to Isis in his treatise *On Isis and Osiris* (56, 374B3–8):

> Isis is sometimes named *Mouth* and sometimes *Athyri* and *Methyer*. The first name means 'mother', the second 'the cosmic house of Horus', or as Plato also says (*Tim.* 52D-53A), 'the place and receptacle of creation'; the third is a compound of 'full' and 'good' etc.[24]

The name *mouth* (from the ancient Egyptian *mwt*, 'mother') does not occur in any alchemical treatise,[25] so the proposed identification remains a tentative hypothesis. We must observe, however, that Isis does appear as the author of an alchemical recipe book in other late Byzantine

[22] This recipe book was not included in Berthelot and Ruelle's (1887–8) pioneering edition of the Greek alchemical writings; it has been mentioned, however, by Lebègue in *CMAG* I.130.

[23] See Du Cange (1688) I.197, s.v. βίσσιον; II.1333, s.v. σαραντάρι; II.168, s.v. σατουνίτζιν.

[24] Translation by Gwyn Griffiths (1970: 209). On the Egyptian terms used by Plutarch see Gwyn Griffiths (1970: 101–10) and Froidefond (1988: 305).

[25] We must note, however, that, according to the *Chronography* of Synkellos, ed. Mosshammer (1984) 14.5, a treatise attributed to Zosimus of Panopolis was entitled *Imouth* ('Ἰμούθ'), usually interpreted as a Greek transcription of Imhotep: see Mertens (1995: XCIII–XCVI).

manuscripts, such as MS Parisinus gr. 2327 (ff. 256r, line 12–258r, line 16), where she delivers to her son Horus a set of procedures described as secret instructions for the 'preparation of gold and silver' (*kataskeuē chrysou kai argyrou*).[26]

A fictional Egyptian framework for our recipe book handed down in MS Parisinus gr. 2314 is confirmed by the other two figures mentioned in its title: Orpheus and Cleopatra. The Ptolemaic queen Cleopatra, renown for her expertise in fields such as cosmetics and gynaecology,[27] was also credited with at least two technical writings included in Byzantine alchemical collections: a short text, *On Weights and Measures*, which largely overlaps with the tenth chapter of a longer treatise on the same topic attributed to Galen;[28] an alchemical dialogue with the 'philosophers' (i.e. the alchemists), among whom the Persian magus Ostanes, alleged master of Democritus, stands out.[29] On the other hand, Orpheus' alchemical expertise is confirmed by a short text that a few fifteenth-century manuscripts transmit under the title of 'Agathodaimon's collection (?) and commentary on the oracle of Orpheus'.[30] This short exegetical work is interestingly presented as a letter that the mythical Agathodaimon addressed to the Egyptian god Osiris, Isis' husband and father of Horus. Moreover, its Egyptian setting is further confirmed by other details scattered through the text: Memphis is mentioned as the place where Agathodaimon was at work, where two Egyptian months (*mechir* and *pharmouthi*)[31] represent the best moment to carry on the preliminary treatment of the ores used for the dyeing procedures. Orpheus is here presented as the author of an alchemical oracle (*chrēsmos*) that, despite its emphasis on making gold, was actually devoted to making silver as well. Agathodaimon explains, in fact, that both yellowing (i.e. how to make base metals yellow and thus transform them into gold) and whitening (i.e. how

[26] See ed. Berthelot and Ruelle (1887–8) II.28–33. See also Martelli (2014: 8–9).

[27] See, for instance, Marasco (1998) and Totelin (2017: 114–18).

[28] Cleopatra's text is edited in Hultsch (1864) I.253–7; Ps-Galen's text in Kühn (1821–33) XIX.748–81. See Martelli (2019b: 578–80).

[29] Greek text edited in Reitzenstein (1919: 14–20). We must note that another alchemical text, usually referred to as the *Teaching of the Philosopher Komarios to Cleopatra*, features the Egyptian queen as a main character: see Reitzenstein (1919: 23–5) and Lagercrantz (1934: 400–3).

[30] See ed. Berthelot and Ruelle (1887–8) II.268–71. The title reads: 'Ἀγαθοδαίμων, εἰς τὸν χρησμὸν Ὀρφέως συναγωγὴ καὶ ὑπόμνημα'. The earliest witness of this short text is MS Parisinus gr. 2327, ff. 262r–264r.

[31] Memphis is mentioned in Berthelot and Ruelle (1887–8), II.268.8; the two Egyptian months ('μεχίρ' and 'φαρμουθί') in II.270.3. These months are also referred to by the alchemist Olympiodorus in his commentary on Zosimus' alchemical work: see, for example, Berthelot and Ruelle (1887–8) II.69.15 and 72.1.

to whiten base metals and transform them into silver) were dealt with by Orpheus.

Both dyeing procedures are explored in the recipe book of MS Parisinus gr. 2314, which is divided in two parts, each including five recipes. In fact, despite the explicit mention of *chrysopoiia* ('the making of gold') in the title, only the second part, introduced by the subtitle 'On Gold' (*Peri chrysou*), is devoted to this topic. The first part, on the contrary, deals with the making of silver, which is referred to at the end of each recipe included in this section. This gives to our text a clear-cut structure, different from other late Byzantine alchemical recipe books, such as the aforementioned 'Explanation of the most noble and illustrious art of goldsmiths', which tends to accumulate a larger number of recipes without organising them according to transparent criteria. In a way, the recipe book ascribed to Isis, Orpheus, and Cleopatra is closer in structure to the earliest alchemical works, such as Pseudo-Democritus' four books on dyeing: the first book, in fact, was entirely devoted to the making of gold, and the second to the making of silver. Our recipe book reverses this order, starting from the less precious metal. A certain debate on the correct sequence of the alchemical procedures and their description in alchemical writings already emerges in late antique authors, such as in Synesius' commentary on Pseudo-Democritus' alchemical work (fourth century). Framed as a dialogue between the master Synesius and his pupil Dioscorus (a priest of the *Serapeion* in Alexandria), the work features the following discussion:

(DIOSCORUS) . . . What is the first operation of the Art, whitening or yellowing?
SYNESIUS. Whitening, to be sure.
DIOSCORUS. So why did he (i.e. Democritus) first speak about yellowing?
(SYNESIUS) Because gold is more valued than silver.
(DIOSCORUS) So must we work following this order, Synesius?
(SYNESIUS) No, Dioscorus, but he (i.e. Democritus) chose this order with the intent of training our mind and intellect etc.[32]

Pseudo-Democritus decided to open his work by dealing with the most precious metal, namely gold. However, according to a correct understanding of the alchemical art, any practitioner was expected to start with the making of silver (by whitening base metals), and then to change it into gold (by dyeing silver yellow). This whitening-yellowing sequence is classical, so to speak, and was encapsulated in a short precept attributed to the mythical Agathodaimon in MS Marcianus gr. 299 (f. 95v): 'after purifying,

[32] See Synesius alch., *Notes on Democritus' Book*, 8, in ed. Martelli (2013) 132.7–8.

blackening and, at last, whitening copper, then there will be a stable yellowing'.[33] This 'rule' was often repeated, with slight variations, by Byzantine authors, such as Stephanos of Alexandria and the philosopher Christianos,[34] and it seems to have been followed by the compiler of our recipe book ascribed to Isis, Orpheus, and Cleopatra.

On the other hand, if these elements anchor our short text to an ancient and well-established tradition, the language of the recipes, in terms of grammar, syntax, and nomenclature, clearly points to a quite later date of composition. Our recipe book, indeed, is quite similar to the aforementioned late Byzantine alchemical compendia, such as the collections included in MSS Parisinus gr. 2419 and Holkhamicus gr. 109 recently edited by Colinet (2010).[35] Moreover, the described procedures sometimes also overlap. For instance, our compendium ascribed to Isis, Orpheus, and Cleopatra is opened by a recipe on the making of silver, which makes use of a specific device: the dyeing substances are put in a closed vessel that has been pierced on the top; the vessel is set on fire and a metal knife covers the hole so the alchemist can check the state of the 'reaction' by looking at the chromatic transformations of the knife exposed to the vapours of the dying ingredients (especially mercury). The same technique is described in a recipe of Cosmas' *On Chrysopoiia*, which is preserved in two slightly different versions in Byzantine manuscripts.[36] Furthermore, the recipe book handed down in MS Holkhamicus gr. 109 prescribes squill to dye copper:[37] likewise, in our text ascribed to Isis, Orpheus, and Cleopatra, the same ingredient is used to treat tin (rec. 2). Among plants, our recipe book also mentions laserwort (*silphion*; rec. 5 and 8), which rarely enters alchemical procedures. Other techniques, on the other hand, involve various minerals as main dyeing ingredients that were added to different melted metals.

After the last recipe on the making of gold, a second contemporary copyist added a detailed description of how to prepare a *glykysma*, a kind of dessert or cake, in our case prepared with green walnuts and honey as its main ingredients. The recipe seems to respond to a purely gastronomical

[33] See ed. Berthelot and Ruelle (1887–8) II.115.7–8: 'Μετὰ τὴν τοῦ χαλκοῦ ἐξίωσις καὶ μέλανσιν καὶ εἰς ὕστερον λεύκωσις, τότε ἔσται βεβαία ξάνθωσις.'

[34] See Stephanos alch., *The Great Art*, 2.68–9, in ed. Papathanassiou (2017) 163.9–10; for Christianos, *On Chrysopoiia* see ed. Berthelot and Ruelle (1887–8) II.417.21–2. On the still debated chronology of Christianos see Letrouit (1995: 62) and Martelli (2019a: 11–12).

[35] Specific terms and grammatical/syntactical features are discussed in the footnotes to the Greek text and translation in the appendix.

[36] See Cosmas, *On Chrysopoiia*, rec. 10, in ed. Colinet (2010) 71–4.

[37] See Rec. H2, in ed. Colinet (2010) 21–2 (see note 51).

interest and its inclusion in the recipe book is difficult to account for apart from the traditional links between alchemical practices and cooking techniques.[38] If we take into account the second recipe of the section on silver making, the use of sea squills to be filled in was probably known in Byzantine kitchens (where, however, we may presume that minerals and metals were not the usual filling!). However, this recipe with walnuts, the *glykysma*, is not included in other (published) Byzantine sources, such as the *Geoponika* or dietary treatises approaching food from a medical perspective. On the other hand, we must observe that different types of *glykysma* feature prominently in the medical dispensatory of Demetrios Pepagomenos,[39] physician of Manuel II Palaiologos (1391–1425) and copyist of MS Parisinus gr. 2256, a massive anthology of medical texts including, among others, works by Hippocrates, Aetios of Amida, and John Zacharias Aktouarios.[40]

11.3 Medicine and 'Chemistry': Cross-Contamination in Manuscripts

The Parisinus gr. 2256 manuscript does not include alchemical sections. Technical recipes, on the contrary, are embedded in an almost contemporary medical manuscript, MS Bononiensis 1808 (fourteenth–early fifteenth century),[41] which belonged to another physician working at the court of Manuel II Palaiologos: Nikephoros Doukas Palaiologos Malakes. His exchange of letters with Manuel Holobolos, court secretary of the emperor, closes the satirical dialogue usually referred to as *Mazaris' Journey to Hades* (AD 1414–15), where Demetrios Pepagomenos is mentioned as well, mocked as a 'certified killer'.[42] Nikephoros Malakes signed folio 301r of the Bologna manuscript and left a few scattered marginal

[38] See, for example, Leontsini and Merianos (2016: 215–22).

[39] See Demetrios Papagomenos, *Medical Dispensatory* (*recensio L*), chapters 21, 32, 45, 74–5, 78, 103, and so forth, in ed. Capone Ciollaro (2003) 54–6, 59, 66–8, 75, and so forth. On the interrelationship between food and medicines with a focus on Arabic cookbooks and pharmacopoeias see Chipman (Chapter 10) in this volume. In Byzantine medical recipe books the term 'γλύκυσμα' is also used for sweet pharmaceutical dosage forms, usually potions (the equivalent Greek term for the Arabic جوارشن/*jawārishn*). See Bouras-Vallianatos (2021: 1000, n. 188). I thank Petros Bouras-Vallianatos for pointing this meaning out to me.

[40] *RGK* II, n. 133. On Demetrios Pepagomenos see also Lazaris (2006: 252–6).

[41] This massive pharmacological compendium has not attracted the attention of many scholars since Alessandro Olivieri described it: see Olivieri and Festa (1895: 389–96); De Gregorio (2019: 252–3).

[42] *Mazaris' Journey to Hades*, ed. Barry, Share, Smithies, and Westerink (1975) 40.23–4 (see also 34.26). On the satire against doctors in this text see Garland (2007: 199–200). The identification of Mazaris has been much debated; Krallis (2016: 90–1) has recently argued that Nikephoros Malakes himself might have been the real author of the dialogue.

notes:[43] in particular, at folio 54r, he both wrote 'with saffron, galbanum' (upper margin) and copied (right margin) a recipe that already occurs in a section on saffron-based medicines of Aetios' medical encyclopaedia, book 12 (chap. 27).[44]

Aetios of Amida (sixth century) indeed represents an important source of the pharmacological collection handed down in the Bologna manuscript,[45] which also includes excerpts from later medical writings, such as the epitomes of a dispensatory (*De remediis*; ff. 1r–4v) and of a handbook on therapeutics (*De curatione morborum*; f. 69r–v), both compiled by the Byzantine physician Theophanes Chrysobalantes (tenth century).[46] Sandwiched between a lexicon of plants (ff. 38r–41v)[47] and a treatise on weights and measures (ff. 63v, line 7–66r), folia 42r–63v transmit hundreds of recipes that also feature the description of ten procedures for making metallic, black, and coloured inks, a field of expertise often associated with alchemy in the many premodern collections preserved in different languages (Greek, Syriac, Latin).[48] This section of the Bologna manuscript is mainly medical. It is opened by three recipes of medicinal 'salts' (f. 42r, line 1–42v, line 19), some of which also occur in various manuscripts of book 9 of Aetios' encyclopaedia; at the end, a section is devoted to digestive medicines.[49] However, these recipes were not included in Zervos' edition of Aetios' book, where we only find a short reference to 'salts' (*halatia*) at the very end of chapter 24: 'It (i.e. an oxymel-based medicine) is suitable for

[43] See MS Bononiensis 1808, f. 301r (upper margin): '† νϊκηφόρος δούκας ὁ μαλάκης' (*Nikēphoros Doukas ho Malakēs*); see Cataldi Palau (2010: 370, n. 15). In the same folium Nikephoros also wrote a cursive sigma inscribed in an omicron, perhaps a kind of ex-libris. On Nikephoros Doukas Malakes see *PLP* VII, n. 16454.

[44] See MS Bononiensis 1808, f. 54r (upper margin): '† τὸ διὰ κρόκου· χαλβάνης'; (right margin): 'κρόκ(ου) < ις΄, ἀμωνιακοῦ θυμιάματος < μη΄, κηροῦ < ϟς΄, πίσσης ξηρᾶς < φος΄, ἐλαίου ῥοδίνου < μη΄, ὀξους λευκοῦ δριμυτάτ(ου) κοτύλ(ας) α΄', ('saffron, 36 drachmae; incense of ammoniac gum, 48 drachmae; wax, 96 drachmae; dry pitch, 576 drachmae; rose oil, 48 drachmae, very sharp white vinegar, 1 *kotylae*'). See Aetios of Amida, *Medical Books*, 12.27, 33–8, in ed. Kostomoiris (1892) 51.10–14. Marginal notes by Nikephoros also occur at folios 209r and 332v.

[45] For instance, at f. 61r, we read the heading: 'Various medical treatments from Aetios' medical book' ('Ἐκ τῆς ἰατρικῆς βίβλου τοῦ αἐτίου ἰατρεῖαι διάφοροι'). Excerpts from Aetios have been detected in Olivieri and Festa (1895: 389–96).

[46] Sonderkamp (1987: 90–1). On the relationships between Aetios' medical books and Theophanes' writings see Capone Ciollaro and Galli Calderini (1999). On *De remediis* see also Felici (1981–2).

[47] See Touwaide (1999: 215). For other examples of similar dictionaries of *materia medica* see Delatte (1927–39): II.272–454, and Bouras-Vallianatos (2018) with further up-to-date bibliography.

[48] The recipes of inks have been recorded by Zuretti in *CMAG* II.143–4.

[49] For instance, MS Laur. Plut. 75.2 (ff. 32v–33r, twelfth century) hands down recipes of salts attributed to King Ptolemy and to Iamblichus along with the formula of the 'twelve gods' salt; this selection is expanded in MS Parisinus suppl. gr. 631 (f. 133r–133v, fourteenth century), which adds salts attributed to the apostle Luke and the prophet Elijah. I owe this information to Dr Irene Calà, whom I warmly thank for her help. On Luke's salt see Ideler (1841: I.297).

such cases, as well as the great remedy that lasts for years, Archigenes' remedies with citron and wine from Skybela, and the salts, whose preparations will be explained in a moment.'[50]

Then the Bologna manuscript describes a medical treatment for those who have accidentally swallowed gold, copper, iron, or similar substances (f. 43r, line 1–43v, line 2), who were prescribed to take evacuating drugs according to the instructions of the physician Antyllos (second century AD). In all likelihood, the text is taken from Aetios' book 9, chapter 42, where the Byzantine physician deals with the same topic.[51] Aetios' *Medical Books* also represent the main source for the next recipes on the uses of various medicinal plants (ff. 43v, line 2–46r, line 19).[52]

Two recipes on silver writing – that is, on the making of silver inks prepared either with or without the precious metal – seamlessly follow the aforementioned medical prescriptions:

> f. 46v, lines 1–4: Περὶ ἀργυρογραφίας. Ἀργυρογραφίας ἐπιστήμη· λαβὼν ῥίνισμα ἀργύρου, τρῖψον μετὰ ὑδραργύρου εἰς θυίαν ψήφινον· καὶ μίξας κόμμι ἀρκοῦν γράφε.
>
> On writing in silver letters. Explication of how to write in silver letters. Take silver filings and grind with mercury in a marble mortar; then mix enough Arabic gum and write.
>
> f. 46v, lines 4–6: Ἀργυρογραφίας ἐπιστήμη. Τοῦ μολίβδου τὸ ἀπόκαυμα λαβὼν ὠοῦ τὸ λευκὸν (λεπτὸν cod.) βρέξας καὶ τρίψας γράφε.
>
> Explication of how to write in silver letters. Take calcined lead, wet with egg white and grind, then write.

Recipes on the making of metallic inks are scattered through Byzantine manuscripts, especially recipes on chrysography.[53] Less frequent are formulas for the preparation of silver inks (argyrography), which often occur in collections traditionally linked to alchemy, in particular the so-called *Leiden papyrus* (third–fourth century AD), the *Mappae clavicula* identified with the Latin translation of a (lost) Greek alchemical recipe book, and the collection of recipes that opens the Syriac alchemical manuscript Mm. 6.29

[50] See Aetios of Amida, *Medical Books*, 9.24,114–17, in ed. Zervos (1911) 324.32–325.3: 'Ἐπιτήδειον δέ ἐστι τοῖς τοιούτοις, τό τε μέγα πολυετὲς καὶ τὸ διὰ κιτρίου καὶ τὸ διὰ σκυβελίτου Ἀρχιγένους καὶ τὰ ἁλάτια, αἱ δὲ συνθέσεις αὐτῶν μετ' οὐ πολὺ ῥηθήσονται.'

[51] See Aetios of Amida, *Medical Books*, 9.42,282–93, in ed. Zervos (1911) 387.6–18.

[52] The recipes are taken from Aetios of Amida, *Medical Books*, 3.19 ('Ἴσχαιμον'); 3.22 ('Περὶ βδελλῶν'); 1.89 ('Δάφνης κτλ.'); 1.145 ('ἐρέβινθος') and 1.146 ('ἕρπυλλος'). See ed. Olivieri (1935–50) I.276.3–8; I.277.19–29; I.51.16–20; I.71.23–72.19.

[53] See Alexander (1964); Schreiner and Oltrogge (2011).

(fifteenth century, Cambridge University Library).[54] In this last witness a recipe points to the close link between silver and golden inks: in order to write with silver letters, it prescribes mixing silver filings with mercury and proceeding as has been already explained for gold.[55] The addition of mercury probably facilitated the grinding of the silver, which then was to be mixed with a glue such as Arabic gum. The use of lead, on the contrary, seems less frequent in Latin and Syriac sources, where tin is rather preferred.[56] In one case, lead is melted with tin: the alloy is then ground and mixed with a glue.[57]

After these two technical recipes we have a section entitled *On Husbandmen* (*Peri gēponōn*; ff. 46v, line 7–47r), which includes the description of four methods to farm and treat grapevines (*ampelos*) as well as a section on how to protect them against grasshoppers (*akrides*). If these texts pertain to agriculture, medicine is again the main interest of the next recipes, which are grouped in short paragraphs, each introduced by general headings loosely arranged in alphabetical order: a group of three recipes *On Scurf* (*Peri achōras*, f. 47r, line 15–47v, line 3) opens the section, which is closed by four recipes on chrysography (f. 54v, lines 1–14): golden inks are prepared by grinding various metals (iron, lead, electrum) and minerals (mainly orpiment). Then come chapters on hunting and fishing (ff. 54v, line 15–56r, line 13): apples filled with soda (sodium carbonate), for instance, are used to hunt boars and deer. Among these texts we also find a recipe on how to prepare a black paint (f. 56r, line 13–56v).[58] Finally, after a few chapters on various animals (e.g. bees or mice) and many medical recipes, folio 62 features recipes on chrysography as well as the preparation of yellow vegetal paints (*barzion*) and red paints (*lacha*).[59]

A certain interest in practical applications of the properties of natural substances seems to hold together all these short texts and recipes dealing with an intriguing variety of subjects, from medicine to agriculture, from hunting to ink and paint making. A compilation that somehow reminds of

[54] See *Leiden papyrus*, rec. 60, 77, in ed. Halleux (1981) 99, 102; see also *Mappae clavicula*, rec. 82–3, 103–9, in ed. Baroni, Pizzigoni, and Travaglio (2013) 132–4, 146–9. On the origins of *Mappae clavicula* see Halleux and Meyvaert (1987); Syriac collection, rec. 24–8 (unedited), partially translated in Berthelot and Duval (1893) 207.

[55] Mm. 6.29, f. 8v.

[56] See *Mappae clavicula*, rec. 83, 103, 108, in ed. Baroni, Pizzigoni, and Travaglio (2013) 134.

[57] See *Mappae clavicula*, rec. 109, in ed. Baroni, Pizzigoni, and Travaglio (2013) 148.

[58] See also Schreiner and Oltrogge (2011: 43).

[59] The recipes on *lacha* ('λαχᾶ') have been edited in Benedetti (2014: 452–4).

Iulius Africanus' *Cesti*, which combined chemistry, agriculture, medicine, and warfare and gained great popularity in Byzantium.[60]

On the other hand, sometimes medical recipes were also copied in manuscripts mainly devoted to alchemy. This is the case with MS Vaticanus gr. 1174 (fourteenth–fifteenth century), which transmits a rich anthology of alchemical texts.[61] Indeed, on folio 49v (left blank by the first copyist), a second scribe interestingly combined a short alchemical recipe book with the formula for a medicinal salt:

> Περὶ κιμίας κατασκευή.
>
> Ἵνα ποιήσῃς ἄργυρον (☾ cod.). Λαβὼν ὑδράργυρον ὅσον βούλ(ει) καὶ θεῖον ἄπυρον τὸ ἴσον βάλε αὐτὰ εἰς ἄγγειον χων(ίον) καὶ θὲς εἰς πῦρ πραέον ὅσον τὴν θέρμην τοῦ ἡλίου (☉ cod.) καὶ σάλευε αὐτὸ συχνάκις καὶ μετὰ τὸ λαβεῖν τῆς ἑνώσεως τὴν πῆξιν καὶ στεγνῶσαι, λαγάρισον αὐτὸ μετὰ τοῦ μολίβδου, καὶ γίνεται ἄργυρος (☾ cod.) λαμπρός. Καὶ ἐὰν ἔστι σκληρὸς καὶ θέλεις μαλακίσαι, ῥῖψον εἰς τὸ χων(ίον) χάλκανθον Ἀλεξανδρινόν.
>
> Εἰς τὸ ποιῆσαι χρυσόν (☉ cod.) λευκόν· θεῖον ἄπυρον πότισον μετὰ ἐλαίου ἐρυθροῦ τῶν ᾠῶν καὶ ποίησον αὐτὸ κατὰ τοὺς (τὰς s.l.) ἄνωθεν διδασκαλίας καὶ ποίησον χρυσόν (☉ cod.) λαμπρόν.
>
> Εἰ δὲ βούλει ποιῆσαι τὸν χρυσόν (☉ cod.) τὸν κοινὸν ἐρυθρόν· τρῖψον ὄστρακον ἐρυθρὸν καὶ βράσον μετὰ ὕδατος τοῦτον καὶ λαμπρυνθήσεται.
>
> Ἐὰν δὲ καὶ τὴν σελήνην (☾ cod.) τὴν νοθευομένην βούλει λαμπρῦναι καὶ γενέσθαι σελήνην (☾ cod.) εἶδος καθαροῦ, τρῖψον στύψιν καὶ σὺν ὕδατι βράσον, καὶ λευκανθήσεται ὁ κίβδηλος.[62]
>
> Σκευασία ἅλατος σκευασθεῖσα ὑπὸ τοῦ ἁγίου Γρηγορ(ίου) τοῦ θεολόγ(ου).
>
> Ὑσσώπου Κρητικοῦ οὐγγίας δ', σκαμμωνίας οὐγγίαν α' καὶ ἥμισυ, ἀμμωνιακοῦ οὐγγίας β', κυμίνου, σκίλλης, ζιγγιβέρεως, πεπέρεως, σελίνου, ἀνὰ οὐγγίαν α', γλήχωνος ὀρεινοῦ οὐγγίας γ', σμύρνης, σιλφίου οὐγγίαν α', ἅλατος κοινοῦ οὐγγίαν α', φύλλ(ου) οὐγγίας γ'.

> On the preparation of alchemy.
>
> In order to make silver. Take as much mercury as you want and unburnt sulphur, the same quantity, put them in a vessel, [i.e.] a crucible, and set on a gentle fire as warm as the heat of the sun and stir it often; after reaching the solidification of the mixture and letting it get dry, purify it with lead and it will become shining silver. If it is hard and you want to soften it, throw Alexandrian vitriol in the crucible.
>
> To make gold white. Moisten the unburnt sulphur with red oil of eggs and proceed according to the instructions given above; make gold shining.

60 For a recent analysis of the extant fragments of the *Cesti*, edited and translated, see Wallraff, Scardino, Mecella, and Guignard (2012).

61 See *CMAG* II.61–8; Colinet (2010: CXXXIV); Martelli (2011: 46–54).

62 A preliminary transcription of these alchemical recipes is provided by Heiberg in *CMAG* II.332.

If you want to make the common gold red, grind a red potsherd, boil it in water and it will be polished.

If you want to polish the adulterated silver [lit. moon] so that the silver becomes a kind of pure (silver), grind alum, boil with water, and the adulterated coin will become white.

Preparation of the salt prepared by Saint Gregory the Theologian.

Cretan hyssop, 4 unciae; scammony, 1 uncia and a half; ammoniac salt, 2 unciae; cumin, squill, ginger, pepper, celery, 1 uncia each; pennyroyal of the mountains, 3 unciae; myrrh, laserwort, 1 uncia (each); common salt, 1 uncia; dog's mercury, 3 unciae.

The first four recipes are mainly metallurgical and describe the treatment of various metals which were dyed with different ingredients. The text is opened by a short description on how to combine mercury and sulphur to make artificial cinnabar, a technique that was quite popular in Byzantium.[63] Pseudo-Democritus' alchemical book *On the Making of Gold* also includes a clear reference to how to solidify mercury and use it to make metals white and yellow.[64]

Then the scribe added the formula for a medicinal salt. A similar recipe was already edited by Ideler[65] and is included in the first book of the *Dynameron*, an influential handbook of pharmaceutics by the Byzantine medical author Nicholas Myrepsos (fourteenth century).[66] The first book is divided into four sections describing uses and preparations of four types of remedies, whose names begin with the letter alpha. The section on 'salts' (*halatia*) features the recipe of Gregory the Theologian's *halation*, which is introduced by a short description of its medical applications: it was mainly used to treat eye diseases, preventing ophthalmia until old age and sharpening the sight.[67]

Similar recipes, with slight variations in term of ingredients (both in their number and in their order of appearance) are scattered in various Byzantine manuscripts dating to between the fifteenth and sixteenth centuries, in particular therapeutic handbooks (the so-called *iatrosophia*).[68] Bononiensis 1808 includes Gregory's formula in its section on salts (f. 42r, line 13–42v, line 6); another fifteenth-century manuscript of

[63] Colinet (2010: LXXXIII–XCI).

[64] See Pseudo-Democritus, *On Natural Secrets* (*Physika kai mystika*), 5, in ed. Martelli (2013) 86–7.

[65] Ideler (1841) I.297–8.

[66] His traditional identification with Nicholas *aktouarios*, a physician working at the court of Emperor John III Vatatzes (1222–54), is uncertain and has been questioned: see Ieraci Bio (2017: 301–2), Valiakos (2019: XLIX–L), and Bouras-Vallianatos (2020: 26, n. 156) with further bibliography.

[67] See Nicholas Myrepsos, *Dynameron*, 1.2 (*halatia*), rec. 14, in ed. Valiakos (2019) 234.1–12. On the *Dynameron* see Ieraci Bio (2017).

[68] On *iatrosophia* see Ieraci Bio (1982), Touwaide (2007), Valentino (2016: 15–18), and Zipser (2019).

the Bologna University Library (MS 3632) lists 'the *halation* of Saint Gregory the Theologian' as the first recipe of a section on the preparation of salts that features ten different prescriptions.[69] We also find salts ascribed to King Ptolemy and the apostle Luke.[70] Likewise, the *iatrosophion* of the Turin MS B.VII.18 (ff. 1r–67r, sixteenth century) includes a 'salt prepared by the Saint Apostle Luke' (rec. 250) followed by 'another salt prepared by Saint Gregory the Theologian' (rec. 251).[71] Finally, Gregory's formula was even put into verses in MS.MSL.60 (fifteenth century) held by the Welcome Library.[72]

These remedies were used to treat eye problems, and professional groups could also benefit from their applications. In the section on *halatia* Nicholas Myrepsos includes a recipe (n. 17) of a 'marvellous salt that is used by copyists (*kalligraphoi*), when they become dim-sighted: in fact, it cleanses the vision and makes the sight sharp'.[73] It mainly includes the same ingredients mentioned in Saint Gregory the Theologian's recipe. Moreover, earlier medical sources confirm that some recipes were targeted at specific groups of craftsmen. Goldsmiths, in particular, could benefit from eye salves (*kollyria*), as already emerges from Oribasios' *To Eunapios* (fourth century AD). This pharmacological handbook describes preparations that are ranked among the easily available remedies or *euporista*: they were made of cheap and common ingredients, which were always at hand for laymen (with a very limited medical training) who, when travelling in the countryside, could not rely on the expertise of professional physicians.[74] In book 4 (chap. 24), Oribasios provides formulas for compound medicines against eye diseases, among which we also find the recipe of an eye salve called *oxyderkes*, which was particularly suitable for painters (*zōgraphoi*), engravers of gems (*daktylioglyphoi*), and goldsmiths (*chrysochooi*).[75]

69 MS Bononiensis 3632, f. 229r–v. The section is introduced by the general heading (in red ink) 'On various salts' ('Περὶ ἁλατίων διαφώρων') and opened by the recipe of Saint Gregory's salt (f. 229r1–6) with the title (in red ink): 'ἁλάτιον τοῦ ἁγί(ου) Γριγωρίου [*sic*] τοῦ θεολόγ(ου)'.

70 MS Bononiensis 3632, f. 229r, lines 6–10 (title in red ink): 'ἁλάτ(ιον) ὃ προσήνεγκε Πτολωμέων [*sic*] ὁ βασιλεύς' ('Salt that was administered by the king Ptolemy'); 229r, lines 10–18 (title in red ink) 'ἁλάτ(ιον) τοῦ ἁγίου ἀσποστόλου Λουκᾶ ὃ καὶ δοδεκάθεων [*sic*] λέγεται' ('salt of the Saint Apostle Luke, that is also called "of the twelve gods"').

71 See Anonymous, *Iatrosophion*, rec. 250, in ed. Valentino (2016) 170. 13–172.2: 'ἁλάτιον σκευασθὲν παρὰ τοῦ ἁγίου ἀποστόλου Λουκᾶ'; rec. 251, in ed. Valentino (2016) 172.3–10: 'ἕτερον ἁλάτιον σκευασθὲν παρὰ τοῦ ἁγίου Γρηγορίου τοῦ Θεολόγου'.

72 Bouras-Vallianatos (2015: 293, 295).

73 See Nicholas Myrepsos, *Dynameron*, 1.2 (*halatia*), rec. 17, in ed. Valiakos (2019) 235.3–8.

74 See Eijk (2010: 529–32).

75 See Oribasios, *Books to Eunapium*, 4.24, 8–11, in ed. Raeder (1926) 447.22–8.

The same formula is included in book 7 of Aetios' medical encyclopaedia, which is mainly devoted to ophthalmology.[76] In the same book Aetios also provides the recipe of an 'eye-salve called the goldsmith's testament': the medicine is said to have been called after a goldsmith, who, before dying, deposited its formula in the Ephesians' temple in order to help patients left untreated by professional physicians. Then the recipe – Aetios continues – was rediscovered by Emperor Hadrian (AD 76–138).[77] We cannot rule out that the salt of Saint Gregory the Theologian, as a medicine used to improve vision and prevent eye problems, was also particularly valued by craftsmen working with precious metals. For this reason, it might have been copied in MS Vaticanus gr. 1174 after a short recipe book on metallurgical alchemy.

Conclusion

The sources discussed so far point to a wide circulation of alchemical and technical recipes during the Palaiologan era. Recipe books were usually part of larger compendia of alchemical texts or, in some cases, they were included in less specialised anthologies. Medical or even cooking recipes could sometimes complement alchemical collections, thus revealing entangled trajectories of texts pertaining to various areas of expertise: these experts, indeed, despite the differences of their trade, shared tools, procedures, and habits of hands.

A certain interest in alchemical recipes is already well documented in tenth-century Byzantium, as emerges from the letter on the making of gold that the Byzantine scholar and natural philosopher Michael Psellos (1018–78) addressed to his patron, Michael I Keroularios, Patriarch of Constantinople (1043–59).[78] Psellos first frames alchemy as a set of techniques that can lead to marvellous achievements (the production of gold, gemstones, glass, and pearls), which, however extraordinary they may be, like natural wonders, do obey the transformations of the four elements.[79] Then he explicitly claims to narrow the scope of his inquiry to recipes for the making of gold: he collects eleven recipes on this topic, said to

[76] See Aetios of Amida, *Medical Books*, 7.101,4–14, in ed. Olivieri (1935–50) II.350.22–351.2.

[77] Aetios of Amida, *Medical Books*, 7.117,53–65, ed. Olivieri (1935–50) II 395.10–396.5. The recipe is introduced by the title 'κολλύριον ἡ διαθήκη ἐπικαλούμενον τοῦ Χρυσοχόου'. See also Nicholas Myrepsos, *Dynameron*, 9.60 (*kollyria*), in ed. Valiakos (2019) 679–80.

[78] See ed. Bidez (1928) 26–43. See also Albini (1988).

[79] See Magdalino and Mavroudi (2006: 18); Katsiampoura (2018: 124–7).

summarise all the wisdom of Democritus, one of the founders of the alchemical art.[80]

Without ever severing the bond with the ancient fathers of alchemy, Byzantine alchemical compilers did not avoid exploring more recent and multilingual sources of information. The number of Arabic, Latin, and even Italian loanwords scattered in late recipe books, such as the compendium ascribed to Isis, Orpheus, and Cleopatra discussed in this chapter, best exemplify this tension between tradition and innovation.[81] Along with new terms, substances, and technologies, new texts expanded on the earlier tradition. For instance, an anonymous treatise usually referred to as *Work of the Four Elements* describes a fractional distillation of eggs believed to isolate the four elements.[82] The described procedures heavily depend on the third book of the so-called *Book of Seventy* attributed to the famous Arabic alchemist Jābir ibn Ḥayyān (eight–ninth century).[83] Moreover, recipes based on Latin sources are scattered in alchemical manuscripts,[84] along with Greek translations of Latin alchemical treatises, such as Albertus Magnus' *Semita recta* and an excerpt from a treatise attributed to Arnaldus de Villanova.[85] These translations are macroscopic examples of much deeper and thorough influences which left their marks in each single recipe of compendia copied in fourteenth- and fifteenth-century manuscripts. These marks require our full attention as crucial pieces of evidence for the cross-cultural forces that shaped late Byzantine science and technology.

Appendix

Edition and translation of the recipe book in MS Parisinus gr. 2314, ff. 274r–278v

In editing the text, I have tacitly normalised the spelling of various words which feature many orthographical variations between long and short

80 See Michael Psellos, *On the Making of Gold*, 14.1–2, in ed. Bidez (1928) 40.6–7.

81 On the use of terms of ingredients in various languages in the same text see also Käs (Chapter 1), Walker-Meikle (Chapter 3), and Mavroudi (Chapter 4) in the present volume.

82 Greek text edited in Berthelot and Ruelle (1887–8) II.337–42 under the general title of 'Travail de quatre éléments'.

83 See Kraus (1942: 39); Colinet (2000); Roberts (2022: 572–4).

84 Colinet (2010: LXXXVII–XCI), for instance, has shown that a recipe on the making of artificial cinnabar edited by Berthelot and Ruelle (1887–8): II.383–4 from MS Parisinus gr. 2327 (f. 332r) depends on Latin sources, perhaps a recipe included in MS Sélestat, Bibliotheque Humaniste, 17 (ff. 24r and 213v).

85 On Albertus Magnus' text, preserved in MS Parisinus gr. 2419 (ff. 279r–288v), see Colinet (2010: XV, CV); for Arnaldus' Greek text see Zuretti's transcription in *CMAG* V.95–6. On Albertus Magnus see also Rinotas (Chapter 12) in this volume.

vowels (e.g. ο/ω and η/ε) or vowels and diphthongs that had the same pronunciation (η/υ/ι/ει, αι/ε). For instance, the copyist writes 'ἀσίμην' for 'ἀσήμιν', 'χονεύω' for 'χωνεύω', 'χρύω' for 'χρίω', and 'χάλκομαν' for 'χάλκωμαν'. When noteworthy, I have recorded the spellings of the manuscript in brackets or discussed them in the footnotes.

[274r] Εὕρεσις (Ἔβρεσις cod.) ἐκ τῆς χυμευτικῆς (χυμα- cod.) βίβλου τῆς χρυσοποιΐας τῆς χρύθ (*sic*, μοῦθ in marg.) καὶ τοῦ Ὀρφέως καὶ Κλεοπάτρας.

(1) Λαβὼν ὑδράργυρον ὅσον θέλ(εις) βάλον (βαλλὸν cod.)[86] τοῦτον εἰς τζουκάλιν καινούργιον ἄθικτον· καὶ πλήρωσον αὐτήν (i.e. τζουκάλην), τουτέστιν γέμισον ἐλαῖον καθαρόν· καὶ χρῖσον αὐτήν ἄνωθεν μετὰ πηλοῦ ἄσπρου ὅπου ποιοῦσιν (ποιῶσην cod.) τὰ χωνία καλά. ποίησον δὲ ἀπάνω τρύπαν μικρὴν ὅσον βελόνην (-ώνιν cod.)· καὶ μετὰ τοῦτο (-ω cod.) σκέπασον ταύτην μετὰ μαχαιρίου ἢ ἑτέρου τινὸς σιδήρου καθαροῦ· καὶ βράσον καλῶς ἕως ἂν καῇ (-εῖ cod.) ὅλον τὸ ἔλαιον· σήκωνε (σίκοναι cod.) γοῦν τὸ σίδηρον καὶ βλέπε αὐτό· καὶ εἰ (ἡ cod.) μὲν ἐξέρχεται ὑγρώτης ποσός, καὶ ὑγραίνεται τὸ σίδηρον, ἄφες αὐτὸ καυθῆναι καλῶς. [274v] ἐπὰν δὲ ἴδῃς (εἴδης cod.) <ὅτι> εἶναι λευκός, οἷον (ἧον cod.) ὁ τόπος τοῦ μαχαιρίου ἢ τοῦ σιδήρου, ἐν ᾧ σκεπάζει (-η cod.) τὴν τρύπαν, τότε χρῖσον καὶ αὐτὴν τὴν τρύπαν καλῶς ἐκ τοῦ αὐτοῦ πηλοῦ. Καὶ μετ' ὀλίγον ἄνοιξον καὶ ἔχε τεάφην ἄσπρην τριμμένην καὶ ῥῖψον ἀπέσω· καὶ τάραξον αὐτὴν καλῶς· καὶ ἄφες αὐτήν, ἵνα κρυώσῃ (κριῶσι cod.) καὶ οὕτως πηγνύει καὶ γίνεται (γύναισται cod.) ἀσήμιν.

(2) Ἄλλο. Κασ<σ>ίτηρον χώνευσον· εἶτα βάψον αὐτὸν εἰς ζουμίν, ὀπτοῦ μορίου καὶ εἰς ὀρὸν (ὄρος cod.) κυνὸς εἰκοσάκις· εἶτα σχίσας σχέλαν (i.e. σκίλλαν) ὅ ἐστιν σκιλλοκρόμμυον (σκηλοκρόμιον cod.), ἔνθες ἔνδον αὐτὸ καὶ ἐπάνω μαρκάσιταν τριμ<μ>ένον, καὶ χρῖσον (χρύ- cod.) τὴν σχέλαν μετὰ κο<κ>κίνου πηλοῦ, καὶ θὲς ταύτην εἰς μεγάλην ἀνθρακιάν, κεῖσθαι (κέεσθαι cod.?) ἡμέρας β΄· καὶ εὑρήσεις (-ις cod.) ἀσήμιν [275r] πλὴν ἡ ἐπιφάνεια ἔσται μέλαινα· κρούσας δὲ ταύτην μετὰ σφύρας, πεσεῖται τὸ μέλαν· ἔνδον δὲ ἔσται ἀσήμιν καθαρόν.

(3) Ἕτερον [in marg.]. Νίτρον, ψιμίθιν καὶ γάλα, βράσον ὁμοῦ· εἶτα ἔπαρον σίδηρον καθαρόν, καὶ βράσον ὁμοῦ καλῶς· καὶ βάψον εἰς τὸ αὐτὸ γάλα, σαραντάκις· εἶτα λαβὼν ἐξ αὐτοῦ ἐξάγιον ἕν, καὶ ἀσήμιν καθαρόν, ἐξάγιον ἕν, χώνευσον ὁμοῦ· καὶ χώνευσον ὁμοῦ καὶ χῦσον, καὶ ἔσται ἀσήμιν καθαρόν.

[86] The endings of present and second aorist imperatives can be either -ον or -ε; see Colinet (2010: XXXVII).

(4) Ἕτερον. Λαβὼν ἀρσενίκιν (-ην cod.) ἀναβασμένον ἐξάγιον ἕν· χάλκωμαν ῥινισμένον, ἐξάγια ιε′· τρῖβε τοῦτο μετὰ λευκοῦ λινελαίου (λυναιλαῖου cod.) καλῶς· καὶ πότιζε ἕως ἑπτάκις· εἶτα χώνευσον (χό- cod.) καὶ χῦσον· καὶ πάλιν χώνευσον καὶ χῦσον· [275v] ἔνθες (ἐνθῆς cod.) καὶ ἀσήμιν, ἐξάγια ε′· καὶ ἔκτοτε πάλιν τοῦτο χῦσον, εὑρήσεις (εὐρίσις cod.) δοκιμώτατον ἀσήμιν.

(5) Ἕτερον [in marg.]. Σίλφιον, ἀμμωνιακόν (ἀμον- cod.),[87] χαλβάνην, καὶ ὑάλην βοράχην (βαρά- cod.), ἀνὰ οὐγγίαν μίαν· τρῖψον ταῦτα μετ᾽ ὄξους καὶ λῦσον· καὶ λαβὼν χάλκωμα Ἱσπανικὸν ῥινισμένον, καὶ τουτίαν, ἀνὰ οὐγγίαν μίαν, καὶ σύκα λιπαρά, ζύμωσον ἅπαντα τὰ ῥηθέντα ὁμοῦ· καὶ βαλὼν ταύτα ἐν χωνίῳ, σκέπασον αὐτὰ μεθ᾽ ἑτέρου χωνίου, καὶ χρῖσον τὴν ἁρμογὴν αὐτῶν ἐν πηλῷ πυριμάχῳ· εἶτα λαβὼν ἐξ αὐτοῦ ἐξάγια ε′, καὶ ἀσήμιν καθαρὸν ἐξάγιον ἕν, χώνευσον ὁμοῦ καὶ χῦσον· καὶ ἔσται σοὶ καθαρὸς ἄσημος.

Περὶ χρυσοῦ

(6) [276r] Ὄξος ἐξάγια ν′, ἀρασούκτην, ἐξάγια ιε′, τρίψας καλῶς θὲς ὁμοῦ ἐν βικίῳ ὑαλίνῳ· καὶ θὲς αὐτὸ εἰς ἥλιον δυνατόν, ποιῆσαι ἡμέρας ἑπτά· καὶ τοῦτο τάραττε ἑπτάκις τῆς ἡμέρας· μετὰ τοῦτο ἀνελόμενος, χῶσον αὐτὸ ἐπὶ κοπρέαν ἀλόγων θερμήν· καὶ ἂς ἕνι (ἀσένι cod.) χωσμένον ἡμέρας (-αν cod.) κα′· καὶ μετὰ τοῦτο ἐκβαλὼν αὐτό, λάβε κινάβαριν, οὐγγίας ε′, καὶ τρίβων αὐτὴν πότιζε τοῦ ἐν τῷ βικίῳ κατολίγον, ἕως οὗ πίει τὸ ὅλον τοῦ βικίου ἐν μίᾳ ἡμέρᾳ· εἶτα φρῦξον τοῦτο ἐπὶ ἥλιον θερμόν, ἀνέμου μὴ πνέοντος· τρίψας οὖν πάλιν ὡς ἄλευρον, ἔνθες ἐπὶ μολιβδίνου ἀγγίου καὶ φύλασσε αὐτό· καὶ ὁπόταν θελήσῃς (ὅποτα -σις cod.) [276v] ποιῆσαι μάλαγμα, λάβε ῥινισμένον ἄσπρον χάλκωμαν καὶ ἐκ τῆς <σ>κευασίας (κεβα- cod.) ἐξίσου καὶ λύσας, ἔσται σοι καθαρόν.

(7) Ἕτερον. Λαβὼν σατουνίτζιν (*lege* σαπου- ?), καὶ θεῖον, καὶ ἀρσενίκιν (-ην cod.) κό<κ>κινον, ἀνὰ οὐγγίας β′· ἐμβαλὼν εἰς ἄγγος ὕδωρ καὶ ἔλαιον καθαρόν, καὶ βράσον ὁμοῦ τὰ ῥηθέντα· εἶτα λαβὼν ἄργυρον (☾ cod.) οὐγγίας β′· πύρωνε[88] αὐτό, καὶ τὸ βάνε[89] εἰς τὸ βράσμα, καὶ τύπτε μετὰ σφύρας, καὶ οἱ[90] ἐξ αὐτοῦ πηδῶσαι (πηδοῦ- cod.) λεπίδες· ἀντισταθμήσας, ἕνωσον μαλάγματι ἐξίσου· καὶ λύσας τοῦτο διπλασιάσεις (-σις cod.).

[87] The MS reads 'σίλφιον ἀμονιακόν· χαλβάνην κτλ.' with no semicolon between the first two terms; however, I could not find other mentions of an 'ammoniac laserwort' in Byzantine literature. I have then interpreted 'ἀμονιακόν' as a second, distinct ingredient.

[88] From the Byzantine verb 'πυρώνω' (= πυρόω). [89] From the Byzantine verb 'βάνω' (= βάλλω).

[90] On this form of the feminine article see Colinet (2010: XXX).

(8) Ἕτερον. Λαβὼν χάλκωμαν Ἱσπανικὸν ῥινισμένον, οὐγγίας ὅσας θέλεις, καὶ τουτίαν ἴσην (ἧσιν cod) · ἔτι τε καὶ σύκα λιπαρά· κοπάνισον αὐτά ὑγραίνων (ὑγρένον cod.) τὸ κόπανον ἔλαιον καθαρόν· ἐὰν (ἣν cod.) κοπανίσας,[91] ἕνωσον μετὰ τῶν σύκων πάντα, καὶ βάλον (-ων cod.) εἰς χωνίον [277r] σκεπάσας αὐτὸ καλῶς εἰς τὸ μὴ ἐξατμίζειν (-τμήζην cod.) ποσῶς (-ός cod.)· ἔνθες οὖν πρῶτον ἐπάνω αὐτῶν καὶ σίλφιον, καὶ χώνευσον· καὶ μετὰ τοῦτο ἐκβαλὼν αὐτό, καθὲς (καθὴν cod.) ἐν ἑτέρῳ χωνίῳ τὸ χωνευόμενον (χονεβό- cod.), νὰ ἔνῃ (ἔνι cod.) δὲ τὸ χωνίον πάνυ καθαρόν· βάλον καὶ χρυσόν, ἐξάγιον ἕν, καὶ χύσας κάπνισον αὐτὸ τεάφην, καὶ ἔσται σοι χρυσὸς καθαρός (-ὸν cod.).

(9) Ἕτερον. Ποίησον φοῦρνον, ὡς <τὸ> τοῦ ῥοδοστάγματος, καὶ λαβὼν βικίο (-ω cod.), χρῖσον αὐτὸ (χρύσον αὐτῶ cod.) μετὰ πηλοῦ τῶν χωνίων ἄχρι τῆς μέσης· καὶ ἔνδον βάλον τὸν χρυσόν, ὅνπερ ἐποίησας, καὶ λαβὼν χύτραν κενήν, βάλον (-ων cod.) ἐν αὐτῇ στάκτην, ἕως τὴν μήσην· καὶ ἐν αὐτῇ θὲς τὸ βικίο (-ήω cod.), καὶ αὐτὴν τὴν χύτραν θὲς μετὰ τοῦ βικίου ἐν τῷ τοῦ φούρνου στομίῳ, κάτωθεν δὲ τῆς χύτρας βαλὼν πῦρ ἰσχυρότατον [277v]· καὶ χωνευθὲν (χονευθείς cod.) γενήσεται καθαρὸν μάλαγμα.

(10) Ἕτερον. <Λ>αβὼν λινέλαιον, ἐξάγια μ′, καὶ χάλκωμαν ῥινισμένον, ἐξάγια ιε′, ἔνθες καὶ βικίο (-ω cod.)· καὶ θάψον αὐτὸ (-ῶ cod.) εἰς κόπρον ἵππου νεαράν, καὶ ἂς π<ο>ιήση (-οι cod.) ἡμέρας μ′· εἶτα χώνευσον καὶ χῦσον, καὶ ἔσται σοι χρυσὸς καθαρός.

Σκευασία (σκεβα- cod.) καρυδίνου (καρι- cod.) γλυκύσματος (γλυκή- cod.)· ἠτινοζάω (? *sic*).[92]

ἔπαρον τὰ κάρυα τρυφερὰ καὶ κόψον αὐτὰ ἀπὸ τὴν μύτην τρίγωνιν (?)·[93] καθάρισον (-ω cod.) δὲ καὶ τὸ πιάδιν (?)·[94] εἶτα ἔχε σουγλὴν καὶ τρύπα αὐτὰ σταυροειδῶς καὶ βάλε εἰς τὸ ὕδωρ· καὶ ἄ<λ>λα<σ>σε τα (*lege* το ?)[95] ἡμέρας η′· ἐκ τοῦ ὕδατος ἔκβαλε ταύτα καὶ καθάρισον αὐτά· ἔκτοτε πάλιν βάλο<ν> αὐτὰ εἰς ὕδωρ, καὶ ἄς ποιήσουν[96] ἡμέρας ς′· ἄ<λ>λα<σ>σον τὸ ὕδωρ· ἔπειτα βάνε εἰς τὰς τρύπας καρεόφαλον καὶ τζιτζίβερ· βράσον δὲ μέλιν καὶ ἐξάφρισε το καὶ βάλε τὰ κάρυα μετ᾽ αὐτό· ἔχε σπέτζαν ἐὰν (ἤαν

91 On ‘ἐὰν’ + participle see Colinet (2010: XLIV).

92 A slightly different title is copied again in the margin: ‘σκεβασία τοῦ γληκήσματος τ(ὸν)[?] καρηδήον’.

93 The text is conjectural (I am indebted to Petros Bouras-Vallianatos for this valuable conjecture); the MS reads: ‘αποτ(ὴν) μή τῖν τριγόνιν’.

94 The MS reads: ‘καθάρισω δὲ κετοπιάδιν’.

95 I would have expected a pronoun that refers back to water (rather than to walnuts).

96 Imperative form typical of modern Greek.

cod.) θέλη̣ς τριμ<μ>ένην· καὶ ὅταν τα ποιήση̣ς (-σις cod.), να ἀλλάσση̣ς τὸ μέλιν μέχρις ἄν [α]νοήση̣ς ὅτι παντελῶς ἐξέλθη̣ (-ήλθεν cod.) ἔξω του τὸ ὕδωρ· καὶ ἐν<ωθ>ὲν τὸ μέλιν παστι<λ>λόμενον εἰς αὐτά, τότε πάσον αὐτὰ τὴν σπέτζαν· ἔχε γοῦν μέλιν καλὰ παστι<λ>λόμενον καὶ βάλε τὰ κάρυα εἰς τζουκάλιν καὶ ἐπάνω τὸ μέλιν· καὶ σκέπασον μετὰ χάρτου.

Findings from the alchemical book on the making of gold by Isis (?), Orpheus, and Cleopatra.

(1) Take as much mercury as you want and put it in a newly made, untouched vessel; fill it, I mean, make it full of pure oil, and smear its upper part with the white clay that is used to make good crucibles. Make a hole as small as a needle above, then cover it with a small knife or something else of pure iron. Boil it well until all the oil is burnt, lift the iron, and look at it. If a bit of humidity comes out and the iron is wet, let it burn well. If you see that it is white – I mean the part of the knife or of the iron object, which closes the hole – carefully smear this hole as well with that clay. Shortly after, open it, take ground white sulphur and throw it in the crucible. Stir it well, let it get cold: thus, it gets solid and becomes silver.

(2) Another [recipe]. Melt tin, then dip it in a juice, if it is roasted [dip it] in serous milk of a dog for twenty times. Then chop a *schelan*,[97] that is a sea squill, put the tin in it with ground marcasite[98] on the top; smear the sea squill with red clay and set it on a big charcoal fire; let it rest for two days. You will find silver, except for its black surface. If you strike it with a hammer, it will lose its black colour: it will be pure silver inside.

(3) Another [recipe]. Soda, white lead and milk, boil them together. Take pure iron and boil it well with these substances; dip it in that milk for seventy times. Then take 1 *exagion*[99] of it, 1 exagion of pure silver, and melt them together. Melt together and pour them: it will become pure silver.

(4) Another [recipe]. Take distillate of orpiment, 1 *exagion*; copper filings, 15 *exagia*; grind them well with white linseed oil and moisten them up to seven times. Melt them and pour, then melt them again and pour; put silver as well, 5 *exagia*. Thereafter pour it again, and you will find the noblest silver.

97 Perhaps a late spelling for 'σκίλλα' ('squill'); see Colinet (2010: 22, n. 21).

98 Du Cange (1688) I.879, s.v. μαρκασήτα. See the Arabic term *marqashīthā* (مرقشيثا), with many Latin transliterations, such as *marc(h)as(s)ita*: Käs (2010: II.992–7). It also occurs in the fourteenth-century anonymous treatise on metals first discovered by Zuretti (the so-called *Anonimo di Zuretti*): see the *index verborum* in Colinet (2002: 361–2 and 409): μαρκασίθα, μαρκασίτα, μαρκεσίθα / *marcassita*, *marchasida*, *margasita*, and so forth.

99 Unit of weight (from Latin *exagium*).

(5) Another [recipe]. Laserwort, ammoniac salt, galbanum, and borax-glass, 1 uncia each; grind them with vinegar and make them liquid; take fillings of Spanish copper, cadmia,[100] 1 uncia each, and fatty [juicy] figs, knead all the ingredients mentioned above together, put them in a crucible, cover it with another crucible, and smear their joints with fire-proof clay. Take 5 *exagia* of this product, 1 *exagion* of pure silver, melt them together and pour; you will have pure silver.

On gold

(6) Vinegar, 50 *exagia*; calcined copper,[101] 15 *exagia*; grind them well and put them together in a glass vessel; expose it to strong sunlight, keep it for seven days and shake it seven times a day. Then collect it, cover it with warm dung of a horse, and keep it covered for 21 days. Then take it out and add cinnabar, 5 unciae; having ground the cinnabar, wet it with the content of the vessel little by little, so that it absorbs all the content of the vessel in a day. Then roast it by the heat of the sun, when no wind blows; grid it again like flour, put it in a lead vessel and keep it. If you want to make an alloy, take filings of bright copper and the same quantity of this preparation, and make it liquid: you will have it clean.

(7) Another [recipe]. Take soap,[102] sulphur, and red orpiment, 2 unciae each; pour water and clear vinegar in a bowl and boil the above-mentioned ingredients together; then take silver, 2 unciae, fire it and add it to the boiling matter; strike with an hammer, and [there will be] metal flakes peeling off from it; counterbalance [this loss?] and mix the same amount with the alloy; make it liquid and you will double it.

(8) Another [recipe]. Take filings of Spanish copper, as many unciae as you want, and the same amount of cadmia, and even fatty [juicy] figs; pound them while watering the pestle with clear vinegar; after pounding, mix everything with the figs and put in a crucible, covering it well so that it will not evaporate in large quantities. First, put laserwort as well over these [ingredients] and melt; after this, cast it

100 Zinc oxide; see Du Cange (1688) II.1592, s.v. τουτία. See the Arabic term *tūtiyā* (توتيا, from the Persian دود), which was often transliterated in Latin as *t(h)utia*: Goltz (1972: 259–61); Käs (2010: I.361–72).

101 See Cosmas, *On the Making of Gold*, rec. 9, in ed. Colinet (2010) 70–1. According to this Byzantine recipe book, after being calcined with sulphur in a closed earthen pot, copper becomes the so-called *rhasouktē* or *rhasoukhtē*. The term, of Persian origin, comes from the Arabic *(al-)rūsakhtaj* (روسختج), 'burnt copper', also spelled *rāsukhtaj*: Goltz (1972: 262–3); Käs (2010: I.594–7); see also Lagercrantz (1924: 33) and Colinet (2010: XLVI and 121 n. 35).

102 Du Cange (1688: II.168, s.v. σατουνίτζιν) argues to read 'σαπουνίτζιν' ('soap').

out of [the crucible], and pour the melted [substance] in another crucible, so that the crucible is completely clean. Add gold as well, 1 *exagion*, melt while exposing it to the smoke of sulphur, and you will have pure gold.

(9) Another [recipe]. Built an oven like the one [used to make] distillate of rose,[103] take a little jar and smear it with the clay of crucibles up to the middle [of the jar]; put the gold that you have prepared inside, and taking an empty earthen pot, fill half [the pot] with ashes. Lay the little jar on it [the pot] and put the pot with the jar in the mouth of the oven; make a very strong fire under the earthen pot. After melting, it will become a pure alloy.

(10) Another [recipe]. Take linseed oil, 40 *exagia*; filings of copper, 15 *exagia*; also take a little jar, put it under fresh horse dung and keep it for 40 days. Then melt it and pour; you will have pure gold.

How to prepare a dessert of green walnuts or [?][104]

Take soft walnuts, cut off a little triangular piece from their top [?],[105] and also clean the *piadin* [?].[106] Then, take a skewer, pierce them like a cross, and put them in water; change it [the water] in the course of 8 days; remove from the water and clean them. Then, put them again in water, and let them stay for 6 days; change the water. Then, put clove and ginger[107] in their holes, boil some honey, remove its froth, and mix the walnuts with it.

[103] The term 'ῥοδόσταγμα' refers to an extract of rose often mentioned in late antique and Byzantine medical texts; the production of distillates of rose is typical in Arabic and medieval alchemy and also appears in late Byzantine texts, such as the recipe books ascribed to Nikephoros Blemmydes or the fourteenth-century anonymous treatise on metals discovered by Zuretti (the so-called *Anonymous of Zuretti*): see, for example, Blemmydes, *On Egg-chrysopoia*, rec. 21, in ed. Steiner (2022) 440.13: 'καὶ κτῖσον (*sic*) εἰς φουρνάκιον ὡς τὸ τοῦ ῥοδοστάγματος'; see *Anonymous of Zuretti*, § 67, in ed. Colinet (2002) III.22 (and n. 473): 'ποίησον κατασταλάξαι ὡς ῥοδόσταμαν (*sic*)'.

[104] The manuscript reads 'ἠτι$^{\nu}$οζάω', which I could not interpret properly. This corrupted form might refer to another name of the cake or its main ingredient.

[105] The Greek text 'ἀπὸ τὴν μύτην' is conjectural. The Byzantine term 'μύτη' means 'nose' and is also used to refer to the extremity ('τὸ ἄκρον') of objects, such as the sharp ending of a knife in alchemical recipes: see Colinet (2010: 135, s.v. μύτη). Our recipe describes how to prepare a dessert that is similar to the 'γλυκό καρυδάκι', a traditional Greek sweet: modern recipes prescribe to remove a small triangular piece from the top and the bottom of green walnuts before soaking them in water for eight days. See, for example, the section on local recipes in the Cyprus Tourism Portal (www.visitcyprus.com, accessed 15 March 2020).

[106] It is unclear to me whether the term refers to a part of the walnuts or to kitchenware – for example, a 'πατί(ο)ν' ('dish'), or a πανί(ο)ν, 'a cloth'. Traditional recipes for γλυκό καρυδάκι usually prescribe to peel the green walnuts (an instruction that does not seem to be mentioned in our recipe).

[107] On the various spellings of 'καρεόφυλλον' (such as 'γαρόφαλον', 'καρόφυλλον' or 'καρυόφυλλον'), see Trapp (1994–2017: 765, s.v. καρεόφυλλον); 'τζιτζίβερ' is a Byzantine spelling for forms such as 'ζιγγίβερ', 'ζιζίβερι', and 'ζιγγίβερις': see Trapp (1994–2017, s.v. ζιγγίβερ), Du Cange (1688: II.1571, s.v. τζιτζίπερ).

Also take some spice,[108] after grinding it if you prefer. When you have done this, rework [lit. change] the honey until you notice that the water has fully come out of it. When the honey made into a paste has been mixed with them, then springe the spice over them. Take then the honey well made into a paste, put the walnuts in a vessel[109] and [pour] the honey over them; cover with paper.

REFERENCES

Albini, F. ed. 1988. *Michele Psello, la crisopea ovvero come fabbricare l'oro*. Genoa: Edizioni culturali internazionali.

Alexander, M. 1964. 'Medieval Recipes Describing the Use of Metals in Manuscripts', *Marsyas* 12: 34–53.

Bandt, C. ed. 2007. *Der Traktat 'Vom Mysterium der Buchstaben': Kritischer Text mit Einführung, Übersetzung und Anmerkungen*. Berlin: De Gruyter.

Baroni, S., Pizzigoni, G., and Travaglio, P. eds. 2013. *Mappae clavicula: Alle origini dell'alchimia in Occidente*. Saonara: il Prato.

Barry, J. N., Share, M. J., Smithies A., and Westerink, L. G. eds. 1975. *Mazaris' Journey to Hades: Or Interviews with Dead Men about Certain Officials of the Imperial Court*. Buffalo: State University of New York at Buffalo Press.

Benedetti, L. 2014. 'Ricette bizantine del XII secolo per tinture e inchiostri', *Aevum*, 88: 443–54.

Berthelot, M., and Duval, R. eds. 1893. *La chimie au Moyen Âge: 2. L'alchimie syriaque*. Paris: Imprimerie nationale.

Berthelot, M., and Ruelle, C. E. eds. 1887–8. *Collection des anciens alchimistes grecs*. 3 vols. Paris: Georges Steinheil.

Bidez, J. et al. 1924–32. *Catalogue des manuscrits alchimiques grecs*. 8 vols. Brussels: Union Académique Internationale (=*CMAG*).

Bidez, J. ed. 1928. *Michel Psellus, Epître sur la Chrysopée, opuscules et extraits sur l'alchimie, la météorologie et la démonologie* (*CMAG* VI). Brussels: Lamertin (Union Académique Internationale).

Bouras-Vallianatos, P. 2015. 'Greek Manuscripts at the Wellcome Library in London: A Descriptive Catalogue', *Medical History* 59.2: 275–326.

Bouras-Vallianatos, P. 2018. 'Enrichment of the Medical Vocabulary in the Greek-Speaking Medieval Communities of Southern Italy', in B. Pitarakis and G. Tanman (eds.), *'Life Is Short, Art Long': The Art of Healing in Byzantium. New Perspectives*. Istanbul: Istanbul Research Institute, 155–84.

Bouras-Vallianatos, P. 2020. *Innovation in Byzantine Medicine: The Writings of John Zacharias Aktouarios (c.1275–c.1330)*. Oxford: Oxford University Press.

[108] For the term 'σπέτζα' (or 'σπέτσα'), from the Italian 'spezia' ('spice'), see Du Cange (1688: II.1421, s.v. σπετζίαις).

[109] For the term 'τζουκάλι' (or 'τσουκάλι'), from the Italian 'zucca' ('pumpkin'), see Colinet (2010: XLV).

Bouras-Vallianatos, P. 2021. 'Cross-Cultural Transfer of Medical Knowledge in the Medieval Mediterranean: The Introduction and Dissemination of Sugar-Based Potions from the Islamic World to Byzantium', *Speculum* 96.4: 963–1008.

Capone Ciollaro, M. ed. 2003. *Demetrio Pepagomeno, Prontuario medico, testo edito per la prima volta, con introduzione, apparato critic e indice*. Naples: Bibliopolis.

Capone Ciollaro, M., and Galli Calderini, I. G. 1999. 'Aezio Amideno in Teofane Nonno-Crisobalante', in A. Garzia and J. Jouanna (eds.), *I testi medici greci: Tradizione ed ecdotica. Atti del III Convegno Internazionale (Napoli, 15–18 ottobre 1997)*. Naples: M. D'Auria Editore, 29–50.

Cataldi Palau, A. 2010. 'Mazaris, Giorgio Baiophoros e il monastero di Prodromo Petra', *Νέα Ῥώμη* 7: 367–97.

Colinet, A. 2000. 'Le travail des quatre éléments ou lorsqu'un alchimiste byzantin s'inspire de Jabir', in I. Draelants, A. Tihon, and B. van den Abeele (eds.), *Occident et Proche-Orient: Contacts scientifiques au temps des croisades*. Turnhout: Brepols, 165–90.

Colinet, A. ed. 2002. *Les alchimistes grecs,* x: *L'Anonyme de Zuretti ou L'art sacré et divin de la chrysopée par un anonyme*. Paris: Les Belles Lettres.

Colinet, A. ed. 2010. *Les alchimistes grecs,* xi : *Recettes alchimiques (Par. gr. 2419; Holkhamicus 109). Cosmas le hiéromoine, Chrysopée*. Paris: Les Belles Lettres.

De Gregorio, G. 2019. 'Un'aggiunta su copisti greci del secolo XIV. A proposito di Giovanni Duca Malace, collaboratore di Giorgio Galesiota, nell'Athen. *EBE* 2', *Νέα Ῥώμη* 16: 161–276.

Delacenserie, E. 2014. 'Le traité de diététique de Hiérophile: Analyse interne', *Byzantion* 84: 81–103.

Delatte, A. ed. 1927–39. *Anecdota Atheniensia*. 2 vols. Paris: Droz.

Du Cange, C. 1688. *Glossarium ad scriptores mediae et infimae Graecitatis*. 2 vols. Lyon: Anisson; Posuel; Rigaud.

Eijk, P. J. van der 2010. 'Principles and Practices of Compilation and Abbreviation in the Medical "Encyclopedias" of Late Antiquity', in M. Horster and C. Reitz (eds.), *Condensing Texts: Condensed Texts*. Stuttgart: Franz Steiner, 519–54.

Eijk, P. J. van der, Geller, M., Lehmhaus, L., Martelli, M., and Salazar, C. 2015. 'Canons, Authorities and Medical Practice in the Greek Medical Encyclopaedias of Late Antiquity and in the Talmud', in E. Cancik-Kirschbaum and A. Traninger (eds.), *Wissen in Bewegung. Institution – Iteration – Transfer*. Wiesbaden: Harrassowitz, 195–221.

Felici, L. 1981–2. 'L'opera medica di Teofane Nonno in manoscritti inediti', *Acta medicae historiae Patavina* 28: 59–74.

Festugière, A.-J. 1950². *La révélation d'Hermès Trismégiste, vol. 1: L'astrologie et les sciences occultes*. Paris: J. Gabalda.

Froidefond, C. ed. 1988. *Plutarque, Oeuvres morales, Tome V – 2ᵉ partie: Isis et Osiris*. Paris: Les Belles Lettres.

Gamillscheg, E., Harfinger, D., Hunger H., and Eleuteri, P. 1981–97. *Repertorium der griechischen Kopisten 800–1600*. 3 vols in 9 pts. Vienna: Verlag der Österreichischen Akademie der Wissenschaften (=*RGK*).

Garland, L. 2007. 'Mazaris' Journey to Hades: Further Reflections and Reappraisal', *Dumbarton Oaks Papers* 61: 183–214.

Goltz, G. 1972. *Studien zur Geschichte der Mineralnamen in Pharmazie, Chemie und Medizin von den Anf den Anfängen bis Paracelsus*. Wiesbaden: F. Steiner.

Gwyn Griffiths, J. ed. 1970. *Plutarch's De Iside et Osiride*. Cardiff: University of Wales Press.

Halleux, R. ed. 1981. *Les alchimistes grecs, vol. 1, Papyrus de Leyde, papyrus de Stockholm, fragments de recettes*. Paris: Les belles lettres.

Halleux, R., and Meyvaert, P. 1987. 'Les origines de la *Mappae clavicula*', *Archives d'histoire doctrinale et littéraire du Moyen Âge* 62: 5–58.

Hultsch, F. ed. 1864–6. *Metrologicorum scriptorum reliquiae*. 2 vols. Leipzig: Teubner.

Ideler, J. L. ed. 1841–2. *Physici et medici Graeci minores*. 2 vols. Berlin: G. Reimer.

Ieraci Bio, A. M. 1982. 'I testi medici di uso strumentale', *Jahrbuch der Österreichischen Byzantinistik* 32: 33–43.

Ieraci Bio, A. M. 2017. 'La sistematizzazione della farmacologia a Bisanzio', in L. Lehmhaus and M. Martelli (eds.), *Collecting Recipes: Byzantine and Jewish Pharmacology in Dialogue*. Berlin: De Gruyter, 301–14.

Käs, F. 2010. *Die Mineralien in der arabischen Pharmakognosie*. 2 vols. Wiesbaden: Harrassowitz.

Katsiampoura, G. 2018. 'The Relationship between Alchemy and Natural Philosophy in Byzantine Times', in E. Nicolaidis (ed.), *Greek Alchemy from Late Antiquity to Early Modernity*. Turnhout: Brepols, 119–29.

Kostomoiris, G. A. ed. 1892. *Ἀετίου λόγος δωδέκατος*. Paris: C. Klincksieck.

Krallis, D. 2016. 'Harmless Satire, Stinging Critique: Notes and Suggestions for Reading the *Timarion*', in D. Angelov and M. Saxby (eds.), *Power and Subversion in Byzantium: Papers from the Forty-Third Spring Symposium of Byzantine Studies, University of Birmingham, March 2010*. London: Routledge, 221–46.

Kraus, P. 1933. 'Zu Ibn al-Muqaffa'', *Rivista degli studi orientali* 14: 1–20.

Kraus, P. 1942. *Jābir ibn Ḥayyān. Contribution à l'histoire des idées scientifiques dans l'Islam, vol. II: Jābir et la science grecque*. Cairo: Imprimerie de l'IFAO.

Kühn, C. G. ed. 1821–33. *Claudii Galeni opera omnia*. 20 vols. in 22 pts. Leipzig: Knobloch.

Lagercrantz, O. ed. 1924. 'Les recettes alchimiques du *Codex Holkhamicus*', in *CMAG* III.30–81.

Lagercrantz, O. 1932. 'Über das Verhältnis des Codex *Parisinus* 2327 (= A) zum Codex *Marcianus* 299 (= M). Fortsetzung von Catalogue II 341–358', in *CMAG* IV.399–432.

Lazaris, S. 2006. 'La production nouvelle en médecine vétérinaires sous les Paléologues et l'oeuvre cynégétique de Dèmètrios Pépagôménos', in M. Cacouros and M.-H. Congourdeau (eds.), *Philosophie et sciences à Byzance de 1204 à 1453 : Les textes, les doctrines et leur transmission*. Leuven: Uitgeverij Peeters, 225–67.

Leontsini, M., and Merianos, G. 2016. 'From Culinary to Alchemical Recipes: Various Uses of Milk and Cheese in Byzantium', in I. Anagnostakis and A. Pellettieri (eds.), *Latte e Latticini: Aspetti della produzione e del consumo nelle società mediterranee dell'Antichità e del Medioevo*. Lagonero: Grafica Zaccara, 205–22.

Letrouit, J. 1995. 'Chronologie des alchimistes grecs', in D. Kahn and S. Matton (eds.), *Alchimie: Art, histoire et mythes*. Paris: S.É.H.A/Arché, 9–93.

Magdalino, P., and Mavroudi, M. eds. 2006. *The Occult Sciences in Byzantium*. Geneva: La Pomme d'Or.

Marasco, G. 1998. 'Cléopâtre et les sciences de son temps', in G. Argoud and J. - Y. Guillaumin (eds.), *Sciences exactes et sciences appliquées à Alexandrie*. Saint-Étienne: Université de Saint-Étienne, 39–53.

Martelli, M. ed. 2011. *Pseudo Democrito, Scritti alchemici con il commentario di Sinesio*. Paris: S.É.H.A/Archè.

Martelli, M. ed. 2013. *The Four Books of Pseudo-Democritus*. Leeds: Maney.

Martelli, M. 2014. 'The Alchemical Art of Dyeing: The Fourfold Division of Alchemy and the Enochian Tradition', in S. Dupré (ed.), *Laboratories of Art: Alchemy and Art Technology from Antiquity to the 18th Century*. London: Springer, 1–22.

Martelli, M. 2018. 'Byzantine Alchemy in Two Recently Discovered Manuscripts in Saint Stephen's (Meteora) and Olympiotissa's (Elassona) Monasteries', in E. Nicolaidis (ed.), *Greek Alchemy from Late Antiquity to Early Modernity*. Turnhout: Brepols, 99–118.

Martelli, M. 2019a. *L'alchimista antico: Dall'Egitto greco-romano a Bisanzio*. Milano: Editrice Bibliografica.

Martelli, M. 2019b. 'Galen in Late Antique, Byzantine, and Syro-Arabic Alchemical Traditions', in P. Bouras-Vallianatos and B. Zipser (eds.), *Brill's Companion to the Reception of Galen*. Leiden: Brill, 577–93.

Mavroudi, M. 2002. *A Byzantine Book on Dream Interpretation: The* Oneirocriticon of Achmet *and Its Arabic Sources*. Leiden: Brill.

Merianos, G. 2017. 'Alchemy', in A. Kaldellis and N. Siniossoglou (eds.), *The Cambridge Intellectual History of Byzantium*. Cambridge: Cambridge University Press, 234–51.

Mertens, M. ed. 1995. *Les alchimistes grecs. Tome 4, 1ère partie, Zosime de Panopolis: mémoires authentiques*. Paris: Les Belles lettres.

Mioni, E. 1981. *Bibliothecae divi Marci Venetiarum, Codices Graeci manuscripti. Thesaurus antiquus, vol. 1: Codices 1–299*. Rome: Istituto polografico e zecca dello Stato, Libreria dello Stato.

Mosshammer, A. A. ed. 1984. *Georgius Syncellus: Ecloga chronographica*. Leipzig: Teubner.

Olivieri, A. ed. 1935–50. *Aetii Amideni Libri medicinales*. 2 vols. Leipzig: Teubner.

Olivieri, A., and Festa, N. 1895. 'Indice dei codici greci bolognesi delle biblioteche Universitaria e Comunale di Bologna', *Studi italiani di filologia classica* 3: 385–494.

Omont, H. 1888. *Inventaire sommaire des manuscrits grecs de la Bibliothèque Nationale. Seconde partie, Ancien fonds grec: Droit–Histoire–Sciences*. Paris: Alphonse Picard.

Papathanassiou, M. K. ed. 2017. *Stephanos von Alexandria und sein alchemistisches Werk: Die kritische Edition des griechischen Textes eingeschlossen*. Athens.

Raeder, J. ed. 1926. *Oribasii Synopsis ad Eustathium, Libri ad Eunapium*. Leipzig: Teubner.

Reitzenstein, R. 1919. 'Zur Geschichte der Alchemie und des Mystizismus', *Nachrichten von der Königlichen Gesellschaft der Wissenschaften zu Göttingen*, s.n.: 1–37.

Roberts, A. M. 2020. 'Framing a Middle Byzantine Alchemical Codex', *Dumbarton Oaks Papers* 73: 69–102.

Roberts, A. M. 2022. 'Byzantine Engagement with Islamicate Alchemy', *Isis* 113: 559–80.

Romano, R. ed. 1999. 'Il calendario dietetico di Ierofilo', *Atti della Accademia Pontaniana* 47: 197–222.

Saffrey, H. D. 1995. 'Historique et description du manuscrit alchimique de Venise *Marcianus Graecus* 299', in D. Kahn and S. Matton (eds.), *Alchimie: Art, histoire et mythes*. Paris: S.É.H.A/Arché, 1–10.

Schreiner, P., and Oltrogge, D. eds. 2011. *Byzantinische Tinten-, Tuschen- und Farbrezepte*. Vienna: Österreichischen Akademie der Wissenschaften.

Sonderkamp, J. A. M. 1987. *Untersuchungen zur Überlieferung der Schriften des Theophanes Chrysobalantes (sog. Theophanes Nonnos)*. Bonn: Dr. Rudolf Habelt GMBH (Freie Universität Berlin byzantinisch-neugriechisches Seminar).

Steiner, S. ed. 2022. 'Nikephoros Blemmydes: Concerning Gold Making', in F. Spingou (ed.), *The Visual Culture of Later Byzantium (c. 1081–c.1350)*. Cambridge: Cambridge University Press, 432–44.

Totelin, L. 2017. 'The Third Way: Galen, Pseudo-Galen, Metrodora, Cleopatra and the Gynaecological Pharmacology of Byzantium', in L. Lehmhaus and M. Martelli (eds.), *Collecting Recipes: Byzantine and Jewish Pharmacology in Dialogue*. Berlin: De Gruyter, 103–22.

Touwaide, A. 2007. 'Byzantine Hospital Manuals (*Iatrosophia*) As a Source for the Studies of Therapeutics', in B. Bowers (ed.), *The Medieval Hospital and Medical Practice*. Aldershot: Ashgate, 147–74.

Touwaide, A. 1999. 'Lexica medico-botanica byzantina: Prolégomènes à une étude', in L. Pérez Castro, F. Adrados, and L. de Cuenca (eds.), *Tês filiês tade dôra: Miscelánea léxica en memoria de Conchita Serrano (Manuales y Anejos de 'Emerita', XLI)*. Madrid: National Foundation for Scientific Research, Center of Humanities, 211–28.

Trapp, E. 1994–2017. *Lexikon zur byzantinischen Gräzität, besonders des 9.-12. Jahrhunderts*. 8 vols. Vienna: Verlag der Österreichischen Akademie der Wissenschaften.

Trapp, E., Walther, R., and Beyer, H.-V., eds. 1976–96. *Prosopographisches Lexikon der Palaiologenzeit*. 12 vols. Vienna: Verlag der Österreichischen Akademie der Wissenschaften (=*PLP*).

Ullmann, M. 1972. *Die Natur- und Geheimwissenschaften im Islam*. Leiden: Brill.

Valentino, D. ed. 2016. *Das Iatrosophion des Codex Taur. B.VII.18*. Munich: Ars Una Neuried.

Valiakos, I. ed. 2019. *Das Dynameron des Nikolaos Myrepsos*. Heidelberg: Propylaeum.

Viano, C. 2018. 'Byzantine Alchemy, or the Era of Systematization', in P. T. Keyser and J. Scarborough (eds.), *The Oxford Handbook of Science and Medicine in the Classical World*. Oxford: Oxford University Press, 943–64.

Wallraff, M., Scardino, C., Mecella, L., and Guignard, C. eds. 2012. Iulius Africanus, Cesti, *translated by William Adler*. Berlin: De Gruyter.

Zervos, S. ed. 1911. 'Ἀετίου Ἀμιδηνοῦ Λόγος Ἔνατος', *Ἀθηνᾶ* 23: 265–392. [Reedited in *Aetius aus Amida, über die Leiden am Magenmund, des Magens selbst und der Gedärme, Buch IX der Sammlung zur ersten Mal nach den Handschriften veröffentlicht*. Athens: P. D. Sakellarios, 1912.]

Zipser, B. ed. 2009. *John the Physician's Therapeutics: A Medical Handbook in Vernacular Greek*. Leiden: Brill.

Zipser, B. 2019. 'Galen in Byzantine *Iatrosophia*', in P. Bouras-Vallianatos and B. Zipser (eds.), *Brill's Companion to the Reception of Galen*. Leiden: Brill, 111–23.

CHAPTER 12

Making Connections between the Medical Properties of Stones and Philosophy in the Work of Albertus Magnus

Athanasios Rinotas

12.1 Introduction

In the early Middle Ages Isidore of Seville (570–636) depicted the character of medicine[1] as follows:

> Medicine is the art that protects or restores the body's health; its subject matter concerns illnesses and wounds. To medicine belong not only things practiced by the skill of those properly called physicians (*medicus*), but also matters of food and drink, clothing and shelter.[2]

In a similar manner, at the end of his account, the medieval scholar touches upon a crucial question, which continued to be asked up to the end of the high Middle Ages and which concerns the epistemological status of medicine:

> Some people ask why the art of medicine is not included in the other liberal disciplines. It is for this reason: the liberal disciplines treat individual topics, but medicine treats the topics of all. Thus the physician ought to know grammar, so that he can understand and explain what he reads. Similarly he must know rhetoric, so that he is capable of summing up the cases he treats with true arguments. He must also know dialectic in order to scrutinize and cure the causes of disease with the application of reason. So also arithmetic, to reckon the number of hours in the onsets of illness, and their periods of days. Likewise with geometry, so that from his knowledge of the qualities of regions and the location of places, he may teach what a person should attend to there. Then, music will not be unknown to him, for we read of many things that have been accomplished for sick people by way of this discipline – as we read of David who rescued Saul from an unclean spirit with the art of

[1] There are many excellent introductions to medieval medicine – for example: Riddle (1974), Ottosson (1984), Siraisi (1990), Wallis (2005a, 2005b), Jacquart (2013), and Park (2013).

[2] Isidore of Seville, *Etymologies*, trans. Barney et al. (2006) 109.

> melody. The physician Asclepiades also restored a certain victim of frenzy to perfect health through harmonious sounds. Finally, he will be acquainted with astronomy, through which he may observe the logic of the stars and the change of seasons. For, as a certain physician says, according to their mutations our bodies are also changed. Thus medicine is called the Second Philosophy, for each discipline claims for itself the entire human: by philosophy the soul is cured; by medicine, the body.[3]

This description stresses from the very beginning medicine's dependency on the liberal arts, or, to put it in another way, on 'officially institutionalised' knowledge. Nevertheless, at the end it is called the 'second philosophy', thus alluding to the strong ties between the two disciplines. Yet, as Jacquart has noted,[4] medicine had a long way to go before it could be said to be a 'Second Philosophy'. Many factors contributed to hindering the acknowledgement of medicine as an academic discipline up to the tenth century, and it was not until the thirteenth century that it became a university discipline in the universities of Paris, Montpellier, and Bologna, and thus established strong ties with philosophy.[5]

It is precisely in the milieu of the thirteenth century that we find Albertus Magnus (1200–80). The Dominican master did not see himself as a *medicus* per se and therefore we shall not come across any book by him dedicated to medicine. However, this does not mean that Albertus was indifferent to the *scientia medica*, since he commented on various subjects connected to the theory of humours, the notion of *complexio*, and especially discrepancies highlighted by the Aristotle-Galen controversy.[6] But Albertus, a wide-ranging thinker, connected medicine with other doctrines of ambiguous character like magic and alchemy and, moreover, in *On Minerals* he seems to be trying to create real links between the three disciplines. This brings us to the central focus of this chapter. Briefly, the aim of this chapter is to examine how the medical properties of stones are related to certain philosophical doctrines of Albertus. Two questions are going to guide the reasoning in this chapter. First, does Albertus account

[3] Isidore of Seville, *Etymologies*, trans. Barney et al. (2006) 115.

[4] Jacquart (1998a: 199).

[5] Talbot (1978: 396–402); Ottosson (1984); Jacquart and Micheau (1990); Lindberg (1992: 317–25); Jacquart (1998b); Nutton (2013).

[6] Albertus' commentaries on Aristotle's natural works dealt with topics that overlapped with Galenic medical doctrines and therefore discrepancies between the two authorities emerged. These included, for example, the question of whether the heart or the brain is the source of our nervous system, while another controversial topic pertained to generation and its connection to male and female sperm. Siraisi (1980: 399–403) noted that, in general, Albertus tried to reconcile the two authorities, but on 'major issues' he favoured Aristotle. However, in his recent study Asúa (2013) showed that Albertus mostly attempted to mediate between and reconcile the two authorities rather than aligning himself with Aristotle.

for the 'magical properties' of stones philosophically? Second, when Albertus says that *celidonius* can be used against epilepsy, is this something he has adopted from past authorities, or can we find some sort of justification for this claim in his philosophical work or at least some compatibility with his philosophical thinking? In approaching this topic I will first give an introduction to Albertus' attitude towards medicine and then I will answer the first question by showing how the Dominican master accounts for the properties of stones. In the second part of this chapter I will take two case studies, one on melancholy and one on epilepsy, conditions that were thought to be susceptible to treatment by certain stones. My aim here is to show that Albertus' theories with regard to melancholy and epilepsy provide some evidence that can relate them philosophically with the properties of stones. Finally, I would like to stress that, in terms of methodology, this chapter will not deal with any external sources that might have influenced Albertus on the subject, but will attempt an 'internal study', considering various works by Albertus that pertain to the topic under examination.

12.2 Albertus Magnus' Medical Thought and Learning

Albertus Magnus' references to medicine are scattered throughout almost his entire work, but it is especially in the books that describe the 'natural sciences' that he deals in depth and in detail with medical issues. Already in his *Physica*, which was the first of his Aristotelian paraphrases, written a little after 1250,[7] Albertus states his attitude towards medicine:

> Augustine is to be preferred rather than the philosophers in case of disagreement in matters of faith. But if the discussion concerns medicine, I would rather believe Galen or Hippocrates, and if it concerns things of nature, Aristotle or anyone else experienced in natural things.[8]

This passage introduces two key words which are very important if we are to understand its content: *disagreement* and *authorities.* From a very early point in his project of commenting on Aristotle, Albertus became aware that there were many 'grey areas' of knowledge between the disciplines of philosophy, theology, and medicine due to overlapping subjects and

[7] Concerning the dates of Albertus Magnus' works I follow Weisheipl (1980: 565–77).

[8] Albert the Great, *On the IV Books of the Sentences*, 2.13.2, ed. Borgnet (1893) I.246b: *Unde sciendum, quod Augustino in his quae sunt de fide et moribus plusquam Philosophis credendum est, si dissentiunt. Sed si de medicina loqueretur, plus ego crederem Galeno, vel Hipocrati: et si de naturis rerum loquatur, credo Aristoteli plus vel alii experto in rerum naturis.* English translation taken from Siraisi (1980: 382).

therefore he was ready to accept certain figures as authorities in their field. Yet one should bear in mind some things about Albertus' medical background. In 1220 Albertus was in Padua, which was a centre of medical learning. Despite his stay there and the evidence for the availability of medical teaching in the Italian city, we have no substantial evidence that Albertus studied medicine there and, as Siraisi has shown, the only thing that we are sure of is that by that time there were many men who were well versed in medicine in Padua.[9] The Dominican master seems to have acquired his medical knowledge through his personal reading over a long period of time. As a result, the important question that emerges is what kind of books Albertus consulted. Again Siraisi has cast some light on the matter by adducing that Albertus' main source was Ibn Sīnā (Avicenna), whereas the absence of references or even allusions to Hippocrates in his work is quite striking.[10] Even for Galen, it is very difficult to prove which Galenic books he had read and whether Albertus had them in his possession. In all probability it was through Ibn Sīnā that Albertus became acquainted with Galen.

In light of this, Albertus' reference to Hippocrates should be mostly understood in terms of his acknowledging a traditional medical authority. Galen, on the other hand, is a different matter. In fact, due to the Arabo-Latin translation movement, Galen had become better known and was established as an important medical authority. But as his works became more widely disseminated and studied, it became evident that he overlapped with Aristotelian doctrines on some medical topics. This was also noticed by Albertus, who seriously engaged with the task of highlighting, explicating, and amending the differences between the two authorities. As Asúa has suggested, even though Albertus was a natural philosopher he did not necessarily come down on the side of philosophy, but rather he tried to reconcile the two disciplines by making use of certain techniques and exegetical tools.[11] So, what, in fact, was Albertus' thinking on the relationship between medicine and philosophy? A preliminary answer is attempted in his *On Sense and What Is Sensed*:

> It is no part of *physica* to treat of sickness and health, but only of first principles and causes. However, the principles of life are the same as those of health and the principles of death the same as those of sickness . . . therefore in considering the principles of life one has to consider those of health, and in considering the principles of death one has to consider the first principles of sickness and from them the causes of disease. And therefore many of the *physici* and the more skilled among the medici who use the philosophical art

[9] Siraisi (1980: 386–7). On Albertus' medicine, see also Schipperges (1980).
[10] Siraisi (1980: 389–91). [11] Asúa (2013).

> to the greatest extent end up at the same point (*terminantur adinvicem*). For the *physici*, coming from first principles to their consequences and from universal considerations to particulars, end their thoughts about living things by reaching matters which have to do with medicine, namely the particular causes of health and sickness. But those physicians (*medici*) who use the art of *physica* ascend from particular diseases to general signs and causes and *accidentia*; for they do not cure the disease unless they remove its causes and draw out the causes of health.[12]

In the aforementioned work by Albertus, written around 1256, he points out that, while both disciplines deal with the first principles and causes of life and death, philosophy fulfils its goal by 'descending' from these first principles to the particulars, whereas medicine attains its end by going in the opposite direction – that is, by 'ascending' from the particular to the first principles and causes. This text has caused some modern scholars to regard Albertus as an innovative scholar for the thirteenth century, who acknowledged medicine as a science.[13] As tempting as this conclusion might seem, one should look deeper into the sources in order to describe more accurately the Dominican master's attitude towards the two disciplines. Some years later, around 1258, Albertus wrote his *Questions concerning Aristotle's* On Animals, in which he examines the question of whether this book was only about animals and here he clearly asserts that medicine is subordinate to philosophy. In particular, he stresses:

> Besides, an animal is composed of body and soul. Therefore, any treatment of animals can be threefold: either in terms of the soul, in terms of the body or in terms of the soul as it is related to the body. But the soul is treated in the book 'on the soul'. Moreover, the body is sufficiently treated in the book the 'Physics' and in other subordinate sciences like medicine.[14]

[12] Albert the Great, *On Sense and What Is Sensed*, 1.1, ed. Borgnet (1890a) 2b: *ed de sanitate et infirmitate non est physici considerare, sed tantum prima principia et causas. Sunt etenim eadem principia vitae et sanitatis et mortis et infirmitatis. Quod autem physici sit considerare de primis principiis et causis istorum, patet ex eo quod sanitas et infirmitas non accidunt carentibus vita: et ideo considerans principia vitae, considerare habet principia sanitatis: et considerans principia mortis, considerare habet principia infirmitatis prima, et de ipsis causis aegritudinis. Et ideo plurimi physicorum et peritiores eorum medicorum qui maxime philosophica arte utuntur, terminantur ad invicem. Physici enim venientes a primis in posteriora, et ab universalibus in particularia, terminant considerationes suas de animatis ad ea quae sunt medicinae, quae sunt causae sanitatis et infirmitatis particulares. Medici autem physicae arte utentes a particularibus aegritudinibus in signa et causas et accidentia communia ascendunt: eo quod morbum non sanant nisi remota causa morbi, et inducta causa sanitatis.* English translation taken from Siraisi (1980: 382).

[13] In fact, Siraisi (1980: 382) spoke of 'a highly positive appraisal of learned medicine as an intellectual discipline', while Reynolds (1999: 135–6) argued that the two disciplines 'meet half way'.

[14] Albert the Great, *Questions concerning Aristotle's* On Animals, 1.1, ed. Filthaut (1955) 77: *Praeterea, animal componitur ex corpore et anima. Ergo consideratio de animali potest esse tripliciter: vel ratione animae vel ratione corporis vel ratione animae comparatae ad corpus. Sed consideratio de anima traditur*

In this text Albertus treats medicine as a science, but as a subordinate one, and therefore it seems that he is not yet convinced of medicine's efficacy and status. A plausible explanation for his attitude could be his personal experience of and contact with physicians through which he had been able to see and evaluate the average 'scientific' level of medicine's representatives. For instance, in the same book Albertus refers to his refuting of a physician in Cologne, who was accustomed to regard urine as a simple body.[15] Extrapolating from this, it is perhaps for this reason that Albertus refers to the *perfectus medicus* (perfect physician) in his *On Animals*, written between 1260 and 1261. In fact, according to Albertus, the perfect physician uses prudent judgement to ascertain first causes, which signify in turn the causes of death and disease, and says that it was due to his ascertaining these first causes that he would become the perfect physician.[16] In general, Albertus' zoological books are the ones which are most closely connected with medicine and therefore one could say that it was in these books that the Dominican master treated the relationship between the two fields most intensively. And it was probably at that stage that he grasped medicine's practical weakness in sometimes being unable to fully ascertain the first principles and causes of things. Following this line of thinking, one can explain Albertus' scorn towards those physicians who were ignorant of philosophy and reason and yet gave their opinion on Galen and philosophy when it was not appropriate for them to do so.[17] However, this should not be considered as a shift in Albertus' opinion of medicine in general and his remarks in this respect in *On Sense and What Is Sensed*. In my opinion in that book Albertus describes the potential of medicine and the theoretical status it could achieve if practised with 'prudent judgement', whereas in the zoological books he mostly refers to the actual state of medicine – that is, a discipline which was largely scientific but had not yet accomplished its full potential. Yet, it is also in his zoological books that Albertus introduces the notion of the 'perfect physician' and thus he also leaves room for medicine to fulfil its higher purpose.[18]

in libro de anima. Consideratio autem de corpore sufficienter traditur in libro physicorum et in aliis scientiis subalternis, ut medicina. English translation is taken from Resnick and Kitchell (2008: 13).

15 Albert the Great, *Questions concerning Aristotle's* On Animals, 1.1, ed. Filthaut (1955) 168: *Et per istam distinctionem quondam medicum Coloniae confudi, qui dicebat urinam esse simpliciter corpus simplex.*

16 Albert the Great, *On Animals*, 10.1.2, ed. Stadler (1916) I.740: *Si enim homo per aestimationem prudentem investiget de causis mortis aut infirmitatis et aliorum quaecumque nomine et ratione conveniunt istis, oportet ipsum pervenire ad primas causas istorum et ad accidentia quae significant ea: et tunc erit perfectus medicus.*

17 Albert the Great, *On Animals*, 3.2.8, ed. Stadler (1916) I.345: *Medici autem quidam ignari rationis et philosophiae, Galieni praeferunt sententiam, licet non ad eos pertineat de uno vel de alio proferre iudicium.*

18 Asúa (2013: 288 and 296) draws on Albertus' zoological works in order to argue that the Dominican master 'had adopted an epistemological distinction between the physicians who followed the

12.3 Accounting for the Medical Properties of Stones through Philosophy

Having seen how Albertus conceived of the ties between philosophy and medicine, it is time to turn to a more specific aspect of Albertus' thought, which concerns the medical properties of stones and how they could be related to and explained through his philosophy. In order to deal more comprehensively with this question I will first present a short account of Albertus' natural philosophical theory of stones, which will serve as an intellectual basis from which to proceed with the special case studies of those stones that are supposed to treat or influence 'mental' diseases, such as epilepsy and melancholy.

Albertus provides an extensive treatment on the subject of stones in the first two chapters of his *On Minerals*.[19] Apart from the stones as such he extends his study to other topics relevant to them like their 'magical powers' and the sigils that were purported to enhance these powers through the influence of celestial bodies. From the very beginning of the book, the Dominican master notes that he does not have the Aristotelian books on minerals at his disposal but only some chapters from Ibn Sīnā, which in turn offer only an inadequate treatment of the subject.[20] A bit later in this text Albertus' focus is centred on the traditional authorities who have spoken of stones, like Hermes Trismegistus, Dioscorides, and Pliny the Elder. But their works are also insufficient, though Pliny's is the most deficient because he does not treat the common causes of the stones 'in a wise way'.[21] Thus Albertus signalled the method with which he is going to handle and present his material – that is, by making use of the four Aristotelian causes as explanatory means of the 'physics' of stones.[22]

appearances and the philosophers who aspire to reach the ultimate truth of things'. Thus, Asúa gives the impression that this is a fixed distinction in Albertus' mind. However, in my opinion, Albertus' notion of *perfectus medicus* leaves room for the aforementioned distinction to be reconsidered, provided that the 'perfect physician' can reach the ultimate truth of things by attaining the first causes through prudent judgement.

19 For general studies on Albertus' *On Minerals* see Riddle and Mulholland (1980), Angel (1992), and Jeck (1998).

20 Albert the Great, *On Minerals*, 1.1.1, ed. Borgnet (1890b) 1a: *De his autem libros Aristotelis non vidimus, nisi excerptos per partes. Et hoc quae tradidit Avicenna de his in tertio capitulo priori sui libri quem fecit de his, non sufficiunt.*

21 Albert the Great, *On Minerals*, 1.1.1, ed. Borgnet (1890b) 2: *Sunt autem quidam maximae auctoritatis in philosophia viri, qui non de omnibus, sed de quibusdam lapidum generibus tractatum facientes, sufficientem se dicunt de lapidibus fecisse mentionem, quales sunt Hermes Cuates rex Arabum, Diascorides, Aaron, et Joseph, qui de lapidibus tantum pretiosis tractantes, non de genere lapidum tractaverunt. Minus autem sufficientem notitiam tradidit Plinius in Historia naturali, non sapienter causas lapidum in communi assignans.*

22 On Albertus' methodology on minerals, see Asúa (2001: 389–93, 397–400).

In general, stones for Albertus are *commixta*, which means simple mixtures of elements, and thus the material cause of them is either a form of earth or a form of water:

> We say in general that the material of a stone is either some form of Earth or some form of Water. For one or the other of these elements predominates in stones; and even in stones in which some form of Water seems to predominate, something of Earth is also important.[23]

In this excerpt Albertus establishes the direct relation of the stones to the elements. Moreover, the elements of Earth and Water are always interrelated in stones and, depending on which one is dominant over the other, the results will be different. In particular, the stones made of Earth have Water in the form of moisture as a factor of coherence within the stone. Alternatively, the stones made of Water have Earth as a determinant of their transparency. Turning to the efficient cause, the Dominican master introduces the notion of mineralising power, which is responsible for the formation not only of stones, but also of metals. Yet he admits that, since there is no certain name for it, he will have to describe it by analogy.[24] In order to clarify his line of thought, he creates a parallel with the seed of an animal, which contains a certain power by which animals are produced. In a similar manner, the mineralising power works as a seed through which stones are formed. However, as regards its efficacy, this power is influenced by the power of the stars and the place in which it acts. Consequently, the mineralising power uses heat and moisture as its tools for forming stones – that is, the qualities of Earth and Water that we have already seen. Finally, Albertus attributes the formal cause to the Mover who sets the celestial bodies in motion, which is how they exert their influence on the beings of the sublunary world and therefore also on the places where the stones are produced. Albertus sums up his account by saying:

> It should also be added that the power of the elements is the material cause, and the power of the heavens is the efficient cause, and the power of the

[23] Albert the Great, *On Minerals*, I.I.I, ed. Borgnet (1890b) 2b: *in genere dicimus omnis lapidis materiam esse aut speciem cujusdam terrae, aut speciem quamdam aquae. Vincit enim in lapidibus alterum istorum elementorum, et in his etiam in quibus quaedam species aquae dominari videntur, est etiam aliquid terrae simul dominans*. Translation taken from Wyckoff (1967: 12). All the translations I use from *On Minerals* are from her book.

[24] Albert the Great, *On Minerals*, I.I.I, ed. Borgnet (1890b) 7: Nos autem ex omnibus his sententiam veram colligentes, dicimus causam verissime generativam esse *virtutem mineralem lapidis formativam. Virtus enim mineralis quaedam communis virtus est efficiens et lapides et metalla, et ea quae sunt media inter haec. Et ideo addimus, quod sit lapidis formativa, ut efficiatur lapidi propria: et quia propria nomina hujus virtutis non habemus, ideo per similia oportet declarare quae sit illa virtus.*

> Mover is the formal cause; and the result of all these is the power that is poured into the material of stones and the place where they are formed, as has been adequately stated in earlier chapters.[25]

Up to this point Albertus' account on stones is quite philosophical and characterised by Aristotelian influence. Yet, towards the end of the second book of *On Minerals*, Albertus says that he must talk about the sigils of stones – a doctrine connected with necromancy, astrology, and magic – noting that most people cannot understand their true meaning.[26] Without doubt the Dominican master had wide-ranging knowledge of stones and, appropriately, he seemed open to accepting new doctrines, even if they were controversial in nature.[27] But his willingness to accept such a doctrine also has a philosophical basis, since the influence of the celestial bodies and the material structure of precious stones were key factors for the efficacy of the sigils. The important thing for us in relation to the subject of this chapter is that the sigils augmented and enhanced the properties of the precious stones on which they were impressed and therefore any medical properties attached to them became even stronger. In fact, Albertus adduces many cases of precious stones which could cure eye diseases, dropsy, epilepsy, and other illnesses, if the appropriate kinds of sigils were engraved on them. In a similar manner, in his lapidary he speaks of numerous other cases of stones, which also had medical properties, and it is therefore worth looking into whether and how such special cases are philosophically justified in his work.

12.3.1 Precious Stones and Epilepsy

In the second book of his *On Minerals* Albertus presents his famous lapidary in alphabetical order. As Wyckoff has suggested, Albertus Magnus made little or no direct use of the ancient authorities, such as

[25] Albert the Great, *On Minerals*, 1.1.1, ed. Borgnet (1890b) 13: *Sicut autem diximus de terra, sic intelligendum est fieri de qualitatibus omnium elementorum: et adjiciendum quod virtus elementi sit materialis, et virtus coelestis instrumentalis, et formalis sit virtus motoris: et quod ex omnibus resultant, est virtus infusa materiae et loco lapidum, sicut satis in antehabitis dictum est.*

[26] Albert the Great, *On Minerals*, 1.1.1, ed. Borgnet (1890b) 48b: *De imaginibus autem lapidum et sigillis post haec dicendum est: licet enim pars ista sit pars necromantiae secundum illam speciem necromantiae quae astronomiae subalternatur, et quae de imaginibus et sigillis vocatur: tamen propter bonitatem doctrinae, et quia illud cupiunt a nobis scire nostri socii, aliquid de hoc hic dicemus, omnino imperfecta et falsa reputantes quidquid de his a multis scriptum invenitur. Antiquorum enim sapientium scripturam de sigillis lapidum pauci sciunt, nec sciri potest nisi simul et astronomia et magica et necromantiae scientiae sciantur.*

[27] On Albertus and astrological images, see Thorndike (1923: 555–8), Weill-Parot (2002: 260–80), and Rutkin (2013: 451–97).

Pliny the Elder, Dioscorides, and so forth, and most of his material was drawn from Arnold of Saxony (fl. 1225) and Thomas of Cantimpré (*c.*1200–*c.* 1270).[28] Yet, from the very beginning of the lapidary, Albertus clarifies how he intends to deal with the stones and their corresponding authorities:

> Let us now list below the names of the most important precious stones and their powers, as they have come down to us, either by experience or from the writings of authorities. But we shall not report everything that is said about them because this is of no advantage to science. For it is [the task] of natural science not simply to accept what we are told but to inquire into the causes of natural things.[29]

So, according to this passage, Albertus does not seem satisfied with merely accepting the word of the authorities because this goes against natural science, which enquires into the causes of things. Following this line of thinking, one could explain Albertus' heavy reliance on experience when it comes to the powers of stones. There are many instances throughout the lapidary where Albertus accounts for the powers and other miraculous properties of stones by asserting that this is something that has been proven by experience.[30] But he also uses experience in order to confirm the extraordinary powers of stones. The Dominican master seems to have struggled to account for certain powers allegedly possessed by the stones, such as their capacity for counteracting poison, winning a victory, and other similar outcomes, which are described as wonderful (*mirabilia*). In order to explain and justify such powers he seems to have adopted Ibn Sīnā's notion of specific form, as described in the *Canon of Medicine*. Likewise, Ibn Sīnā alleged that certain effects of compounds and medicines were due to their specific form and thus he brought together all the cases that could not be explained by the elemental qualities of these compounds under the umbrella of a specific form. As Chandelier notes, the attribution of the powers of stones to a specific form and their justification could be known only by experience.[31] This opinion is something that Albertus also adopts. When Albertus was in Padua around 1220, the *Canon of Medicine* was already known in northern Italy.[32] Of course it cannot be proved that

[28] Wyckoff (1967: 264–71); Draelants (2005: 229–38).

[29] Albert the Great, *On Minerals*, 2.2.1, ed. Borgnet (1890b) 30b: *Supponamus autem nomina praecipuorum lapidum, et virtutes secundum quod ad nos aut per experimentum, aut ex scripturis Auctorum devenerunt. Non autem omnia quae de eis dicuntur referemus, eo quod ad scientiam non prodest. Scientiae enim naturalis non est simpliciter narrata accipere, sed in rebus naturalibus inquirere causas.* Wyckoff (1967: 68–9).

[30] Riddle and Mulholland (1980: 209–10). On the role of experience in the use of amulets, see Lieberman (Chapter 8), who examines the case of Moses Maimonides.

[31] Chandelier (2017: 434). [32] Chandelier (2017: 37).

Albertus was himself familiar with it by that time, but we know for sure that by around 1240 he was acquainted with the *Canon of Medicine*.[33] Given that his *On Minerals* was probably written almost fifteen years later, there was arguably quite enough time for the Dominican master to become well acquainted with its material and adopt some of its content in his own texts. Albertus' approach to the subject of the powers of stones with respect to their specific form[34] is well illustrated in the case of sapphires, where he holds that the power of its specific form is something which is self-evident once experienced and almost impossible not to believe in. He explicitly says:

> Furthermore, it is proved by experience that some sapphires cure abscesses, and we have seen one of these with our own eyes. This is a widespread belief; and it is impossible that there should not be some truth at least in what is a matter of common report . . . For it would be ridiculous if we were to say that the primary qualities [hot, cold, moist, dry] have strong effects and yet the substantial forms[35] which are set as their natural limits, as being divine and best, have no effect at all.[36]

This text is important because it shows, on the one hand, Albertus' fervent belief in the power of the specific form and, on the other, his openness to the notion of the efficacy of the elements via their primary qualities.[37] In the third chapter of the second book, Albertus becomes even clearer on the subject of the elements when he discusses the wrong opinions of others concerning the powers of the stones. There he says:

> To this the objection may be raised that the elements do not act except through the primary qualities [hot, cold, moist, dry], and the actions of stones cannot be reduced to these primary qualities. The reply [that is made to this] is that the elements have certain actions in themselves and certain others when they are in a mixed [body]; because in a mixed [body] an elementary quality is moved and acts as an instrument; and then it is able to effect many things which it could not do by itself.[38]

33 Siraisi (1980: 393).

34 See Jeck (2000) for a discussion on Albertus' notion of specific form in stones.

35 For Albertus the substantial form of the stones is their specific form.

36 Albert the Great, *On Minerals*, 2.1.1, ed. Borgnet (1890b) 24: *Adhuc autem expertum est saphiros aliquos anthraces fugare, et unum tale videmus oculis nostris. Hoc etiam ab omnibus vulgatum est, et non potest esse quin in toto vel in parte sit verum quod ab omnibus communiter est dictum . . . Risibile enim esset valde, quod diceremus qualitates primas vehementes habere operationes, et formas substantiales ipsis rebus ut fines naturae datos sicut divinum et optimum, omnino nullas habere operations.* Wyckoff (1967: 56, 58).

37 On the subject of medicine and elements in the eleventh and twelfth centuries, see McKeon (1961); on Albertus and elements, see Baldner (1999).

38 Albert the Great, *On Minerals*, 2.1.1, ed. Borgnet (1890b) 25: *Quidam autem dixerunt ab elementis componentibus lapides tales inesse virtutes, quibus cum objicitur, elementa, non operari nisi qualitatibus*

The Dominican master's main objection is that the elements do not act per se but only through their primary qualities. In fact, it is in a mixed body, like stones, that the qualities gain 'instrumental' character and can affect things that otherwise they could not. This kind of qualitative effect allows to draw some lines of connection between the power of stones and the case of epilepsy.

In the Middle Ages epilepsy was known by various names, but the most well known were *epilepsia* (epilepsy) and *caduca* (falling-down sickness).[39] From an early stage the understanding of epilepsy oscillated between rationalism and magic or superstition. On the one hand, Galenism provided a rational approach concerning its study and explanation, whereas, on the other, epilepsy's supposed links with demonic possession and the moon triggered a great deal of literature associated with magic and supernatural elements.[40] Albertus' references relate mostly to the idiopathic kind of epilepsy, the one caused by excessive phlegmatic humours in the brain.[41] The fact that the phlegm contains humidity made Albertus posit a sort of connection between epilepsy and the state of sleep; thus he claimed that epilepsy was some kind of sleep.[42] So, if we put these two sources together, Albertus' theory of epilepsy would entail an excessive quantity of humidity which ascended to the head and then, on its descent, obstructed the veins and caused suffocation. Yet, humidity and cold, which are the qualities of phlegm, are the key factors causing epilepsy and, as we will see, properties of stones could be applied to remedy this.

Albertus' catalogue comprises several stones supposed to prevent or cure epilepsy, but, for lack of space, we will limit ourselves to the cases of *Celidonius* and *Echites*. Concerning these stones Albertus states:

> *Celidonius* (swallowstone) has two varieties. One is black, the other reddish brown; but both are taken from the stomach of a swallow. The reddish one,

primis, et operationes lapidum ad qualitates primas non posse reduci. Respondent elementa quasdam habere operationes per se, quasdam autem in mixto: quia in mixto qualitas elementaris operatur mota sicut instrumentum, et tunc habet multa operari quae per se non operatur. Wyckoff (1967: 59).

39 Temkin (1971: 85–6). 40 Temkin (1971: 86–101); Kemp (1990: 140–4).

41 Albert the Great, *On Man*, 27.2, ed. Anzulewicz and Söder (2008) 347: *Epilepsia enim provenit ex subito motu proveniente ex superfluitate humoris et spiritus infrigidatis in cerebro, quae postea 'descendendo venas tumefaciunt', ut dicit Philosophus in primo de somno quae tumefactae 'coartant porum, ubi respiration fit', hoc est vocativam arteriam, in tantum quod etiam quandoque suffocantur.*

42 Albert the Great, *On Sleep and Wakefulness*, 1.2.8, ed. Borgnet (1890c) 150b: *Haec etiam est causa, quod frequenter pueri epileptici sunt propter multum humidum quod fertur ad caput eorum: somnus enim simile aliquod est ita causa epileptiae: et ipse somnus quaedam epileptia videtur esse.* For a modern evaluation of Albertus' theory of epilepsy connected to sleep, see Theiss (1997: 248).

> if wrapped in a linen cloth or a calfskin and worn under the left armpit, is said to be good against insanity and chronic weakness and lunacy. And [Costa ben Luca/Qusṭā ibn Lūqā] says that it is good against epilepsy, if worn in the manner described above.[43]
>
> Echites (eaglestone) is the best of gems. It is of a dark red colour and it is called by some *aquileus* and by others *erodialis* ... It is reported that, suspended on the left arm, it strengthens pregnant women, prevents abortion, and lessens the dangers of childbirth. And some say that it prevents frequent attacks in epileptics.[44]

As we have already seen, at the beginning of his lapidary Albertus signals that the ancient authorities are not to be followed slavishly and that it is necessary to inquire into the causes of things. Albertus was not a physician and therefore he was not interested in the application of a cure. Needless to say, his interest is purely in the theoretical aspect of medicine, something that was connoted through his notion of the 'perfect physician'. All these things account for the lack of references in Albertus' work to the actual performance of a remedy. This does not mean, however, that one cannot find any texts which would serve themselves as an explanatory basis with respect to how a stone could act against epilepsy. The two stones in the case under examination have their red colour in common, and this is significant in Albertus' theory of stones.

In particular, in *On Minerals* again, Albertus discusses the causes of different colours in precious stones and thus he refers to the occurrence of red in stones. After exploring the white and black colours in stones he refers to the intermediate hues, which include red.

> The intermediate colours are reds, greens, and blues, and different shades of these. And, as will be said in the book on *The Senses*, there will be red when a luminous transparency is covered by a thin burning smoke. This colour is found in certain stones which are called 'water jacinths' and in the three kinds of carbuncles; and therefore Aristotle says that these are all hot by nature.[45]

[43] Albert the Great, *On Minerals*, 2.2.3, ed. Borgnet (1890b) 33: *CELIDONIUS duas habet species. Unus est niger, alter rufus invenitur: trahuntur autem ambo de ventre hirundinis. Rufus autem involutus panno lineo vel corio vitulino et sub sinistra ascella gestatus, dicitur valere contra insaniam et antiquos languores et lunaticam passionem. Et Constantinus dicit eum valere contra epilepsiam praedicto modo gestatum*. Wyckoff (1967: 80).

[44] Albert the Great, *On Minerals*, 2.2.4, ed. Borgnet (1890b) 35: *ECHITES gemmarum optima est, colore puniceo, et vocatur a quibusdam aquileus, et ab aliis erodialis ... Fertur autem quod suspensus sinistro lacerto, confert vires praegnantibus, impedit abortum, et periculum parturitionis mitigat. Et aiunt quidam, quod caducorum hominum prohibet frequentem casum*. Wyckoff (1967: 87–8).

[45] Albert the Great, *On Minerals*, 1.2.2, ed. Borgnet (1890b) 15b: *Medii autem colores sunt rubeus in genere, viridis, et flavus, et differentiae ipsorum. Et sicut dicetur in libro de Sensibilibus rubeus erit*

According to this text the redness of a stone indicates its hot nature, and Albertus repeats this with respect to *granatus*, which is again red and of a hot and dry nature.[46] In both cases Albertus cites Aristotle as his source – that is, his lapidary – perhaps with the aim of linking philosophical allusions to his description. As we saw, Albertus explained epilepsy in terms of humoral theory and therefore a connection between epilepsy and the two stones in respect of qualities would not be irrelevant in the context of his work. The key idea here is that the red stones, thanks to their hot and dry qualities, can counter the coldness and humidity of epilepsy. In short, the action of stones, through their opposite qualities, could be seen as regulators or inhibitors of, for example, humidity in the human body, a common therapeutic practice in the Middle Ages in order to restore balance in the human organism.[47] Apart from this reference, which is of a contextual character, Albertus gives us another insight into treating epilepsy through opposite qualities in his *On Plants*, where he speaks of *salvia* (sage), and asserts that it is hot and dry and beneficial to those who suffer from epilepsy.[48] This reference shows that the qualities of sage are cited as a means of treating epilepsy and therefore the herb could act in the same way as the stones in our case – that is, as a regulator of humidity by virtue of its opposite qualities.

Yet we still need to ascertain whether we have any hint in Albertus' work concerning the application of therapy. To my knowledge, Albertus does not refer to or describe the application of precious stones to the human body as a means of therapy. However, in another case relating to a precious stone, which is again reddish and is supposed to be effective against epilepsy, Albertus stresses that, if it is worn around the neck, it is good against epilepsy.[49] This remark is pertinent to his theory of epilepsy. In *On Sleep and Wakefulness* he describes how one could be fatally suffocated by epileptic vapours, and the neck seems to play a crucial role in this process. Specifically, he stresses that, as evaporations descend from the veins of the neck and the throat, they make the veins swell and obstruct the channels through which respiration occurs and as a result suffocation ensues.[50] So,

quando super perspicuum luminosum infunditur fumus tenuis succensus. Et iste invenitur in quibusdam lapidibus, qui vocantur hyacinthi aquatici, et in tribus generibus carbunculorum: propter quod ab Aristotele omnes illi calidi secundum naturam esse dicuntur. Wyckoff (1967: 40).

[46] Wyckoff (1967: 96). [47] Wallis (2005b: 335).

[48] Albert the Great, *On Plants*, 6.2.17, ed. Meyer and Jessen (1867) 569: *Salvia est autem calida et sicca, consumens et confortans, et confert paraliticis et epilepticis.*

[49] Wyckoff (1967: 81).

[50] Albert the Great, *On Sleep and Wakefulness*, 1.2.8, ed. Borgnet (1890c) 150b: *cum enim multus spiritus evaporationis tam in somno quam in epileptia feratur sursum ad caput, descendens per venam colli et*

from this description one may infer the central role of the neck since it is through the channel of the neck that evaporations descend from the head and thus suffocation may head potentially causing suffocation. Following this train of thought, connecting the anti-epileptic stones with the neck starts to make some sense as the aim of the 'therapy' would be to moderate and regulate the qualities which bring about epilepsy in the part of the body which is pivotal for the progress of the disease. If the veins of both neck and throat are susceptible to swelling and can get obstructed and cause suffocation, suspending the stones from the neck as a means of prevention would seem quite logical.[51]

12.3.2 Precious Stones and Melancholy

The medieval scholars of the thirteenth century inherited a Galenic-Avicennian definition of melancholy, according to which it was an illness connected to the four known humours and occurred either due to an excess of black bile or due to the combustion of yellow bile.[52] Usually the term *melancholia* was used to signify both black bile and the mental disease caused by an excess of the former. The writings of Constantine the African and of Ibn Sīnā undoubtedly played an important role in the dissemination of theories on melancholy. The former focused on the notions of fear and sorrow and how they could produce a distressed state of mind, which was occupied with imaginative fears, hallucinations, and suspicious thoughts that could in turn affect the person suffering from these thoughts.[53] Ibn Sīnā defined melancholy as a disorder of the cerebral organs inasmuch as it concerned their proper function.[54] Furthermore, he distinguished between *melancholia naturalis* and *innaturalis*; the former was harmless and was associated with the natural function of black bile, whereas the latter was concerned with the pathological aspect of melancholy through combustion of the humours.[55] The fact that Ibn Sīnā had associated melancholy with cerebral areas and their proper function bestowed a philosophical character on the disease because some medieval thinkers, including Albertus, discussed melancholy in terms of the doctrine of the soul and of the internal senses. Finally, the image of the *melancholicus* (a melancholic person) was divided into two categories. On the one hand, we have the melancholic,

gutturis, facit intumescere venas, et illis intumescentibus coarctatur et praefocatur porus cannae per quem fit respiratio, et sic suffocatur.

[51] Cf. Riddle and Mulholland (1980: 213–14). [52] Klibansky et al. (1964: 67).

[53] Klibansky et al. (1964: 98–102); Jackson (1986: 60–1); Kemp (1990: 117–18).

[54] Gilon (2018: 80). [55] Klibansky et al. (1964: 87–8).

who is the representative of the 'bad' version of melancholy and is characterised by fearful and unstable behaviour and, on the other, we have the 'good' version, the one which derives from Pseudo-Aristotle's *Problems* and presents a melancholic of a heroic and quite gifted nature.[56] The connection between *acedia* and melancholy is made in a similar moral context. In particular, *acedia* was produced either by excessive phlegm or black bile and it was synonymous with the state of sorrow. Religious people who were suffering from *acedia* were being punished for their past sins or 'tormented' in a way that was designed to avert any future transgressions.[57]

Turning to Albertus Magnus and his notion of melancholy, it is noticeable that he uses the word *melancholia* to connote either black bile or the mental disease which was usually associated with a cerebral disorder. In general terms he follows Constantine the African and Ibn Sīnā and distinguishes between *melancholia naturalis et innaturalis* (natural and non-natural/unnatural melancholy). With respect to the former, he defines natural melancholy as dregs of blood, whereas the non-natural/unnatural one is the result of combustion of the four known humours and has four types.[58] Albertus' acquaintance with the Pseudo-Aristotelian text *Problems* influenced his conception of the melancholic.[59] The melancholics with natural melancholy are described as sad, sombre, and suffering from terrible visions, while the heaviness, coldness, and horror of the melancholic blood are responsible for the aforementioned state of these melancholics.[60] In contrast, the melancholics of unnatural melancholy were supposed to have well-supported convictions and regulated passions and be characterised by the greatest of virtues. All these traits could appear only if the melancholy was not severely combusted.[61]

[56] Klibansky et al. (1964: 18–43). [57] Klibansky et al. (1964: 77–8); Jackson (1986: 69–77).

[58] Albert the Great, *On Animals*, 3.2.3, ed. Stadler (1916) I.329: *Haec igitur melancolia naturalis faex sanguinis est, sicut diximus, nec potest esse aliqua naturalis melancolia quae sit faex et ypostasis aliorum humorum . . . Haec igitur innaturalis melancolia est quadruplex*. For more, see Resnick and Kitchell (1999: 401–4).

[59] Note that the Latin text of the *Problems* goes back to a translation made between 1258 and 1266 and yet Albertus seems to have had some excerpts of the text. See Klibansky et al. (1964: 67–8) and Gilon (2018: 90–2).

[60] Albert the Great, *On Animals*, 3.2.3, ed. Stadler (1916) I.47: *Melancolicos enim tristes et graves dicimus et terribiles ymagines patientes et detineri in hiis propter sanguinis melancolici gravitatem et frigiditatem et horrorem, quia ymagines receptae in horrido efficiuntur horribiles.*

[61] Albert the Great, *On Animals*, 3.2.3, ed. Stadler (1916) I.330: *In hominibus autem etiam diversimode participatur humor iste: quoniam si non sit multum adusta . . . tunc illa melancolia erit habens multos et stabilitos et confirmatos spiritus: quia calidum eius bene movet et humidum eius cum ypostasi terrestri non incinerata optime movetur propter quod tales habent stabilitos conceptus et ordinatissimos affectus et efficiuntur studiosi et virtutum optimarum.*

Albertus' attempt to harmonise the exceptional melancholic men of the *Problems* with the general medical doctrines of his period indicates his intention of establishing a medico-philosophical approach to melancholy. This approach also entails differences in the way the two kinds of melancholy operate and therefore, as far as his explanations are concerned, there are noticeable nuances. For instance, in natural melancholy, Albertus notes that black vapours ascend to the head and because of them terrible images are impressed on the brain, while these vapours lack sufficient heat to warm the heart and the blood.[62] So, in this case cold is the key to the generation of terrible images in the head. However, in *On Memory and Reminiscence* Albertus describes a different process with respect to unnatural melancholy or, as he sometimes calls it, accidental melancholy. According to this process heat or warmth (*calidum*) acts as a catalyst for the images to move to the highest degree (*maxime*) and in combination with humidity this triggers an incessant flow of memory, which may be ended and linked to such emotions as wrath and fear.[63] This example shows that the opposite qualities are of importance for the manifestation of melancholic symptoms – that is, heat and moisture.

These explanations hinder us from making any connection between Albertus' description of stones and certain conditions or types of melancholy because Albertus does not use the sort of terminology in *On Minerals* that would allow us to understand which type of melancholy he is referring to. Despite these difficulties I believe that expressions used and remarks Albertus made in certain parts of his text could render us capable of distinguishing between the types of melancholy with relatively great possibilities of success. The most interesting and intriguing case is that of onyx. In his description of it Albertus states:

> Onyx is said to be a gem of a black colour; there is found a better kind of it which is black, streaked with white veins. It comes from Media and Arabia. Five varieties are found, based on differences in their veining and colours. They say that, worn around the neck or on the finger, it induces sorrow and fear and terrible dreams in sleep; and it is reported to increase sorrows and dissensions; and they say that it increases saliva in children. But sard, if present, restrains the onyx and keeps it from doing harm. If [onyx] really has all these [properties], surely this is because it has the power of affecting black

[62] Albert the Great, *On the IV Books of the Sentences*, 4.29.3, ed. Borgnet (1893) I.206b: *Cum enim melancholia sit terrea frigida, habet evaporationes nigras ad cerebrum lucidum, quibus imprimuntur terribilia phantasmata: et est in eis calor non sufficiens ad calefactionem cordis et sanguinis.*

[63] Albert the Great, *On Memory and Reminiscence*, 2.7, ed. Borgnet (1890d) 117a–118a. See also Theiss (1997: 251).

> bile, especially in the head; for all these disorders come from the motion and vapour [of black bile].[64]

In this excerpt Albertus comes across as being quite sure about the property of onyx in affecting the black bile. In the last part of his description Albertus becomes thoroughly expressive with respect to the stone's effect and therefore we can understand which type of melancholy he is talking about. The Dominican master locates black bile's action in the head and consequently he explains that these disorders come from the motion and vapour of black bile. Judging by the description Albertus is referring to natural melancholy, the one which is *terrea frigida* – that is, earthly cold.[65] But why is onyx likely to affect the black bile? The answer to this question lies again in Albertus' theory of colours. Onyx is black in colour and, as such, Albertus informs us:

> A black colour in stones is most frequently caused by burnt earthy [material]; and therefore black stones are frequently very hard, and capable only of being polished but not cut. For this colour is caused merely by lack of transparency in the mixture, as will appear when the science of colours is discussed.[66]

So, according to this text, the blackness of a stone is due to its burnt earth constituent, which in turn signifies the presence of the qualities of coldness and dryness. In *On the Causes of the Properties of the Elements* Albertus discusses the four humours in terms of their elemental composition. It is there he states that melancholy is cold and dry and therefore has the qualities of earth.[67] Given that both onyx and melancholy are of the same elemental complexion, one can understand why Albertus was so willing to affirm the negative effect of onyx on black bile. In the same context we could explain why sard – that is, sardinus – a stone of a dense

64 Albert the Great, *On Minerals*, 2.2.13, ed. Borgnet (1890b) 42a: *ONYX gemma esse perhibetur, nigri coloris, invenitur melius genus ejus nigrum albis venis variatum. Venit autem de Media et Arabia. Invenitur autem quinque diversitatum propter varietatem venarum et colorum. Aiunt quod collo vel digito suspensus, excitat tristitiam et timores et in somno phantasias terribiles, et multiplicare fertur tristitias et lites. Dicunt autem quod auget salivam pueris. Si autem sardinus sit praesens, ligatur onyx et suspenditur a nocumento. Haec autem omnia si habet, profecto habet ideo, quia virtutem habet movendi melancholiam praecipue in capite: ex motu enim illius et vapore omnia ista procedunt.* Wyckoff (1967: 108–9).

65 See note 62.

66 Albert the Great, *On Minerals*, 1.2.2, ed. Borgnet (1890b) 15b: *Niger autem color in lapidibus frequentissime causatur ex terrestri combusto: propter quod etiam ut frequenter lapides nigri durissimi sunt, et magis polibiles quam secabiles sunt. Hic enim color non causatur nisi ex privatione perspicui in commixtione, sicut patebit cum de scientia colorum tractabitur.* Wyckoff (1967: 40).

67 Albert the Great, *On the Causes of the Properties of Elements*, 1.1.2, ed. Hossfeld (1980) 52: *Et invenitur alia quae est ex cholera nigra, quae melancholia vocatur, quae est frigida et sicca, virtutes habens terrae.*

red colour, can mitigate the effects of the cold nature of onyx. As we have already seen in the Albertinian theory of stones, the red ones are hot in nature and therefore a red stone could act against a cold one by virtue of its contrariety, a concept that was by no means alien to Albertus' work.[68]

Conclusion

Albertus Magnus' relation with medicine was always filtered through philosophy. Even when Albertus seems to be critical of physicians, this is not for the most part because the Dominican master has lost faith in medicine. Actually, he wishes to amend the erroneous practices of physicians and render them 'perfect physicians' by putting them back on track to seek the first principles and causes. Turning to the medical properties of stones, as described in *On Minerals*, one cannot claim that there is an obvious and evident link between the stones and the illnesses they are purported to treat. The lack of this evident link may have encouraged Albertus to adopt Ibn Sīnā's specific form in an attempt to explicate all the extraordinary properties of stones using one common model. Yet the medical properties of stones with respect to epilepsy and melancholy could be reduced to the explicatory formula of colours and their qualitative significance, a possibility which Albertus neither explicitly stressed nor rejected. So, in the case of epilepsy the hot and dry nature of red stones and the cold and moist nature of epilepsy allows the former to act as a regulator or inhibitor of humidity and frigidity in the human body. Furthermore, Albertus' reference to the herb salvia, which has the same qualities as red stones, as a means of preventing epilepsy adds weight to my initial argument. Consequently, the idea of hanging a stone around the neck of an epileptic patient does not seem out of place in the work of Albertus Magnus, since, according to Albertus' theory of epilepsy, the veins of the neck were the pivotal channels through which travelled the evaporations that could cause suffocation. In the case of melancholy, it is harder to create the same connections because Albertus is vague and ambiguous about what he means by the term *melancholy*. In particular his distinction between natural and unnatural melancholy is absent from the description of those stones that were supposed to deal with melancholy and therefore one cannot be sure about the type of melancholy a stone is supposed to

[68] Albert the Great, *Ethics*, 14.4.12, ed. Kübel (1972) 275: *Praeterea, contrarium in contrario citius exstinguitur; sed ira est ut calidum quoddam movens; ergo videtur, quod in melancholicis, qui sunt frigidi, citius exstinguatur ira.*

treat. However, the way in which Albertus expresses himself in the case of onyx allows us to infer that he is referring to natural melancholy and to understand how the stone might affect black bile. By applying his theory of colour to the blackness of onyx, it is apparent that the stone is characterised by the same qualities as melancholy and thus onyx would augment and enhance the symptoms of melancholy. Taking all of this into account one can assert that Albertus did not act as a mere compiler or a slavish preserver of authoritative knowledge with respect to the properties of stones. The Dominican master sought to philosophise this knowledge, and this has been shown to happen to some extent in the cases presented in this chapter.

REFERENCES

Angel, M. 1992. 'Propriétés accidentelles des pierres: couleur, dureté, fissilité, porosité et densité selon Albert le Grand', *Travaux du Comité français d'Histoire de la Géologie* 6: 87–92.

Anzulewicz, H., and Söder, J. R. eds. 2008. *De homine*. Munster: Aschendorff.

Asúa, M. de. 2001. 'Minerals, Plants and Animals from A to Z: The Inventory of the Natural World in Albert the Great's *Philosophia Naturalis*', in W. Senner (ed.), *Albertus Magnus: Zum Gedenken nach 800 Jahren. Neue Zugänge, Aspekte und Perspektiven*. Berlin: Akademie Verlag, 389–400.

Asúa, M. de. 2013. 'War and Peace: Medicine and Natural Philosophy in Albert the Great', in I. M. Resnick (ed.), *A Companion to Albert the Great: Theology, Philosophy and the Sciences*. Leiden: Brill, 269–97.

Baldner, S. 1999. 'St. Albert the Great and St. Thomas Aquinas on the Presence of Elements in Compounds', *Sapientia* 54: 41–57.

Barney, S. A. et al. trans. 2006. *The Etymologies of Isidore of Seville*. New York: Cambridge University Press.

Borgnet, A. ed. 1890a. *Alberti Magni opera omnia: De sensu et sensate*. Paris: L. Vivès.

Borgnet, A. ed. 1890b. *Alberti Magni opera omnia: De mineralibus*. Paris: L. Vivès.

Borgnet, A. ed. 1890c. *Alberti Magni opera omnia: De somno et vigilia*. Paris: L. Vivès.

Borgnet, A. ed. 1890d. *Alberti Magni opera omnia: De memoria et reminiscentia*. Paris: L. Vivès.

Borgnet, A. ed. 1893–4. *Alberti Magni opera omnia: Super IV libros Sententiarum*. 2 vols. Paris: L. Vivès.

Chandelier, J. 2017. *Avicenne et la médecine en Italie*. Paris: Honoré Champion.

Draelants, I. 2005. 'Échanges dans la *Societas* des naturalistes au milieu du XIIIe siècle: Arnold de Saxe, Vincent de Beauvais et Albert le Grend', in D. James-Raoul, D. Jacquart, and O. Soutet (eds.), *Par les mots et les textes . . . Mélanges de langue, de littérature et d'histoire des sciences médiévales offerts à Claude Thomasset*. Paris: Presses de l'Université Paris-Sorbonne, 219–38.

Filthaut, E. ed. 1955. *Quaestiones super de animalibus*. Munster: Editio Coloniensis.

Gilon, O. 2018. 'Savoirs médicaux et traditions philosophiques: Le cas de la mélancholie au XIIIe siècle', in Z. Kaluza and C. Dragos (eds.), *Regards sur les traditions philosophiques (XIIe–XIVe siècles)*. Leuven: Leuven University Press, 69–97.

Hossfeld, P. ed. 1980. *De causis proprietatum elementorum*. Munster: Aschendorff.

Jackson, S. V. 1986. *Melancholia and Depression*. New Haven, CT: Yale University Press.

Jacquart, D. 1998a. 'Medical Scholasticism', in M. D. Grmek (ed.), *Western Medical Thought from Antiquity to the Middle Ages*. Cambridge, MA: Harvard University Press, 197–240.

Jacquart, D. 1998b. *La médecine médiévale dans le cadre parisien*. Paris: Fayard.

Jacquart, D. 2013. 'Anatomy, Physiology, and Medical theory', in D. C. Lindberg and M. H. Shank (eds.), *The Cambridge History of Science. Volume 2: Medieval Science*. Cambridge: Cambridge University Press, 590–610.

Jacquart, D., and Micheau, F. 1990. *La médecine arabe et l'occident médiéval*. Paris: Maisonneuve et Larose.

Jeck, U. R. 1998. 'Albert der Grosse über die Natur der Steine', *Zeitschrift* 47: 206–11.

Jeck, U. R. 2000. 'Virtus Lapidum: Zur philosophischen Begründung der magischen Wirksamkeit und der physikalischen Beschaffenheit kostbarer Mineralien in der Naturphilosophie Alberts des Grossen', *Early Science and Medicine* 5.1: 33–46.

Kemp, S. 1990. *Medieval Psychology*. New York: Greenwood Press.

Klibansky, R. et al. 1964. *Saturn and Melancholy: Studies in the History of Natural Philosophy, Religion and Art*. London: Nelson.

Kübel, W. ed. 1972. *Super Ethica*. Munster: Aschendorff.

Lindberg, D. C. 1992. *The Beginnings of Western Science: The European Scientific Tradition in Philosophical, Religious, and Institutional Context, 600 B.C. to A.D. 1450*. Chicago: University of Chicago Press.

McKeon, R. 1961. 'Medicine and Philosophy in the Eleventh and Twelfth Centuries: The Problem of Elements', *Thomist: A Speculative Quarterly Review* 24.2: 211–56.

Meyer, E. and Jessen, C. eds. 1867. *De vegetabilibus libri VII*. Berlin.

Nutton, V. 2013. 'Early-Medieval Medicine and Natural Science', in D. C. Lindberg and M. H. Shank (eds.), *The Cambridge History of Science. Volume 2: Medieval Science*. Cambridge: Cambridge University Press, 323–40.

Ottosson, P. G. 1984. *Scholastic Medicine and Philosophy: A Study of Commentaries on Galen's Tegni (ca. 1300–1450)*. Naples: Bibliopolis-Edizioni di filosofia e scienze.

Park, K. 2013. 'Medical Practice', in D. C. Lindberg and M. H. Shank (eds.), *The Cambridge History of Science. Volume 2: Medieval Science*. Cambridge: Cambridge University Press, 611–29.

Resnick, I. M., and Kitchell, K. F. trans. 1999. *Albertus Magnus On Animals: A Medieval Summa Zoologica*. 2 vols. Baltimore, MD: Johns Hopkins University Press.

Resnick I. M., and Kitchell, K. F. trans. 2008. *Albert the Great: Questions concerning Aristotle's* On Animals. Washington DC: Catholic University of America Press.

Reynolds, P. L. 1999. *Food and the Body: Some Peculiar Questions in High Medieval Theology*. Leiden: Brill.

Riddle, J. M. 1974. 'Theory and Practice in Medieval Medicine', *Viator* 5: 157–84.

Riddle, J. M., and Mulholland, J. A. 1980. 'Albert on Stones and Minerals', in J. A. Weisheipl (ed.), *Albertus Magnus and the Sciences: Commemorative Essays*. Toronto: Pontifical Institute of Mediaeval Studies, 203–34.

Rutkin, D. H. 2013. 'Astrology and Magic', in I. M. Resnick (ed.), *A Companion to Albert the Great: Theology, Philosophy and the Sciences*. Leiden: Brill, 451–505.

Schipperges, H. 1980. 'Das medizinische Denken bei Albertus Magnus', in G. Meyer and A. Zimmermann (eds.), *Albertus Magnus: Doctor Universalis 1280/1980*. Mainz: Grunewald, 279–94.

Siraisi, N. G. 1980. 'The Medical Learning of Albertus Magnus', in J. A. Weisheipl (ed.), *Albertus Magnus and the Sciences: Commemorative Essays*. Toronto: Pontifical Institute of Mediaeval Studies, 379–404.

Siraisi, N. G. 1990. *Medieval and Early Renaissance Medicine: An Introduction to Knowledge and Practice*. Chicago, IL: University of Chicago Press.

Stadler, H. ed. 1916–20. *De animalibus Libri XXVI*. 2 vols. Munster: Ascendorff.

Talbot, C. H. 1978. 'Medicine', in D. C. Lindberg (ed.), *Science in the Middle Ages*. Chicago, IL: University of Chicago Press, 391–428.

Temkin, O. 1971. *The Falling Sickness: A History of Epilepsy from the Greeks to the Beginnings of Modern Neurology*. Baltimore, MD: Johns Hopkins University Press.

Theiss, P. 1997. 'Albert the Great's Interpretation of Neuropsychiatric Symptoms in the Context of Scholastic Psychology and Physiology', *Journal of the History of the Neurosciences* 6.3: 240–56.

Thorndike, L. 1923. *History of Magic and Experimental Science*, vol. II. New York: Columbia University Press.

Wallis, F. 2005a. 'Medicine, Practical', in T. Glick, S. J. Liveley, and F. Wallis (eds.), *Medieval Science, Technology, and Medicine*. New York: Routledge, 335–6.

Wallis, F. 2005b. 'Medicine, Theoretical', in T. Glick, S. J. Liveley, and F. Wallis (eds.), *Medieval Science, Technology, and Medicine*. New York: Routledge, 336–40.

Weill-Parot, N. 2002. *Les 'images astrologiques' au Moyen Âge et à la Renaissance: Spéculations intellectuelles et pratiques magiques (XIIe–XVe)*. Paris: Honoré Champion.

Weisheipl, J. A. ed. 1980. *Albertus Magnus and the Sciences: Commemorative Essays*. Toronto: Pontifical Institute of Mediaeval Studies.

Wyckoff, D. trans. 1967. *Albertus Magnus: Book of Minerals*. Oxford: Clarendon.

CHAPTER 13

Healing Gifts

The Role of Diplomatic Gift Exchange in the Movement of Materia Medica *between the Byzantine and Islamicate Worlds*

Koray Durak

Frequent references to medicinal drugs of South Asian and African provenance in Byzantine sources, as well as mention of drugs of Byzantine provenance in medieval Arabic sources, point to a lively exchange of *materia medica* between the Byzantine Empire and the Islamicate Near East in the early Middle Ages. Various genres of Byzantine literature attest to the use of aromatic substances of Eastern origin as drugs, spices, and perfume in Byzantium. In a letter to a certain Alexios the twelfth-century poet John Tzetzes asked for agarwood/aloeswood, while in a military manual attributed to Emperor Constantine VII (r. 913–59), the emperor's personal baggage on a military expedition included 'ointments, various perfume/medicinal vapours, incense, mastic, frankincense, sugar, saffron, musk, ambergris, moist and dry aloeswood, cinnamon of the first and second quality, cinnamon wood, and other unguents'.[1] Saints' Lives attest to the use of herbs and spices for treatments, such as pepper, which was used to cure a fleshy growth on a patient's nose.[2] However, the richest type of evidence is found in medical sources, including medical recipes/formularies, calendars of diet, works on properties of foodstuffs (such as the *Treatise on the Capacities of Foodstuffs* of Symeon Seth), medical lexica, and copies of canonical texts such as *De materia medica* by Dioscorides.[3] The eleventh-century physician

This research has been supported by Bogazici University's (BU) Research Fund Grant no. 11921, BU's Byzantine Studies Research Center and the Mellon Foundation.

[1] John Tzetzes, *Letters*, 29, ed. Leone (1972) 45. Constantine Porphyrogennetos, *Three Treatises on Imperial Military Expeditions*, (c).210–39, ed. Haldon (1990) 108. All translations are my own unless otherwise stated.

[2] Magoulias (1964: 148).

[3] On annotations related to *materia medica* in Greek and Arabic manuscripts of Dioscorides, see Mavroudi (Chapter 4) in this volume.

Symeon Seth describes a large number of plants and animals of Eastern origin (ambergris, balsam, ginger, cinnamon, cloves, nutmeg, camphor, frankincense, musk, aloe, and pepper) for pharmaceutical and dietary use. Likewise, Dioscorides' *De materia medica*, which was consulted for practical purposes in the Byzantine period, contains 'exotic' ingredients whose uses are attested in Byzantine medical sources such as Leo the Physician's *Synopsis of Medicine* from the eighth/ninth centuries and John the Physician's *Iatrosophion* from the thirteenth century.[4]

Medieval Arabic sources too provide abundant information on *materia medica* originating in Byzantine territories that were employed for treatments in the Islamicate world. For instance, writers of geographies and *adab* (*belles-lettres*) works agree that mastic, Lemnian earth, and storax were three most famous Byzantine products.[5] Medical lists of simples/synonymic treatises such as *Qānūn fī al-ṭibb* (*Canon of Medicine*) by Ibn Sīnā (d. 1037), as well as medical formularies/recipe books such as the medical regimen book for the pilgrims of Qusṭā Ibn Lūqā, confirm this. Chios was associated with mastic to such an extent that Ibn Sīnā called the island 'the land of mastic'.[6] Quoting Cato, al-Bīrūnī writes in *Kitāb al-jamāhir fī maʿrifat al-jawāhir* (*Sum of Knowledge about Precious Stones*) that the best variety of mastic came from Chios. Then he quotes the tenth-century poet Kushkī, who explains '[it is] a resin of a tree from the *Bilād al-Rūm*; it is brought through al-Jazīra [i.e. northern Mesopotamia], the Syrian border, and the region of Armenia'.[7] This last statement shows the complex nature of the networks through which drugs were traded.

13.1 Major Mechanisms for the Exchange of *Materia Medica*

What mechanisms were employed for the transfer of *materia medica* from the ninth to the twelfth centuries between the two worlds? The majority of

4 Symeon Seth, *Treatise on the Capacities of Foodstuffs*, ed. Langkavel (1868). Riddle (1992). Touwaide (2002a). Durak (2018).

5 Al-Iṣṭakhrī, *Kitāb al-masālik wa-l-mamālik* (*Book of Routes and Realms*), ed. de Goeje (1967a) 69. Ibn Ḥawqal, *Kitāb ṣūrat al-arḍ* (*Book of the Shape of the Earth*), ed. de Goeje (1967b) 204. Al-Thaʿālibī, *Laṭāʾif al-maʿārif* (*Book of Curious and Entertaining Information*), ed. de Jong (1867) 125.

6 Ibn Sīnā, *Qānūn fī al-ṭibb* (*Canon of Medicine*), ed. Al-Kash and Zayur (1987) I.542. For Lemnian earth see Ibn Sīnā, *Qānūn fī al-ṭibb* (*Canon of Medicine*), ed. Al-Kash and Zayur (1987) I.539–40. Qusṭā Ibn Lūqā, *Risālāh fī tadbīr safar al-ḥajj* (*Medical Regimen for the Pilgrims to Mecca*), ed. Bos (1992) 31, 49, 51 (on storax and mastic). Sābūr ibn Sahl, *al-Aqrābādhīn al-ṣaghīr* (*Small Dispensatory*), trans. Kahl (2003), recommends storax fourteen times (no. 5, 280, 299, 32, 34, 41, 65, 171, 259, 264, 266, 273, 311, 315), solid storax three times (no. 5, 280, 299), and Lemnian earth three times as an ingredient (no. 52, 171, 173).

7 Al-Bīrūnī, *Kitāb al-jamāhir fī maʿrifat al-jawāhir* (*Sum of Knowledge about Precious Stones*), (1936) 348–56.

the cases discussed in this chapter date to the ninth and tenth centuries when the Byzantine Empire and the Abbasids (followed by the Buyids) established hegemony over the eastern Mediterranean region. The eleventh and twelfth centuries saw the continuation of Byzantine rule under the Komnenian dynasty, having diplomatic relations with the Fatimids in Egypt and the Great Seljuk Empire in the Near East. One does not see a significant break either in the tradition of diplomatic exchange or in the drug lore, justifying the treatment of this long period from the ninth to the twelfth centuries as a unity. As one might expect, commerce constituted the principal type of exchange involved in the procurement of foreign drugs in the eastern Mediterranean. The *Kitāb al-tabaṣṣur bi-al-tijārah* (*Book of Insight into Commerce*), a commercial treatise attributed to the famous *adab* writer Pseudo-Jāḥiẓ and written in the late ninth/tenth century, clearly states the significance of the Byzantine Empire as a source of drugs for the Islamicate east:

> From the Byzantine Empire (*al-Rūm*) [are imported] gold and silver utensils, dinars of pure gold, drugs (*ʿaqāqīr*), *buzyūn* [i.e. a fine silk], *al-abrūn* [?], brocade, fast horses, female slaves, rare brass utensils, unpickable locks, lyres, hydraulic engineers, agricultural experts, marble workers, and eunuchs.

Pseudo-Jāḥiẓ specifically singles out *materia medica* (*ʿaqāqīr*), alongside textiles, utensils, and craftsmen, as among the most important Byzantine exports.[8] At around the same time and in the same region, the geographer Ibn al-Faqīh defines four major categories of products that the Byzantines possessed: livestock, textiles, slaves/eunuchs, and aromatics ('perfume, storax and mastic').[9] The central role Byzantium played as the source of certain drugs sold in Eastern markets continued uninterrupted into the eleventh and twelfth centuries. In the Genizah archive, which contains the largest collection of medieval Jewish manuscripts describing not only the religious, but also the social and economic life of the Jewish community in Fustat from the eleventh century onwards, Byzantium appears as a source of medicinal plants and textiles.[10] Transfer of medicinal drugs was not a one-way affair. In the period when the *Kitāb al-tabaṣṣur bi-al-tijārah* was written down, Jewish merchants (*al-Rādhāniyyah*) were travelling from Egypt to bring, in the

[8] More specifically, *ʿaqāqīr* meant simple – as opposed to compound – drugs. Pseudo-Jāḥiẓ, *Kitāb al-tabaṣṣur bi-al-tijārah* (*Book of Insight into Commerce*), ed. ʿAbd al-Wahhāb (1966) 34. The *Kitāb al-tabaṣṣur* most likely meant the Byzantine Empire by the term *bilād al-Rūm*. Pellat argues that the work was produced in an Iranian cultural milieu, which was geographically very close to Byzantium (Pellat 1954: 153).

[9] Ibn al-Faqīh, *Kitāb al-buldān* (*Book of the Countries*), ed. de Goeje (1967c) 148.

[10] Goitein (1967: I.46).

geographer Ibn Khurradādhbih's words, 'musk, aloeswood, camphor, cinnamon, and other products that are brought from these regions [i.e. Sind, India, and China]' to Constantinople.[11] The sea route, used by *Rādhāniyyah* Jews in the ninth and tenth centuries to connect Constantinople with Egypt, was still in use in the eleventh and twelfth centuries. According to Genizah documents, Byzantine merchants bought pepper, aloe, cinnamon, ginger, and indigo in Egypt and the Levant.[12] The *Book of the Eparch* – a Byzantine legal work of the early tenth century regulating certain aspects of the economic life of Constantinople from a government perspective – lists almost the same group of products mentioned by Ibn Khurradādhbih as imports from the Islamicate world. In the chapter on the *myrepsoi* (drug/perfume/dye dealers) we read that the guild of aromatics dealt with 'pepper, spikenard, cinnamon, aloeswood, ambergris, musk, frankincense, myrrh, balsam, indigo, lac, lapis lazuli, yellow wood, *zygaian*[13] and all other such things that constitute aromatics and dyestuffs'. These commodities arrived in Constantinople via Chaldia (modern Iraq), Trebizond and 'Syria' (the core territories of the Abbasid Empire, i.e. greater Syria and Iraq).[14]

Alongside commercial exchange, looting and taking tribute played a certain role in the transfer of drugs and medical knowledge between the Byzantine and Islamicate worlds. Known examples of looting and taking tribute are limited but suggestive. Even though they were not the primary target of invading armies or raiders and pirates, aromatics were sometimes among the spoils. In 853, the Byzantine attack on Damietta in Abbasid Egypt resulted in the seizure of raw sugar (*qand*), which was destined for Iraq.[15] *Qand* or *sukkar qand* referred to raw sugar solidified from the juice of sugar cane. It was also called red sugar (*sukkar aḥmar*). When the raw sugar was refined, it became white and was then called *sukkar*. Sugar (*sukkar*/*sachar*) was a ubiquitous item used as a simple in both Near Eastern and Byzantine

[11] Ibn Khurradādhbih, *Kitāb al-masālik wa-l-mamālik* (*Book of Routes and Realms*), ed. de Goeje (1967d) 153–4.

[12] Goitein (1967: I.44); Gil (1997: 243); Simonsohn (1997: I.314); Jacoby (2000: 43–4).

[13] Freshfield translates 'ζυγαίαν' as caper (*Capparis spinosa*) while Koder (1991: 111) prefers 'things that are weighed by scales' – that is, as opposed to by steelyard. Freshfield (1938: 30). *Book of the Prefect*, 10.1–2, ed. Koder (1991) 110. Dalby (2007: 54–5) identifies *zygaian* as storax (*Liquidambar orientalis*). He bases his argument on the observations of the twelfth-century Russian pilgrim Daniel, who speaks of a resin in Caria produced from two trees – *styuryaka* (storax?) and *zygia*. On the other hand, an anonymous, late medieval Byzantine botanical glossary defines *zygaia* as a resin and associates it with mastic (see ed. Delatte (1927–39) II.418). Cf. LSJ, s.v. ζυγία: 'maple tree resin'. *Zygaia* was most likely a resin product.

[14] *Book of the Prefect*, 5.1, 10.1–2, ed. Koder (1991) 94, 110. On the definition of Syria see Durak (2011).

[15] Al-Ṭabarī, *Ta'rīkh al-rusul wa al-mulūk* (*The Annals of the Prophets and Kings*), ed. de Goeje et al. (1964–5), series 3, III.1418.

medicine. In the Islamicate world, sugar was famous for its cleansing and soothing effects on the stomach, chest, and throat. A brief look at the entries on *sukkar* in Ibn al-Bayṭār's *al-Jāmiʿ li-mufradāt al-adwiyah wa-l-aghdhiyah* (*Collector of Simple Drugs and Foodstuffs*) (entry no. 4) or Ibn Sīnā's *Qānūn fī al-ṭibb* show how many varieties of sugar there were and how widely they were used for medicinal purposes.[16] Sugar abounds in medical recipes. For instance, Sābūr ibn Sahl, the court physician of the Abbasid caliph al-Mutawakkil in the ninth century, recommends white sugar (*fānīdh*) thirteen times, sugar (*sukkar*) seventeen times, and sugar cane juice, sugar-water, and *sulaymānī* sugar once each for various ailments in his dispensatory. More specifically, al-Kindī, another court physician and philosopher from ninth-century Baghdad, employs red sugar, in other words *qand*, in two clysters in his *Aqrābādhīn* (*Dispensatory*).[17] The raw sugar looted in the Byzantine attack of 853 on Damietta must have found its way into the markets as well as the imperial storehouses or even the palace in Byzantium. In any case, Byzantine physicians certainly employed sugar in their treatments. Symeon Seth emphasises the cleansing and diaphoretic qualities of sugar, John the Physician recommends it in a compound drug for *phthisis* (possibly tuberculosis), and the anonymous writer of the Mangana *xenōn* in eleventh-/twelfth-century Constantinople includes it in the diet of a patient suffering from a sore throat/inflammation of the larynx.[18]

A few centuries later, another case of pillaged aromatics is mentioned in a letter from the Byzantine emperor Isaac II Angelos to the Genoese authorities. In November 1192 Isaac complains about the piratical activities of Genoese captains who had captured ships carrying gifts sent by Salah ad-Din, the founder of the Ayyubid dynasty. The ships were carrying

[16] Ibn al-Bayṭār, *al-Jāmiʿ li-mufradāt al-adwiyah wa-l-aghdhiyah* (*Collector of Simple Drugs and Foodstuffs*) 4, ed. Sezgin (1996) III-IV.22–3. Ibn Sīnā differentiates between *sukkar aḥmar*, *sukkar sulaymānī*, *sukkar ṭabarzad* and *sukkar al-ʿaṣr*. See Ibn Sīnā, *Qānūn fī al-ṭibb* (*Canon of Medicine*), ed. Al-Kash and Zayur (1987) I.648–50.

[17] Al-Dīnawarī, *Kitāb al-nabāt* (*Book of plants*), ed. Hamidullah (1973) 211–12. For more on *qand*, see Sato (2014: 2, 43, 46–7, 91–104, 186) and Dozy (1968: II.417). On the sugar cane industry in Egypt see Ibn Ḥawqal, *Kitāb ṣūrat al-arḍ* (*Book of the Shape of the Earth*), ed. Goeje (1967) 142. For more on sugar in the medieval Mediterranean see Ouerfelli (2008). For an extensive discussion of the use of sugar in Byzantine medicine, see Bouras-Vallianatos (2021). On sugar cane (*qand*) see Ibn al-Bayṭār, *al-Jāmiʿ li-mufradāt al-adwiyah wa-l-aghdhiyah* (*Collector of Simple Drugs and Foodstuffs*), ed. Sezgin (1996) 227 (*ṭabarzad*), 193 (*sukkar*), 297 (*qand*). On the use of *qand* by Ibn Sīnā see Ibn Sīnā, *Qānūn fī al-ṭibb* (*Canon of Medicine*), ed. Al-Kash and Zayur (1987) II.1125, 1495. See also Sābūr ibn Sahl, *al-Aqrābādhīn al-ṣaghīr* (*Small Dispensatory*), trans. Kahl (2003), passim; al-Kindī, *Aqrābādhīn* (*Dispensatory*), ed. Levey (1966) 210, 160. Sugar is categorised with drugs in Maimonides' glossary of drug names. See Moses Maimonides, *Glossary of Drug Names*, trans. Rosner (1995) 221.

[18] Symeon Seth, *Treatises on the Capacities of Foodstuffs*, ed. Langkavel (1868) 96. John the Physician, *Iatrosophion*, ed. Zipser (2009) 126. Bennett (2003: 395).

diplomatic gifts, including ambergris, to Constantinople.[19] Ambergris (*ʿanbar* in Arabic), which is a substance produced in the biliary tract of sperm whales in the Indian Ocean, was used as a simple in Islamicate medicine as well as in perfumery and cooking. Ibn Sīnā devotes an entry to ambergris in his list of *materia medica*, while Sābūr ibn Sahl in the ninth century and al-Samarḳandī in the thirteenth include ambergris in their medical recipes.[20] Putting aside the mention of ambergris in Aetios of Amida's sixth-century *Medical Books*, which might be a later addition, we encounter the use of ambergris in the Byzantine medical tradition in both the middle and late Byzantine periods.[21] In a commentary on Hippocrates' aphorisms, Damaskios (who lived in the middle Byzantine period) provides a recipe containing ambergris for a medical fumigation to aid conception, while John Zacharias Aktouarios, from the first half of the fourteenth century, recommends its use three times in his *Medical Epitome*.[22] Plunder created opportunities for the procurement not only of drugs, but also of medical books. In a letter from the Genizah archive dated 1137, a Jewish doctor from Seleukeia in Byzantine Asia Minor tells his relative that he has asked the Byzantine army generals to bring him any medical books 'which might fall into their hands' during their campaigns in Aleppo and Damascus.[23]

Large amounts of portable wealth were transferred between eastern Mediterranean polities through tribute in the form of gold, captives, or textiles. For example, Edessa paid an annual tribute of fifty pounds of gold to Byzantium in Romanos III's reign. A Muslim governor of Sicily attacked the Byzantine town of Butira in Sicily and received 6,000 Muslim prisoners as tribute, while the Byzantine empress, Irene, delivered 30,000 pounds of goat-hair textiles, called *mirʿizzā*, to the Muslims as tribute at the beginning of the ninth century.[24] The economic value of

[19] Ed. Miklosich and Müller (1865) III.37.

[20] Durak (2018: 201–25). Ibn Sīnā, *Qānūn fī al-ṭibb* (*Canon of Medicine*), ed. Al-Kash and Zayur (1987) I.664–5. Sābūr ibn Sahl, *al-Aqrābādhīn al-ṣaghīr* (*Small Dispensatory*), tr. Kahl (2003) 62, 66. Al-Samarqandī, *Aqrābādhīn* (*Dispensatory*), tr. Levey and al-Khaledy (1967) 77, 135. I was not able to consult these last two works in the original Arabic, only in English translation.

[21] For the complicated tradition of the transmission of *Medical Books* see Garzya (1984: 250–4). For a more detailed discussion of ambergris in *Medical Books* see Durak (2018: 15–16).

[22] Damaskios, *Scholia on Hippocrates and Galen*, ed. Dietz (1834) II.477. John Zacharias Aktouarios, *Medical Epitome*, in MS.MSL.112, The Library at Wellcome Collection, London, ff. 172, 150, 173. Bouras-Vallianatos (2020: 30–1).

[23] Goitein (1964: 300).

[24] John Skylitzes, *Synopsis of Byzantine history*, 18.16, ed. Thurn (1973) 388. Ibn al-Idārī in Canard and Grégoire (1935: 376). Al-Ṭabarī, *Taʾrīkh al-rusul wa al-mulūk* (*The Annals of the Prophets and Kings*), ed. de Goeje (1964–5), series 3, III.505.

these tributes was not negligible. However, the transfer of drugs as tribute does not seem to have been a common practice. The only reference to this, though indirect and disputable, comes from a passage in Leo the Deacon's *History*. After Emperor John Tzimiskes had captured Mayyafarikin in northern Syria from the Hamdanids in 974, from which 'he carried off numerous beautiful gifts in gold, silver and cloth woven with gold, which he demanded from its inhabitants', he went on towards Iraq. Due to the inhospitable conditions he encountered,

> he packed up gifts brought to him by the Agarenes, which amounted to three million [nomismata?] in gold and silver, and he returned to Byzantium; there he displayed in a triumphal procession through the market place the gold and silver and the cloths and the perfumes (*arōmata*) from the Seres [i.e. Chinese] and the other gifts that he received from the Agarenes.[25]

Although the writer of the text describes the items in question as gifts (*dōra*), the context of a successful invasion by the Byzantine armies and the reference to these 'gifts' having been 'demanded' blur the line between gift and tribute. Following the textbook definition of tribute as a transfer of wealth as an acknowledgement of the superiority of the recipient and submission of the sender, it is more plausible to see the gifts submitted by the Agarenes (Muslims) as tribute. The fact that the people of Iraq (or more specifically those living in the area between Nisibis and Baghdad) brought aromatics (*arōmata*) allow us to make two important observations. First, the area must have been on a spice route. Second, one should not rule out the possibility that aromatics were sometimes included in the payment of tribute.

13.2 Diplomacy As an Occasion for the Movement of *Materia Medica*

Compared to looting and tribute, gift exchange seems to have been a more common means of transfer during the period in question.[26] Drugs and medical books were likely transferred between the two realms via gifts

[25] Leo the Deacon, *History*, ed. Hase (1828) 162–3. For the translation, see Talbot and Sullivan (2005: 204).

[26] Currently, there is no modern work on the relationship between diplomacy and medicine for the period under investigation, apart from Magdalino's translation of and commentary on a diplomatic letter sent from the son of the Fatimid caliph to [Byzantine] Emperor Romanos II (Magdalino (2015)). The only other work specifically devoted to this subject that I am aware of is Blockey (1980), but he focuses on the late antique period. Blockey examines the case of three Byzantine doctors, who

exchanged between individuals – that is to say, outside the network of diplomatic gifts. Proof of this comes from the letter from the Jewish doctor mentioned earlier in this chapter. Writing from Byzantine Seleukeia, he complains that he had previously sent some letters to his relative in Fustat accompanied by gifts of 'mulberries, ribes, barberries, gentian leaves and essence, absinth, and other medical plants'. However, they had not arrived because, he claims, 'every letter accompanied with a gift never arrives', referring to the stealing of gifts and discarding of letters by couriers or other third parties. Despite being aware of the possibility of gifts getting lost on the way, the Seleucian doctor still asks the same relative to send him 'a quarter of a dirham of seeds of mallow, mandrake, and althaea', which were not available in Cilicia. He also asks his relative to bring his (the Seleucian doctor's) medical books if he travels from Fustat to Seleukeia.[27] This episode shows that individuals connected by kinship or community ties exchanged drugs and medical books via correspondence and travel. The quantities must have been small in each case, but the frequent movement of letters and people in the eastern Mediterranean might justify seeing exchange at the individual or community level as a possible means of transferring drugs and medical books.

Nevertheless, written sources reveal more examples of drug transfer in the sphere of diplomatic gift exchange than in any other context. The Byzantine and Islamicate polities were not the only states to send *materia medica* as diplomatic gifts to each other. Aromatics and medicinal drugs (more specifically, *Schisandra chinensis* seeds, theriac – *tiryāq* in Arabic, gold essence, rose water, camphor) played an important role in Sino-Islamic relations from the seventh to the eleventh centuries. Similarly, balsam oil, theriac, skink, sugar, various aromatics such as aloeswood, benzoic resin, and the 'usual drugs' were among the gifts Mamluks sent to neighbouring states.[28]

The earliest example of a drug being exchanged between Byzantium and the Islamicate Near East as a diplomatic gift dates to the early ninth century. According to the historian al-Ṭabarī, Emperor Nikephoros I (r. 802–11) sought a truce and agreed to pay tribute to the Abbasid caliph, Hārūn al-Rashīd, when the caliph captured Herakleia in 806. Nikephoros also sent a letter to Hārūn al-Rashīd requesting, in addition to perfumes and royal tents, a specific Herakleian girl taken captive by the Abbasids, whom

were sent as envoys to the Sassanid court in the sixth century not only because of their skills as doctors, but also due to their training as philosophers and orators.

[27] Goitein (1964: 299–301).

[28] Bielenstein (2005: 369–73); Behrens-Abouseif (2014: 64, 113, 137, 146–50).

Nikephoros wanted to marry to his son. The caliph not only granted the emperor his requests for gifts, but also sent him dates, desserts, raisins, and theriac (*tiryāq*). In exchange, the emperor dispatched money, expensive garments, falcons, hunting dogs, and horses to the caliph.[29] All the gifts exchanged were elements of a courtly life that the ruler would put to personal use. Theriac was a very famous panacea and antidote against venomous poisons. Employed as far back as the Hellenistic period, it became especially popular, becoming a subject of scientific interest to Galen, as reflected in his writings (i.e. *On Theriac to Piso*, attributed to Galen) and his promotion of theriac as a cure-all. Theriac was a compound drug composed of up to eighty plant, animal, and mineral substances. It was produced as solid particles, in liquid form, or as ointment and was preserved in containers. The wide range of exotic, difficult-to-find ingredients involved and the necessity of adhering to strict rules in its production made theriac an expensive drug. As the twelfth-century doctor Moses Maimonides writes in his *Treatise on Poisons and Their Antidotes*, local preparation of theriac was extremely difficult due to the difficulty of procuring its herbal ingredients.[30] The writer of the thirteenth-century *Itinerarium peregrinorum et gesta regis Ricardi* (*Journey of the Crusaders and Deeds of King Richard*), a Latin history of the Third Crusade, refers to theriac as an expensive antidote for reptile bites that only the wealthiest nobles could access.[31]

We know that theriac was a gift exchanged among Byzantines, especially members of the political elite, as an antidote against poisons. In a letter addressed to the Nicaean emperor Theodore Laskaris (r.1205–21), Byzantine writer Michael Choniates compares the humoral qualities of the hare and the theriac sent to him by the emperor. A certain Potamiates, who was among the *oiketai* of Emperor John VI Kantakouzenos (r. 1347–54), was ordered by the emperor to poison himself, but he escaped death by consuming theriac. Manuel Philes, a Byzantine poet of the early fourteenth century, even dedicated a poem to a 'theriac jar' (*Eis thēriakarion*), in which he praises the object as 'the golden basket' that can bring back heat to the

[29] Al-Ṭabarī, *Ta'rīkh al-rusul wa al-mulūk* (*The Annals of the Prophets and Kings*), ed. de Goeje (1964–5), series 3, II.710.

[30] Watson (1966: 1–10); Fabbri (2007: 248). On Maimonides' statement, see Leiser and Dols (1987: 210). On the history of theriac, see Holste (1976), Stein (1997), Boudon-Millot (2002), and Mayor (2014: 20–3). On the use of theriac in medieval Europe, see Rubin (2014). On theriac containers, see Ciaraldi (2000), and Vladimirova-Aladzhova (2012). On theriac in the medieval al-Shām, see Amar, Serri, and Lev (Chapter 5) in this volume.

[31] *Itinerarium peregrinorum et gesta regis Ricardi* (*Journey of the Crusaders and Deeds of King Richard*), ed. Stubbs (1864) 254.

veins in the human body because 'it has a saving heat'.[32] In addition to the references in non-medical sources, theriac was described as a drug in numerous medical sources. The great medical compilers of the late antique period such as Aetios of Amida and Paul of Aegina as well as medical writers, such as Paul of Nicaea and Leo the Physician, from the middle Byzantine period recommended theriac very frequently.[33] As inheritors of classical medicine, Muslims in the medieval period not only included theriac in their pharmacopeia, but also improved the knowledge of it. A number of treatises were penned on this compound drug, such as *Maqālah fī adwiyat al-tiryāq* (*Treatise on the Medicaments Used in Theriac*) by Ibn Juljul from the tenth century and *Maqālah fil-tiryāq* (*Treatise on Theriac*) by Ibn Rushd from the twelfth. For instance, scholars of the Islamicate world discussed the health benefits of theriac and the timing and frequency with which it should be taken prophylactically.[34]

It was common practice among the political and religious elite of the Middle Ages to present theriac as a diplomatic gift. An early example dates to 667 when Byzantine envoys brought a gift of theriac (*diyejia*) to the rulers of the Tang dynasty in China. From this date period onwards, theriac was recorded in Chinese medical literature, although the use of theriac was limited to the imperial court in the early stages of its introduction to Chinese pharmacological lore.[35] Two centuries later, at the other end of Eurasia, the patriarch of Constantinople, Ignatios, sent *theriacam probatissimam* (most approved theriac) to Pope Adrian II in 871 along with many other gifts of liturgical objects. Likewise, another patriarch, Elias II of Jerusalem, sent theriac as gift to the Saxon king of England, Alfred the

[32] Michael Choniates, *Letter* 179, ed. Lampros (1880) 2. John Kantakouzenos, *History*, ed. Schopen (1831) II.598. Manuel Philes, *Poems*, ed. Miller (1857) 186.

[33] Aetios of Amida, *Medical Books*, 5.84.78, ed. Olivieri (1950) II.64 et passim. Paul of Aegina, *Epitome*, 3.13.4, ed. Heiberg (1921) I.155 et passim. Paul of Nicaea, *On Medicine*, ed. Ieraci Bio (1996) 85, 113, 122 (on lycanthropy, consumption, and plague). Leo the Physician, *Synopsis of Medicine*, ed. Ermerins (1840) 163, 175, 97, 189 (on consumption, dysentery, quartan fever, and oedema). On the use of theriac in a post-Byzantine medical recipe collection from Crete see Clark (2011: 86).

[34] Ullmann (1970: 321–42). 'Sum' in *Encyclopaedia of Islam* (1997: IX.872). Ricordel (2000a). Ricordel (2000b). For an analysis of the illustrations of a 1199 copy of *Kitāb al-tiryāq* (*Book of Antidotes or Theriac*) attributed to Galen, see Pancaroğlu (2001). On the afterlife of *On theriac to Piso* attributed to Galen in the Islamicate world see Boudon-Millot (2017). See also the recent volume by Boudon-Millot and Micheau (2020) with several contributions on theriac. On the Galenic corpus as studied and taught in Constantinople in the fourteenth and fifteenth centuries, see Touwaide (1997). On the many types of theriac that Ibn Sīnā recommends, ranging from theriac of opium to *tiryāq al-kabīr*, *tiryāq al-arba'*, and *tiryāq farrukhī*, see Ibn Sīnā, *Qānūn fī al-ṭibb* (*Canon of Medicine*), ed. Al-Kash and Zayur (1987), books 2, 3, passim.

[35] Nappi (2009); Dobroruka (2016); Chen (2019: 14, 28).

Great (r. 871–*c.*886), in the late ninth century.[36] In the twelfth-century *Chanson de Girart de Roussillon*, a Byzantine emperor gave Westerners sacs of theriac.[37] In short, expensive and elaborate recipes for theriac belonged exclusively to the political elite, who were willing to share it with one another.

Half a century after al- Rashīd sent theriac to the Byzantine emperor, the Abbasid caliph al-Mutawakkil sent Nasr ibn al-Azhar as an envoy to Emperor Michael III in 859 (861?) as part of the negotiations for a prisoner exchange. The historian al-Ṭabarī writes that the envoy brought '1000 musk bags, silk garments, much saffron, and exquisite pieces' with him to present to the emperor.[38] Saffron was exchanged frequently between Islamicate courts. Governors or rulers from Iran and the Maghreb (north-west Africa) around the same period were inclined to include it among the gifts they sent since the saffron from these two regions was famous in the medieval world. Al-Ṭabarī describes the quantity of saffron sent to the Byzantine emperor simply as 'much' – that is, a lot. It is hard to guess the amount in question. However, the reference to the 1,000 bags of musk that accompanied the saffron gives a hint as to the quantity involved. Moreover, similar cases of saffron sent as diplomatic gifts between Muslim potentates, such as 'a hundred camel loads of saffron' and '3000 *mann* of saffron', point to very large amounts.[39] That saffron was a worthy gift for Byzantine rulers is demonstrated by its inclusion in the

[36] Schreiner (2004: 272). Schreiner translates *theriacam* in *theriacam probatissimam* as a theriac container, but I prefer to translate the term as 'most approved theriac' due to the adjective *probatissimam. Leechdoms, Wortcunning, and Starcraft of Early England*, ed. Cockayne (1863) II.288–91. For the three poison-detecting birds sent from Bertha, queen of the Franks, to the Abbasid caliph al-Muktafi, see *Kitāb al-dhakhā'ir wa al-tuḥaf* (*Book of Gifts and Rarities*), attributed to Rashīd ibn al-Zubayr, ed. Hamidullah (1959) 48–59. Muhammad Hamidullah identifies the author as a certain Ibn al-Zubayr. On the other hand, Ghada Qaddumi (1996: 11) does not find this identification convincing. She argues that the anonymous work was written sometime after 1070, based on internal evidence.

[37] Girart de Roussillon, *Chanson de geste*, trans. Meyer (1884) 10 and Dalby (2010: 111). A few centuries later the Venetians sent theriac regularly to the Mamluks in addition to clothes, harness for horses, perfumes, and porcelain as a tribute for the possession of Cyprus until Egypt was taken over by the Ottomans in 1517. From then on, the Venetians paid the same tribute to the Ottomans (Setton 1969: 409, n. 160). For other examples of the Mamluk dispatch of theriac as diplomatic gifts, see Behrens-Abouseif (2014: 148–9).

[38] Al-Ṭabarī, *Ta'rīkh al-rusul wa al-mulūk* (*The Annals of the Prophets and Kings*), ed. de Goeje et al. (1964–5), series 3, III.1450. For the translation into English, see Kraemer (1989) 168.

[39] *Kitāb al-dhakhā'ir wa-l-tuḥaf* (*Book of Gifts and Rarities*), attributed to Rashīd ibn al-Zubayr, ed. Hamidullah (1959) 28, 69, 74. According to Ibn Ḥawqal, the yellow saffron that made clothes red came from the city of Barqa in central North Africa. Ibn Ḥawqal, *Kitāb ṣūrat al-arḍ* (*Book of the Shape of the Earth*), ed. de Goeje (1967b) 66. He adds later that Sabiba, on the route between Fez and sub-Saharan Africa, produced saffron. Ibn Ḥawqal, *Kitāb ṣūrat al-arḍ* (*Book of the Shape of the Earth*), ed. de Goeje (1967b) 87. As a unit of weight one *mann* weighed between 816.5 grams and

contents of the Byzantine emperor's personal baggage on a military expedition in the tenth century.[40] In medieval Islamicate culture saffron was consumed either as a simple in the preparation of drugs or as an ingredient in cooking for colouring and flavouring. Medieval medical compilations from the Islamicate world are unanimous about the medicinal properties of saffron. Ibn Sīnā and Ibn al-Bayṭār recommend saffron for eye problems, as well as cardiac and respiratory problems. They claim that it increases sexual desire and relieves urinary tract ailments and is useful for the treatment of female genito-urinary system disorders.[41] In a tenth-century cookbook from Baghdad, saffron is counted among the ten most popular aromatics used in cooking. Cooks added it to many types of dishes from beef stews to fish dishes, but primarily employed it to give colour to the food.[42] One finds saffron in Byzantine medicine and cooking too. Medical writers from the late antique Oribasios to John Zacharias Aktouarios in the fourteenth century, who employed it thirty-one times in the last two books of his *Medical Epitome*, recommend it frequently.[43] The *xenōn* (hospital) texts dating to the later centuries of Byzantium distinguish between common and true saffron, referring indirectly to a more expensive species.[44] It is a perfect example of food-cum-medicine appearing in works on the properties of food; for example, 'a sweet-and-sour saffron dish' was prepared in twelfth-century Constantinople.[45] In addition to the 1,000 bags of musk and 3,000 *mann* of saffron sent from the Abbasid caliph al-Mutawakkil to Emperor Michael III in 859, we can attest the following items among the diplomatic gifts sent from representatives of Islamicate polities to the

6,656 grams (Rebstock 2008: 2261). *Mann-i Sharʿī* was 833 grams while *mann-i Tabrīz* was 2.97 kilograms (Lambton 1988: 358).

40 Constantine Porphyrogennetos, *Three Treatises on Imperial Military Expeditions*, (c).210–39, ed. Haldon (1990) 108.

41 Ibn Sīnā, *Qānūn fī al-ṭibb* (*Canon of Medicine*), ed. Al-Kash and Zayur (1987) I.499. Ibn al-Bayṭār, *al-Jāmiʿ li-mufradāt al-adwiyah wa-l-aghdhiyah* (*Collector of Simple Drugs and Foodstuffs*), ed. Sezgin (1996) 3–4: 172–3 and Javadi et al. (2013: 2).

42 Ibn Sayyār al-Warrāq, *Kitāb al-ṭabīkh* (*Book of Dishes*), ed. Samiri and Kadhat (2012) 79, 128–9, 187–8, 211–13 and Nasrallah (2007) 138, 180–1, 230, 249. On this cookbook see also Lewicka (Chapter 9) in this volume.

43 Oribasios, *Medical Collections*, 5.33, ed. Raeder (1928) I/1.151–3. John Zacharias Aktouarios, *Medical Epitome*, in MSL, 112, Wellcome Library for the History of Medicine, London, passim. On Paul of Nicaea's use of saffron see Paul of Nicaea, *On medicine*, ed. Ieraci Bio (1996) 175, 369, 370. For the medicinal use of saffron in antiquity, see Goubeau (1993).

44 For the *Prostagai* texts (eleventh century to 1204), see Bennett (2003: 345–6, 351–2). On the same distinction in Θ text, see Bennett (2003: 410).

45 Symeon Seth, *Treatise on the Capacities of Foodstuffs*, ed. Langkavel (1868) 58. For a late- or post-Byzantine text entitled *Peri trophōn dynameōs* (*On the Capacity of Foodstuffs*) with a section on saffron, see ed. Delatte (1927–39) II.476. On this dish, see *Ptōchoprodromika*, 2.46, ed. Eideneier (1991) 112.

Byzantine capital city: 'ten scent baskets lined with leather [full] of camphor and aloeswood' from the Seljuk sultan Tughrul beg to the Byzantine emperor in 1057; and 'two masts of Indian aloeswood' of very large dimensions, weighing eight and forty *mann* each, from the Hamdanid ruler of Syria, Naṣr al-Dawla, to Emperor Romanos IV Diogenes in 1071.[46] Just as saffron was used in cooking and medicine, musk, aloeswood, and camphor were medicinal drugs in medieval pharmacology and equally cherished as raw materials for making perfume.[47]

The last example of *materia medica* sent from an Islamicate court to a Byzantine one is another wonder drug that healed broken bones. In a diplomatic letter dated to between 958 and 961, the son of the Fatimid caliph al-Muʿizz wrote to the son of the Byzantine emperor Romanos II that there was a certain medicinal substance (*eidos*) among the gifts dispatched by the caliph, called *moumie* in Greek. The son of the caliph claimed that the substance healed fractured limbs. The Fatimid prince warns his counterpart that this gift, being very rare and valuable, should not be lost among the other gifts sent by his father, al-Muʿizz. He supports his claim about the rarity of the drug by explaining how difficult it was for his father to obtain it and how merchants counterfeited it. He claims that the Abbasid rulers occupied the location where the substance oozed like tears from a rock. They could extract only a limited amount of it over a long period, but men close to the Fatimids sent the Fatimid caliph a small piece of this *moumie*. The tone of the letter is extremely amicable and courteous, dotted with words of endearment and concern. There seems to be some connection between the writer's concern for his correspondent's health and the choice of gift. After all, as the prince writes, 'for gems only provide delight for the eyes of the men, whereas this heals the sick and drives away many diseases from men'.[48]

The information al-Bīrūnī and Ibn al-Bayṭār provided confirms the claims of the letter writer. Ibn al-Bayṭār, quoting various medical authorities from Dioscorides to al-Raḍī, associates *moumie* with pittasphaltus (pitch-asphalt) and speaks of a number of varieties of it, such as that coming from Yemen and the 'bitumen of the Jews', found in great profusion in Egypt, especially in ancient tombs. His list of ailments that can be

[46] *Kitāb al-dhakhāʾir wa-l-tuḥaf* (*Book of Gifts and Rarities*), attributed to Rashīd ibn al-Zubayr, ed. Hamidullah (1959) 79–80, 85. For translations, see Qaddumi (1996: 112, 116).

[47] Ibn al-Bayṭār, *al-Jāmiʿ li-mufradāt al-adwiyah wa-l-aghdhiyah* (*Collector of Simple Drugs and Foodstuffs*), ed. Sezgin (1996) 3–4, 155–6 (musk), 143 (aloeswood), 42–4 (camphor). Symeon Seth, *Treatise on the Capacities of Foodstuffs*, ed. Langkavel (1868) 58–9, 66, 74–5.

[48] Magdalino (2015: 245–6).

healed by *moumie* is very similar to the list provided by the son of the caliph. The story of the specific type of *moumie* that we encounter in the letter from the caliph's son is presented in much more detail in al-Bīrūnī's work. Al-Bīrūnī mentions a cave in a mountain in Iran, protected by soldiers, which would be opened at specific times by the officials who supervised the collection of the *moumie* from the rock inside the cave. The substance oozed from the rock and was separated from the liquid using a filter. The officials would be given pieces of the *moumie* before leaving. The men 'close to the Fatimid caliph', mentioned in the letter, must have been among the Abbasid officials present at the extraction process described in Bīrūnī's account.[49]

The only case of a drug sent as a diplomatic gift from a Byzantine to an Islamicate court that I have been able to identify from the period in question was 'a medium-sized stone of dusty colour and triangular shape, which was useful for the disease of dropsy' sent by Emperor Basil II to the *amīr* of Sicily under the Fatimids, Abu al-Futūḥ ibn Abu al-Ḥusayn, sometime between 989 and 1020.[50] The antiquated term *dropsy* (*hyderos/*

[49] Ibn al-Bayṭār, *al-Jāmi' li-mufradāt al-adwiyah wa-l-aghdhiyah* (*Collector of Simple Drugs and Foodstuffs*), ed. Sezgin (1996) 3–4: 169–70. For *moumie* in Ibn al-Bayṭār's commentary on *De materia medica* of Dioscorides see 1.71. ed. Dietrich (1991) 61. Al-Bīrūnī, *Kitāb al-jamāhir fi ma'rifat al-jawāhir* (*Sum of Knowledge about Precious Stones*), (1936) 329–35. Al-Bīrūnī, *Kitāb al-ṣaydanah fi al-ṭibb* (*Book of Pharmacy in Medicine*), ed. Kahya (2011) 123–4. Ibn Sīnā, *Qānūn fi al-ṭibb* (*Canon of Medicine*), ed. Al-Kash and Zayur (1987) I.606. For more on *moumie*, see 'Mumiya' in *Encyclopaedia of Islam* (1993: VII.556), Pommerening (2007: 194, 196), Manjarrés (2010: 163–97) and Bryer and Winfield (1985: I.171).

[50] See ed. Hamidullah (1959), 83–4. On al-Raḍī's treatment of oedema with great cardamom and turmeric, see Meyerhof (1935: 343). Stern, quoting from Qāḍī al-Nu'mān ibn Muḥammad's tenth-century work *al-Majālis wa-l-musāyarāt* (*Book of Audiences and Voyages*), refers to a case of drug exchange in a diplomatic context. According to Stern's translation, a Byzantine envoy arrived at the Fatimid court in 957–8 carrying 'vessels of gold and silver inlaid with jewels, embroidery, silk, nard (*nardūn*), and other precious articles which they gave' as gifts (Stern 1950: 244, 253). See also Tibi (1991: 91). *Nardūn* in the work of Qāḍī al-Nu'mān cannot be the plant nard (*Valeriana* spp.) or spikenard (*Nardostachys jatamansi*). The terms *nārdus* and *nārdīn* referring to nard occur in some Islamicate pharmacological texts, but first they are not related in terms of grammar to *nardūn* in the work of Qāḍī al-Nu'mān; second, they are transliterations from Greek whose equivalent was *sunbul*, which was the term used for nard/spikenard in medieval Arabic. For instance, in his commentary on Dioscorides' *De materia medica*, Ibn al-Bayṭār lists Dioscorides' Indian/Syrian, Celtic, and mountain spikenards as *nārdus safārītīkī*, *nārdīn iklītīkī*, and *nārdīn ūrīnī* respectively, but explains that they are all varieties of *sunbul*. For Ibn al-Bayṭār's commentary on *De materia medica* of Dioscorides: ed. Dietrich (1991) 40–1. For cases of *sunbul* as the regular term for nard/spikenard in Islamicate pharmacological literature see Ibn al-Bayṭār, *al-Jāmi' li-mufradāt al-adwiyah wa-l-aghdhiyah* (*Collector of Simple Drugs and Foodstuffs*), ed. Sezgin (1996) 3–4: 36–7. Ibn Sīnā, *Qānūn fi al-ṭibb* (*Canon of Medicine*), ed. Al-Kash and Zayur (1987) I.650. Qadi al-Numan would have used *sunbul* rather than *nārdus* in his account, if he meant nard. In the work of Qāḍī al-Nu'mān *nardūn* should be translated as 'backgammons'. *Nard* meant backgammon in medieval Arabic (Dozy 1968: II.663). Al-Zamakhsharī, *Asās al-balāghah* (*Foundation of Eloquence*), ed. Naīm and Maarri (1998) 820. On backgammon in the Islamicate world, see Walker (2005: 88–9) and Rosenthal (1975). On

hydrōps in Greek and *istisqā*ʾ in Arabic), more or less equivalent to oedema, refers in very general terms to an abnormal accumulation of fluid in the body, and 'could correspond to a broad spectrum of modern diseases characterised by oedema and ascites, such as liver, renal, and heart diseases, including chronic heart failure'.[51] Since the term *dropsy* encompassed a wide range of diseases, we find it quite frequently in the medieval written sources. The Byzantine emperor Herakleios (r. 610–41) died in 641 suffering from dropsy (*hyderiasas*); [Leo III] suffered a fatal case of dropsy in 741; Emperor Alexios Komnenos' stomach and feet swelled up before he died, just like Michael IV the Paphlagonian (r. 1034–41), whose hands became very swollen due to 'sickness of the internal organs'.[52]

Hippocratic medicine provides a relatively detailed account of the aetiology and treatment of dropsy. The Galenic corpus has a great deal of discussion about dropsy but largely articulates what Hippocrates had already said. Galen provided a long list of solutions, ranging from bloodletting and drainage to drugs that contained simples such as ox dung or elaterium. Late antique compilers (such as Aetios of Amida and Paul of Aegina) and the medieval Islamicate medical corpus mostly repeat what the aforementioned authors had already explained.[53] Thābit ibn Qurra in *Kitāb al-dhakhīrah fī ʿilm al-ṭibb* (*Treasury of Medicine*) writes that a disease of the liver caused dropsy (*istisqā*) and recommends a fruit-rich diet and diuretics as a treatment. Ibn Sīnā too points to liver disease as the cause of dropsy.[54] Most of the remedies offered for the treatment of dropsy were plant-based. Leo the Physician recommends theriac for oedema, while John the Physician from the late Byzantine period lists plant-based

backgammon found in the eleventh-century shipwreck of Serçe Limanı in south-western Turkey, see Bass et al. (2009: 338–9).

[51] Riva et al. (2017: 187–9).

[52] Theophanes the Confessor, *Chronographia*, ed. de Boor (1883) I.341. Nikephoros, Patriarch of Constantinople, *Short History*, 64, ed. Mango (1990) 132; Anna Komnene, *Alexias*, 15.11,4–10, in ed. Reinsch and Kambylis (2001) 495–7; Michael Psellos, *Chronographia*, 4.50, in ed. Reinsch (2014) 77–8; and Lascaratos and Zis (2000: 914–16).

[53] Identifying it mainly as a disease of the liver or spleen, Hippocrates describes three types of dropsy: hydrops (fluid accumulation in the abdomen), anasarca (fluid build-up in the whole body), and tympanites (accumulation of gas rather than fluid in the abdomen). He recommends laxatives and venesection. Celsus distinguishes between generalised dropsy, curable by incisions in the skin, and ascites, where the fluid is drained by a metal tube. See Comrie (1928: 228–9) and Aronson (2003). See also Paul of Aegina, *Epitome*, 3.48, ed. Heiberg (1921) I.255–8. For a review of references to dropsy by late antique and early medieval medical doctors, see Adams (1844) I.569–76.

[54] Although al-Raḍī disagrees with his source on a number of points, he follows the Galenic knowledge closely on the different types of dropsy: ascites (*istisqā zikkī*), an unusual accumulation of fluid in the abdomen; anasarca (*istisqā laḥmī*), the build-up of fluid all over the body; and hydrothorax (*istisqā ṭablī*), accumulation of fluid in the lungs. See Meyerhof (1930: 67), Iskandar (1975: 44), and Ozaltay and Köşe (2001: 13).

recipes containing ground nettle, celery, mare's tail, hazelwort, and wormwood, in addition to theriac.[55] It is difficult to find in Byzantine sources a mineral drug that would fit the definition of a triangular, dusty-coloured, medium-sized stone that Emperor Basil II gave to the Sicilian emir. However, there are a number of possible candidates. First, Aetios of Amida describes jasper-like agate (*iaspachatēs*) as a remedy for thirst and dropsy.[56] Second, lodestone (*lapis magnes*) or magnetite is presented as a dark blue magnetic stone that cures dropsy in the *Alphabet of Galen*, an early medieval list of *materia medica* in Latin derived from classical sources. Dioscorides had already drawn attention to its magnetic qualities and claimed that it drew out thick masses from the body when given with hydromel. From Galen to Paracelsus, magnets were employed as purgatives to cure dropsy. For instance, the author of the fifteenth-century Peterborough Lapidary (Cambridge University Library MS Peterborough Cathedral 33) describes lodestone (defined as *magnes*) as a purgative against dropsy.[57] Stones for combatting dropsy seem to be in common use as gifts among members of the Muslim ruling elite too. The mother of the Fatimid caliph al-Mustanṣir's prime minister presented a similar stone to the mother of the caliph, who was suffering from dropsy. The white stone in the shape of a bead was supposed to be regularly tied around the belly at night in order to dry up the liquid in the abdomen.[58] The entry on the white stone sent to the mother of the caliph in *Kitāb al-dhakhāʾir wa-l-tuḥaf* comes right before the entry on Basil II's gift of a dusty-coloured stone to the Sicilian *amīr*. This textual juxtaposition shows that healing gifts could be exchanged among the Mediterranean elite regardless of their political and religious affiliations.

[55] Leo the Physician, *Synopsis of Medicine*, 6.2, ed. Ermerins (1840) 189. John the Physician, *Iatrosophion*, ed. Zipser (2009) 92. On the use of squill in the treatment of dropsy, see Stannard (1974). The few mineral remedies that Paul of Aegina recommends (sulphur, pyrite, nitre, alum, and flakes of copper) do not take the form of a dusty-coloured stone. Paul of Aegina, *Epitome*, 3.48, ed. Heiberg (1921) I.255–8.

[56] Aetios of Amida, *Medical Books*, II.37, ed. Olivieri (1935–50) I.168. For additional classical references to jasper-like agate in the treatment of dropsy, see *Medicina Plinii*, ed. Hunt (2020) 261.

[57] Pseudo-Galen, *The alphabet of Galen*, ed. Everett (2011) 271. *The Peterborough lapidary*, ed. Young (2016) 61–3. Dioscorides, *De materia medica*, 5.130, ed. Wellmann (1914) III.96. See also Frei (1970: 36) and Mills (2004). Other candidates for the stone used to combat dropsy are jet stone, a lignite and mineraloid; and amber, a fossilised resin. On jet, see Alexander Neckam's *De naturis rerum* (*On the Nature of Things*) from the late twelfth century in Coulter (2015: 110). On amber, see Arnold of Saxony's *De finibus rerum naturalium* (*On the Boundaries of Nature*) from the late twelfth and early thirteenth centuries in Duffin (2013: 18). The subject needs further investigation, especially of the Greek sources from the classical and Byzantine periods.

[58] *Kitāb al-dhakhāʾir wa-l-tuḥaf* (*Book of Gifts and Rarities*), attributed to Rashīd ibn al-Zubayr, ed. Hamidullah (1959) 82–3.

Conclusion: Gifts for Making Friends

Materia medica constitute a relatively small category in the gifts exchanged between the Byzantines and the Islamicate polities in the early Middle Ages. In the period between 639 and 750, which precedes the period under investigation in this chapter, sources that mention diplomatic exchanges between the Byzantine and Umayyad courts do not often refer to specific gifts, but, when they do, the gifts in question are gold, horses, garments, as well as building material and manpower for a number of construction sites in the Islamicate Near East (columns, mosaic pieces, and mosaic workers), with only one reference to pepper (worth 20,000 dinars), which al-Walīd (705–15) planned to send to the Byzantine ruler, though he ultimately failed to do so for some unknown reason.[59] The sources provide more detail on diplomatic gifts in the ninth to the eleventh centuries. Among the twenty-nine accounts of specific diplomatic gifts sent from the Byzantine court to various Islamicate courts from 806 to 1071, only one medicinal substance can be identified, and that is the previously discussed stone used to treat dropsy.[60] There seems to have been more *materia medica* moving in the opposite direction. Of the nine cases of diplomatic dispatches from the Abbasid and post-Abbasid Islamicate courts to Byzantium during the same period, there are six instances of aromatics and drugs as gifts (saffron, theriac, *moumie*, musk, aloeswood, and camphor).[61] The imbalance is understandable since a large proportion of the aromatics originated from South Asia and Africa, regions that were in touch with the Byzantine world only through the agency of Islamicate intermediaries. Moreover, many of the items that have been defined as *materia medica* in this chapter were also employed as spices and perfumes. Saffron was both a drug and an ingredient used to colour and flavour food in cooked dishes. Pepper, musk, aloeswood, and camphor were utilised in food, perfumes, and drugs. Only theriac, *moumie*, and the stone used for dropsy were genuinely and solely medicinal in purpose and use.

However, when we compare the Byzantine-Islamic diplomatic gifts with the diplomatic gifts exchanged between the Byzantines and their other neighbours, we realise that *materia medica* were not a negligible gift category in Byzantine-Islamic interactions. In Byzantine–Western European diplomatic exchanges in the early Middle Ages, Western polities

[59] Kaplony (1996: 175, 181, 201, 366–7, 377–8).

[60] For these accounts, see Durak (2018: 256–61).

[61] On the nine cases, see Durak (2018: 261). Al-Ṭabarī, *Taʾrīkh al-rusul wa al-mulūk* (*The Annals of the Prophets and Kings*), ed. de Goeje (1964–5), series 3, II.710; Magdalino (2015). For a catalogue of Byzantine-Abbasid diplomatic exchanges, see Vaiou (2002).

sent cheap objects such as hunting animals, livestock, arms, slaves, and eunuchs, while the Byzantine Empire dispatched gifts of a more luxurious nature such as expensive textiles, relics, books, spices, and exotic animals (such as lions and camels). In this 'asymmetric exchange' the ratio of *materia medica* to other types of gifts is low. Peter Schreiner lists only five cases of aromatics (*pigmenta*, *aromata multa*, *balsamum*, *aleipta* [ointments in Greek]) sent by the Byzantine emperors as gifts in fifty-six cases of gift-giving in the period between 800 and 1200. None of these aromatics served purely medicinal purposes; rather they were more often used as spices or for religious rituals. When the religious nature of the accompanying gifts in the same consignments, such as relics and encolpia, are taken into account, it seems likely that the balsam and ointments included among the gifts were more probably for ritual than medical use.[62] In short, not a single gift can be identified as having a solely medical function in Byzantine-Western European diplomatic relations. Interestingly, according to studies by Günter Prinzing and Yusuf Ayönü, there is not a single case of an aromatic substance sent as a gift in the diplomatic relations of the Byzantines, neither with the Eastern and South-eastern European polities nor with the Seljuks of Anatolia.[63] One might wonder whether the high ratio of drugs employed/[drugs] sent as diplomatic gifts between the Byzantines and the Islamicate Near East is a reflection of the intensive transfer of medical knowledge between these two cultures, an exchange accomplished partly through the transfer of books in their original languages or in translation.[64]

The overwhelming majority of the gifts exchanged between Byzantine and Islamicate states belong to the category of what we might call the fundamentals of court life. This courtly context was created with the help of gifts that contributed to: a) the decoration of the interior (textiles,

62 Schreiner (2004: 264–6, 273, 274, 278, 280, 282). On Byzantine–Western European diplomatic gifts, see Lounghis (1980: 163–7), Nerlich (1999: 163–74), and Tinnefeld (2005: 127, 129, 134). On the concept of asymmetry in diplomatic exchanges, see Grabar (1984). On the medicinal and ritual use of balsam, see Truitt (2009).

63 Prinzing (2005); Ayönü (2015). China appears to be the only exception. Out of the nine known cases of Sino-Byzantine diplomatic contacts, we have specific information about gifts in five cases. In one of these exchanges, which took place in 667, Byzantine envoys brought theriac to the Chinese court. See Bielenstein (2005: 367).

64 On the translation of medical texts from medieval Greek to Arabic and vice versa, see Touwaide (1995, 2002b, 2011). Diplomatic gift-giving was a means by which the Muslims acquired books from Byzantium. In 948 Constantine VII sent a copy of Dioscorides' *De materia medica* to the Spanish Umayyad caliph al-Naṣr ʿAbd al-Raḥmān al-Muḥammad as part of a diplomatic mission. Ibn Abī Uṣaybiʿah, *ʿUyūn al-anbāʾ fī ṭabaqāt al-aṭibbāʾ* (*Sources of Information on the Classes of Physicians*), ed. Jahier and Noureddine (1958) 38. For more on this exchange, see Cardoso (2015: 145–50) and Codoñer (2004).

utensils, gems, fragrances), b) the beautification and preservation of the human body (garments, gems, medicinal/cosmetic products, food), c) service and attendance on the elite (human labour, slaves), d) hunting (birds, dogs, horses), e) demonstrating the cultural or military might of the sending party (books, arms, prisoners), and f) amazing the recipient (exotic animals and objects).[65] In the Middle Ages diplomatic gifts fulfilled multiple functions, two of which have been emphasised by modern scholars. On the one hand, by appealing to the sensory pleasures of a leisurely class, diplomatic gifts exhibited common aesthetics and collective memoires, contributing to the creation of a shared courtly culture around the medieval Mediterranean. On the other hand, they functioned as ideological and cultural challenges to the authority of the recipient.[66] When exchanged as gifts, the aromatics and drugs discussed here established bonds between political actors, creating mutual ties. As I have attempted to show, saffron and theriac were pan-Mediterranean gifts exchanged among members of the political and religious elite, regardless of their political affiliations. As objects aimed at preserving the health of royal figures, gifts of drugs were much more personal than gifts of wall hangings or gold coins. They saved lives. For instance, theriac was a panacea against poison. The gifts sent by Hārūn al-Rashīd – dates, desserts, raisins, and theriac – seem to have been selected for the personal use of the recipient, almost as if inviting him to a feast. The friendly discourse in the letter of the Fatimid caliph al-Muʿizz's son to the son of the Byzantine emperor Romanos II and the gift of *moumie* accompanying the letter are not the usual ways of showing/demanding submission symbolically to/from the person on the receiving end. Besides, medicinal gifts did not function as 'objects of display'. Lacking the element of magnificence, small medicinal gifts could not be paraded like the golden brocades or captives received as gifts or tribute. Neither could they act as vehicles for artistic media like the gifts of silver vessels exchanged between Sassanians and Byzantines.[67] What attracted the attention of the writer of *Kitāb al-dhakhāʾir wa-l-tuḥaf* was not the stone to treat dropsy, but the casket in which it was carried.

[65] Durak (2008: 242–3).

[66] Grabar (1997: 116, 126). Cutler (1996) sees gift items as a means of showing the opulence of the donor court and feeding the recipient's desire for the exotic. In interpreting diplomatic gifts, Walker (2005: 127, 130) proposes that gifts articulated the power dynamics between the sender and the recipient and 'evoked mutually recognised indices of royal authority'. While emphasising the nature of these gifts as shared courtly objects, she also views them as 'precious and exceptional', a view that coincides with Cutler's argument.

[67] Cutler (2005, 2008).

Nevertheless, no gift comes with a single message. Although the friendly aspect of medicinal gifts was more pronounced, the rarity and cost of some drugs or the sheer amount of others may have transformed them into gifts intended to impress the recipient and make him/her grateful, and therefore indebted to the sender. The stone used against dropsy and the *moumie* were extremely rare objects, theriac prepared according to complicated recipes with rare ingredients was a necessarily expensive item, and, finally, the 3,000 *mann* of saffron or the 'two masts of Indian aloeswood' of very large dimensions sent to Constantinople would have cost a fortune. A story in the Miracles of Saints Cyrus and John in the late antique period shows very clearly how gifts burdened the recipient with an obligation to return the favour: when Empress Sophia approached the Sassanian ruler, Chosroes II, for peace, she reminded him how, when he had been seriously ill, he had been saved by the intervention of Byzantine doctors she had sent.[68] Staking a claim to superior medical knowledge in international relations was not only accomplished through possessing the best doctors at a royal court. *Materia medica*, whether sent as gifts or grown for local consumption, could be transformed into occasions for reaffirming one culture's superiority over the other. The tenth-century writer Ibn al-Faqīh relates a story about an envoy sent by the eighth-century Abbasid caliph al-Mansur to the Byzantine emperor. During the negotiations, the emperor took ʿUmāra ibn Ḥamza, the Abbasid envoy, to an enclosed field full of tamarisk trees. The emperor asked ʿUmāra whether he knew the tree. ʿUmāra answered in the negative, curious as to the emperor's reaction. The emperor responded by saying that the smoke of tamarisk wood was employed against ulcers. The envoy said to himself: 'If the emperor only knew that tamarisk is a cheap firewood for us.' Then the emperor took ʿUmāra to another garden where there was a caper bush. Upon being asked to identify the bush, the envoy said that he could not. When the emperor explained the medicinal uses of caper, ʿUmāra said to himself: 'If he only knew that this plant exists only in the most desolate places and the deserts in our country.'[69] These anecdotes are most likely literary constructions, not an exact reflection of what really happened, but they show that neither the Byzantines nor their eastern neighbours missed any opportunity to humiliate or impress the other in a confrontation fought with words, gestures, and objects. As rare and costly means of healing, medicinal substances could offer opportunities for both rapprochement and boasting in the theatre of diplomacy.

[68] Magoulias (1964: 129).
[69] Ibn al-Faqīh, *Kitāb al-buldān* (*Book of the Countries*), ed. de Goeje (1967) 138.

REFERENCES

ʿAbd al-Wahhab, H. H. ed. 1966. Al-Jāḥiẓ: *Kitāb al-tabaṣṣur bi-al-tijārah*. Beirut: Dār al-Kitāb al-Jadīd.

Adams, F. trans. 1844. *The Seven Books of Paul of Aegina*. 3 vols. London: Sydenham Society.

Aronson, J. 2003. 'When I Use a Word Dropsy', *British Medical Journal* 326.7387: 491.

Ayönü, Y. 2015. 'Bizans'tan Selçuklulara Gönderilen Hediyeler', in *Türk Kültüründe Hediye Sempozyumu [Symposium on Gifts in Turkish Culture]*. Istanbul: M.Ü. Türkiyat Uygulama ve Araştırma Merkezi.

Bass, G. F. et al. eds. 2009. *Serçe Limani, vol. 2: The Glass of an Eleventh-Century Shipwreck*. Austin: Texas A&M University Press.

Behrens-Abouseif, D. 2014. *Practising Diplomacy in the Mamluk Sultanate: Gifts and Material Culture in the Medieval Islamic World*. London: I. B. Tauris.

Bennett, D. 2003. 'Xenonika: Medical Texts Associated with Xenones in the Late Byzantine Period'. University of London: PhD thesis.

Bielenstein, H. 2005. *Diplomacy and Trade in the Chinese World, 589–1276*. Leiden: Brill.

Al-Bīrūnī. 1936. *Kitāb al-jamāhir fī maʿrifat al-jawāhir*. Hyderabad: Jamʿīyat Dāʾirat al-Maʿārif al-ʿUthmānīyah.

Blockey, R. C. 1980. 'Doctors As Diplomats in the Sixth Century A.D.', *Florilegium* 2: 89–100.

Boor, C. de. ed. 1883. *Theophanis chronographia*, vol. I. Leipzig: Teubner.

Bos, G. ed. and trans. 1992. *G. Qusṭā Ibn Lūqā's Medical Regime for the Pilgrims to Mecca: The Risālā fī tadbīr safar al-Ḥajj*. Leiden: Brill.

Boudon-Millot, V. 2002. 'La thériaque selon Galien: Poison salutaire ou remède empoisonné', in F. Collard and E. Samama (eds.), *Le corps à l'épreuve: Poisons, remédes et chirurgie: aspects des pratiques médicales dans l'Antiquité et au Moyen Âge*. Langres: Gueniot, 45–56.

Boudon-Millot, V. 2017. 'La tradition orientale du traité pseudo-galénique *Sur la thériaque à Pison (De theriaca ad Pisonem)*', *Galenos* 11: 17–30.

Boudon-Millot, V., and Micheau, F. eds. 2020. *Histoire, transmission et acculturation de la Thériaque. Actes du colloque de Paris (18 mars 2010)*. Paris: Beauchesne.

Bouras-Vallianatos, P. 2020. *Innovation in Byzantine Medicine: The Writings of John Zacharias Aktouarios (c.1275–c.1330)*. Oxford: Oxford University Press.

Bouras-Vallianatos, P. 2021. 'Cross-cultural Transfer of Medical Knowledge in the Medieval Mediterranean: The Introduction and Dissemination of Sugar-based Potions from the Islamic World to Byzantium', *Speculum* 96.4: 963–1008.

Bryer, A., and Winfield, D. 1985. *The Byzantine Monuments and Topography of the Pontos*. 2 vols. Washington, DC: Dumbarton Oaks.

Canard, M., and Grégoire, H. 1935. *La dynastie d'Amorium (820–867), Byzance et les Arabes*, vol. I. Brussels: Edition de l'Institut de Philologie et d'Histoire Orientales et Slaves.

Cardoso, E. R. F. 2015. 'Diplomacy and Oriental Influence in the Court of Cordoba (9th–10th Centuries)'. University of Lisbon: PhD thesis.

Chen, M. 2019. '"The Healer of All Illnesses": The Origins and Development of Rûm's Gift to the Tang Court: Theriac', *Studies in Chinese Religions* 5.1: 14–37.

Ciaraldi, M. 2000. 'Drug Preparation in Evidence? An Unusual Plant and Bone Assemblage from the Pompeian Countryside, Italy', *Vegetation History and Archaeobotany* 9: 91–8.

Clark, P. A. ed. and trans. 2011. *A Cretan Healer's Handbook in the Byzantine Tradition*. Farnham: Ashgate.

Cockayne, T. O. ed. 1863. *Leechdoms, Wortcunning, and Starcraft of Early England*. 2 vols. London: Longman.

Codoñer, J. S. 2004. 'Bizancio y Al-Andalus en los siglos IX y X', in P. B. de la Peña and I. P. Martín (eds.), *Bizancio y la Península Ibérica: De la Antigüedad tardía a la Edad Moderna*. Madrid: Consejo Superior de Investigaciones Científicas, 177–245.

Comrie, J. D. 1928. 'Remarks on Historical Aspects of Ideas Regarding Dropsy', *British Medical Journal* 2.3527: 229–32.

Coulter, C. 2015. 'Consumers and Artisans: Marketing Amber and Jet in the Early Medieval British Isles', in G. Hansen et al. (eds.), *Everyday Products in the Middle Ages: Crafts, Consumption and the Individual in Northern Europe c. AD 800–1600*. Oxford: Oxbow Books, 110–24.

Cutler, A. 1996. 'Les échanges des dons entre Byzance et l'Islam', *Journal des Savants* 1: 51–66.

Cutler, A. 2005. 'Silver across the Euphrates: Forms of Exchange between Sassanian Persia and the Late Roman Empire', *Mitteilungen zur spätantiken Archäologie und byzantinischen Kunstgeschichte* 4: 9–37.

Cutler, A. 2008. 'Significant Gifts: Patterns of Exchange in Late Antique, Byzantine, and Early Islamic Diplomacy', *Journal of Medieval and Early Modern Studies* 38: 79–102.

Dalby, A. 2007. 'Some Byzantine Aromatics', in L. Brubaker and K. Linardou (eds.), *Eat, Drink, and Be Merry (Luke 12:19). Food and Wine in Byzantium: Papers of the 37th Annual Spring Symposium of Byzantine Studies*. Burlington: Ashgate, 51–8.

Dalby, A. 2010. *Tastes of Byzantium*. London: Phrase Book.

Delatte, A. ed. 1927–39. *Anecdota Atheniensia et alia*. 2 vols. Paris: Droz.

Dietrich, A. ed. 1991. *Die Dioscorides-Erklärung des Ibn al-Baitār, Ein Beitrag zur arabischen Pflanzensynoymik [!] des Mittelalters*. Gottingen: Vandenhoeck & Ruprecht.

Dietz, F. R. ed. 1834. *Scholia in Hippocratem et Galenum*. 2 vols. Konigsberg: Regimontii Prussorum.

Dobroruka, V. 2016. 'Theriac and Tao: More Aspects on Byzantine Diplomatic Gifts to Tang China', *Journal of Literature and Art Studies* 6.2: 170–7.

Dozy, R. P. A. 1968. *Supplement aux dictionnaires Arabes*. 2 vols. Beirut: Librairie du Liban.

Duffin, C. 2013. 'Lithotherapeutical Research Sources from Antiquity to the Mid-18th Century', in C. J. Duffin, R. T. J. Moody, and C. Gardner-Thorpe (eds.), *A History of Geology and Medicine*. London: The Geological Society, 7–43.

Durak, K. 2008. 'Commerce and Networks of Exchange between the Byzantine Empire and the Islamic Near East from the Early Ninth Century to the Arrival of the Crusaders'. Harvard University: PhD thesis.

Durak, K. 2011. 'The Location of Syria in Byzantine Writing: One Question, Many Answers', *Journal of Turkish Studies* 36: 45–55.

Durak, K. 2018. 'Dioscorides and Beyond: Imported Medicinal Plants in the Byzantine Empire', in B. Pitarakis (ed.), *Life Is Short, Art Long: The Art of Healing in Byzantium*. Istanbul: Istanbul Research Institute, 152–60.

Eideneier, H. ed. 1991. *Ptochoprodromos: Einführung, kritische Ausgabe, deutsche Übersetzung, Glossar*. Cologne: Romiosini.

Ermerins, F. Z. ed. 1840. *Anecdota medica graeca e codicibus MSS. Expromsit*. Leiden: S. et J. Luchtmans.

Everett, N. ed. and trans. 2011. *The Alphabet of Galen: Pharmacy from Antiquity to the Middle Ages*. Toronto: University of Toronto Press.

Fabbri, C. N. 2007. 'Treating Medieval Plague: The Wonderful Virtues of Theriac', *Early Science and Medicine* 12: 247–83.

Frei, E. H. 1970. 'Medical Applications of Magnetism', *C R C Critical Reviews in Solid State Sciences* 1.3: 381–407.

Freshfield, E. H. 1938. *Roman Law in the Later Roman Empire, Byzantine Guilds, Professional and Commercial, From the Book of the Eparch*. Cambridge: Cambridge University Press.

Garzya, A. 1984. 'Problèmes relatifs à l'édition des livres IV–XVI du *Tétrabiblon* d'Aétios d'Amida', *Revue des Études Ancienne* 86.1: 245–57.

Gibb, H. A. R. et al. eds. 1960–2007. *Encyclopaedia of Islam*. 12 vols. Leiden: Brill.

Gil, M. 1997. *A History of Palestine 634–1099*. Cambridge: Cambridge University Press.

Goeje, M. J. de. ed. 1967a. Al-Iṣṭakhrī: *Kitāb al-masālik wa l-mamālik*. Bibliotheca geographorum Arabicorum, pars 1. Leiden: Brill.

Goeje, M. J. de. ed. 1967b. Ibn Ḥawqal: *Kitāb ṣūrat al-arḍ*. Bibliotheca geographorum Arabicorum, pars 2. Leiden: Brill.

Goeje, M. J. de. ed. 1967c. Ibn al-Faqīh: *Kitāb al-buldān*. Bibliotheca geographorum Arabicorum, pars 5. Leiden: Brill.

Goeje, M. J. de. ed. 1967d. Ibn Khurradādhbih: *Kitāb al-masālik [wa-] al-mamālik*. Bibliotheca geographorum Arabicorum, pars 6. Leiden: Brill.

Goeje, M. J. de. et al. eds. 1964–5. Al-Ṭabarī: *Taʾrīkh al-rusul wa al-mulūk*, 3 series. Leiden: Brill.

Goitein, S. D. 1964. 'A Letter from Seleucia (Cilicia): Dated 21 July 1137', *Speculum* 39.2: 298–303.

Goitein, S. D. 1967–93. *Mediterranean Society: The Jewish Communities of the Arab World As Portrayed in the Documents of the Cairo Geniza*. 6 vols. Berkeley: University of California Press.

Goubeau, R. 1993. 'De quelques usages médicaux du crocus dans l'Antiquité', in M.-Cl. Amouretti and G. Comet (eds.), *Des hommes et des plantes: Plantes méditerranéennes, vocabulaire et usages anciens, édité par, table ronde d'Aix- en-Provence, Mai 1992*. Aix-en-Provence: Service des Publications de l'Université, 23–6.

Grabar, A. 1984. 'L'asymétrie des relations de Byzance et de l'Occident dans le domaine des arts au moyen âge', in I. Hutter (ed.), *Byzanz und der Westen: Studien zur Kunst des Europäischen Mittelalters*. Vienna: Verlag der Österreichischen Akademie der Wissenschaften, 9–24.

Grabar, O. 1997. 'The Shared Culture of Objects', in H. Maguire (ed.), *Byzantine Court Culture from 829 to 1204*. Washington, DC: Dumbarton Oaks, 115–29.

Haldon, J. F. ed. 1990. Constantine Porphyrogennetos, *Three Treatises on Imperial Military Expeditions*. Vienna: Verlag der Österreichischen Akademie der Wissenschaften.

Hamidullah, M. ed. 1959. *Kitāb al-dhakhā'ir wa-l-tuḥaf*, attributed to Rashīd ibn al-Zubayr. Kuwait: Dā'irat al-Maṭbū'āt wa-l-Nashr.

Hamidullah, M. ed. 1973. *Al-Dīnawarī: Kitāb al-nabāt*. Cairo: al-Ma'had al-'Ilmī al-Faransī lil-Athār al-Sharqīyah.

Hase, K. B. ed. 1828. *Leonis Diaconi Caloënsis Historiae Libri Decem*. Bonn: Weber.

Heiberg, J. L. ed. 1921–4. *Paulus Aeginita*. 2 vols. Leipzig: Teubner.

Holste, T. 1976. *Der Theriakkrämer: Ein Beitrag zur Frühgeschichte der Arzneimittelwerbung*. Pattensen: Horst Wellm.

Hunt, Y. ed. and trans. 2020. *The Medicina Plinii: Latin Text, Translation, and Commentary*. Abingdon: Routledge.

Ieraci Bio, A. M. ed. 1996. Paolo di Nicea: *Manuale Medico*. Naples: Bibliopolis.

Iskandar, A. Z. 1975. 'The Medical Bibliography of al-Razi', in G. Hourani (ed.), *Essays on Islamic Philosophy and* Science. Albany: State University of New York Press, 41–6.

Jacoby, D. 2000. 'Byzantine Trade with Egypt from the Mid-Tenth Century to the Fourth Crusade', *Thesaurismata* 30: 25–77.

Jahier, H., and Noureddine, A. eds. 1958. Ibn Abī Uṣaybi'ah: *'Uyūn al-anbā' fī ṭabaqāt al-aṭibbā' = Sources d'informations sur les classes des médecins: XIIIe chapitre*. Alger: Ferraris.

Javadi, B. et al. 2013. 'A Survey on Saffron in Major Islamic Traditional Medicine Books', *Iranian Journal of Basic Medical Sciences* 16.1: 1–11.

Jong, P. de. ed. 1867. Al-Tha'ālibī: *Laṭā'if al-ma'ārif*. Leiden: Brill.

Kahl, O. trans. 2003. *The Small Dispensatory by Sābūr Ibn Sahl*. Leiden: Brill.

Kahya, E. ed. 2011. Al-Biruni: *Kitabü's-saydana fi't-tıb*. Ankara: Kültür ve Turizm Bakanlığı.

Kaplony, A. 1996. *Konstantinopel und Damaskus, Gesandtschaften und Vertrage Zwischen Kaisern und Kalifen 639–750*. Berlin: Klaus Schwarz.

al-Kash I., and Zayur, A. eds. 1987. Ibn Sīnā, *Qānūn fī al-ṭibb*. 4 vols. Beirut: Ṭab'ah jadīdah muḥaqqaqah.

Koder, J. ed. 1991. *Das Eparchenbuch Leons des Weisen*. Vienna: Verlag der Österreichischen Akademie der Wissenschaften.

Kraemer, J. L. trans. 1989. *The History of al-Tabari, Incipient Decline: The Caliphates of al-Wathiq, al-Mutawakkil, and al-Muntasir A.D. 841–863/A.H. 227–248*, vol. XXXIV. New York: State University of New York Press.

Lambton, A. K. S. 1988. *Continuity and Change in Medieval Persia*. New York: Persian Heritage Foundation.

Lampros, S. P. ed. 1879–80. *Μιχαὴλ Ἀκομινάτου τοῦ Χωνιάτου. Τὰ σωζόμενα*. 2 vols. Athens: Ek tou typographeiou Parnassou.

Langkavel, B. ed. 1868. Symeon Seth: *Syntagma de alimentorum facultatibus*. Leipzig: Teubner.

Lascaratos, J., and Zis, P. V. 2000. 'The Epilepsy of Emperor Michael IV, Paphlagon (1034–1041 A.D.): Accounts of Byzantine Historians and Physicians', *Epilepsia* 41.7: 913–17.

Leiser, G., and Dols, M. 1987. 'Evliyā Chelebi's Description of Medicine in Seventeenth-Century Egypt: Part I: Introduction', *Sudhoffs Archiv* 71.2: 197–216.

Leone, P. ed. 1972. *Ioannis Tzetzae epistulae*. Leipzig: Teubner.

Levey, M. ed. and trans. 1966. *The Medical Formulary of Aqrābādhīn of al-Kindī*. Madison: University of Wisconsin Press.

Levey, M. and al-Khaledy, N. trans. 1967. *The Medical Formulary of al-Samarqandi and the Relation of Early Arabic Simples to Those Found in the Indigenous Medicine of the Near East and India*. Philadelphia: University of Pennsylvania Press.

Liddell, H. G., Scott, R., and Jones, H. S. eds. 1996. *A Greek-English Lexicon* [9th ed. 1940; with a revised supplement edited by P. G. W. Glare]. Oxford: Clarendon [LSJ].

Lounghis, T. C. 1980. *Les ambassades byzantines en occident depuis la fondation des Etats barbares jusqu'aux Croisades (407–1096)*. Athens: Typographia.

Magdalino, P. 2015. 'Pharmaceutical Diplomacy: A New Document on Fatimid. Byzantine Gift Exchange', in Th. Antonopoulou, S. Kotzabassi, and M. Loukaki (eds.), *Myriobiblos: Essays on Byzantine Literature and Culture*. Berlin: De Gruyter, 245–51.

Magoulias, H. J. 1964. 'The Lives of the Saints As Sources of Data for the History of Byzantine Medicine in the Sixth and Seventh Centuries', *Byzantinische Zeitschrift* 57.1: 127–50.

Mango, C. A. ed. and trans. 1990. *Nikephoros Patriarch of Constantinople, Short History: Text, Translation and Commentary*. Washington, DC: Dumbarton Oaks.

Manjarrés, M. Á. G. 2010. 'Presencia de mumia en la medicina medieval (siglos XI–XIV)', in A. P. Bagliani (ed.), *Terapie e guarigioni*. Florence: Edizione Nazionale La Scuola Medica Salernitana, 163–97.

Mayor, A. 2014. 'Mithridates of Pontus and His Universal Antidote', in *History of Toxicology and Environmental Health*, vol. I. Waltham, MA: Academic Press, 21–34.

Meyer, P. trans. 1884. Girart de Roussillon, *Chanson de geste*. Paris: Champion.

Meyerhof, M. 1930. 'The "Book of Treasure", an Early Arabic Treatise on Medicine', *Isis* 14.1: 55–76.

Meyerhof, M. 1935. 'Thirty-Three Clinical Observations by Rhazes (Circa 900 A.D.)', *Isis* 23.2: 321–72.

Miklosich, F., and Müller, J. eds. 1865. *Acta et diplomata graeca medii aevi sacra et profana*. 6 vols. Vienna: Crolus Gerald.

Miller, E. ed. 1857. *Manuelis Philae Carmina*. Paris: Kessinger.

Mills, A. A. 2004. 'The Lodestone: History, Physics, and Formation', *Annals of Science* 61.3: 273–319.

Naīm, M., and Maarrī, S. eds. 1998. Jār Allāh Maḥmūd ibn ʿUmar al-Zamakhsharī: *Asās al-Balāghah*. Beirut: Maktabat Lubnān Nāshirūn.

Nappi, C. 2009. 'Bolatu's Pharmacy, Theriac in Early Modern China', *Early Science and Medicine* 14: 737–64.

Nasrallah, N. trans. 2007. Ibn Sayyār al-Warrāq: *Annals of the Caliphs' Kitchens: Ibn Sayyār al-Warrāq's Tenth-Century Baghdadi Cookbook*. Leiden: Brill.

Nerlich, D. 1999. *Diplomatische Gesandtschaften zwischen Ost- und Westkaisern 756–1002*. Bern: Peter Lang.

Olivieri, A. ed. 1935–50. *Aëtii Amideni Libri Medicinales*. 2 vols. Leipzig: Teubner.

Ouerfelli, M. 2008. *Le sucre: Production, commercialisation et usages dans la Méditerranée médiévale*. Leiden: Brill.

Ozaltay, B., and Köşe, A. 2001. 'On the Etymology and the Semantics of the Medical Term: Istiska', *Yeni Tıp Tarihi Arastirmaları* 7: 11–15.

Pancaroğlu, O. 2001. 'Socializing Medicine: Illustrations of the Kitāb al-diryāq', *Muqarnas* 18: 155–72.

Pellat, Ch. 1954. 'Gahiziana, I. Le Kitab al-Tabassur bi-l-Tigara attribue Gahiz', *Arabica* 1: 153–65.

Pommerening, T. 2007. 'Mumia: Vom Erdwachs zum Allheilmittel', in A. Wieczorek, M. Teilenbach, and W. Rosendahl (eds.), *Mumien: Der Traum vom ewigen Leben. Ausstellungskatalog der Reiss-Engelhorn-Museen*. Mainz: Zabern, 191–200.

Prinzing, G. 2005. 'Zum Austausch diplomatischer Geschenke zwischen Byzanz und seinen Nachbarn in Ostmittel- und Südosteuropa', in *Mitteilungen zur spätantiken Archäologie und byzantinischen Kunstgeschichte* 4: 139–71.

Qaddumi, G. H. trans. 1996. *Book of Gifts and Rarities (Kitāb al-hadāyā wa al-tuḥaf)*. Cambridge, MA: Harvard University Center for Middle Eastern Studies.

Raeder, J. ed. 1928–33. *Oribasii Collectionum medicarum reliquiae*. 4 vols. in 3. Leipzig: Teubner.

Rebstock, U. 2008. 'Weights and Measures in Islam', in H. Selin (ed.), *Encyclopaedia of the History of Science, Technology, and Medicine in Non-Western Cultures*. Berlin: Springer, 2255–67.

Reinsch, D. ed. 2014. *Chronographia Michaelis Pselli Chronographia*. Berlin: De Gruyter.

Reinsch, D., and Kambylis, A. eds. 2001. *Annae Comnenae Alexias*. Berlin: De Gruyter.

Ricordel, J. 2000a. 'Ibn Djuldjul: Propos Sur la Thériaque', *Revue d'Histoire de la Pharmacie* 48.325: 73–80.

Ricordel, J. 2000b. 'Le traité sur la thériaque d'Ibn Rushd (Averroes)', *Revue d'Histoire de la Pharmacie* 48.325: 81–90.

Riddle, J. M. 1992. 'Byzantine Commentaries on Dioscorides', in J. M. Riddle (ed.), *Quid pro Quo: Studies in the History of Drugs*. Hampshire: Variorum Prints, 95–102.

Riva, M. A. et al. 2017. 'The "Thirsty Dropsy": Early Descriptions in Medical and Non-medical Authors of Thirst As Symptom of Chronic Heart Failure', *International Journal of Cardiology* 245: 187–9.

Rosenthal, F. 1975. *Gambling in Islam*. Leiden: Brill.

Rosner, F. trans. 1995. Moses Maimonides: *Glossary of Drug Names*. Haifa: Maimonides Research Institute.

Rubin, J. 2014. 'The Use of the "Jericho Tyrus" in Theriac: A Case Study in the History of the Exchanges of Medical Knowledge between Western Europe and the Realm of Islam in the Middle Ages', *Medium Aevum* 83.2: 234–53.

Samiri, I. Z., and Kadhat, M. A. eds. 2012. Ibn Sayyār al-Warrāq: *Kitabü't-tabîh*. Beirut: Dar al-Sadr.

Sato, T. 2014. *Sugar in the Social Life of Medieval Islam*. Leiden: Brill.

Schopen, L. ed. 1831. *Ioannis Cantacuzeni Eximperatoris Historiarum Libri IV*. 3 vols. Bonn: Weber.

Schreiner, P. 2004. 'Diplomatische Geschenke zwischen Byzanz und dem Westen ca. 800–1200: Eine Analyse der Texte mit Quellenanhang', *Dumbarton Oaks Papers* 58: 251–82.

Setton, K. M. 1969. 'Penrose Memorial Lecture: Pope Leo X and the Turkish Peril', *Proceedings of the American Philosophical Society* 113.6: 367–424.

Sezgin, F. ed. 1996. Ibn al-Bayṭār: *Al-Jāmiʿ li-mufradāt al-adwiyah wa-l-aghdhiyah*. 4 vols. Frankfurt: Institut für Geschichte der Arabisch-Islamischen Wissenschaften.

Simonsohn, S. 1997. *The Jews in Sicily*. 18 vols. Leiden. Brill.

Stannard, J. 1974. 'Squill in Ancient and Medieval Materia Medica, with Special Reference to Its Employment for Dropsy', *Bulletin of the New York Academy of Medicine* 50/6: 684–713.

Stein, M. 1997. 'La thériaque chez Galien: Sa préparation et son usage thérapeutique', in A. Debru (ed.), *Galen on Pharmacology: Philosophy, History and Medicine. Proceedings of the Vth International Galen Colloquium, Lille, 16–18 March 1995*. Leiden: Brill, 199–209.

Stern, S. M. 1950. 'An Embassy of the Byzantine Emperor to the Fatimid Caliph al-Muʾizz', *Byzantion* 20: 239–58.

Stubbs, W. ed. 1864. *Itinerarium Peregrinorum et Gesta Regis Ricardi*. London: Longman.

Talbot, A.-M., and Sullivan, D. F. 2005. *The History of Leo the Deacon: Byzantine Military Expansion in the Tenth Century*. Washington, DC: Dumbarton Oaks Research Library and Collection.

Thurn, J. ed. 1973. *Ioannis Scylitzae Synopsis Historiarum*. Berlin: De Gruyter.

Tibi, A. 1991. 'Byzantine–Fatimid Relations in the Reign of Al-Muʾizz Li-Din Allah (r. 953–957 A.D.) As Reflected in Primary Arabic Sources', *Graeco-Arabica* 4: 91–107.

Tinnefeld, F. 2005. '"Mira varietas": Exquisite Geschenke byzantinischer Gesandtschaften in ihrem politischen Kontext', *Mitteilungen zur Spätantiken Archäologie und Byzantinischen Kunstgeschichte* 4: 121–37.

Touwaide, A. 1995. 'L'intégration de la pharmacologie grecque dans le monde arabe: Une vue d'ensemble', *Medicina nei Secoli* 7.1: 259–89.

Touwaide, A. 1997. 'Une note sur la thériaque attribuée à Galien', *Byzantion* 67: 439–82.

Touwaide, A. 2002a. 'Arabic *Materia Medica* in Byzantium during the 11th Century A.D. and the Problems of Transfer of Knowledge in Medieval Science', in M. R. Ansari (ed.), *Science and Technology in the Islamic World (Proceedings of the XXth International Conference of History of Science, Liège, 20–26 July 1997 vol. XX.* Turnhout: Brepols, 223–46.

Touwaide A. 2002b. 'Arabic Medicine in Greek Translation: A Preliminary Report', *Journal of the International Society for the History of Islamic Medicine* 1: 45–53.

Touwaide, A. 2011. 'Arabic into Greek: The Rise of an International Lexicon of Medicine in the Medieval Eastern Mediterranean?', in R. Winowsky, F. Wallis, J. C. Fumo, and C. Fraenkel (eds.). *Vehicles of Transmission, Translation, and Transformation in Medieval Textual Culture.* Turnhout: Brepols, 195–222.

Truitt, E. 2009. 'The Virtues of Balm in Late Medieval Literature', *Early Science and Medicine* 14.6: 711–36.

Ullmann, R. 1970. *Die Medizin im Islam.* Leiden: Brill.

Vaiou, M. 2002. 'The Diplomatic Relations between the Byzantine Empire and the Abbasid Caliphate: Methods and Procedures'. Oxford University: PhD thesis.

Vladimirova-Aladzhova D. 2012. 'Lid for Theriac Drug Jars from Melnik (Southwest Bulgaria)', in E. Paunov and S. Filipova (eds.), *Herakleous Soteros Thasion: Studia in honorem Iliae Prokopov Sexagenario ab Amicis et Discipulis Dedicata.* Sofia: Veliko Tŭrnovo, 641–8.

Walker, P. E. 2005. 'Backgammon', in J. W. Meri (ed.), *Medieval Islamic Civilization: An Encyclopedia.* London: Routledge.

Watson, G. 1966. *Theriac and Mithridatium: A Study in Therapeutics.* London: Wellcome Historical Medical Library.

Wellmann, M. ed. 1914. *Pedanii Dioscuridis Anazarbei, De Materia Medica Libri quinque*, vol. III. Berlin: Weidmann.

Young, F. ed. and tr. 2016. *A Medieval Book of Magical Stones: The Peterborough Lapidary.* Cambridge: Texts in Early Modern Magic.

Zipser, B. ed. and tr. 2009. *John the Physician's Therapeutics: A Medical Book in Vernacular Greek.* Leiden: Brill.

Index

Printed in the United States
by Baker & Taylor Publisher Services